COMPLETE FAMILY HEALTH GUIDE

New
Medicine

COMPLETE FAMILY HEALTH GUIDE

New Medicine

how to integrate complementary & conventional medicine
for the safest and most effective treatment

EDITOR-IN-CHIEF Professor David Peters

MB, ChB, DRCOG, DMSMed, MF Hom, FLCOM

TED SMART

London, New York, Munich, Melbourne, Delhi

For my colleagues at the University of Westminster

Project Editors Kathy Fahey, Pip Morgan
Science Writer Erica Bower
Picture Research Suzanne Williams
Picture Librarian Romaine Werblow
Illustrator Philip Wilson
Senior Art Editor Rosamund Saunders
Design Schermuly Design Co.
Managing Editors Penny Warren, Stephanie Farrow
Managing Art Editor Marianne Markham
Art Director Carole Ash
Publishing Director Mary-Clare Jerram
DTP Designer Sonia Charbonnier
Production Joanna Bull, Stuart Masheter

First published in Great Britain in 2005 by
Dorling Kindersley Limited
80 Strand, London WC2R 0RL
A Penguin Company

This edition produced for The Book People Ltd, Hall Wood Avenue, Haydock, St. Helens WA11 9UL

IMPORTANT
If you have symptoms of illness, do not diagnose the problem yourself from this book. It is essential that you also consult your doctor. If you use complementary therapies, do not stop taking prescribed medication without first seeking medical advice. Always inform both your doctor and your complementary practitioner of all the treatments, remedies and nutritional supplements you are taking or using. See also pp.46, 69 and 111.

A CIP catalogue record for this book is available from the British Library.

ISBN 1 4053 0283 6

Colour reproduced by GRB, Italy
Printed and bound in Singapore by Star Standard

Discover more at **www.dk.com**

Editor-in-Chief

Professor David Peters MB, ChB, DRCOG, DMSMed, MFHom, FLCOM is a highly respected practitioner in the field of integrated medicine. A medical doctor who is trained in osteopathy and homeopathy, he is currently Chair of the British Holistic Medical Association. He is also the Clinical Director of the School of Integrated Health at the University of Westminster, which has a comprehensive programme of complementary therapy degrees, and he is a Board member of the Prince of Wales Foundation for Integrated Health. He is a consultant to various NHS complementary health projects and research initiatives.

Professor Peters is a contributing editor for the journal *Complementary Therapies in Medicine* and is the author of a number of books, including *The Complete Guide to Integrated Medicine* (2000) and *Encyclopedia of Natural Healing* (1997). For more information, visit his website at www.integrativehealthcare.co.uk.

Contributors

Dr John Briffa, BSc (Hons) MB BS (Lond) (Nutritional Therapy) works in private practice specialising in the nutritional management of nutrition and disease. Formerly the natural health columnist for the *Daily Mail*, he is now the *Observer*'s nutrition and well-being columnist. His most recent book is *Natural Health for Kids*.

Leon K. Chaitow, ND DO (Bodywork Therapies) is a consultant naturopath and osteopath, and a honorary fellow at the School of Integrated Health, University of Westminster, London. He is the author of over 60 books including *Conquer Pain the Natural Way*.

Andrew B. Chevallier BA (Hons), PGCE, FNIMH (Western Herbal Medicine) is a past president of the National Institute of Medical Herbalists and a senior lecturer in herbal medicine at Middlesex University. His publications include *Encyclopedia of Medicinal Plants*.

Dr Peter Fisher FRCP, FFHom (Homeopathy) is Clinical Director, Royal London Homoeopathic Hospital. He also edits the journal *Homeopathy*.

Dr Adrian Hemmings, DPhil CPsychol AFBPsS UKCP (Psychological Therapy) is a lecturer and counsellor at the University of Sussex.

Dr Randy Horwitz, MD PhD (Environmental Health) is a Lecturer at the Program in Integrative Medicine, University of Arizona College of Medicine, Tucson, Arizona.

Dr David S. Kiefer, MD (Environmental Health) is Clinical Assistant Professor of Medicine, Program in Integrative Medicine, University of Arizona College of Medicine, Tucson, Arizona.

Professor George Lewith, MA DM FRCP MRCGP (Acupuncture) is a Senior Research Fellow and Honorary Consultant Physician at the School of Medicine, University of Southampton. He is a partner at the Centre for Complementary Medicine in Southampton.

Michael McIntyre MA, FNIMH, FRCHM, MBAcC (Western and Chinese Herbal Medicine) is a past President of the National Institute of Medical Herbalists and chairs the European Herbal Practitioners' Association. His books include *Herbal Medicine for Everyone*.

Dr Kenneth R. Pelletier, PhD MD (Mind–Body Medicine) is Clinical Professor of Medicine at the University of Maryland School of Medicine and the University of Arizona School of Medicine. He is also Chairman of the American Health Association. His publications include *Alternative, Complementary and Integrative Medicine – An Evidence-Based Approach* and *The Best Alternative Medicine: What Works? What Does Not?*

Dr Penny Preston, MB ChB MRCGP (Conventional Medicine) is an experienced family doctor and now a full-time medical writer. She writes extensively both for the medical profession and for the general public.

Contents

HORMONAL SYSTEM

WOMEN'S HEALTH

PREGNANCY & CHILDBIRTH

MEN'S HEALTH

CHILDREN'S HEALTH

MIND & EMOTIONS

ALLERGIES & SYSTEMIC DISORDERS

Foreword

Conventional Western medicine used to mean taking the body apart and analysing it down into ever smaller components. But examining a piston can't tell you how an engine works. We cannot explain the mind by dissecting the brain, nor understand a person by doing chemical tests. And living organisms are quite different from mechanisms: they self-assemble, and the whole has a huge effects on its parts. The healthy body is an infinitely intricate three-dimensional jigsaw, which is continually breaking itself apart, even down at the molecular level, and then reconstructing itself.

A new medicine is emerging that realises you cannot predict how a complex system functions just by studying its parts. So it aims to work with the body as a whole, to trigger the awesome capacity for self-healing. This means tapping into a spectrum of complementary and conventional treatments and mind–body medicine to maintain health and well-being. Medical science is rediscovering the power of self-healing processes, an area where traditional systems, such as acupuncture, massage or herbal medicine, may have a lot to offer.

We should consider health as having three "realms": structural, biochemical and psychological (*see p.14*). Conventional medicine tends to focus on one or other of the three dimensions. For example, drugs target biochemical aspects, surgery focuses on the body's structure and counselling on the mind. But since many health problems are complex, conventional medicine can offer no single "magic bullet", and its existing treatments have limited success or cause side-effects. In painful, stress-related illnesses such as migraine, or in recurring disorders like arthritis, psoriasis and eczema single-level approaches fall short. In chronic fatigue or persistent pain syndromes where standard tests detect no changes in body tissues, drug treatment alone often proves unsatisfactory. New medicine comes into its own where there is no single well-defined cause, and various factors – biochemical, structural and pyschosocial – are involved. Avoiding single solutions, new medicine adopts a holistic approach, looking at temperament, bodily tension, breathing, coping style, lifestyle and diet, and explores complementary therapies' potential to trigger vitality.

New medicine is increasingly driven by patients' needs. Doctors though, realise self-care and patient choice are crucially important. Increasing collaboration between conventional and complementary practitioners, and the rise of mind–body therapies are supported by promising research results. We present some of them in this book. While doctors are catching up with new medicine, individuals need to make special efforts to stay well and understand the spectrum of treatments available. This book has been written to support all those who share these aims.

David Peters

Integrated

Medicine

Well-Being and Health

DR DAVID PETERS

When we are healthy, we can adapt to change. If our bodies and minds get what they need and are not overwhelmed, they can successfully meet challenges. Like a spinning gyroscope, we stay upright provided we have enough energy, but lose our balance if we are pushed too far. So what do we mean by "energy", how do we get and keep it, and how does the body manage to maintain the balance and harmony that add up to well-being?

These are the questions that new medicine has to ask. They are different from the questions medical science has asked until now, and they are important because medicine is in crisis. The crisis has to do with rocketing costs and a widespread disillusionment among the public with scientific medicine's obsession with molecules, drugs and technology at the expense of serving the whole person. It is an aspect of a worldwide concern with sustainability and the side-effects, whether global or medical, of technological solutions to complex problems. Fortunately, science is becoming more holistic as it realises the limitations of a fragmented approach to solving problems and starts to understand complexity. Curiously, the scientific picture emerging today has a lot in common with truths known to the world's oldest healing traditions. The new medicine will integrate this timeless knowledge about self-healing and whole person care with 21st-century science. It is even possible, as complexity is further explored and understood, that traditional notions such as "life-force" and "energy-body" could find their way into mainstream medicine.

The Body in Flux

The new medicine requires a new way of thinking about the body. The body is alive and constantly on the move, constantly changing. The body is also constantly healing and renewing itself – cells die and are replaced, food is processed and oxygen pours in to fuel the biochemical furnaces that give us energy. Physical and mental demands are met by continual adjustments in our internal systems. On the one hand, these demands may be as straightforward as those involved in taking this book off the shelf, sitting down with a cup of coffee and reading; or they may be demands that the body finds hard to deal with. These difficult challenges could involve something as tiny as abnormal genes, chemical toxins or disease-causing germs, or something much larger, such as the constant strain of an uncomfortable working position, the effects of an injury, or widespread hardening of the arteries. More subtle kinds of distress, such as the emotional strain of a difficult relationship, financial pressures or the death of a loved one, can also present the body with challenges.

Common sense tells us that how well we feel must influence our approach to life, and that when negative influences outweigh the natural resilience of our body and mind, we become ill. Science bears these ideas out. The latest research shows that the connection between mind and body is complete; one influences the other. It is also clear that the mind–body has built-in healing responses of its own that we can tap into. Many scientists and doctors suspect that natural healing techniques can mobilise this self-healing response to prevent illness and promote better health and well-being, even in someone who has a chronic disease. Some people are convinced that the future of medicine depends on our learning how to make use of the response. Modern medicine, although skilled in waging war on disease, has lost its knowledge of self-healing. Various people have compared medical science to war: weapons can backfire and wars tend to increase the enemy's aggressiveness. Looking at medicine today, we can see how the "arms race" between science and disease has led to over-reliance on technology, high costs and side-effects, and more resistant infections.

What is missing is a way of building up the mind–body's natural defences. This is something the world's traditional medical systems know about. These systems have had to rely not on scientific research but on their traditional knowledge and skills to trigger self-healing through touch, words, movement, art, the products of nature, food, exercise and harmonious living.

Three Mind–Body Levels

We can think of the human mind–body as comprising three interdependent levels: biochemical, structural and psycho-social (*see box, p.14*). These levels provide a framework for thinking about aspects of our health. They are interrelated, so an impact on one level affects the others. The holistic nature of complementary medicines aims to encompass all three levels, although clearly some types of therapy are directed at a particular level: herbal medicines and nutritional supplements are more biochemical in their effect than structural therapies, such as chiropractic and massage, while cognitive behavioural therapy and other talking therapies act mainly on the psycho-social level.

In regulating itself, the body draws on all three levels: the biochemical level that fuels body processes; the structural level that supports the organs and body systems; and the psycho-social level that governs thoughts, desires, actions and emotions. For example, after an exhausting and stressful day, a good night's sleep allows the biochemical furnace to cool down, the body's structures to rest and relax, and the mind to assimilate the day's events. If challenges become intense, unrelenting or too frequent, the body and mind's extraordinary capacity to adapt can be overwhelmed. Coping relies on energy and order, but if

REALMS OF BODY AND MIND

Integrated medicine seeks to encompass the whole person when treating a disease or disorder. Instead of looking only at symptoms and a specific disease, integrated medicine practitioners take into account a patient's lifestyle, personality type and social environment as well as their general health and medical history. This holistic approach means that treatment of many diseases is more effective.

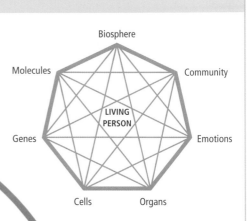

Our body, and therefore our health, is intimately connected at every level to cells, organs and our living processes, but also to the external influences around us. For example, our genes influence the way we respond to pollutants in the biosphere, our emotions alter the way we interact with people in our community, and our emotions affect our immune cells.

Health is controlled by three interdependent "realms" – psycho-social, structural and biochemical. They are underpinned by a fourth realm, "life force" or "energy".

"LIFE FORCES"

Encompassing and acting on all three realms, this concept is variously described by therapists as "regulatory forces", "vital forces", "energy" and "Qi".

Treatments include high-potency homeopathic remedies, traditional Chinese acupuncture, traditional herbalism and spiritual healing.

PSYCHO-SOCIAL

The psycho-social realm includes thoughts and feelings, relationships, social environment, community, workplace, and culture.

Treatments include psychotherapies, behavioural approaches, health promotion information, social work, hypnotherapy, meditation.

STRUCTURAL

The structural realm includes muscles, bones, nerves, blood vessels, movement and the physical environment.

Treatments include physiotherapy, osteopathy, chiropractic, massage, medical acupuncture, and surgery.

BIOCHEMICAL

The biochemical realm includes cells, hormones, enzymes, chemical processes, digestion and respiration, the chemical environment and pollution.

Treatments include drugs, nutritional supplements, low-potency homeopathic remedies, dietary changes and herbal medicines.

a person's resources are depleted then the ability to maintain balance is undermined. Defence and repair systems may begin to fail if the integrity of cell chemistry, body structures and mind are threatened.

The underlying factors upsetting self-regulation can be obvious or subtle, intense or diffuse, short-lived or prolonged. They can include a short-term, severe injury, for example from a car accident, a bereavement triggering depression, a spell of rushed working lunches resulting in bouts of indigestion, or flu caught from exposure to an infected person. In their own important ways, the resulting ill-effects tell us something vital about how well we are adapting to the demands placed on us; they are a message about things we need to attend to, and changes that we might have to make.

Challenges affect all three levels – psycho-social, structural and biochemical – and, since they are entwined, when there is a problem in one, it can affect how the other two work. For example, a biochemical disorder such as a nutritional deficiency or food sensitivity may have psychological consequences, such as depression. Loneliness, depression, bereavement and inner conflicts can undermine immune system defences, while a structural injury might cause pain that then undermines well-being and relationships.

The implications are obvious: give your body what it needs to work well and avoid the things that harm it. This may include taking up yoga, meditation or dance, giving up smoking, seeing friends or making dietary changes. Do whatever you need to do to nourish yourself intellectually, emotionally and spiritually.

Complexity and Medicine

Complexity is the name for the universal tendency of parts to organise themselves into more complex wholes. We humans are so much a part of our world that we often take many of its properties and qualities for granted. We fail to

New medicine views the body as a complex system through which information flows. A shoal of fish is an excellent example of this type of complexity. Although each is a separate animal, when fish come together in a shoal they behave as a single entity.

remember that weight, water, light and warmth, although totally familiar to us, are also rather mysterious. Complexity can be seen at the most basic level: who could predict, for instance, that bringing the gases hydrogen and oxygen together would give you something to drink! Complexity operates too on the biggest scale of all. After the Big Bang, when time and space first began, our pattern-forming universe produced stars and galaxies; planets formed. Life – miraculously it seems, but also quite naturally – emerged out of this universal process. Organisms are alive precisely because the whole is always greater than the sum of its parts.

Medical scientists until now have tried to understand life by isolating its biochemical properties in a test tube, or by examining dead tissues. While this approach has certainly proved very useful in understanding how the human body works, it can only reveal our chemical nature. Modern technology now lets us see into the intricate design and workings of the living body. As science discovers how the parts communicate, form wholes and self-organise, medicine will change quite profoundly. It is too soon to know what medicine would look like if it were based on mind–body connectedness and the flow of information that keeps us well, but there are similarities between such an approach and the traditions that gave birth to complementary medicine. These traditions all include notions of mind–body wholeness, energy flow, harmonious living and therapeutic relationships, along with knowledge of how to encourage self-healing. Science is becoming increasingly interested in this territory and the possibility that complementary therapies might provide us with further clues about human health.

Complex processes are not like sequential ones, where A causes B, which causes C. Whole-system processes are networked; they happen all at once, and communication is across the whole system in all directions, so C influences A even as B influences Z – and back! This realisation has enormous practical implications: scientists developing artificial intelligence, or predicting weather patterns or ecological consequences, need to know how to predict whole-system behaviour. It is of even greater relevance for medicine to understand how the processes of life interweave, and how the whole and the part continually reshape one another.

The Intelligent Body

We tend to think of the brain as being intelligent, and that the brain controls the body, while the body is just dumb flesh. Indeed, the brain is a network of almost infinitely interconnected neurons; it has been called the most complex object in the known universe. But the whole body is a network too, which is why the psychologist Michael Hyland has put forward his "intelligent body" hypothesis. Dr Hyland takes further the idea that there is no strict division between brain and the rest of the body. He proposes that intelligence is not confined to the brain, but rather it is distributed throughout the body in an extended network.

Medicine, if it is to get to grips with health rather than just confront disease, must comprehend the living body's extraordinary ability to maintain conditions stable enough for life to happen at all. Too hot or too cold, too acid or too alkaline, too many waste products or not enough nutrients, and we die. The same goes for the body's internal architecture and outer form, for they are not fixed, but are constantly broken down and rebuilt. The sense of self, too, although it seems stable, is formed out of a whirl of sense impressions and memories.

At a biochemical level, the properties that emerge from the network provide its ability to self-organise, control the myriad chemical reactions that provide energy and produce the living tissues. At the structural level, these so-called "emergent" properties allow the body to move through space and constantly reconstruct itself; at the level of awareness they give us the ability to sense, respond to, and reflect on our experiences.

When systems go wrong

Moderate challenges to the mind–body generally lead to recovery and even to improved resilience. Challenges that are successfully met result in better immunity, improved fitness and more appropriate coping styles.

However, the information system can go wrong and develop less efficient modes of working. These states of "dys-regulation" prepare the ground for disease to take hold. They may arise because the challenge to the body is too great or too persistent, or the person is vulnerable psychologically (various styles of thinking and feeling can undermine recovery), biochemically (due to genetic,

nutritional and ecological factors), or structurally (because of deep patterns of tension, a lack of fitness or flexibility). The system may be overwhelmed because a person fails to notice the body's messages of distress and change habits that prevent recovery. It is the seamless mind–body network – not just brain-based intelligence – that adapts to changing internal and external conditions. The new medicine will recognise this. Faced with an illness, an injury or a social crisis, the new medicine, which aims to unite the best of complementary therapies and conventional medicine, will aim to re-establish balance.

Michael Hyland's theory that disease begins as an information error suggests a new and important way of thinking about health. There are two kinds of "error" in the mind–body. One is the type that conventional Western medicine deals with when it looks at the body as a biological machine, identifying a biological disease such as diabetes, cancer, heart disease or arthritis. Conventional treatment involves fixing the "broken part" or removing it. This might involve replacing a missing hormone, killing bacteria with antibiotics, reducing blood pressure with a drug, suppressing inflammation with steroids, replacing a blocked artery with an artificial graft, or cutting away a cancerous tumour.

There is another type of error affects the information in the whole network. In this case, no single organ or biochemical system can be targeted and repaired, because the information that produces health and healing processes is spread over the entire network.

In the case of the latter error, approaches that aim to create health or to trigger healing responses by acting on the mind–body as a whole are most likely to be effective. And, just as networks can take in many different kinds of information, so the mind–body can respond to diverse kinds of input – diet, botanical medicines, movement and touch. So too can it pick up more refined information – from art, communication with a therapist, and perhaps even the subtle information conveyed by a homeopathic medicine or the effect of an acupuncture needle. The entire mind–body could be influenced by lifestyle choices that have an impact on the biochemical, structural and mental information systems.

We can imagine the whole system of information flow – the body's intelligence – as a choir of myriad voices. But it is a choir without a score or a conductor. The parts sing themselves and each voice hears the entire chorale and responds more or less harmoniously. The voices are biochemical and electrical messages, structural impulses, communications from the conscious and unconscious mind. This is an example of complexity in action: the information flow emerges from the interweaving of biochemical, the structural and mental information systems, but it simultaneously forms and shapes them all.

Perhaps the information flow that makes complexity possible is what the traditional healers refer to as "life

TWELVE STEPS TO WELL-BEING

There are many things you can do to improve the quality of your life. Some of them are material things, such as eating well and getting exercise, but many of them are psychological. Learning to treat yourself well and to interact well with the people around you can improve the quality of your life immensely.

THE STEPS	WHY TRY THEM?	PUT THEM INTO PRACTICE
1 Eat fresh food; it's a better source of vitamins and minerals than even the best supplements.	Antioxidants mop up free radicals (super-reactive chemicals) that can damage the body's cells.	Get serious about healthy eating and choose a diet high in fibre and antioxidants and low in fat.
2 Incorporate exercise into your daily routine — you'll feel better for it.	Exercise makes bones and heart stronger and lifts mood.	Take the stairs rather than the lift; walk as much as you can; find a sport you enjoy and do it regularly.
3 Relax regularly and take time to appreciate the good things you have in your life.	Relaxation prevents the body staying in "emergency mode" due to stress.	Make time to relax each day, even if only for 15 minutes. Use a relaxation tape, or try yoga or massage.
4 Be aware of stress in your life and minimise it as much as you can.	Stress puts strain on body systems and contributes to many health problems.	Keep a stress diary to help you identify where your stress is coming from. Then work to minimise or eliminate it.
5 Appreciate yourself. Dwell on your positives, not on your negatives.	People with high self-esteem cope better with life's challenges.	Try positive affirmations, such as "I am peaceful" and "I can organise my life". Sounds corny, but it works.
6 Think positively.	Optimism and humour have been shown scientifically to benefit health.	Let go of old hurts, which can drag you down psychologically. Use counselling to do this if necessary.
7 Make yourself understood. Clear communication is important in all spheres of life.	Communicating your needs and thoughts clearly can prevent stressful misunderstandings and conflicts.	Say what you think, as pleasantly and politely as possible. Listen fully to what the other person actually says.
8 Build your confidence. Believe your contribution is of value.	Being confident gives you control. People also feel more comfortable with confidence than insecurity.	Try acting with assurance, which often brings real self-confidence.
9 Build close relationships. You don't need many but you do need a few.	Having a sense that you value others and are valued yourself is essential to mental well-being.	Be open with people. Don't allow distance to grow between you and the people you love.
10 Find things to appreciate every day. It's often the little things that make life enjoyable.	Small things can be very uplifting and can help you get through difficult days.	Observe the world around you and appreciate giving and receiving kindnesses.
11 Be generous. Generosity and compassion feel better than selfishness and cynicism.	Altruism is healthy, science has shown.	Be charitable and try not to let the pace of modern life make you unkind.
12 Be thankful.	You are a living miracle and you have a right to be here, as do all people.	At the end of each day, count its blessings, no matter how small. Let the bad things go and give tomorrow another chance.

force". If this is the case, then the body's intelligence may correspond to complementary medicine's "energy body", but it would probably be more accurate to call it the "information body".

Expectation, relationships and healing

The information body may be particularly affected by the relationship between practitioner and patient. Positive belief and expectations on the part of both the therapist or caregiver and patient can have a strong influence on the course of a condition, regardless of the type of treatment involved. This effect has been attributed to the placebo effect (*see Clinical trials, p.23*). A positive relationship between therapist and patient fuels this effect and can be a powerful force for healing. This healing effect was demonstrated in a famous study at Massachusetts General Hospital in Boston in 1964. Patients undergoing surgery who received a pre-operative visit from a warm and sympathetic anaesthetist had far less post-operative pain, so needed fewer painkillers, than other patients undergoing similar surgery who were not visited.

It also seems that the patient has responsibilities to cultivate a good relationship with their caregivers. In another Boston study, patients with chronic illnesses such as diabetes, rheumatoid arthritis and high blood pressure were coached to ask relevant questions of their doctor. Afterwards they reported more satisfaction with their visit and even enjoyed better health than those who had not been coached to ask questions.

The strong healing forces triggered by expectation can also work in a negative way. People who have insensitive treatment from nurses, doctors or other practitioners often complain of feeling worse. This is known as the "nocebo" effect – the opposite of the placebo. The power of a positive therapist–patient relationship is the key reason why you should choose a therapy (and a therapist) which you trust.

How the Mind Influences the Body

Future research into mind–body processes will reveal a great deal more than we know now about how mind–body differences – differences in temperament, for instance – affect individual susceptibility to illness and response to treatment. Research shows that emotional states such as loneliness and grief can depress the immune system, leaving people susceptible to disease. When psychologists, immunologists and endocrinologists began to pool information in the 1980s, they found they could track chemical pathways linking brain activity to physiological processes in the body. It had long been understood that the stress hormones adrenaline and cortisol suppressed the

production of antibodies, the body's defence against disease. But studies in 1977 and 1983 showed how white blood cells (a key part of the body's immune system) were temporarily paralysed in bereaved men, possibly accounting for deaths from so-called "broken-heart syndrome".

The brain and central nervous system are control centres for both conscious and automatic life processes. In evolutionary terms we have three brains. The first, the cortex, is the most recently developed and allows us rational thought and language. Traditional psychotherapy or talk therapy aims to influence this "conscious" brain. The left side of the cortex processes information in a linear fashion and coordinates aspects such as language and numerical skills; the other side is more concerned with non-linear spatial relations, metaphor and music. Recent research has hinted that emotional closeness in the first months of life triggers the development of an area in the forebrain called the neocortex, which allows us to deal with emotion, respond sensitively to others, and experience feelings of pleasure and beauty.

Beneath the forebrain is the second, older brain, which we share with other mammals and which is involved with non-linear and non-rational aspects, emotions, memory and feelings. This part of the brain is a rich source of what Candace Pert (who discovered the endorphins and enkephalins) calls "molecules of emotion". These "molecules of emotion" are not confined to the brain, though, because all the body's cells are coated with receptors that constantly scan for them, while also sending out their own messenger molecules to communicate with sites in the brain.

We share the third brain with the reptiles. The medulla oblongata, which is found at the base of the skull, is the seat of instincts and unconscious body-control processes such as breathing.

Science is realising that well-being is not just "all in the mind" and that the mind is not confined to the brain. So individual temperament is physical as well as psychological, for both brain and body play their crucial part. But is temperament something we inherit or do we learn to be the way we are? A study was done in which 2,000 people were asked to rate their levels of well-being. It showed that people with high well-being ratings usually said they had a happy childhood, are usually optimistic, feel that others think well of them and that they have life under control. Are people born this way, or does upbringing and learning mould their sunny outlook? Both factors probably come into play. Yet curiously, the science of well-being is revealing how even happiness has its physical components. The way we respond to life's demands and how we express feelings depends at least partly on genetic make-up, body make-up and brain chemistry. It is not simply that genes programme our personality, but rather that our personal style of dealing with the world around us – how we think, feel, learn – has a definite bodily basis.

Neuroscientists now say there's a biological foundation for the temperaments, based on how the brain works and the amounts of different chemical messengers there are. The latest evidence shows how positive feelings boost activity in the left frontal lobe of the brain – for if you offer someone an incentive this part of the brain starts to work harder; even small babies show this pattern when they gaze at their mother. The current theory sees this part of the brain as a sort of psychological accelerator pedal, which psychologists call the behavioural approach system – BAS for short. It's more active in people who are extrovert, impulsive and sensation-seeking, but much quieter in the brain scans of more introverted people. So if temperament is shaped by the way individual brains work and how the body responds, this will influence what we need for our own individual style of well-being.

The Cellular Level

The entire body is built from cells and connective tissue. Each cell is an incredibly complex structure carrying out the processes of life. Cells turn food molecules into energy and building materials; they deal with toxins, enlarge and divide to make your body grow, heal wounds and replace cells that have died. The various kinds of cell have different natural lifespans, a natural limit to the number of times they can divide and reproduce. For example, red and white blood corpuscles can divide millions of times, but most nerve cells do not reproduce at all. Once a cell has reached its natural limit, it withers and dies. When enough of our cells die, so do we. Some kinds of cell do not age; bacteria keep on dividing forever, unless killed by some outside event. Cancer cells are immortal too, dividing endlessly, unless treatment kills them or the person dies.

Cells communicate with one another by chemical messengers in the intra-cellular fluids, but they are also intricately connected to the spinal cord and brain through the finest filaments of the nerve fibres that reach each one of them. Inside the cell specialised zones in the outer layer (the cytoplasm) produce energy, or secrete specific molecules that give an organ a specialised function: for instance, liver cells produce large amounts of enzymes, catalysts that speed up the chemical processes of detoxification; fibroblasts produce the skin's supportive matrix of collagens and elastin and have a role in wound healing. As new and ever more powerful microscopes probe the minute detail of cells' internal architecture, science has realised that each cell has its own cytoskeleton. This acts as a

scaffolding, steadying the nucleus (the cell's central control system) and holding up the cell membrane. The cytoskeleton also provides a communication web within the cell, through which physical forces (pressure and stretching) are transmitted to the nucleus. The cytoskeleton's extension links with those from other cells.

The old idea was of the body as a stack of separate cells awash in fluids; the new image is of a network of cells intricately connected and inter-penetrated by fibrils and nano-fibres, all embedded in connective tissue that positively hums with vibrant energetic and chemical messages. As well as involving the brain, nervous and endocrine systems, this information flow takes place in the connective tissues that hold the organs in place and gives the body its flexible firmness.

Genes, chromosomes and health

In recent years, medical science has come to realise the vital role that genetic make-up plays in human health. The human genome, or complete set of genes, has now been mapped and further genetic research will no doubt provide insight into many health problems. But what are these somewhat mysterious things called genes? A gene is one stretch of DNA that contains instructions for making a

Chromosomes, such as this X-chromosome, are made up of genes – segments of DNA that code for many of our physical and psychological characteristics, such as eye colour, stature, sex and possibly some aspects of personality. Human cells each contain 23 pairs of chromosomes.

particular protein, one of the key molecules that make up your body. Genes store and process biochemical information that evolved as Earth itself was changing from a cloudy swamp into a blue planet. For aeons, genes have evolved both as parts of whole organisms and in response to the organisms' relationship with the environment.

Thus, our genes record not only our parents' heredity, but also our evolutionary past. Just as our threefold brain connects us to our reptilian ancestors, so too do our genes contain the immense accumulated biochemical intelligence of the evolutionary process. The information they carry is an important aspect of the intelligent body.

Genes are arranged along chromosomes – neatly packaged strings of DNA that hold the genetic instructions controlling your biochemical make-up and determining many physical aspects of who you are. The nucleus of each cell that makes up your body contains 46 chromosomes – 23 inherited from each parent. This set of chromosomes, which each of us has, is estimated to contain about 90,000 pairs of genes. Inheriting 23 chromosomes from each parent means that we have two copies of most genes. This has a bearing on our health, because if one gene is defective, we usually have another to fall back on.

However, in some cases we may have just one copy of a gene. Only 22 of the 23 pairs of chromosomes in each cell are matching. The sex chromosomes may be different. Women have two "X" chromosomes, one inherited from their mother and one from their father. Men, on the other hand, have just one "X" chromosome, inherited from their mother, and a "Y" chromosome, inherited from their father. This means that many of the genes on the X chromosome have no back-up copy in men, and accounts for the fact that genetic conditions due to faulty genes on the X chromosome, such as red–green colour blindness and haemophilia, are more common in men than women.

An Integrated Approach to Health

Most diseases do not have a single specific cause. For example, smoking may cause lung cancer, but there are smokers who live into their 90s without any apparent ill-effects. Whether or not we succumb to illness and our recovery rate are all dependent on a multitude of inter-related factors that affect our self-regulation.

Illness is not the same as disease. Someone with a headache may feel ill, for example, without having a diagnosable disease. A doctor makes a diagnosis based on the patient's story and clinical signs (observable changes) and then prescribes treatment. Complementary practitioners consider signs and symptoms differently and may suggest treatments to stimulate the self-healing processes. The integrated approach seeks to use conventional treatments if a clear diagnosis and safe, effective treatments are available, and to explore the role of complementary treatments depending on their appropriateness and availability. Very often, this approach will explore what triggered the problem now, made you susceptible or undermined your resilience; and also what may be preventing you from getting better. An integrated approach will call for motivation to change something: diet, exercise or perhaps a way of thinking; or it may mean learning a self-healing practice.

The risks of integrated medicine

As natural products – herbs and nutritional supplements – become more popular, there has been much publicised concern about their side-effects and interactions. Experts are advising caution when prescribing natural products

MAKING A DIAGNOSIS

	CONVENTIONAL DIAGNOSIS	COMPLEMENTARY DIAGNOSIS	THE INTEGRATED APPROACH
Conventional and complementary practitioners both diagnose illness, but they tend to take different approaches. Conventional practitioners rely on symptoms and signs, possibly with tests, to make a diagnosis. Complementary practitioners spend more time discussing your lifestyle and medical history.	● A doctor asks you about symptoms and refers to your medical notes. ● He examines you for clinical signs of disease, such as a raised temperature, a rash, lumps, enlarged liver, or abnormal heart beat. ● You may have blood and urine tests and X-rays. ● You might be referred for further tests, such as ultrasound or MRI. ● Depending on the diagnosis, treatment might include drugs, physiotherapy, surgery etc.	● A practitioner takes a full case history and asks about your lifestyle. ● Depending on the therapy type, the practitioner may run diagnostic tests. ● The explanation given may bear no relationship to conventional medical diagnosis. ● The diagnosis will usually imply certain biochemical, structural or psycho-social causes. ● Treatment is likely to be tailored to suit the individual.	In integrated medicine, diagnosis and treatment is based on both conventional and complementary approaches to treat the whole person.

alongside conventional drugs. So should we be concerned about herb–drug interactions? Yes, we should, because they may be more common than we know; reporting systems for complementary therapies are not yet very effective. However, so far, many nutritional supplements and herbs have excellent safety records, while there are sizeable known health risks associated with many medications. Vitamin E, omega-3 fatty acids and ginkgo, for instance, all have a slight anticoagulant effect, so they could in theory increase the blood-thinning effects of aspirin and warfarin. Their interaction could therefore increase the tendency to bleed. Perhaps further research will confirm these interactions are truly significant. However, the greatest risk of adverse interaction with conventional medicines comes from food, rather than from vitamin supplements or herbs. Grapefruit enhances the effects of many drugs, among them certain antihistamines, calcium-channel blockers (for reducing blood pressure) and some statin drugs (also used to reduce blood pressure). Some vegetables, including garlic, onions, and broccoli, have the opposite effect, enhancing drug breakdown by boosting the liver's detoxification enzymes.

St John's wort, which has a similar effect on the liver to these vegetables, reduces the effectiveness of certain drugs, particularly oral contraceptives and the antibiotic cyclosporin. Coenzyme Q10 and hawthorn (*Crataegus*), both of which improve heart function, may mean that heart patients need to reduce any prescribed heart stimulants, such as digitalis (*see Using herbs safely, p.69*).

There are also some real risks associated with other complementary therapies. The biggest risk by far is the danger that a harmful but conventionally treatable condition might be missed. This is far less likely to happen when conventional doctors and complementary practitioners are working together. Other rare risks include stroke and damage to arteries in the neck after manipulation of the cervical spine. Massage has few adverse effects, although it would be best avoided where deep vein thrombosis, burns, skin infections, eczema, open wounds, bone fractures, advanced osteoporosis and lymphoma are involved. Acupuncture is extremely safe when performed by a skilled practitioner, even though it involves needles. One survey of doctors and physio-therapists who performed acupuncture reported no serious adverse events and only 671 minor adverse events per 10,000 consultations. Only 14 of these minor events were said to have been significant. The danger of cross-infection through needles is negligible if disposable needles are used, as they always should be.

Integrating conventional medicine and complementary therapies

Complementary therapies can work well in conjunction with conventional ones, to reinforce effectiveness of conventional treatments, to strengthen the body and aid recovery, or to ease symptoms or side-effects of treatment.

However, conventional and complementary therapists may often have totally different approaches to your health care.

Differences in use of language and concepts can cause communication problems. Conventional medical practitioners tend to have a highly scientific approach, which treats the body or the symptoms as a set of separate, discrete entities. Disease is usually ascribed to a fault in one or more measurable physical or biochemical systems. On the other hand, complementary therapists tend to make their diagnosis using a very different interpretation of the patient's body, the patient's experiences and the illness. For example, an acupuncturist might attribute a certain type of headache to "stagnation in the gallbladder meridian"; this is clearly not a diagnosis that any conventional doctor will understand.

Such different approaches can make it difficult to see compatible therapeutic aims between your conventional doctor and complementary practitioner. Perhaps you have found a practice where doctors and complementary practitioners are working together. If so, you are fortunate indeed, for such projects are still rather unusual. However, there is a powerful trend towards collaboration, driven by promising research results in some areas, particularly acupuncture, nutrition, herbal medicine and mind-body medicine. For most people, taking an integrated approach to health will mean that you as the patient will have to co-ordinate the various therapies you are using. This means taking responsibility for communicating between therapists and ensuring that your treatments are compatible.

Integrated medicine in practice

Taking an integrated approach to managing your healthcare involves thinking and working on several levels. The three key factors are: maintaining self-regulation and building up resilience; using self-help and conventional medicine when necessary and using complementary approaches appropriately.

Although many GP practices provide access to some form of complementary therapy, the availability of integrated treatment, and the amount you may have to pay for it, varies widely among regions. The most commonly used therapies available within the UK's National Health Service are acupuncture, aromatherapy, chiropractic, homeopathy, hypnotherapy and osteopathy. There are also five homeopathic hospitals in the UK (in Bristol, Glasgow, Liverpool (Mossley Hill), London and Tunbridge Wells) which offer outpatient complementary therapy services.

Hospitals, hospices, palliative care services and some pain clinics are increasingly using complementary therapies to give patients a wider choice of therapies. Many charities and community health services, such as those for people with alcohol or drug-related problems, mental health issues, cancer or HIV, also offer complementary therapies as part of their programme.

Most complementary therapists run their own private practices. They may work from home or be based in complementary health clinics. Information on associations and regulatory bodies can easily be found on the internet (*see Useful addresses and websites, p.486*).

Choosing a therapy and a practitioner

In choosing a therapy, you need to examine your attitude to health. Do you believe in making an effort to stay in good health, or do you prefer not to think about it? It is also important to consider your attitude to the treatment itself and what it will involve. For example, do you dislike being touched? Are you organised enough to take pills regularly? Are you comfortable talking about your life with someone else? All of these things have a bearing on the type of therapy that might work for you.

Once you have chosen the therapy/therapies that you feel most likely to help your condition, it is important that you also find a practitioner that you feel comfortable with. You should be sure to check that they have appropriate training, qualifications and facilities to help you with your condition (*for details of regulatory bodies, see Useful addresses and websites, p.486*).
If you feel unwell and are planning to see a complementary therapist, it is also important that you see your doctor first. The doctor can rule out any dangerous or life-threatening conditions and can discuss treatment options with you.

Doctors may send blood or tissue samples to a laboratory, where they will be examined to determine the nature of a disease.

You should always try to discuss your decisions about using complementary therapies with your conventional practitioners (GP, midwife, etc).

Questions you many want to ask include the following:
- Is the practitioner regulated by a professional body?
- What do they charge for a treatment? Does the first appointment cost more?
- Is the treatment available in an NHS clinic or through a GP practice?
- Have they treated people with your condition before?
- How many treatments might be needed?
- Is there anything you should do before before treatment, such as fasting for a short time, or wearing special clothes?
- How will you feel after treatment? Are there any precautions you should take straight after a treatment?
- Are there any possible side-effects or risk factors? If you are not entirely happy, say so.
- Tell your doctor and practitioners about any over-the-counter medication or complementary remedies or treatments you are taking.
- Tell your practitioner and your doctor whether a treatment worked. Feedback is always appreciated.

Managing health and illness

Research shows that when people take responsibility for their healthcare, symptoms often improve and quality of life is enhanced. The first stage involves gaining knowledge, so it is important to learn as much as possible about all the factors that influence your health. If you are prone to, or already have, a health problem, understanding how you can compensate for this susceptibility will help to minimise its impact. Knowing about causes, symptoms and the range of available treatment options is obviously empowering. You can begin your research by looking up your condition in the relevant section of this book and then doing some further reading or research on the internet.

Overly optimistic expectations about your condition can lead to a roller-coaster of emotional highs and lows that does nothing to aid your recovery from illness. Beware of practitioners who say they have a definite cure for a chronic condition, or of advertisements for products that make exaggerated claims; you should even be cautious of reports of scientific breakthroughs (whether made or about to be), for they rarely turn out to be the wished-for "magic bullet"; all to often the silver lining comes with a grey cloud of side-effects. Particularly for people with chronic disease, it is crucial to have realistic expectations and it helps to develop an understanding of these claims and how research is conducted (*see right*) so that you can make judgements about the quality of the information that you are presented with. However, bear in mind that even if many useful therapies can only control or ameliorate symptoms, their value in improving quality of life should not be under-estimated.

Research and Evidence

Any treatment that you receive should be safe and effective, therefore there should be evidence for its safety and efficacy. However, the general understanding of the safety and efficacy of treatment options is not always as good as it could be. For example there is a widespread belief that "chemicals" are bad, while "natural" is good for you. (Snake poison is entirely natural!)

Research to obtain this evidence is not always straightforward and easy to conduct, and interpreting the results from research can be equally complex. Even when good experiments have been conducted, getting the information in an appropriate and unbiased form to patients and practitioners can be slow and difficult. One of the key difficulties facing a medical researcher is that people are all different. Not only do we look different from those around us, we also respond differently as a disease progresses, and to the treatments that we might be using. This means that even if you have the same disease or condition as your neighbour, it may not follow exactly the same course, and a treatment that works for your neighbour may not work for you. Researchers have to use large numbers of people in their studies to untangle real effects from this background variation. Another factor to be taken into account is that patients have "good days" and "bad days". A researcher also needs to know if an improvement in a condition is the result of treatment, or just part of this natural variation. Therefore, large numbers of patients in a study, and an appropriate timescale for the tests, may be important factors when testing for efficacy.

Alternatives to research and evidence do not provide proof that treatments are safe and effective. Anecdotes (stories) of cures may be coincidences or due to natural variability of conditions and people. People also have a natural tendency to report only positive stories ("miracle cures") rather than those where not much happened. Even less reliable is "knowing" or a "gut feeling" that something works. What is "known" to be true by one person can just as easily be "known" to be false by another. Long-term use of a therapy (e.g. over centuries) does instill confidence in its effectiveness, but safety issues may be harder to establish, especially where problems occur over many months or years making it difficult to pinpoint their true cause.

Medical research attempts to distinguish real effects from random events, tease out bias and detect unexpected or unwanted outcomes.

Clinical trials

The main method for testing a treatment is the clinical trial. These were originally devised to test pharmaceutical drugs and treatments in conventional medicine, and now they are also being used to investigate complementary therapies such as herbal medicines.

A clinical trial aims to test whether a treatment works, but one of the main problems with testing any therapy is the act of providing the therapy (or even just talking about it in positive terms) can cause a person's condition to improve, whether the therapy has any true activity or not. This is a natural and widely documented response known as the placebo effect.

Placebo-controlled trials are conducted to distinguish between the placebo effect and a true response. In a placebo-controlled trial, the therapy under test is compared with a seemingly identical treatment. The patients are split into two groups and one is given the test therapy (e.g. the medication in pill form) while the other group is given a "control" (.e.g. an inactive sugar pill that looks the same as the test pill). For the treatment to be deemed to have worked, patients in the experimental group must perform significantly better than those taking the placebo.

For ethical reasons, particularly in life-threatening conditions, the "control" is often the best available current medication, as giving patients a non-active treatment could mean their condition worsens. The "control" can also be the current standard treatment, or the drug of a competing pharmaceutical company, depending on what the researcher is trying to demonstrate. In clinical trials, enough people are tested to minimise bias due to natural variation in people and their illness. Further risks of bias are ruled out by assigning patients at random to the groups.

More recently research has demonstrated that even subtle cues given unconsciously by therapists or experimenters can influence the outcome. To counteract these subtle effects, researchers use double-blind methods (where a clinician randomly assigns patients to either group, then codes the treatments so that neither the patient nor the experimenter knows who is getting which treatment). This makes the randomised double-blind trial the ultimate test.

However, testing complementary therapies using standard randomised controlled methods can be difficult, as it can be hard to provide a realistic control. Some complementary therapies have been tested using placebo-controls, for example, acupuncture methods have been tested by using needles on patients either in the correct acupuncture locations, or at sham non-acupuncture sites. However, if you want to test the benefits of massage, how do you give the control group a dummy treatment that is convincingly similar to massage? The personalised nature of many complementary therapies means that clinical trials need to be carefully adapted.

Finally meta-analyses or systematic reviews are useful tools. These are ways of collecting and analysing the results of a number of studies in the same area to give a more accurate picture of the total research evidence available.

Throughout this book the authors have endeavoured to base treatment recommendations on reliable scientific evidence, combined with practitioner experience of what is particularly effective (*see p.111 for how treatments are rated*).

CONVENTIONAL MEDICINE

DR PENNY PRESTON

Conventional medicine views the body as a number of interdependent systems that can be affected by a variety of diseases. The aim of conventional medicine is to treat existing medical conditions while also promoting a healthy way of life. Doctors and other healthcare workers often make recommendations on lifestyle and other measures with the aim of reducing the risk of developing diseases. In addition, screening, for example for pre-cancerous changes of the cervix through cervical smears, is part of the remit of conventional medicine.

Doctors and Diagnosis

Different medical specialities tend to focus on particular systems. Thus, apart from the family doctor (general practitioner – GP), there are doctors who specialise in treating problems with the ears, nose and throat; doctors who specialise in obstetrics and gynaecology; doctors who specialise in treating problems with the heart; and so on. Some specialities deal only with specific conditions, such as cancer, while others, such as radiology and haematology, concentrate mainly on diagnosis. In some instances, the combined expertise of several specialist doctors may be needed to treat a condition or an injury successfully. Specialists are normally based in hospitals.

In addition to specialists, many other medical professionals deliver healthcare. These include nurses, health visitors, physiotherapists, occupational therapists and counsellors.

The role of the GP

The GP plays a key role in the delivery of medical treatment, being the usual first port-of-call for people who are ill. GPs have a broad knowledge base and expertise in diagnosing a wide range of illnesses. In many cases they can recommend the appropriate treatment, whether it is lifestyle measures (such as reducing stress), drugs or other treatments. Sometimes, a GP will recommend referral to a specialist or to another member of the medical team, such as a counsellor or speech therapist.

Complementary therapies in general practice

Doctors increasingly recognise the value of complementary therapies and a GP may aim to incorporate them into his treatment plan. The relative roles of these treatments may depend on several factors, including the condition to be treated, the patient's wishes and the treatment options available to the doctor. For certain conditions, such as cancer, schizophrenia or coronary artery disease (CAD), the GP will generally recommend that conventional drugs and procedures take a predominant role, but for other disorders complementary therapies may be a preferred first option. Complementary therapies can often work hand-in-hand with conventional treatments to relieve symptoms, reduce underlying stress and improve general well-being.

Making a diagnosis

Key to making appropriate recommendations for treatment is making a diagnosis whenever possible. The GP will look for patterns of symptoms that may suggest particular disorders. For example, certain types of chest pain may be characteristic of coronary artery disease. He or she will take your medical history, which involves not only asking about your symptoms but also about other issues. This may include a discussion of any previous illnesses, lifestyle habits (such as alcohol intake, exercise and whether you smoke) and the health of relatives. If stress may be contributing to or causing your symptoms, the GP will ask about work, conflicts, worries, relaxation and sleep patterns. He or she may then carry out a physical examination. All of this information will guide the GP to make a diagnosis and to select appropriate treatment, or to recommend further tests or referral to a hospital specialist if necessary.

Hospital medicine

Hospital doctors are specialists who have additional training in their chosen area. For example, an oncologist specialises in cancer and an urologist in disorders of the urinary tract. In some cases, hospital doctors "super-specialise", concentrating on one particular aspect of a speciality. For example, an endocrinologist (a specialist in diseases affecting the hormone system) may have a particular interest in diabetes mellitus.

Visiting a hospital specialist can seem daunting, but it is worth remembering that his or her aims are the same as your GP's: to make a diagnosis, which may involve ordering some tests, and to recommend treatment that will cure or relieve your condition while causing the fewest possible side-effects. Be as open as possible; feel free to ask any questions you have and discuss any concerns.

In some cases, specialists will prescribe drugs or recommend a treatment and then hand the patient's care back to the GP; in other cases, they will wish to see the patient on a regular basis to monitor progress and to make changes to the treatment plan as necessary.

Tests and investigations

Where further tests or investigations are required, your doctor may arrange them directly or refer you to a hospital specialist, who will organise the appropriate procedures. Tests and investigations can range from simple blood tests to highly sophisticated imaging tests, such as MRI and radionuclide scanning. The tests you will have depend on the nature of the condition that is suspected. Some of the more common tests and investigations are described below.

COURSE OF TREATMENT

Your family doctor (GP) is usually the first person you contact when you or a member of your family is ill. He or she will ask you about your symptoms and may examine you physically if necessary. The course of treatment may go something like this:

• Visit to the GP's surgery.

• Examination by GP.

• The GP may prescribe a drug or suggest a treatment, such as a NSAID gel for muscle pain or an antifungal drug for vaginal thrush.

• The GP may arrange further tests, such as blood tests, urine tests, X-rays or ultrasound scans. Some may be done in the surgery.

• Alternatively, the GP may refer the patient to a hospital consultant for further examination.

• The consultant (or a member of his team) will examine the patient and may arrange tests from simple blood tests to more sophisticated procedures, such as CT scans, MRI, or endoscopy.

• The patient's care may then be handed back to the GP, or be arranged and monitored at the consultant's clinic.

Blood tests

These are among the most frequently and easily performed medical tests. The composition of the blood can tell a great deal about the state of someone's health. Blood cell tests look at the number and composition of red and white blood cells and platelets in the blood. They help doctors in diagnosing diseases of the blood, such as anaemia. Blood cell tests can also show evidence of infection because it causes the white blood cell count to rise.

Tests on blood chemistry measure the levels of certain chemicals and minerals in the blood and are particularly used to check the functioning of the kidneys and the liver.

Finally, blood lipid tests measure the levels of certain fatty substances (known as lipids) in the blood. High levels of some lipids cause fatty deposits to develop on the lining of the artery walls, a condition known as atherosclerosis (*see p.252 for more information*).

Urine tests

The substances that are usually checked in a urine analysis include glucose, proteins, some electrolytes and creatinine (a product of protein metabolism). The presence of certain hormones in the urine indicates pregnancy. Testing a urine sample may also reveal blood cells, bacteria or other substances that indicate an underlying problem.

Tissue tests

Tissue tests, often called biopsies, involve taking a small sample of tissue from the body for examination under a microscope. Biopsies may be done for a number of reasons, including confirmation of a diagnosis or in order to

investigate a suspicious lump or area of tissue. In the case of cervical smears, a few cells from the cervix are removed to be examined for pre-cancerous changes.

Patch tests

A dermatologist or allergist can carry out patch tests on the skin to look for evidence of allergic reactions. In these tests, small, diluted amounts of potential allergens are placed on strips or discs, which are then taped to the skin for 48 hours. When the strips or discs are removed, the skin underneath is examined. Skin that is reddened or inflamed indicates an allergic reaction to the substance. Tested areas that show no reaction at first are examined again after a further 48 hours for any delayed reaction.

X-rays

These use high-intensity radiation to form an image on film placed on the other side of the body. Hard structures in the body, such as bones, block the radiation and show up on the film as white areas. X-rays are useful for imaging hard structures but are not very useful for imaging most soft tissues, including liver tissues, since soft tissue does not effectively block the radiation. However, a type of X-ray known as a contrast X-ray may be used to image certain soft tissue structures, such as those in the digestive tract.

Ultrasound scanning

This type of scanning uses sound waves to produce images. The image is formed by the "echo" of the sound waves as they bounce off different parts of the body. The echoes differ in their wavelength according to the density of the area examined. Ultrasound has become an important diagnostic tool, for example to investigate breast lumps in young women and to look for a cause of abdominal pain, such as gallstones. Ultrasound scanning also plays an important part in antenatal testing. A specialised form of ultrasound scanning, known as echocardiography, may be used to assess heart structure and function.

Computerised tomography (CT) scanning

In this technique, X-rays in conjunction with a computer produce images that build up a cross-sectional view of the body. CT scanning makes it possible to gather detailed information about organs and tissues. CT scans are most often taken of the head and the abdomen.

Magnetic resonance imaging (MRI)

Like CT scanning, MRI provides highly detailed cross-sectional images of internal organs and structures. These images are created by a computer using information received from a scanner. Unlike X-rays or CT scanning, MRI does not involve radiation; instead, it uses a magnetic field and radiowaves. MRI may distinguish abnormal soft tissue more clearly than CT scanning, and may be used at a greater range of planes through the body than is possible with CT scanning. MRI is especially useful for imaging the brain and for detecting tumours. It is also valuable for looking at the intervertebral discs and may be used to investigate low back pain.

Radionuclide scanning

In radionuclide scanning a radioactive substance called a radionuclide is introduced into the body (usually by injection) and is taken up by the organ or tissue to be imaged. A counter outside the body detects the radiation that is emitted and this information is in turn transmitted to a computer, which transforms it into images. Radionuclide scans may be used to detect abnormal levels of activity in organs such as the thyroid gland and the kidneys

and is useful for detecting tumours and other disorders in these organs. Another type of scanning, known as thallium scanning, may be used to investigate heart function.

Endoscopy

This procedure allows doctors to look inside the body. A tube-like instrument is inserted into the body. Endoscopes are very fine fibre-optic instruments that allow doctors to view organs and other structures on a monitor. Depending on the area to be viewed, access may be through a natural opening, such as the mouth or anus. Alternatively, it may be through a small incision, which may be made into a joint or the abdominal cavity. Many endoscopic procedures are performed under a general or local anaesthesic.

BLOOD TESTS

When a doctor takes a blood sample from you, it can be used for a range of tests. The blood is usually separated into its different components before testing.

— Plasma

— White cells and platelets

— Red blood cells

How blood separates in a centrifuge

BLOOD COMPONENT	TEST	RESULTS
Plasma The liquid portion of blood that carries dissolved chemicals	Electrolyte (salt) levels	Abnormal: impaired kidney function
	Blood urea nitrogen levels	
	Creatinine levels	
	Liver enzyme levels	Abnormal: impaired liver function
	Blood protein levels	
	Blood sugar levels	High: diabetes
White blood cells Part of the immune system, these cells are involved in the body's defence against disease	Number and type	High: infections, injury or burn, leukaemia, cancer
		Low: impaired bone marrow function. May be a side-effect of certain medication
		Regular cell counts show progress of a condition
Platelets Cell fragments which clump together to initiate blood clotting	Quantity	Low (bleeds too easily and profusely): autoimmune diseases, or leukaemia, viral infections, chemotherapy, and some medicines
		High (blood clots too easily): suggests conditions involving the bone marrow such as leukaemia
Red blood cells Contain haemoglobin – the chemical that carries oxygen around the body	Volume (haemocrit value), measured by spinning the sample very fast in a centrifuge. The red cells are the heaviest, so sink to the bottom.	Low: anaemia High: bone marrow conditions, dehydration
	Microscopic examination	Strange shape: e.g. sickle cell anaemia Abnormal size: e.g. pernicious anaemia
Whole blood	Microscopic examination	Parasites, visible in cases of sleeping sickness or malaria
	Blood culture	Bacteria present: blood poisoning
	Antibody testing	Present: may indicate diseases such as hepatitis

Treatment

Prescribed treatment, such as drugs or physiotherapy, is not always necessary. For some conditions, the most important part of a GP's role may be to offer reassurance that a symptom is not a cause for concern. Many minor health problems cure themselves. In long-term illness, a family doctor can provide crucial support and understanding, often based on a relationship built over years. However, in many cases drug treatment will be recommended, either on a short-term basis to relieve an acute problem (such as antibiotics for a bacterial infection), or for a longer period for a chronic condition (such as drugs for high blood pressure). Other treatments may be recommended to complement prescribed medicines; for example, physiotherapy may be prescribed in combination with non-steroidal anti-inflammatory drugs (NSAIDs) to treat a muscle problem. Sometimes surgery may be necessary to treat a condition and in most cases this involves referral to hospital, unless the surgery is very minor (such as wart removal).

Sometimes, despite many investigations, a definitive cause cannot be found to explain a patient's symptoms. In these circumstances, the GP may recommend measures that aim to relieve symptoms and to address factors that may be contributing to the problem, such as stress.

Why medication is prescribed

Drugs may be given for different reasons. Some cure or control diseases, others relieve symptoms. In addition, there are drugs, including vaccinations, which aim to prevent diseases from developing in the first place. Another example of using drugs for prevention is the prescription of lipid-lowering drugs to reduce blood lipids, thereby lowering the risk of developing coronary artery disease and stroke.

Research continues into improving existing medicines and developing new ones, particularly in key areas such as cancer, HIV and mental health. Drugs are tested extensively before they are marketed. In the UK, for example, all drugs must be approved and licensed by the Committee on Safety of Medicines (CSM). However, side-effects can still be a problem: drugs are given to produce specific desired effects, but they all have the potential to cause unwanted effects in addition, and may also interact with other drugs. If such effects are found to be unacceptable or unnecessarily risky, the CSM can withdraw a drug from the market.

How drugs work
Drugs can have a variety of effects. Some can replace or supplement a substance that is lacking. For example, thyroxine is prescribed to treat an underactive thyroid gland (*see chart opposite*). Some drugs eliminate or prevent the spread of infective organisms, such as bacteria and viruses. Others target a specific type of cell. For example,

certain cancer treatments destroy the rapidly dividing cells of a tumour. Non-steroidal anti-inflammatory drugs (NSAIDs) reduce the production of prostaglandins, chemicals that are released in response to tissue injury and which result in inflammation. Certain other medications are used to oppose unwanted processes, such as muscle spasm and high blood pressure.

Some drugs mimic or block the effect of certain chemicals in the body. Cells have receptors on their outer surface, which are activated by specific chemicals, triggering activities within the cell. Some drugs, called agonists, attach themselves to these receptors and trigger a response by the cell. Agonists often mimic the action of a naturally occurring substance. For example, the painkilling drug morphine is an agonist that mimics endorphins and works by preventing transmission of pain signals in the brain.

Others drugs, known as antagonists, attach themselves to receptors but block the action of the chemicals, so preventing the particular process. Antihistamines are antagonists. The chemical histamine is released by the body in susceptible individuals in response to a substance such as pollen, triggering an allergic reaction. Antihistamines attach themselves to some of the histamine receptors on the surface of certain cells, so reducing the action of histamine and dampening down the allergic response.

Finally, some drugs are useful because of their effect on the nervous system, where impulses are passed from one nerve to another by chemicals called neurotransmitters. Some of these chemicals are reabsorbed into the nerve endings and stored ready to be used again. In depression, the levels of the neurotransmitter serotonin, which acts on brain cells involved in thoughts and mood, are low. Certain antidepressants called selective serotonin re-uptake inhibitors (SSRIs) block some of the reabsorption of serotonin and so increase the amount available to stimulate nerves.

Drug delivery
Drugs can be delivered in various ways. Most are taken orally, but other preparations, such as eye drops, skin creams and inhalers for asthma, bypass the digestive system and deliver the drug to the particular part of the body affected. If rapid effects are required, some drugs can be given by injection directly into the bloodstream. Patches applied to the skin and implants inserted beneath the skin deliver drugs slowly for a more prolonged effect.

Side-effects and interactions
Every drug has the potential to cause side-effects. For example, in addition to lowering blood pressure, beta-blockers may cause fatigue, cold hands and feet and sleep disturbances. Chemotherapy drugs, as well as targeting the rapidly dividing cells of a tumour, can affect other rapidly dividing cells in addition, resulting in hair loss and other side-effects. Drugs may also cause allergic reactions; for example, some people are allergic to the antibiotic

penicillin and must use other antibiotics instead. Most drug side effects are not serious but in some cases doctors have to decide whether the overall benefit outweighs the risk of harmful effects.

Some drugs interact with each other. For this reason, doctors ask about medicines already being taken when prescribing new medication. It is also important to check that any over-the-counter drugs you buy do not interact with your existing medication and to remember that conventional drugs can sometimes interact with nutritional supplements and herbal remedies (*see also pp. 46 and 69*).

If you plan to use herbs or nutritional supplements and you are on medication, check with your doctor first. You should also make sure that your complementary therapist knows which drugs you are taking.

Tolerance and dependence

If certain drugs are taken on a long-term basis, the body may grow accustomed to them in a process known as tolerance. Sometimes, tolerance can be beneficial if some of the side-effects experienced with a drug reduce as the body becomes accustomed to it. However, with a small number

TYPES OF DRUG AND THEIR ACTIONS

Different types of drugs can be categorised according to their mode of action.	TYPE	EXAMPLES	ACTION
	Replacement	Insulin	For diabetes: replaces the insulin that the body no longer produces.
		Thyroxine	For thyroid deficiency: replaces the thyroxine that an underactive thyroid gland is unable to produce.
		Iron	For anaemia: replaces the body's reserves of iron lost through bleeding, poor diet, or when the body fails to absorb iron from food.
	Suppression	Anti-inflammatories	Suppress the body's inflammation response (a natural response to tissue damage). Non-steroidal examples include ibuprofen and diclofenac; corticosteroids include hydrocortisone.
		Antihistamines	Suppress the action of histamine, a chemical that the body releases in an allergic response (e.g. cetirizine, diphenhydramine).
		Painkillers	Prevent pain signals from being produced, or alter the way in which the brain perceives pain. Opioid painkillers include codeine and morphine, non-opioid painkillers include paracetamol and aspirin.
	Elimination	Antibiotics	Kill susceptible bacteria or halt their multiplication, e.g. penicillin.
		Antivirals	Stop viruses from reproducing, e.g. aciclovir.
		Cytotoxics	Kill body cells; used for cancer because the rapidly dividing cancer cells are more susceptible than most of the body's other cells.
	Opposition	Sedatives	Either slow mental activity by reducing the signals between brain cells (e.g. benzodiazepines), or block the action of stress hormones (beta-blockers). Used for anxiety disorders.
		Relaxants	Reduce muscle spasms by reducing transmission of nerve signals from brain and spinal cord to muscles (e.g. baclofen), blocking transmission of nerve signals from nerve endings to muscles (botulinum toxin), or making muscles less sensitive to nerve signals (e.g. dantrolene).
	Immunotherapies	Vaccines	Infectious organisms that have been modified or killed are injected into the body to stimulate the immune system to produce its own antibodies. Or ready-made antibodies are given.
		Allergens	Substances that can cause an allergic reaction, e.g. grass pollen or bee sting venom. To desensitise an allergy sufferer, he or she may be injected with the allergen at intervals, initially with tiny amounts then with a gradually increasing dose.

of drugs, it means that the drug becomes less effective over time and therefore an increasing dose will be needed to achieve the same effect. In some cases, a person develops a physical or psychological need for a drug. This is known as dependence. Sometimes, unpleasant symptoms may develop if the drug is suddenly withdrawn. Various drugs can cause dependence. Benzodiazepines (found in some anti-anxiety drugs and sleeping tablets) have particular dependency-producing potential and can cause dependence within as little as two weeks.

The choice of drug

When considering the choice of prescribed drug, the doctor will discuss the patient's medical history and any existing medication, as well as talking about the potential side-effects of the drugs. When prescribing, the doctor will balance the drug's possible side-effects against its potential benefits. In the ailments section of the book, we mention the side-effects of a few drugs, but it is not possible to give a comprehensive list. It is essential that you discuss possible side-effects with your doctor.

When a doctor makes a recommendation it will be backed up by information from various sources, including information gained from personal experience of use in patients, information from colleagues and data from clinical trials, which may be found in journals, discussed at conferences or presented on recognised websites on the internet, such as the Cochrane Library. The Department of Health has also produced recommendations on the treatment of certain diseases.

Contraindications and cautions

Many drugs are contraindicated (i.e. should not be taken) in certain circumstances, such as during pregnancy or when breast-feeding because they affect the foetus or can be passed via the breast-milk to the baby. Sometimes there are insufficient study data to back the use of the drugs during these times so doctors err on the side of caution and do not prescribe them.

Drugs may also be contraindicated in certain medical conditions. For example, NSAIDs should be avoided by people with peptic ulcers. In some medical conditions certain drugs are not actually contraindicated, but caution may be advised. This means that the drugs are not suitable in certain circumstances or that special monitoring is required. An example would be the use of anticonvulsants for epilepsy during pregnancy, when the risk of the drug to the baby must be weighed against the risk of seizures.

Microsurgery, here on a patient's eye, is one of the increasingly sophisticated techniques used to investigate and treat disease.

It is important to bear all of this in mind when purchasing over-the-counter drugs and to take advice from the pharmacist if you are pregnant, breast-feeding or if you have any medical conditions. Great care must also be taken when giving medication to children. Often the dose of medication is calculated on the basis of a child's weight but it is not precise. Always ask your doctor or pharmacist before giving medicines to children. Many drugs are not licensed for use in childhood.

Surgery

For some conditions, surgery is the most appropriate treatment. Some very minor surgery may be carried out by a GP, but in general it is necessary to go to hospital. Certain operations can be done on an outpatient or a day case basis, so that patients are able to go home the same day, but in other cases a hospital stay is necessary.

Open surgery
In open surgery, an incision is made in the skin large enough to see clearly the internal body parts that require treatment and the surrounding tissues. Open surgery is mainly performed under a general anaesthesic and may leave an obvious scar.

Endoscopic surgery
Endoscopic, or "keyhole", surgery is a relatively new technique that enables various surgical procedures to be performed without making large incisions in the skin. The surgeon makes small incisions and introduces the viewing instrument and surgical instruments into the body through these. Endoscopy on joints (arthroscopy) is often done under local anaesthetic, whereas abdominal endoscopic surgery is usually performed under a general anaesthetic. The length of stay in hospital and recovery time are usually shorter for endoscopic surgery than for open surgery.

Microsurgery
This relatively new form of surgery makes it possible for doctors to operate on extremely small and delicate tissues within the body that are otherwise hard to view. Micro-surgeons use binocular microscopes to view the operating site and specially adapted small operating instruments. Microsurgery can be used to operate on nerves and blood vessels and on small structures in the eye, middle ear and reproductive system. Depending on the operation, it may be performed under a general or a local anaesthetic.

Other treatments

There are many other treatments that a doctor may recommend. Sometimes these are in addition to drug treatment or surgery; for example, physiotherapy may be necessary after an knee or shoulder operation in order to restore a full range of movement to the joint. Psychological therapy may be recommended on its own to treat depression or may be given to patients in combination with antidepressant drugs. In all cases, for the best possible outcome the aim is to put together a treatment package that is appropriate to the individual, taking into account various factors, including patient choice.

The role of complementary therapies in conjunction with conventional medicine is evolving all the time. Many GP practices now have psychotherapists, hypnotherapists, osteopaths, acupuncturists and other complementary practitioners working alongside their teams providing healthcare. Also, many hospital pain clinics use medical acupuncture as well as drugs. As the medical profession's understanding and knowledge of complementary therapies grows, many therapies are likely to play a more prominent role in the care of patients.

Gene therapy and future treatments

New approaches to treating diseases are being researched all the time, some of which are radically different from the treatments we have known in the past. Gene therapy is a good example of an approach that may offer a new way of treating people with a range of conditions.

Genes are made of DNA (deoxyribonucleic acid) which codes for the proteins that make up the body. To a large extent, genes determine who you are. Errors in the genes are responsible for diseases such as some types of cancer and cystic fibrosis. Gene therapy is a technique in which DNA, rather than drugs, is administered to the patient. The new DNA can correct or replace faulty genes, or change the way that genes behave. The most common way for the new DNA to be introduced into the body is through viruses. Viruses normally package and deliver DNA into body cells as part of the infective process. Gene therapists take disease-causing viruses, inactivate them, and put therapeutic genes inside them. The patient is infected with the modified virus so that the new genes will reach body cells and be activated.

Gene therapy is still experimental and is likely only to be appropriate for a few types of diseases. By 2004, over 300 patients had been involved in clinical trials using gene therapy. There have been a number of successes, but also some failures that have highlighted a range of problems. It works best for genetic diseases in which only a single gene is at fault, such as Severe Combined Immunodeficiency Syndrome ("baby in the bubble" syndrome), haemophilia, cystic fibrosis and some cancers. Many common diseases, such as heart disease, arthritis and Alzheimer's disease, have genetic components, but they involve more than one gene and so are more difficult to target.

As with any experimental technique, it will take years of trials before it can be made available to the public. However, gene therapy, new drugs and other technical advances offer real hope for people with as yet unconquered diseases.

NUTRITIONAL THERAPY

DR JOHN BRIFFA

The body is in a state of constant renewal: millions of cells die each second, while others multiply to make good the loss. Food provides the raw materials for building and regenerating the body. Clinical experience and many studies show that dietary changes and nutritional supplements can restore and maintain health and well-being, as well as helping to treat a range of everyday conditions. Nutritional approaches can also be effective in preventing and treating serious conditions such as coronary artery disease, stroke, cancer and diabetes.

Dietary Carbohydrates

Carbohydrates – sugars, starches and fibre – are made of the elements carbon, hydrogen and oxygen. Their main role is to provide a source of energy for the body.

Sugars

The basic building block of all carbohydrates is a single sugar molecule, such as glucose or fructose, known as a monosaccharide. A disaccharide is two monosaccharides joined together – sucrose, for example, contains glucose and fructose. Sugars in fruit and vegetables are "intrinsic" as they are incorporated into the structure of foods, often hidden within cell walls. In some foods, such as biscuits and sweetened cereals, the sugar is not bound into the structure of food and so these are called "extrinsic" sugars. Generally, foods with intrinsic sugars are healthier than those with extrinsic sugars; an apple is healthier to eat than a piece of cake. Foods containing intrinsic sugar tend to release energy more slowly into the bloodstream compared to foods rich in extrinsic sugar.

Starches

Also referred to as complex carbohydrates, dietary starches are made up of chains of sugar molecules. Starch-based foods include vegetables, bread, pasta, rice, potatoes, beans, pulses and breakfast cereals. Starches come in two main forms. Refined starches, as found in white bread, white rice and most commonly available types of pasta, have lost much of their fibre, vitamin and mineral content.

Unrefined starches are richer in fibre and nutrients than their refined counterparts and are therefore considered nutritionally superior. They also tend to give a slower, more sustained release of sugar into the bloodstream, which may be important for health in both the short and long term. Examples of unrefined starches include wholemeal bread, brown rice, wholewheat pasta and rolled oats.

Fibre

Fibre is plant material that is indigestible and is sometimes referred to as non-starch polysaccharide (NSP). Fibre comes in two main forms. Soluble fibre dissolves in the gut to form a thick gel-like substance that slows down the release of some nutrients, particularly sugar, into the bloodstream. It appears to help control the levels of cholesterol in the blood, which may help to reduce the risk of coronary artery disease.

Insoluble fibre does not dissolve in the digestive tract and therefore adds bulk to the faeces. It is useful for preventing constipation and there is evidence that a high-fibre diet is associated with a reduced risk of cancer of the colon. A diet that is rich in insoluble fibre may also reduce the risk of other conditions, including haemorrhoids (piles) and diverticular disease (abnormal pockets on the lining of the colon that can become infected and cause bleeding or perforation of the gut wall).

Good sources of soluble fibre include fruit, vegetables, beans, oats, barley and rye. Good sources of insoluble fibre include wholegrain (unrefined) cereals, such as wholemeal bread, brown rice and wholewheat pasta, as well as beans and pulses, nuts, seeds, and fibrous vegetables, such as carrots, celery and cabbage.

Dietary Proteins

Dietary proteins are composed of amino acids and play a role in the manufacture of many structures and tissues, such as bone, muscle, skin and hair. They are essential for normal growth and development in children. In adults, proteins provide the raw materials needed for cell repair. Cells use amino acids derived from the diet to make DNA and enzymes – molecules with key roles in maintaining healthy structure and function within the body.

Of the 21 amino acids, many can be made in the body and therefore do not, strictly speaking, need to be eaten. However, eight cannot be made in the body and so must be provided in the diet. They are the "essential" amino acids.

It is said that adults need about 0.75–1g of protein for each kilogram of body weight per day. Meat, fish, eggs and dairy products are very good sources of protein, as are non-animal foods, such as beans, peas and nuts. Some grains, such as rice, wheat and maize, can also supply significant quantities of protein. In general, animal-derived proteins are more "complete" in terms of their component amino acids than vegetable sources. Vegetarians should eat a broad range of protein-containing foods, including beans, pulses, nuts, seeds and grains, to ensure amino acid intake.

There is some evidence that too much protein can pose hazards. Excess protein is believed to cause the loss of calcium from bone, predisposing a person to osteoporosis (brittle bones; *see p.38*) and increased risk of fracture. In one study, women who ate more than 95g of protein a day were found to be 20 per cent more likely to have broken a wrist over a 12-year period when compared to women who ate an average amount of protein (less than 68g a day).

Dietary Fats

Fats provide energy and components for some structures, such as cell membranes and certain hormones. The basic building blocks of dietary fats are fatty acids, which consist of chains of carbon atoms with hydrogen atoms attached. There are three main natural forms of fatty acid. Saturated fatty acids are so called because they have as many hydrogen atoms as they can hold. Monounsaturated fatty acids lack a pair of hydrogen atoms per molecule. Polyunsaturated fatty acids lack four or more hydrogen atoms per molecule.

Saturated fatty acids

These are found in animal products, such as butter, cheese, whole milk, ice cream and meat, and in some vegetable oils, such as coconut and palm oils. It is often said that eating a diet rich in saturated fatty acids can raise levels of cholesterol in the blood. However, more than one study has found that this may not be the case. Even the belief that such a diet is a major risk factor for coronary artery disease may be overstated, partly as a result of misquoting and misinterpretation of research studies. Saturated fatty acids may be a factor in weight gain and obesity, although a comprehensive review of the subject concluded that dietary fat is not a major determinant in body weight, and eating less fat is unlikely to bring lasting weight loss.

So, on balance, it appears that saturated fatty acids might be less harmful than is often believed, and that eating them in moderate amounts may not be damaging to health.

Monounsaturated fatty acids

Food rich in monounsaturated fatty acids include olive oil, avocados, nuts and seeds. These fatty acids can lower blood levels of low-density lipoprotein (LDL) cholesterol, the type of cholesterol that is believed to increase the risk of heart disease. They can also raise blood levels of high-density lipoprotein (HDL) cholesterol, which is thought to protect against heart disease. A high intake of mono-unsaturated fatty acids is believed to be one of the reasons certain populations, such as the southern Italians and the Greeks, have relatively low levels of heart disease.

Polyunsaturated fatty acids (PUFAs)

There are two main groups of PUFAs in the diet: omega-6 and omega-3. The major omega-6 fatty acid is linoleic acid – rich sources include plant oils, such as hemp, pumpkin, sunflower, safflower, sesame, corn, walnut and soya oil. Others are gamma linolenic acid (GLA), dihomogamma linolenic acid (DGLA) and arachidonic acid (AA). The major omega-3 fatty acids are alpha-linolenic acid (from plants, such as flaxseed), eicosatetraenoic acid (ETA), eicosapentaenoic acid (EPA) and docosahexaenoic acid (DHA). EPA and DHA are mainly found in oily varieties of fish. Within the body, these fatty acids can be converted into other substances that may affect health.

The omega-6 and omega-3 balance

The omega-3 and omega-6 fatty acids have important roles in many body systems, including the brain, nerves, immune system, cardiovascular system, eyes and skin. They are converted into hormone-like substances called eicosanoids.

Eicosanoids derived from omega-6 fatty acids tend to encourage inflammation, blood-vessel constriction and blood clotting. Therefore, they increase the risk of coronary artery disease and stroke and inflammatory conditions, such as arthritis. Eicosanoids derived from arachidonic acid are particularly potent. Those from omega-3 fatty acids, such as EPA, are less likely to encourage inflammation; some are positively anti-inflammatory. They tend to reduce the risk of clotting and help to relax blood vessels, so helping to reduce the risk of coronary artery disease and stroke as well as inflammatory conditions, such as arthritis.

The roughly opposing actions of omega-3 and omega-6 fatty acids mean that it is important to balance their intake. A ratio of 1:1 is believed to be ideal. Over the past 40 years, however, the proportion of omega-6 to omega-3 in the average diet has increased to roughly six to one. This may be an important factor in the development of many chronic diseases, such as cardiovascular disease and cancer.

To reduce your intake of omega-6 fatty acids and increase your intake of omega-3 fatty acids:

- Limit the intake of vegetable oils, such as sunflower oil, corn oil, rapeseed oil and maize oil, which contain omega-6 fatty acids. Processed foods labelled as containing "vegetable oil" contain these oils.
- Sprinkle flaxseeds on cereals and take flaxseed oil, which is a rich source of omega-3 fatty acids.
- Eat three portions a week of oily fish, such as mackerel, herring, salmon, trout and sardines.
- Take a fish oil supplement each day.

Partially hydrogenated and trans fatty acids

Some margarines and vegetable shortenings (the fats added to many processed foods) are manufactured using a process known as hydrogenation. This can change the structure of fats, creating what are known as trans fatty acids. These are believed to have harmful effects on health, particularly with regard to heart disease. While trans fats do occur naturally in some foods (such as butter), there is evidence that it is only industrially produced, and not naturally occurring, trans fats that have a detrimental effect on heart health. You should consider avoiding margarines and processed foods listing partially hydrogenated oils (or trans fatty acids) as an ingredient.

Water

The body is made up of about 70 per cent water. Water is vital in most of the processes that are integral to health. Even mild dehydration (e.g. losing about 70ml of fluid for

Fats are moved around the body as lipids bound with proteins, to form particles of low-density lipoprotein (LDL). LDLs transport cholesterol (a steroid) from the liver to the tissues of the body. High cholesterol levels are linked to cardiovascular disease, but some cholesterol is vital for the functioning of body cells.

a 70kg adult) can impair essential body processes and cause symptoms such as headaches, appetite loss, fatigue, muscle weakness, light-headedness and dry eyes and dry mouth.

Keeping well hydrated also seems to help reduce the risk of chronic disease. Research indicates, for instance, that low levels of fluid consumption are associated with increased risk of cancers of the kidney, bladder, prostate and testes. Other research has found that increasing fluid intake seems to reduce the risk of bladder and colon cancer. Evidence also suggests that drinking water may reduce the risk of heart disease. In one study, women drinking five or more glasses of fluid each day had a 41 per cent reduced risk of dying from a heart attack compared to women drinking two or fewer glasses each day, and for men the risk was reduced by 54 per cent.

As a rough guide, drink about 30ml of water for each kilogram of body weight. For most people, this equates to 1.5–2.5 litres of water a day. However, individual needs can vary with factors such as outside temperature and activity. A good guide to our state of hydration is the colour of the urine. The aim is to drink enough water to keep the urine pale or very pale yellow during the day.

The quality of the drinking water is important, too. Tap water contains chlorine. This can induce chemical changes which, at least in theory, should increase cancer risk. It seems sensible to drink filtered tap water or mineral water. (*See also Environmental Health, p.86*).

Imbalances and Treatments

The body can be subject to a variety of imbalances that may cause health problems. This section explores the most common ones and explains how to deal with them.

Food intolerance and exclusion diets

Food intolerance occurs when the body has difficulty digesting and using a certain food or group of foods. It is different from food allergy, in which a certain type of food causes an abnormal immune response, such as a rash or swelling. Intolerance, although not usually as dangerous as allergy, can still cause a great deal of discomfort.

Most of what we eat must be broken down by digestion before it can be absorbed via the gut wall into the blood.

However, in some circumstances, incompletely digested food can leak through the wall of the digestive tract (*see p.457*). This can provoke reactions leading to a range of symptoms and conditions. These include fatigue, abdominal bloating, headaches, migraine, irritable bowel syndrome, Crohn's disease, colic, eczema and dermatitis, asthma, rheumatoid arthritis, sinusitis, ear infections, nasal congestion and excessive mucus formation.

If a nutritional therapist suspects a food intolerance, the following tests can help with the diagnosis.

Prick testing

The prick test checks for an allergic response. It involves breaking the outer layer of the skin and introducing a tiny amount of the food or other substance (e.g. animal hair, pollen) to be tested. If the skin becomes inflamed, it is likely that you have a real allergy to the food.

IgG and IgE blood testing

Antibodies are proteins made by the immune system in response to proteins or other compounds that the body recognises as "foreign". One type, the IgG antibodies, are thought to be involved in food reactions. IgG antibodies to specific foods can be detected using biochemical techniques, of which there are two basic types – RAST (radioallergosorbent test) and ELISA (enzyme-linked immunoserological assay). An IgE blood test can measure the levels of a specific form of antibody (Immunoglobulin E) in the blood and also check for allergic response.

Neither prick tests nor IG tests are particularly useful for forms of food intolerance, rather than allergy. Allergies involve the immune system, which recognises food molecules as foreign and attempts to label or attack them with IG antibodies. As food intolerances do not tend to involve an immune reaction, different tests are needed.

THE MICRONUTRIENTS

The diet provides the body with a range of vitamins and minerals that have important roles to play in health and well-being. The major nutrients, along with their dietary sources, key effects and recommended daily amounts (also known as the reference nutrient intakes) are summarised here.

NUTRIENT	MAIN SOURCES	KEY EFFECTS	CURRENT RNI*
Vitamin A	Milk, butter, egg yolk, liver, oily fish As beta-carotene (a precursor of vitamin A) in carrots, tomatoes, dark green/yellow vegetables	● Believed to be cancer protective ● Important for night vision ● Important for cell growth and development ● Important for the health of the skin	600mg per day (women) 700mg/d men
Vitamin B1 (Thiamin)	Cereals, nuts, pulses, wholegrains, green vegetables	● Supplementation may enhance mood and mental alertness ● Important for carbohydrate metabolism ● Important for nervous system maintenance	0.8mg/d women 1.0mg/d men
Vitamin B2 (Riboflavin)	Liver, milk, eggs, green vegetables, yeast extract	● Important for metabolism ● Important for all cell growth and development	1.3mg/d
Vitamin B3 (Niacin)	Liver, beef, pork, fish fortified breakfast cereals, yeast extract	● Important for metabolism ● Essential for the formation of red blood cells ● Important for the nervous and digestive systems	13mg/d women 17mg/d men
Vitamin B5 (Pantothenic acid)	Animal products, cereals, legumes	● A constituent of coenzyme A – essential for metabolism ● Coenzyme A is important for the immune system	No RNI
Vitamin B6	Meat, fish, eggs	● May be important in reducing the risk of heart disease (in combination with folate and vitamin B12) by lowering homocysteine levels ● Is required for the efficient functioning of the immune and nervous systems ● Supplementation may be beneficial in the treatment of pre-menstrual syndrome	1.2mg/d women 1.4mg/d men
Vitamin B12	Liver, meat, eggs, milk, yeast extract	● May be important in reducing the risk of heart disease (in combination with folate and vitamin B6) by lowering homocysteine levels ● Is important for production of red blood cells ● Supplementation may be beneficial in the treatment of pre-menstrual syndrome	1.5mg/d
Vitamin C	Fresh fruit especially citrus fruit, blackcurrants, kiwi fruit, and green vegetables	● Supplementation has been associated with a reduced risk of heart disease (especially in combination with vitamin E) ● Some evidence exists to suggest that vitamin C may be important in cancer prevention	40mg/d
Vitamin D	Oily fish, e.g. mackerel, egg yolk, fortified margarine	● Important for regulating calcium in the body and for bone health ● Evidence suggests that vitamin D supplementation may play a role in cancer prevention (especially colon and breast cancers) ● Evidence suggests that vitamin D supplementation may help prevent heart disease	No RNI for those aged 19–50. After the age of 65 RNI is 10mg/d

*(for those aged 19–50)

THE MICRONUTRIENTS CONTINUED

NUTRIENT	MAIN SOURCES	KEY EFFECTS	CURRENT RNI*
Vitamin E	Nuts, vegetable oils, vegetables, wholegrain cereals, oily fish	● Appears to enhance immune function ● Is associated with a reduced risk of heart disease in some studies ● May reduce the risk of prostate cancer ● May slow the progression of Alzheimer's disease ● Evidence suggests that supplementation (particularly in combination with vitamin C) lowers the risk of developing Alzheimer's disease	No RNI
Vitamin K	Dark green leafy vegetables e.g. spinach	● Evidence suggests supplementation may prevent fractures	No RNI
Folic acid	Liver, orange juice, green vegetables, nuts	● Proven to reduce the risk of neural tube defects such as spina bifida ● Supplementation lowers plasma homocysteine levels – believed to reduce risk of heart disease ● Supplementation may be important in cancer prevention (especially cancers of the colon and breast)	200mg/d
Calcium	Milk, canned fish, pulses, sesame seeds, nuts	● Necessary for the formation and maintenance of strong bones and teeth ● Important for the proper functioning of nerves and muscles	700mg/d
Magnesium	Nuts, pulses, wholegrain cereals	● Important for nerve and muscle function ● May be useful cardiovascular disorders ● Supplementation appears to reduce blood pressure ● Supplementation may reduce the risk of stroke ● Supplementation may be associated with better lung function ● Supplementation may be useful in reducing the symptoms of PMS	270mg/d women 300mg/d men
Zinc	Meat, eggs, milk, fish, wholegrain cereals, pulses	● Important for immune system function ● Supplementation may modulate testosterone levels in men (especially in men who are mildly deficient)	7mg/d women 9.5mg/d men
Selenium	Brazil nuts, fish, liver	● Appears to be cancer protective ● Supplementation may be protective against asthma ● Supplementation may improve immunity ● Supplementation may improve mood	60mg/d women 75mg/d men
Iron	Red meat, cereals, pulses	● Essential for formation of red blood cells ● Important for the immune system ● Essential for brain function ● Essential for the proper functioning of the thyroid	14.8mg/d women 8.7mg/d men
Iodine	Seafood, seaweed, eggs, milk	● Essential for the synthesis of thyroid hormones which regulate metabolic activity	140mg/d
Copper	Meat, wholegrains, nuts, seeds	● Important for the immune system ● Promotes normal formation of red blood cells	1.2mg/d
Potassium	Widespread in food	● Needed for proper nerve function ● Aids in the maintenance of blood pressure	3,500mg/d
Sodium	Widespread in food	● Important for nerve and muscle activity	1,600mg/d

*(for those aged 19–50)

Cytotoxic and ALCAT tests

The cytotoxic test mixes white blood cells with individual food extracts and then ascertains which foods caused reactions in the cells. The ALCAT test (ALCAT stands for antigen leucocyte cellular antibody) is similar except that assessing the reaction of the white cells requires a sophisticated piece of laboratory equipment.

Electro-dermal testing

Practitioners of Chinese medicine believe that energy flows down channels known as meridians in the body. Electro-dermal testing involves measuring the electrical current that flows through an acupuncture point on a meridian, then detecting any changes in the current as the body is challenged with individual foods. Extracts of those foods

DIGESTIVE SYSTEM

The digestive system consists of the digestive tract, which is a tube about 7 metres (24 ft) long from mouth to anus, and its associated organs. Food is digested and the macronutrients (carbohydrates, proteins and fats) are broken down into their constituent components.

ORGAN	FUNCTION
1 Mouth	The teeth and tongue mash food, mixing it with saliva.
2 Salivary glands	Three pairs of salivary glands release saliva. Salivary enzymes begin the digestion process, breaking down starch into simple sugars.
3 Oesophagus	This muscular tube connects the throat to the stomach. At the bottom is a ring of muscle (a sphincter) that relaxes to let food into the stomach.
4 Stomach	The stomach is a muscular bag. Stomach (gastric) juices contain acids and enzymes. The acid kills most bacteria, and enzymes begin to digest protein into amino acids.
5 Liver	The liver produces bile, a digestive juice made from old blood cells. The liver is also where nutrients are modified or stored, and alcohol and other toxins are broken down.
6 Gallbladder	The gallbladder stores bile and releases it into the duodenum.
7 Pancreas	The pancreas produces juices that are powerful digesting agents. Pancreatic juices also neutralise the stomach acids.
8 Small intestine	This is the longest section of the digestive tract, at 5 metres (17 ft), and consists of the duodenum, jejunum and ileum. This narrow, tightly packed tube has a very convoluted lining with millions of microscopic projections that together give a huge surface area for absorption.
9 Large intestine	This section of the digestive tract is around 1.5 metres (5 ft) long, and consists of the caecum, colon and rectum. The tube is wider than the small intestine, and the internal surface is not so wrinkled.
10 Appendix	A blind-ending tube coming off the caecum. In humans it appears to have no digestive function.
11 Rectum	Faeces collect in the rectum before being excreted through the anus.

may be put in the same circuit as the subject being tested – if it changes the current there is a problem with the food.

However, in one reliable study this form of testing failed to identify genuine IgE-type acute food allergy. It has not been fully studied as a way of identifying food intolerance.

The elimination diet

Many practitioners of nutritional medicine regard this as the most accurate way of testing for food sensitivity. Once identified, problem foods can be eliminated for good. Many individuals whose health issues are linked with food intolerance find they experience a sudden improvement in their condition, along with increased energy, enhanced mental clarity and improved digestive function. Foods generally eliminated on such a diet include:

- Wheat (a very common problem food), found in breads, pasta, pastry, pizza, biscuits, cakes, wheat-based breakfast cereals, wheat crackers, breaded food, battered food and anything containing wheat flour.
- Milk, cheese and yoghurt.
- Foods or drinks that are consumed repeatedly, say on four or more days each week (the more often a food is eaten, the more likely it is to be a problem).
- Foods or drinks that are craved (cravings for a particular food can be a sign of intolerance to that food).
- Foods and drinks that are suspected because they seem to induce symptoms.

All likely problem foods are removed from the diet for two to three weeks. If a food sensitivity is at the root of the symptoms, and the problem food has been eliminated, improvement can generally be expected in this time. A good amount of a specific food should be eaten in the morning. Over the next few hours, look out for a return of the original symptoms. Other problems may include headache, itching, depression, fatigue, irritability and foggy thinking. A note should be made of any food that seems to bring on an unwanted reaction and it should be eliminated again from the diet. Foods that do not provoke a reaction after breakfast should be eaten at lunch and dinner. If by the following morning there are still no symptoms, this food can be provisionally added to a list of "safe" foods.

For the next three days, the food should be eliminated again and a watchful eye kept for any symptoms that suggest a food reaction. It is possible that the symptoms of a reaction may come on two or three days after a food or drink is consumed. If there are no symptoms after three days, it is likely that the food being tested is safe to eat. This process can be repeated for all the eliminated foods.

In normal circumstances, it is wise to exclude problem foods for a month, although two or more months may be better. Abstaining from a food for a period of time can make the body more tolerant to it in the long term. However, initial food reactions can be worse, not better, than before – a phenomenon that is referred to as "hypersensitisation". Care should be taken when re-introducing foods, particularly if the condition being treated has an allergic component, such as asthma. When a food is re-introduced, it is best not to eat too much of it too frequently, as this can increase the risk of the original problem recurring.

Improving digestion and food combining

Making sure that foods are fully digested can help reduce food intolerance. Simple steps that can be taken to improve digestion include the following:

Thorough chewing

Chewing mixes food with saliva, which contains an enzyme that starts the digestion of starchy foods, such as bread, potatoes, rice and pasta. It also breaks food up, increasing the surface area available for contact with the digestive juices and enzymes. Each mouthful ideally should be chewed to a cream before swallowing.

Avoid big meals

The larger the meal, the larger the load on the digestive system. Therefore small meals eaten frequently reduce the risk of indigestion.

Avoid drinking with meals

Some people tend to drink fluid with meals in the belief that this helps to "wash food down". The reality is quite the reverse. Drinking with meals dilutes the acid and enzymes that do the digestive work and does nothing to help the process of digestion. On the whole, drinking should be done between meals, not at mealtimes.

Food combining

Proteins and starches are very different chemically and are digested by different enzymes in the gut. Initially, proteins are digested in acid, starches in alkali (quite the opposite). An inability to cope with protein and starch combinations can lead to impaired digestion.

The aim of food combining is to avoid mixing protein and starch at the same meal. This means eating either protein or starch combined with a food that is "neutral" – neither protein nor starch. (For a list of common protein, starch and neutral foods, *see p.40.*)

Examples of healthy meals include: meat or fish with salad or vegetables other than potatoes; pasta with tomato-based sauce (no meat) and salad; vegetable curry and rice; baked potato, ratatouille and salad; meat stew with vegetables and avocado salad sandwiches.

Eating to this pattern can bring tremendous relief to people with indigestion and increase the chances of complete and rapid food breakdown. It may also help to reduce the risk of food sensitivity, and is often very effective in helping improve digestive symptoms such as bloating, indigestion and acid reflux.

Candida overgrowth

Within the gut live about 1–2kg (2–4lb) of gut flora. These "friendly bacteria" have a variety of roles to play, including assisting in digestion, keeping unhealthy organisms at bay and ensuring that the gut lining remains healthy. The yeast organism *Candida albicans* can also inhabit the large intestine and does not usually cause health problems.

However, under certain circumstances, it can overgrow in the small intestine, leading to symptoms that include erratic bowel habits (constipation and/or loose bowel movements); wind and flatulence; abdominal bloating; anal itching; recurrent bouts of thrush (vaginal yeast infection); other fungal infections, including athlete's foot or generalised itching around the groin and/or the inside of the buttocks; recurrent bouts of cystitis and/or problems with vaginal irritation; and cravings for sugar, sugary foods (such as chocolate, biscuits or cakes) or yeasty foods (cheese, bread, alcohol or vinegar). *Candida* overgrowth may also cause vague, unexplained health problems, such as fatigue, pain and mental distress. The overlap between symptoms of gut flora disturbance and depression can be confusing for patients as well as practitioners.

One of the major causes of yeast overgrowth is antibiotic therapy, which can kill the healthy gut organisms that normally help to keep yeast organisms such as *Candida* at bay. Other common underlying factors in yeast overgrowth include stress (which can upset the immune system), the consumption of yeast-encouraging foods, such as sugar, bread, cheese and alcohol, and taking the oral contraceptive pill or hormone replacement therapy (HRT).

Tests for Candida

If *Candida* is suspected, a nutritional therapist may arrange one of the various tests. Yeast analysis of stool samples can be tried, although it can be misleading because *Candida* is normally present in the large intestine. The blood can be tested for the *Candida* antigen – if positive, an ongoing yeast infection may be indicated.

Antibodies are substances the immune system produces in response to antigens. Two types of antibody, known as IgG and IgM, are usually measured in the blood. Raised levels of the antibodies specific for *Candida* may indicate a significant infection. A type of antibody known as secretory IgA is produced by the gut. Measuring the amount of secretory IgA made specifically against *Candida* can be a good guide to the presence of yeast in the gut.

Another test that examines gut fermentation is based on the principle that yeast tends to metabolise sugar into alcohol. After a blood sample is taken, a person is given a measured dose of sugar. One hour later, another sample of blood is taken. Both blood samples are then analysed for various fermentation products. The presence of these in significant quantity can point to the presence of excess yeast in the gut.

FOOD COMBINING		
PROTEIN	**NEUTRAL**	**STARCH**
Meats:	**All green and root**	bread
beef	**vegetables apart**	potatoes
lamb	**from potatoes:**	rice
chicken	asparagus	pasta
turkey	aubergines	cereal
veal	broccoli	
venison	Brussels sprouts	**Foods from flour:**
pork	cabbage	pastries
bacon	carrots	cakes
	cauliflower	biscuits
Fish:	celery	
mackerel	courgettes	**Dried fruits:**
herring	green beans	dates
trout	leeks	figs
salmon	mushrooms	currants
tuna	onions	sultanas
cod	parsnips	raisins
plaice	peas	
skate	spinach	**Other fruit:**
	turnips	bananas
Shellfish:		mangoes
prawns	**Salad vegetables:**	
cockles	avocado	**Sweeteners:**
mussels	cucumber	sugar
crab	tomatoes	maple syrup
lobster	lettuce	honey
	spring onions	
Dairy products:	peppers	
cheese, milk, eggs	radishes	
yoghurt	nuts and seeds	
	Fats and oils:	
Vegetable proteins:	cream, butter	
soya beans	extra virgin olive oil	
soya bean curd	other vegetable oils	
(tofu)		

The anti-Candida diet

The cornerstone of the anti-*Candida* approach is a diet that helps starve yeast out of the system. Foods to be avoided include those that feed yeast directly and those that are yeasty, mouldy or fermented in their own right.

Yeast-feeding foods to avoid include: sugar; sweetening agents, such as maple syrup, molasses, honey, malt syrup; sugar-containing foods, such as biscuits, cakes, pastries, confectionery, ice cream, sugared breakfast cereals, soft drinks and fruit juice; white flour products, such as white bread, crackers, pizza and pasta.

Yeasty, mouldy or fermented foods to avoid include: bread and other items made with yeast; alcoholic drinks, particularly beer and wine, which are very yeasty; gravy mixes (most contain brewer's yeast); vinegar and vinegar-containing foods, such as ketchup (which also contains sugar), mustard, mayonnaise and many prepared salad dressings; pickles, miso, tempeh and soy sauce (all are fermented); aged cheeses, such as cheddar, Stilton, Swiss, Brie and Camembert (cheese is inherently mouldy); peanuts, peanut butter, and pistachios (tend to harbour yeast); mushrooms; dried fruits (these are intensely sugary and tend to harbour mould); prepared soups and pre-packaged foods, which tend to contain yeast.

Foods to eat freely on an anti-*Candida* diet include meat, fish, eggs, beans, pulses, vegetables, nuts (but not peanuts or pistachios), seeds, oats, brown rice.

Views on whether fruit can be eaten on an anti-*Candida* diet vary. Some experts recommend complete exclusion, while others say you can eat it frequently. In general, one or two pieces of fruit a day will be well tolerated, although grapes are generally best avoided because they are very sugary and usually are covered in a mouldy bloom.

Supplements to overcome Candida

In addition to the anti-*Candida* diet, it may help to take specific supplements – probiotics, liver-supporting agents and antifungal supplements – to help restore the full functioning of the digestive system.

Probiotics contain gut bacteria. Those that contain both *Bifidobacterium bifidus* (the predominant bacterium in the large intestine) and *Lactobacillus acidophilus* (the predominant bacterium in the small intestine) can help to restore the balance of organisms in the gut and help combat *Candida* overgrowth.

During the initial phases of an anti-*Candida* regime, it is quite common for the condition to get worse. Lethargy, fuzzy-headedness and flu-like symptoms can start a day or so after the regime starts and generally last from a

few days to a couple of weeks. Liver-supporting agents (*see p.42*) can help reduce these symptoms.

Antifungal supplements can help to combat the *Candida* fungus directly. Oregano contains two important active ingredients, carvacrol and thymol. Studies have shown that oregano can inhibit the growth of *Candida*. In natural medicine, garlic is widely used in the control and eradication of *Candida*. Finally, grapefruit seed extract supplements are also useful as they have the ability to kill *Candida* in the body.

Detoxification

The body is constantly exposed to substances that have the potential to adversely affect health and well-being. Some, such as the pollutants we breathe and the herbicides and pesticides that lace our food, come from outside. Others are the result of the metabolic and physiological processes that go on within the body every day. If the toxic load on the system is large, and/or if there is a problem with detoxification processes, toxins may accumulate, giving rise to fatigue, lethargy, weight gain, headaches, joint and muscle aches, acne, bad breath, body odour and cellulite. Ensuring efficient elimination of toxins from the system is fundamental. The liver is the main organ of detoxification in the body. It contains thousands of lobules, which are tiny blood-

Candida albicans is a type of yeast that lives naturally in the mouth, skin, gut and vagina. One way that it reproduces is by spores. These rounded spores are connected by long thread-like filaments, called hyphae.

processing units just 1mm wide. As the liver takes blood from the digestive tract and from the general circulation it is thus able to neutralise toxins from the diet and the processes of metabolism, and also pollutants from the air taken in through the lungs. It processes these toxins so that they can be removed from the body without causing harm.

Optimising liver function

To improve liver function, try the following:

- Eat plenty of fresh fruit and vegetables. These do not tax or stress the liver, and contain an abundance of nutrients such as vitamin C and carotenoids (e.g. beta-carotene) that can support liver function.
- Limit the amount of dietary fat and protein, as these need substantial processing by the liver. The main foods to avoid are fatty meats, such as beef, lamb and duck; dairy products; hydrogenated vegetable oils present in margarine and many processed, baked and fast foods.
- Avoid artificial additives such as sweeteners, colourings, flavourings and preservatives.
- Avoid alcohol and caffeine, both of which stress the liver and encourage toxicity.
- Drink plenty of water (2 litres a day), which dilutes toxins and speeds their elimination from the body.
- Eat plenty of fibre to avoid constipation, which is believed to increase the risk of toxins being absorbed through the wall of the large bowel.
- Take milk thistle supplements. This herb contains a complex of bioflavonoid molecules known collectively as silymarin, which appears to have the ability to protect liver cells by reducing the take-up and enhancing the removal of harmful toxins. Silymarin also has a powerful antioxidant action and can help in the regeneration of injured liver cells.

Blood-sugar imbalance

The body keeps the level of sugar (glucose) in the blood within a relatively narrow range. Eating carbohydrate-based foods (containing sugars and starches) increases the level of blood sugar, causing the pancreas to secrete insulin, which transfers sugar from the blood into the body's cells and lowers the blood-sugar level. Other hormones, such as glucagon, help to keep blood-sugar levels from falling too low (see p.314).

Some people may have trouble regulating their blood-sugar levels, so that they experience "peaks" and "troughs". Stabilising blood-sugar levels can help to combat a wide variety of symptoms and conditions in the body.

The symptoms of fluctuating blood sugar are most obvious when blood-sugar levels are low (often referred to as hypoglycaemia, although true hypoglycaemia, in which blood-sugar levels fall dangerously low, usually occurs only in people being treated for diabetes). Symptoms of low blood sugar include:

- Fatigue. Low blood-sugar levels can cause energy levels to drop. The mid- to late-afternoon is a common time for fatigue associated with low blood-sugar levels.
- Loss of concentration and/or mood disturbance (especially anxiety and irritability). The brain depends on a ready supply of sugar for normal function. Low blood-sugar levels can provoke loss of concentration, low mood, anxiety, depression and mood swings.
- Sweet cravings. When blood-sugar levels are low, people tend to crave sweet foods, such as chocolate, biscuits, cakes and confectionery.

High levels of blood sugar can damage the body's tissues through a process known as glycosylation; they can also cause the body to produce excessive amounts of insulin that stimulate the conversion of sugar into a starch-like substance called glycogen, which can be stored in the liver. However, when glycogen stores are full, insulin stimulates the production of fat. Excess insulin tends to mean that people accumulate fat around the middle (also known as abdominal obesity), which has been linked with an increased risk of conditions such as coronary artery disease and type 2 diabetes (which usually begins in middle age).

Large amounts of insulin in the circulation affects other parts of the body. It causes the kidneys to retain sodium, which can make an individual prone to high blood pressure and fluid retention over time. Insulin also stimulates the liver to make cholesterol, which is likely to increase the risk of coronary artery disease and stroke.

If the pancreas secretes excess insulin over many years, the body can become less sensitive to insulin's effects. This may lead to a condition known as insulin resistance, which may ultimately lead on to type 2 diabetes.

Balancing blood sugar

Eating patterns and the types of food eaten both influence blood-sugar balance. The best blood-sugar control is achieved by eating unrefined carbohydrates in three meals a day, perhaps with healthy snacks, such as fresh fruit and nuts, in between. This can help control appetite and may prevent overeating, with its corresponding surges in blood sugar and insulin.

In addition to regular, moderately sized meals, it is important to base the diet on foods that give a controlled release of sugar in the body (See glycaemic index foods, opposite). Traditional wisdom dictates that starchy foods release sugar slowly into the blood, because they must first be broken down into sugar before there are absorbed from the gut. It appears that this is not the case for many starch-based foods, including most forms of bread, potatoes, rice and pasta. For the best blood-sugar control, these foods, as well as those containing refined sugar, should be limited in the diet. The best diet for blood-sugar control is one based on meat, fish, eggs (high-protein foods tend to help stabilise blood-sugar levels), beans, pulses, nuts, seeds, fruits and vegetables (other than the potato).

GLYCAEMIC INDEX (GI) FOODS

The speed and extent to which a food increases blood sugar can be quantified using the glycaemic index scale. In this scale, glucose is given an arbitrary glycaemic index (GI) of 100. Other foods are compared to this. In general, the higher a food's GI, the greater its tendency to upset blood-sugar balance. It is wise to choose low GI foods (under 50) as much as possible.
(Adapted from *The Glucose Revolution: The Authoritative Guide to the Glycolic Index* – Jennie Brand-Miller and Thomas Wolever.)

GI INDEX OF COMMON FOODS

Food	GI	Food	GI
Glucose	100	White pitta bread	57
French baguette	95	New potatoes	57
Lucozade	95	Muesli	56
Baked potato	85	Popcorn, brown rice,	55
Cornflakes	83	Sweet corn	55
Rice Crispies	82	Spaghetti made with durum wheat	55
Pretzels	81	Bananas, sweet potatoes	54
Rice cakes	77	Special K	54
Cocopops	77	Kiwi fruit	53
Doughnut	76	Orange juice	52
French fries	75	Pumpernickel	50
Corn chips	74	Porridge	49
Potato – mashed	73	Baked beans	48
Bagel – white	72	Instant noodles	47
Sultana Bran	71	Grapes	46
White bread	71	Oranges	44
Shredded Wheat	69	All-Bran	42
Wholemeal bread	69	Apple juice	41
Croissants	67	Apples	38
Gnocchi	67	Wholemeal spaghetti	37
Pineapple	66	Pears	37
Cantaloupe melon	65	Chickpeas	33
High-fibre rye crispbread	65	Butter beans	31
Couscous	65	Dried apricots	31
Rye bread	64	Soya milk	30
Muffin	62	Kidney beans	29
Muesli bar	61	Lentils	29
Ice cream	61	Grapefruit	25
Pizza with cheese	60	Plums	24
White rice	58	Cherries	22

Supplements for blood-sugar balance

The trace mineral chromium seems to help to regulate the action of insulin in the body. In so doing it helps to ensure that the body handles and metabolises sugar efficiently. The normal recommended dose is 200–800mcg of chromium per day. Other nutrients believed to help blood-sugar metabolism include manganese, vanadium and the B vitamins (particularly vitamin B3).

Diet and the thyroid gland

The thyroid gland sits in the front of the neck just above the top of the breastbone and collarbones. It is essentially the body's thermostat, determining the speed at which it burns fuel. Each cell in the body uses oxygen and sugar to make energy, some of which is released as heat. The speed at which the cells do this, also known as the metabolic rate, is regulated by the thyroid. If, for any reason, thyroid function should falter, all the cells in the body tend not to operate as well as they should. (*For symptoms of low thyroid gland function see Thyroid Problems, p.319.*)

Thyroid blood tests

The thyroid gland produces various hormones including thyroxine (also known as T4), which is converted into a more active hormone called tri-iodothyronine (also known as T3) in the tissues. If the levels of T4 and/or T3 fall, then the pituitary gland at the base of the brain will secrete a hormone called thyroid-stimulating hormone (TSH) which stimulates the production of more thyroid hormones.

There are several tests for levels of thyroid hormones in the blood. Testing for TSH is generally the screening test for thyroid disease, with a raised TSH level generally taken to be a sign of low thyroid function (hypothyroidism).

A HEALTHY DIET

A healthy diet is one that provides the building blocks that your body needs for growth and maintenance, and in appropriate quantities and proportions. It should also be low in substances that can cause harm, or that the body finds difficult to process.

Many of the diseases that are on the increase in developed countries, such as type 2 diabetes (*see p.314*), coronary artery disease (*see p.252*) and some types of cancer, have a strong link with dietary factors. Making changes to improve the health-promoting qualities of your diet will reduce the likelihood of you suffering from these conditions. A good all-round diet also gives you more energy and vitality, and improves your resistance to minor illnesses such as colds and flu.

Base your diet on natural, unadulterated foods

There is a wealth of evidence that shows the most nutritious diet is one based on whole, unprocessed foods. Some of the foods which should form the basis of the diet include meat, fish, seafood, eggs, fruit, vegetables, nuts, seeds, beans and lentils.

Eat plenty of foods rich in healthy fats

Oils and fats are an important part of the diet. Different types of fat, though, have different effects on the body. Oily fish, nuts, seeds, olives, olive oil and avocado are rich in fats that have a range of health-giving properties (*see p.34*).

Avoid eating too much fast and processed food

Fast and processed foods tend to be rich in dietary elements including refined sugar, salt and food additives which can have adverse effects on health. Other ingredients commonly found in fast and processed foods are types of fats known as partially hydrogenated and "trans" fatty acids, which have been strongly linked with coronary artery disease.

Avoid eating too many potatoes and refined grains

Potatoes and refined grains such as white bread, pasta, white rice and many breakfast cereals generally lack nutritional value. They also tend to disrupt blood sugar and insulin levels (*see p.42*). The imbalance that these foods can induce in the body may have adverse effects for short- and long-term health.

Eat regular meals, with healthy snacks in between

Regular meals help to ensure we get the nourishment we need for optimal health. Also, snacking (on foods such as fruit and nuts) can help control appetite and help prevent over-eating. Regular eating also helps stabilise blood sugar and insulin levels.

Drink plenty of water

Water makes up about 70 per cent of the body. We lose water through sweating and urination, so drinking enough to maintain our hydration levels is important for maintaining general well-being and health. You should drink enough mineral or filtered tap water, cordials or juices to keep the urine pale yellow in colour throughout the day. It is better to take drinks between meals, rather than with a meal.

Some practitioners, however, believe that certain people with low thyroid function can have normal TSH readings. Measuring T4 and T3 levels also seems to be important, though in some people with symptoms of low thyroid function, the blood tests may be entirely normal. Anyone who suspects they have low thyroid function is advised to work with a practitioner experienced in this area.

Thyroid function can also be assessed using a simple home test known as the Barnes test. This involves taking the underarm temperature on waking (before rising) with a mercury thermometer (this should be left under the arm for at least 10 minutes). Because pre-menopausal women's temperatures tend to fluctuate with the hormonal cycle, Barnes suggested that the most accurate time to assess temperature was on the third, fourth and fifth day of the period. For non-menstruating women and for men, any days will do as long as there is no sign of infection (this can raise body temperature). The normal underarm body temperature in the morning is between 36.6° and 36.8°C (97.8° – 98.2°F). A temperature of 36.4°C (97.4°F) or less suggests low thyroid function.

Treating a sluggish thyroid gland

Several nutrients may help to support thyroid function. These include iodine, selenium (which helps in the conversion of T4 to T3), vitamin A and the amino acid L-tyrosine. Some doctors recommend supplements that contain actual thyroid tissue. These extracts, which are often referred to as "thyroid glandulars", are usually made from cow or pig thyroid glands. It is believed that the range of hormones available in a glandular supplement is much more likely to have a beneficial effect on hypothyroid individuals than the single hormone conventional treatment, which centres upon thyroxin alone. Thyroid glandulars should only be taken under the supervision of a doctor experienced in their use.

Adrenal weakness

The human body has two adrenal glands. Each sits on top of a kidney and is about the size of an apricot. The adrenal glands secrete a variety of hormones that play important roles in maintaining homeostasis, or balance, in the body. They are also the chief glands responsible for the body's reaction to stress because they produce the hormones adrenaline and cortisol (*see p.409*).

In some individuals, often as a result of long-term stress, adrenal function may be weakened. This condition, which nutritional therapists call "adrenal exhaustion", can have important implications for health.

Symptoms of adrenal exhaustion

- Fatigue. Adrenally weakened individuals tend to be tired, and adrenal exhaustion seems to be a common feature in people with chronic fatigue syndrome.

- Easy fatigue. Adrenally weakened individuals often have little in the way of energy reserves and get tired out quite easily. For people with adrenal exhaustion, any additional stress (of a physiological and/or emotional nature) can cause a significant worsening of the fatigue.
- Low blood pressure. Normal blood pressure is usually around 120–130/70–80mmHg. Adrenally weakened individuals often have a blood pressure of 110/70mmHg or less, which may drop on standing and cause dizziness.
- Salt craving. Some individuals will crave salt, which may reflect the body's need to raise blood pressure.
- The need to eat regularly. Individuals with adrenal exhaustion tend to need to eat regularly to keep them from feeling weak and light-headed.

Laboratory tests for adrenal function

Blood tests designed to diagnose a condition known as Addison's disease, also called "adrenal insufficiency", are available. This condition is characterised by extreme adrenal weakness to the extent that regular doses of steroids, such as cortisol, and perhaps other drugs are necessary to maintain health. Many conventional doctors do not believe in the concept of adrenal exhaustion. However, in practice, some individuals who do not have Addison's disease nonetheless have clinical evidence of impaired adrenal gland function.

Restoring adrenal health

Rest is key to restoring adrenal gland function. Adequate amounts of sleep are important, and it may be necessary to reduce workload or strenuous activity. Techniques designed to reduce demand and promote relaxation (*see p.99*) will also help. In addition, certain supplements may help to restore adrenal gland health, including vitamin C, vitamin B5 and the herbs liquorice and ginseng. However, anyone who may have adrenal exhaustion is advised to work with a practitioner experienced in this health problem.

Immune system health

The immune system is a network of specialised tissues, organs, cells and chemicals, whose chief function is to protect the body against potentially harmful agents including micro-organisms (e.g. bacteria and viruses) and cancerous cells. The lymph nodes, spleen, bone marrow, thymus gland and tonsils all play a role in immune functions, as do blood cells known as lymphocytes and chemicals produced by them known as antibodies.

The immune system uses two main forms of protection: innate and adaptive. Innate immunity is present at birth and provides the first barrier against organisms. It includes the skin, the acid in the stomach, and mucus secreted in the nose and lungs. Adaptive immunity is the second barrier to infection and is acquired later in life. The adaptive immune system may retain a memory of the infecting agent, which means that one infection may be enough to ensure it never happens again (as, for example, with measles and chickenpox). However, some organisms, such as the viruses that cause colds and flu, come in a variety of forms and can infect the body repeatedly.

A weakened immune system may not repel invading organisms efficiently, which makes infections more likely. Dietary approaches to combat this include avoiding sugar and taking supplements. Sugar interferes with the ability of white blood cells to destroy bacteria, and animal studies suggest that a diet high in sucrose (table sugar) may impair some aspects of immune function. Avoiding sugar in the diet may therefore help to improve resistance to infection.

Several nutrients can help increase immune function. Some doctors recommend zinc supplements for people with recurrent infections, suggesting 25mg per day for adults and lower amounts for children (depending on body weight, *see p.46*). Vitamin C stimulates the immune system by elevating the levels of interferon and by enhancing the activity of certain immune system cells.

Diet and mood problems

Mood problems, such as depression and anxiety, can have important links with the diet. Identifying and correcting one or more of the following common imbalances is often very effective in correcting mood-related issues.

- Food sensitivities may give rise to poor concentration, low mood and depression (wheat is a common problem food in this respect). *Candida* overgrowth can cause the same kinds of symptoms.
- Blood-sugar imbalances may give rise to low mood, anxiety and mood swings.
- Adrenal gland weakness can contribute to anxiety (especially when meals are skipped) and depression.
- Hypothyroidism is linked to low mood and depression.

Caffeine and mood

Caffeine is a stimulant with addictive qualities. It can also upset blood-sugar levels and stimulate the adrenal glands to produce adrenaline. One study showed the equivalent of one cup of coffee provoked nervousness and/or anxiety in some individuals prone to these problems. Caffeine may also contribute to insomnia (*see p.448*), which can impact negatively on mood. Reducing or eliminating caffeine from the diet may help to improve mood-related disorders.

Essential fatty acids

Fats play a fundamental structural and functional role in the nervous system. Of particular importance are omega-3 fatty acids (*see p.34*), such as EPA and DHA. People with depression have reduced levels of omega-3 fatty acids. EPA supplements may help depressed people on conventional antidepressant therapy. Omega-3 fatty acids may also help to treat ADHD, manic depression and schizophrenia.

Anaemia, iron deficiency and mood

Iron is important for haemoglobin, the pigment in red blood cells that delivers oxygen to the tissues. A deficiency of iron leads to anaemia (low haemoglobin levels) which may manifest as low mood, mental lethargy, poor attention span and apathy. Iron-deficiency anaemia is quite common in women, vegetarians and vegans. People with persistent fatigue and/or mood disturbance should be tested for both anaemia and for iron levels in the body. The best test for iron measures serum ferritin. If this is low, then increasing iron intake often helps to enhance mood. Iron-rich foods include red meat, fish, dried fruit, nuts and seeds. A doctor should monitor iron supplementation so that it can be adjusted according to a person's serum ferritin level.

Contraindications

The following lists the minerals and vitamins and their contraindications with conventional medications:

Biotin – may improve blood glucose control in diabetics. The dose of a drug that lowers blood sugar (insulin or an oral diabetic medication) may need to be reduced to avoid episodes of low blood sugar.

Bromelain – can increase absorption of amoxicillin and may have a similar effect on other antibiotics. Avoid taking bromelain with antibiotics unless supervised by a doctor.

Calcium – can lower the levels of beta-blockers (for high blood pressure or heart disorders). Avoid taking calcium supplements within two hours of a beta-blocker dose.

Calcium reduces the effectiveness of ciprofloxacin, ofloxacin, doxycycline and tetracycline. Avoid taking calcium supplements within three hours of an antibiotic.

People with kidney failure may develop high blood levels of calcium. Calcium supplements should be avoided in kidney failure unless under the supervision of a doctor.

Calcium may reduce the effectiveness of thyroxine medication (for thyroid problems). Avoid taking calcium supplements within four hours of thyroxine medication.

Coenzyme Q10 – is structurally similar to vitamin K and so may also encourage blood clotting. People on warfarin should not take CoQ10 unless supervised by a doctor.

Folic acid – may increase the frequency and/or severity of seizures. Individuals taking anticonvulsant drugs should consult their doctor before supplementing with folic acid.

Folic acid-containing supplements may interfere with methotrexate therapy for cancer since methotrexate blocks the activation of folic acid. People using methotrexate for cancer treatment should consult their prescribing doctor before using any folic acid-containing supplements.

5-Hydroxytryptophan (5-HTP) – 5-HTP and zolpidem (for insomnia) may increase zolpidem-induced hallucinations.

5-HTP may increase the side-effects of Fluoxetine, Venlafaxine, Fluvoxamine and Paroxetine (antidepressants) and Sumatriptan (for migraines). Avoid taking 5-HTP with these drugs unless supervised by a doctor.

Iron – can reduce the absorption and/or effectiveness of the drugs ciprofloxacin, oflaxacin, tetracycline, doxyclycline, levofloxacin, minocycline and penicillamine. Avoid taking iron supplements within three hours of one of these drugs. People taking deferoxamine (which binds to iron and removes it from the body) should avoid iron supplements. Iron can irritate the stomach, especially if taken with the NSAID indomethacin. Take these separately and with food to reduce this risk.

Iron may reduce the absorption of methyldopa (for high blood pressure). Take methyldopa two hours before or after iron-containing products. Iron can also reduce the absorption of risedronate (for Paget's disease, post-menopausal osteoporosis and osteoporosis brought on by steroids). Avoid taking iron within three hours of a risedronate dose. Iron can reduce the absorption of

White blood cells called macrophages are part of the immune system. They engulf bacteria and clean up cell debris. Macrophages, like many other components of the immune system, work best when there are good levels of vitamin C and other antioxidants in the diet.

sulphasalazine. Avoid taking iron supplements within three hours of taking a sulphasalazine dose.

Iron may decrease the absorption of thyroid hormone medications, such as thyroxine. People taking these prescribed medications should consult their doctor before using iron-containing products.

Iron may reduce the absorption and activity of warfarin. Avoid taking iron within two hours of a warfarin dose.

Magnesium – can reduce the absorption of the antibiotic ciprofloxacin. Take ciprofloxacin two hours after eating dairy products (due to the magnesium content) or taking magnesium-containing supplements.

Spironolactone (a potassium-saving diuretic used for oedema and high blood pressure) may prevent the loss of magnesium (as well as potassium) from the body. People on spironolactone should not take more than 300mg of magnesium per day unless supervised by a doctor.

Magnesium may reduce the activity of warfarin. Avoid taking magnesium within two hours of a warfarin dose.

Omega-3 supplements/Fish oils – the fatty acids EPA and DHA may reduce the clotting ability of blood and the need for warfarin. People on warfarin should not take omega-3 supplements and fish oils unless supervised by a doctor.

Quercetin – may reduce the breakdown of felodipine (for high blood pressure). The subsequent increased blood levels of the drug may lead to side-effects. People taking felodipine should avoid supplementing with quercetin.

Soya products – may reduce the absorption of thyroid hormones when taken at the same time. Avoid taking soya products within three hours of thyroid medication.

Vitamin A – Some people undergoing long-term treatment with HMG-CoA reductase inhibitors may have raised vitamin A levels. These drugs, such as atorvastatin, fluvastatin, lovastatin and pravastatin, block an enzyme the body needs to make cholesterol. Individuals taking the drugs with vitamin A supplements need their vitamin A blood levels monitored.

Isotretinoin/tretinoin (used to treat acne) and vitamin A are structurally similar and have similar toxicities. People taking isotretinoin/tretinoin should avoid vitamin A supplements at levels higher than typically found in a multivitamin preparation (10,000 IU per day).

Vitamin B3/Niacin – Niacin is the form of vitamin B3 used to lower cholesterol. People taking large amounts of niacin with HMG-CoA reductase inhibitors lovastatin or atorvastatin may develop muscle disorders that can be serious. The effect is rare and may extend to other drugs of this type. People taking niacin and HMG-CoA reductase inhibitors should be monitored by a doctor.

Individuals taking niacin with an oral diabetic drug may increase their requirements for the drug.

Vitamin B6 (pyridoxine) – vitamin B6 supplements above 5–10mg per day may reduce the effectiveness of levodopa (used for Parkinson's disease). Combining levodopa with carbidopa prevents this, so vitamin B6 supplements may safely be taken with Sinemet® (carbidopa/levodopa).

Vitamin B6 may reduce blood levels of phenobarbital (used prior to surgery, to combat insomnia and to prevent or treat seizures). Those taking the sedative should avoid taking large amounts of vitamin B6 (50mg a day or more).

Vitamin C – can increase the absorption of antibiotics, though this may not pose problems for the body.

Some reports suggest that vitamin C might increase the activity of the blood-thinning drug warfarin. Individuals taking warfarin should not take more than 500mg of vitamin C a day unless supervised by a doctor.

Vitamin D – may interfere with the effectiveness of verapamil (used for angina, arrhythmia and high blood pressure). People taking verapamil should consult their doctor before using a supplement containing vitamin D.

Vitamin E – may increase the blood-thinning effect of aspirin and warfarin. Individuals taking one or both of these drugs should not take more than 200 IU of vitamin E supplements a day unless supervised by a doctor.

Vitamin K – warfarin inhibits blood clotting by interfering with vitamin K activity. Individuals taking warfarin should avoid a supplement that contains vitamin K unless they are specifically directed by a doctor.

Zinc – long-term zinc supplementation can cause copper deficiency. Take 1mg of copper for every 15mg of zinc.

Zinc may reduce the absorption and/or effectiveness of the drugs tetracycline and ciprofloxacin. Avoid taking zinc supplements within three hours of these antibiotics.

FINDING A PRACTITIONER

The British Association of Nutritional Therapists (BANT) approve courses run by 13 colleges and universities in the UK. Nutritional therapists are professionally insured and are required to abide by the codes of ethics and practice established by BANT. You can find a qualified nutritional therapist in your area by logging on to www.nutripeople.co.uk or by contacting BANT (*see p.486*). In Australia, contact the Australasian College of Nutritional & Environmental Medicine (*see p.486*). Ask about clinical details, procedure and the costs of treatment. Therapists usually run a private practice and will work with you on a one-to-one basis.

BODYWORK THERAPIES

LEON CHAITOW

The musculoskeletal system is the body's largest user of energy. It is through the this system that we walk, talk, run, jump, feed ourselves, paint pictures, perform delicate surgery, make music, war and love, and generally express our human individuality. It is also the "organ" that is most likely to produce symptoms severe enough to take you to a doctor. Bodywork and movement therapies aim to restore harmonious balance to the integrated structures of the musculoskeletal system and to ease restriction, pain and dysfunction.

Structural Framework

The human body has a structural framework of bones, ligaments, tendons, muscles and joints, all held together by connective tissue. The connective tissue framework extends down to the most microscopic level where minute fibres support individual cells and help to carry information – even into the cell nucleus.

The body's central co-ordination depends on the brain and central nervous system and the body's tissues are nourished and oxygenated through the circulation. The structural framework allows us to move freely and painlessly, while also providing space, protection and support for the vital organs and glands that regulate the biochemical activities that fuel and repair the body.

The musculoskeletal system is organised and held together in a structure that is remarkable for its ability to absorb external forces and inner tensions in one part of the body, and to spread the load evenly to the other parts. This flexible ability comes from a quality known as tensegrity, a word derived from "tension" and "integrity" (*see p.53*).

Connective tissue

The most widespread soft tissue in the body is connective tissue, sometimes known as fascia. It forms a thin network or mesh around nerves and between muscles, and a more dense network in cartilage, ligament, tendon and bone. It supports, divides, wraps, connects, invests, separates and gives cohesion to all the other soft tissues of the body.

The connective tissue network is a kind of fascial web that comprises one single continuous tensegrity structure, which reaches from the soles of the feet (plantar fascia) to the inner lining of the skull (the dura). As a result, any distortions and restrictions that occur in one part of the web can influence all the other parts, with body-wide implications. Understanding how connective tissue works helps us to grasp the interconnectedness of the entire body – for example, how fallen arches in the feet can directly influence the neck and head.

Since connective tissue gives shape and cohesion to everything else in the body – including the organs, muscles, blood vessels, nerves and cells – the fascial web can be accurately seen as a single structure. This means that the fascial "sheets" attached to the inside the skull, such as the falx cerebri and the tentorium cerebelli (which divide different parts of the brain and give shape to the structures inside the head), merge with the lining of the skull (the dura). They are connected, without interruption, to the dura surrounding the spinal cord and the fascia of the neck, thorax, diaphragm, lower pelvis, legs and feet. In fact, they are connected to every joint, muscle, tendon and ligament in the body!

It is no surprise that tensions and distortions in any one part can influence the entire network. This influence may range from slight to a great extent, depending on many factors, such as the degree of distortion and the person's age and general state of suppleness and fitness. Many of the progressive changes that tighten, shorten, distort and restrict the fascia and the associated body parts are reversible – either wholly or partially – by means of appropriate treatment and self-care.

Recent research suggests that it is through connective tissue structures – specifically the cleavage planes where the individual muscle groups are separated from each other – that many of the beneficial effects of manual therapy, as well as acupuncture, acupressure and trigger-point deactivation, are achieved.

Form and function of cells

The body's fascial web extends into the connective tissue (cytoskeleton) inside every cell and minute protrusions (integrins) on their surfaces. These two key features have been shown to determine the overall efficiency of a cell's function, and of the way a cell expresses itself genetically.

According to recent research, the fascia of a cell becomes distorted in a gravity-free environment. This effect alters the cell's shape and modifies the way it processes nutrients. Put simply, when the structure of a cell changes, its function changes too, meaning that it cannot absorb and metabolise nutrients properly.

A cell's inability to nourish and ultimately to reproduce itself has enormous implications for the health of the whole body. We do not need to travel in outer space to create changes in our fascial structure, since the processes of adaptation (*see p.53*), compensation, ageing and disease, which affect us all, create localised warping, crowding, compression and distortion of the fascia – right down to a cellular level. Over time, this is potentially harmful to normal cellular life, and therefore to general health and well-being because the changes caused restrict healthy circulation of fluids and the flow of information which organs need to stay healthy.

BIOMECHANICAL AND BODYWORK TISSUES

The body's framework consists of a variety of tissues that rely on biomechanical properties and information networks to perform and coordinate a wide range of movements. These are the tissues on which bodywork and movement therapists focus in order restore health and well-being.

TISSUE	DESCRIPTION
Bone	Bone is hard and strong, but slightly flexible, with an internal structure that absorbs stresses. It is a living tissue that is constantly being rebuilt, even in adulthood.
Joints	Joints are where two bones meet. Most are moveable.
Moveable joints	Moveable joints include the ball-and-socket joint of the shoulder and hip, the hinge joint of the knee, and the pivot joint at the top of the neck. Moveable joints are lubricated by synovial fluid.
Semi-moveable	Semi-moveable joints, such as those in the sacrum (at the base of the spine), are held together by flexible cartilage.
Fixed joints	A few joints are fixed, for example the suture joints in the skull.
Tendons	Tendons are tough, stringy connective tissues that link muscles to bones.
Ligaments	Ligaments are tough bands of connective tissue that support and bind bone to bone at joints.
Cartilage	Cartilage has a smooth protective surface to provide ease of movement where bones meet.
Muscles	Muscle is an elastic tissue that can contract and relax. Each muscle is composed of bundles of fibres surrounded by connective tissue.
Skeletal muscle	● Skeletal muscles are attached to bones. They can be made to contract voluntarily (consciously). They contract swiftly and powerfully, but cannot sustain contractions for long periods of time. ● Different types of muscle fibre have different levels of strength and stamina, and are used in different activities. ● Type 1 fibres ("slow-twitch") have slower contractile speeds, and are used for endurance activities such as long-distance running and maintaining posture. ● Type 2 fibres ("fast-twitch") have faster contractile speeds and are used in more 'high intensity' activities.
Smooth muscle	● Smooth muscle surrounds many of the tubes in the body, e.g. blood vessels and intestines. It contracts in waves (called peristalsis). It is capable of contracting for long periods of time. Smooth muscle contraction is not usually under conscious control.
Connective tissue (fascia)	● The most widespread soft tissue in the body. A thin network, rather like a cobweb, that surrounds nerves, runs between muscles and connects with ligaments, cartilage and bone. It gives cohesion to and interconnects all other tissues in the body.
Spinal cord	● Together with the brain, the spinal cord processes information and keeps the body co-ordinated. The spinal cord runs down a protective tunnel inside the vertebrae (backbones). ● Spinal nerves emerge from gaps between the vertebrae and connect to all parts of the body.
Nerves	● Nerves are bundles of nerve cells. They carry messages from one part of the body to another. The fastest method is via an electrical signal, but chemicals can also be moved along nerve cells. A nerve cell has a rounded body that contains the nucleus and very long, thin extensions called axons. Nerve cells that connect the spinal cord to the toes can be over a metre long.
Cytoskeleton	● Cells are the tiny units that make up all the structures in the body. Each cell contains its own "skeleton" called the cytoskeleton which gives it its shape, holds the nucleus and other organelles ('mini organs') in place, and helps the cell to move. The cytoskeleton is made of chains of protein molecules.

Cartilage, bones and joints

The fascial web of connective tissue is anchored to the bones of the skeleton by elastic tissues (muscles, tendons, ligaments) that form a series of interconnected "poles" and "guy-wires". These allow loads and tensions to be shared by the structure as a whole, of which the bones of the skeleton can be seen as the "struts". Bones seldom actually touch each other in normal conditions. Instead, they "meet" at a joint, which is held in place by ligaments and tied to muscles that move it via tendons.

The primary purpose of semi-moveable joints, such as the sacro-iliac joint in the pelvis, is to provide stability – they are protected by pads or discs of cartilage that absorb the pressure of external loads and forces. Joints that move freely, such as the elbow and knee, offer flexibility and mobility – they are protected and lubricated by synovial membranes and fluid. To some extent, all joints provide both stability and mobility.

Wear and tear, inefficient supporting structures, such as weak muscles and lax ligaments, and the ageing process are the main enemies of joints. These problems are further aggravated by overuse, misuse, disuse and abuse (see p.57). When joint surfaces become irritated, arthritic changes (see Osteoarthritis, p.289) usually begin.

The spine and the rest of the bony skeleton provide a "protective cage" that offers a safe place for the vital organs, such as the heart and liver. The health of these organs can be greatly influenced by distortions and crowding of the skeletal structures. When a slumped posture becomes a habit, for example, it can put stress on the connective tissue around the organs, negatively affecting their nerve and blood supply, as well as their lymph drainage. It may even affect how well the organs actually work.

Tendons

A tendon connects a muscle to a bone, providing the muscle with the anchorage it needs to contract and exert a force. However, tendons can become inflamed or irritated, often when the muscle to which they are attached contracts repetitively or frequently. This can lead to problems such as Achilles tendonitis and many localised painful areas close to joints, especially those prone to overuse (see p.57), such as the knees, wrists and elbows. Trigger points (see p.55) are frequently located in the muscles associated with such irritable, overused tendons.

Ligaments

Ligaments are specialised connective tissue that support and bind joints. They are particularly important (and sometimes vulnerable) in joints that are prone to damage when excessively stressed or strained, such as the knees and ankles. Approximately one person in ten has lax ligaments

(i.e. is "double-jointed"), a condition known as hyper-mobility. In Asian and Arab women, as many as four out of ten may be born with this characteristic. Hypermobile individuals are more likely than others to develop conditions sometimes labelled "soft-tissue rheumatism" (involving muscles rather than bones or joints) and conditions such as fibromyalgia and spinal scoliosis.

Skeletal muscles

These muscles are attached to the various bones of the skeleton and are composed of bundles of fibres that can be made to contract voluntarily. The bundles, or fasciculi, usually lie side by side in a parallel fashion and are individually enclosed in a thin connective tissue sheath known as the endomysium.

There are two types of muscle fibre: type 1 muscle fibres will shorten when continually stressed by overuse, misuse or abuse; type 2 muscle fibres, when similarly stressed, become weak and may lengthen. As a result, imbalances develop between opposing muscle groups, with negative effects on both the muscles and the joints they serve.

For example, the neck and shoulder muscles of someone with a slumped posture and head poked forwards are tense and tight. The deep muscles at the front of the neck (the deep neck flexors) are usually weak and inhibited, putting the joints of the neck under stress and causing awkward movements, usually involving some stiffness and probably discomfort. In time, the nerves emerging from the spine and the discs between vertebrae may become irritated, leading to painful symptoms, both locally and at a distance.

Another example of imbalance is the tight, arched low back of a person who displays a protruding and sagging abdomen. When this is chronic, symptoms of backache and abdominal and pelvic organ dysfunction are likely.

Smooth muscles

Smooth muscles form the circular walls of the bladder, blood vessels, bronchioles and many of the hollow digestive organs, such as the gastrointestinal tract. A smooth muscle has a circular control over the tube it surrounds, often contracting in a wave-like manner – for example, in peristalsis (the action that propels food through the gut).

Tens of thousands of smooth muscle cells are also embedded in the fascial web. When they contract they increase the tension in the connective tissue, sometimes excessively, leading to body-wide stiffness and restriction.

Smooth muscles contract when the blood becomes more alkaline than normal, such as takes place during hyper-ventilation (see p.57). Therefore, people with a tendency to an anxious, upper-chest breathing pattern tend to have an increased degree of tone/tension in the fascia, which may affect the entire musculoskeletal system and probably encourage trigger-point formation (see p.55).

Brain and Nervous System

The brain receives a constant stream of reports (tens of thousands of messages per second) from nerve structures in the limbs, such as Ruffini nerve endings and Pacinian corpuscles, that register motion, temperature, pressure or pain. This information relates to what is happening in the different parts of the body and answers a multitude of questions that the brain asks, such as: Is the left arm moving? If so, how fast and in what direction? What is its temperature? Is anything pressing on it? Is there any pain? In this way, the brain learns what is happening to every bone, muscle, joint, tendon and ligament – even in the furthest reaches of the fascial web.

After interpreting the received information, the brain sends instructions, via the nervous system, that enable us to walk, talk, maintain balance, move, function and live our lives. Some bodily functions, such as digestion, the rhythmic contraction of the heart and breathing, are on "automatic pilot", outside of our conscious control. Other functions, such as walking and talking, are directly influenced by conscious decisions.

Problems may arise as a result of various sources. For example, when the brain either receives inaccurate information from faulty nerves or else misinterprets correct information; when the brain sends inappropriate instructions to the tissues and organs; and when reflex activities are either excessive or diminished.

Reflexes

Many nerve functions are reflexive in nature, which means that responses do not have to be ordered by the brain, but can take place via "short-circuit" pathways in the spine. Perhaps the most familiar example of this is the "knee-jerk" reflex reaction.

When spinal structures are injured or stressed, the normal behaviour of vertebral joints may change. This may irritate or compress the nerves that emerge from it, with the potential to influence the organs and other tissues that they serve. This is known as a somatico-visceral reflex.

Similarly but in reverse, when an organ or tissue is unwell the spinal regions associated with it can become distressed, tense and painful. This is known as a viscero-somatic reflex. A common example is the tense, sensitive region of the upper back (2nd, 3rd and 4th thoracic vertebral areas) frequently noted in people who have heart problems. Some osteopathic and chiropractic practitioners use this knowledge in their work to attempt to modify the negative feedback pathways to the organs.

Although treatment of such spinal areas cannot "cure" organ disease, there is evidence that it brings some benefit. Awareness of these reflex pathways can also help to explain the appearance of many spinal problems that do not have an obvious mechanical cause.

Axonal transportation

Nerves conduct electrical messages and carry "trophic substances", such as proteins, essential fatty acids and neurotransmitters, to and from the target tissues and organs they serve. This movement of substances along nerve pathways is known as axonal transportation.

According to osteopathic research, any interference with nerve function, message conduction or axonal transport, in either direction, can cause a wide range of symptoms. Mechanical deformities, such as compression and stretching, and sustained hyperactivity of nerve cells in sensitised spinal segments can slow down axonal transport. Appropriate mobilisation and manipulation of soft tissues and joints may be able to improve these functions.

Sympathetic and parasympathetic actions

The nervous system can be broadly divided into two parts. The role of the sympathetic nervous system is to mainly stimulate tissues and organs, whereas the parasympathetic nervous system has the opposite effect. It mainly calms, inhibits or damps down the activities of the tissues and organs. These stimulating and calming effects of the nervous system can be hugely affected by both emotions and biochemical factors, such as hormonal balance, diet, drugs and allergies. The nerves of the body are therefore capable of becoming sensitised (hyper-irritable), as well as being potentially inhibited, by biomechanical, psychological and/or biochemical influences.

Central sensitisation

Ultimately, nerves feed into the central nervous system and the brain. At times, this central control mechanism may be responsible for excessive or diminished nerve activity. Just as a local muscle area may become hyper-irritable if repetitively stressed – forming a trigger point, for example – so the central nervous system, or parts of it, including parts of the brain, can become sensitised when bombarded with pain and distress messages, or when biochemically disturbed. This central sensitisation can make the nerve and brain structures far more easily irritated, interfering with accurate interpretation of the messages received from the body and sending inappropriate instructions in response. Central sensitisation is thought to be a major part of what happens in many chronic pain conditions.

Entrapment and compression

Many nerves are vulnerable to mechanical interference because they pass through or around structures, such as muscles and bones, that can trap and/or compress them. Many symptoms result from such situations. Entrapment is usually the excessive pressure that soft tissues place upon a nerve. For example, when the scalene muscles in the neck or the pectoral muscles in the upper chest impinge on and crowd the nerves running towards an arm, a variety of pain and numbness symptoms can be felt in the arm. This is a condition known as thoracic outlet syndrome, or TOS.

An example of compression is when the arch of bones and fascia in the wrist press on the median nerve. This is known as carpal tunnel syndrome (*see p.152*), which is commonly caused and always aggravated by overuse. It may also be partially caused by fluid retention involving swelling of the lower arm or hand.

Self-repair and Adaptation

A fundamental truth should be kept in mind as we explore the many things that can go wrong with the biomechanics of the body: there is an inherent capacity for self-repair, constantly at work, whether this is in response to trauma (broken bones usually heal) or to chronic patterns of overuse and misuse.

If the causes can be reduced or removed and/or the structural integrity of the biomechanical (and, of course, the biochemical and psychological) components of the body can be improved, then self-regulation processes commonly ensure a return of normal function. Many of the symptoms we experience, unpleasant as they may be, should be understood as messages of recovery and repair-in-action – inflammation, for example, may be unpleasant, but without it tissue repair cannot take place.

Other symptoms, such as acute pain, may be understood as vital messages, warning us not to overuse a particular area because to do so would be to aggravate existing damage, or to create a worse situation.

By learning to understand and respect these messages, and to take appropriate action, we can enhance the healing process. Ignoring the symptom's message can be disastrous. For example, inappropriate use of medication that is anti-inflammatory and painkilling can lead to overuse and therefore aggravation of already damaged structures, creating a far worse state of affairs, and delaying recovery.

Does this mean that we should never use anti-inflammatory or painkilling medication? No, but it does suggest that we should only do so if we intend to respect self-healing processes that are going on in the background. The therapeutic measures used for any condition should therefore strike the balance between helping the person to feel more comfortable, while not creating new problems, or retarding the potential for recovery.

Adaptation

The old saying, that there are only two certainties in life – death and taxes – can be accurately expanded to include adaptation. We adapt from the cradle to the grave. We adapt to both internal and external forces as we grow, mature, develop and interact with other people and the

TENSEGRITY

A characteristic feature of the body's musculoskeletal system is its ability to absorb the impact of external stresses and to spread the load of internal tensions without compromising the overall integrity of its structure. This flexible ability evolves from the quality known as tensegrity, which can be found in the structure of both the cell's skeleton and the geodesic dome.

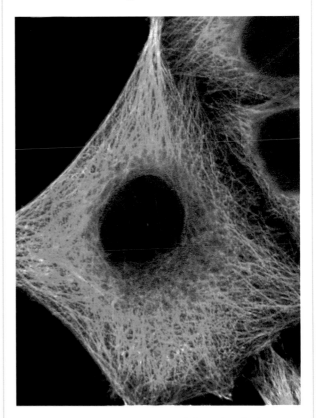

Fluorescent dyes reveal proteins in the cytoskeleton of a cell (*above*). Microtubulin (green) is the main constituent of microtubules, which are important in cell division. Actin (red) is essential to muscle contraction. Golgi protein (blue) is found in the Golgi apparatus, which plays a part in the processing and transport of proteins within the cell.

The word tensegrity was coined in 1961 by the visionary US architect Buckminster Fuller. He wanted to describe the stability that results from the interaction of rigid struts, flexible connecting fibres and filaments, and enclosed fluids under pressure. A suitable architectural example of tensegrity structure is the geodesic dome (*left*), which has no upright pillars.

environment. We adapt to the things we do, the things that happen to us and to the characteristics with which we are born. We adapt physically, biochemically, emotionally and psychologically throughout life. And when we cannot adapt any more, problems become evident.

The pioneer researcher in this area was Hans Selye, a Canadian physiologist who identified adaptation as the main feature that characterises and influences our development. Maladaptation largely determines whether health is good or poor, and ultimately leads to our eventual collapse. On the larger stage, Selye noted that everything that calls for adaptation can be labelled as "stress". By understanding stress in this way (i.e. as an adaptation demand) we can see that it only becomes harmful when we are unable to adapt to the stress factor – i.e. when our capacity for adaptation is overwhelmed.

"As the twig is bent ..."

A simple analogy clarifies what happens when we adapt to the stresses of life, and how the body compensates to the adaptive demands placed on it.

If a living, flexible branch of a tree is bent, it will adapt to the forces applied to it until it cannot absorb any more tension, torsion or distortion – at which moment it breaks or splinters. However, if a milder force is repetitively applied, the living branch will adapt to match the "stress", and will become permanently bent. The fact that it is no longer as nature designed it means that this particular bent twig, although well adapted to the stresses imposed on it, would be unable to perform the same functions that it could when it was straight. In general, adaptation occurs at the expense of the ability to function optimally. The new situation (bent) allows the young twig to survive, but removes some of its original potential.

Research into how blood vessel walls respond and adapt to the stresses imposed on them is an example of how the "bent twig'" analogy applies to the body. Blood vessel walls adapt to the structural strain (high blood pressure), bio-chemical strain (high cholesterol) and psychological strain (hormonal instability caused by a hostile temperament) placed on them by hardening and narrowing. Gradually they become increasingly narrowed and inflexible and eventually the part of the body they supply simply does not receive enough oxygen and nutrients. Angina is the result of not enough oxygen and nutrients reaching the cardiac muscle, while if the coronary arteries block completely a heart attack will probably happen.

Doctors treat the problem by attempting to bring down blood pressure and blood fats with drugs and, if necessary, by replacing the furred-up artery with a vein from somewhere else in the body. In the long term, however, the best medical approach is to address all the structural, biochemical and psychological elements involved in high blood pressure and coronary artery disease in order to reduce the stresses that the blood vessels are being forced

to adapt to. In some parts of the US, cardiac rehabilitation programmes follow up bypass surgery or a heart attack with diet, meditation, yoga and graduated exercise. Such programmes increase fitness and encourage psychological well-being, so improving the patient's ability to cope with stress (*see Coronary artery disease, p.252*).

General and local adaptation

Selye used the terms "general adaptation syndrome" and "local adaptation syndrome". The former describes the effects of stress on the whole person and the latter the effects of stress on a local area, such as the shoulder. Each "syndrome" follows three stages: an initial alarm phase; a period of adjustment, compensation and adaptation, which might last for many years; and a stage of collapse, when adaptive capacity is exhausted.

Examples of local adaptation syndromes include the way specific muscles adapt to new patterns of use – as happens when you take on a new job that involves physical labour or a sustained posture. A general adaptation syndrome involves the whole body. Imagine, for instance, you were born at sea level and relocated to live at altitude. It would take months or years for your body to adapt to the different environmental situation. The changes necessary would involve your heart, lungs, circulation and general metabolic functioning.

Alarm and adjustment phases

Learning a new skill, such as playing tennis, places specific adaptive demands on the body. Generally, the exercise affects the whole body, bringing cardiovascular and muscular changes as the system learns to adapt to the new aerobic activity. Locally, the dominant hand, shoulder and arm has to perform unaccustomed activities, which initially might cause muscular discomfort. This is the "alarm" phase of the adaptation syndrome.

If you continue to play tennis, the initial symptoms (soreness, stiffness) tend to reduce, as the body adjusts to the new demands. However, if you play too much, or too often or for too long, the compensatory demands will become excessive and the adaptive capacity overwhelmed, causing symptoms that may be severe – for example, tennis elbow or repetitive strain injury.

Excessive training of young footballers, gymnasts and other athletes has been shown to produce major structural problems (including early arthritic changes), often ending careers before they begin. In these situations, it is a case of too much activity, for too long, too often and too soon for their immature bodies.

Individual idiosyncrasies

The adaptive demands of work and leisure activities, whether mountain climbing, gardening, gymnastics or watching TV on the sofa, affect us all in different ways. The differences depend on various factors: the type of body and constitution you are born with; the nature of your health history; how "fit" and supple you are (and what you do to maintain this); your age; and how efficiently and non-stressfully you have learned to use the primary machinery of life – the physical body.

The result is that some people adapt without problems to the demands placed upon them, but many do not. In fact few people pass their entire working lives without discomfort and many others experience repetitive strains, aches and pains.

Some people also are born with so-called "inborn stressors" which create adaptive demands. For example, some people have one leg shorter than the other; others have one side of the pelvis that is smaller than the other, leading to a "tilt" of the pelvis and spinal strain; and some people have upper arms that are shorter than usual, which leads to increased sidebending when sitting, in order to gain support when resting on the arms of chair.

Finally, some people are hypermobile (*see p. 51*) and have a tendency to possess lax ligaments (they are "double-jointed"). This tendency causes muscles to overwork in order to protect the "loose" joints. Rehabilitation, learning new and better ways of doing things, and encouraging a more balanced state of the muscles, helps people to overcome such inbuilt problems.

Adaptating to a deskbound occupation

The postural demands of working at a desk in front of a computer terminal for eight hours a day are likely to create adaptive stresses affecting the neck and back. Unless the seating and desk arrangements are ideal and the postural awareness is good, progressive changes occur in overused neck, shoulder and arm muscles. Other muscles will be underused, including the stabilisers of the shoulder blade and the low back, abdominal and leg muscles.

Progressive shortening of some muscles (hip flexors and the pectoral muscles in the upper chest) and weakness in others (abdominal muscles) lead to restrictions in overused joints and in static, underused joints. In the low back and neck, elbows and wrists, localised areas of sensitivity and pain (trigger points) develop, particularly in the overused, shortened muscles. Eventually, background discomfort, pain and restriction become constant, with occasional acute spells of pain whenever irritable muscles (especially in the low back and neck) get even more tense and cramped.

The solutions are obvious. They include: better seating posture and better use of the body, with particular attention to avoiding overuse; stretching and movement strategies to help compensate for being sedentary; and appropriate treatment and self care to loosen and mobilise structures that have become tense and irritable.

TRIGGER POINTS

When cells in part of a muscle persistently receive insufficient blood and therefore oxygen (often because of excessive tension in the muscle), they become irritable. This affects the local nerve supply, producing areas of over-sensitisation known as myofascial trigger points ("myo" relates to muscle and "fascial" to connective tissue).

As tension builds up around this zone, calcium enters the muscle cells, but they lack the energy to pump it out again. This sets up a vicious cycle in which the muscle cells cannot loosen up and the affected muscle cannot relax. A characteristically taut band forms in the muscle, which can be located by a fingertip pressure.

TRIGGER POINT PAIN

Quite commonly, a person with trigger-point pain has not found the tender spot responsible. Sometimes, though, they are aware of a sore point that, when pressed, causes pain that may radiate to other areas. This is characteristic of the pain. The trigger points can cause symptoms some distance away and they become more active when stress, of whatever type, affects the person as a whole.

Trigger points are a common feature of pain. According to leading pain researchers and renowned neurologists, Patrick Wall and Ronald Melzack, there are few, if any, chronic pain problems that do not have trigger-point activity as a major part of the picture. They may not always be a prime cause, but they are almost always a factor that helps to maintain the condition.

Trigger points become self-perpetuating (a cycle in which pain leads to increased muscle tension which leads to pain) and seldom disappear unless they are adequately treated, or unless the reason for their existence, such as overuse or misuse, is removed.

TRIGGER POINT FACTORS

The following factors tend to maintain and enhance trigger point activity:
- Nutritional deficiency (especially vitamin C, B-complex vitamins and iron).
- Hormonal imbalances (for example, low output of thyroid hormones and those imbalances that occur during the menopause or in premenstrual women).
- Persistent, low-grade infections (bacteria, viruses or yeast).
- Food intolerances (wheat and dairy in particular).
- Poor oxygenation of cells and tissues (aggravated by tension, stress, inactivity or poor respiration).

TREATING TRIGGER POINTS

Ways of treating and deactivating trigger points include acupuncture, local anaesthetic injections, direct manual pressure, stretching and ice massage. These treatments will succeed in the long term only if the causes of the trigger points are removed. If muscles are stressed for long periods they tend to undergo fibrotic changes, becoming more "stringy" and less elastic, and more prone to injury when asked to perform new tasks. Regular, moderate degrees of exercise, including stretching, can help to reduce this tendency.

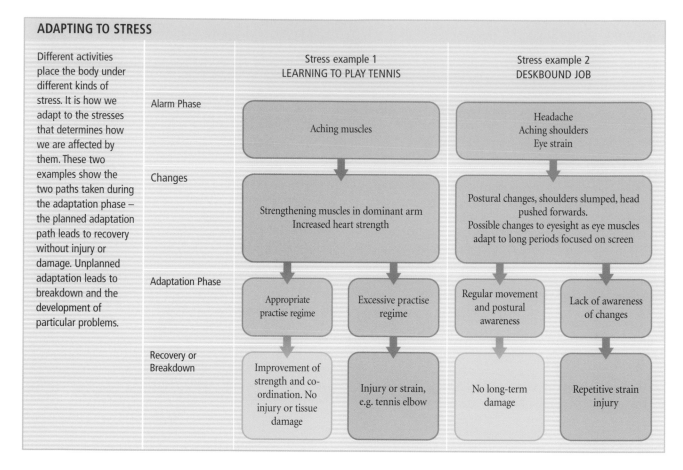

ADAPTING TO STRESS

Different activities place the body under different kinds of stress. It is how we adapt to the stresses that determines how we are affected by them. These two examples show the two paths taken during the adaptation phase – the planned adaptation path leads to recovery without injury or damage. Unplanned adaptation leads to breakdown and the development of particular problems.

Stress example 1
LEARNING TO PLAY TENNIS

Stress example 2
DESKBOUND JOB

Alarm Phase

Aching muscles

Headache
Aching shoulders
Eye strain

Changes

Strengthening muscles in dominant arm
Increased heart strength

Postural changes, shoulders slumped, head pushed forwards.
Possible changes to eyesight as eye muscles adapt to long periods focused on screen

Adaptation Phase

Appropriate practise regime

Excessive practise regime

Regular movement and postural awareness

Lack of awareness of changes

Recovery or Breakdown

Improvement of strength and co-ordination. No injury or tissue damage

Injury or strain, e.g. tennis elbow

No long-term damage

Repetitive strain injury

Planned adaptation

Prolonged sitting results in unplanned adaptation. What happens, however, when adaptation is planned? When someone prepares for a marathon, for example, he or she does not start the process by running the full 26-plus miles! The person trains, gradually increasing the amounts of stress (running and fitness training) so that the body can adapt to the new needs – to be able to run non-stop for 2–3 hours without injury. The adaptation process develops new muscle tissue and changes in responses of the heart, lungs and the whole biochemistry of energy production, as well as psychological adaptation to the discipline of training.

This same process of adaptation occurs in all sports, whether weightlifting or mountain climbing. Planned adaptation (training), therefore, is designed to allow us to do things – and to do them more efficiently – than before. However, just as the "bent twig" on the growing plant would be unable to perform the tasks of a straight twig, so the trained marathon runner could not become a sprinter. Once the body has become specialised to suit one type of sport, it is difficult to adapt to a completely different one.

Factors leading to breakdown

Adaptation leads to specialisation, limiting the potential for further adaptation. This fact is critical to understanding many of the sudden pain events that occur in life. When body structures are unprepared for, or incapable of meeting unexpected demands, such as lifting, stretching or moving suddenly, then tissues fail. Strain occurs and pain and spasm is a frequent consequence.

The limit to how much adaptation is possible is called the point of adaptive exhaustion or breakdown and is brought about by age and condition (of the person or body structure), as well as the kind and duration of stresses to which the person has had to adapt. The addition of a new adaptive demand may also be involved.

One of Selye's great discoveries was that multiple minor stresses have the same cumulative effect on the immune system and general health as one major stressful event. It is therefore extremely important to realise that adaptation is not just a response to external mechanical loads, but also a response to many internal biomechanical, biochemical, emotional and psychological stresses.

Breakdown can cause severe biomechanical symptoms, often involving spinal, pelvic or other joints: slipped discs, nerve impingement, inflamed tissues or other forms of dysfunction, decompensation or maladaptation. Along with actual injuries caused by trauma, falls, etc, these are the problems that keep manipulation therapists busy, as they try in their different ways to restore functionality. However, their efforts will be in vain if the adaptive load that produced the problem is not modified or avoided.

Causes of injuries

Many adaptive changes happen because of overuse, misuse, abuse and disuse. The sorts of problem that arise through sudden or long-term adaptation are often remediable or reversible. Treatment and self-help methods deal with the mechanical and structural changes, the functional changes or both (*see Diagnosis, treatments and therapies, p.59*).

Overuse
Repetitive movements, habitual postures or breathing excessively use certain muscles over and over again. This leads to slow adaptation through multiple changes in the soft tissues and joints. These secondary changes produce new adaptive demands due to muscular irritation and tightness, leading to discomfort, pain and the formation of trigger points. In breathing pattern disorders (*see right*) there is constant overuse of particular breathing muscles.

Misuse
People regularly misuse their musculoskeletal framework when sitting or standing. A slumped, or an excessively "military", posture are two examples. Using the wrong size or design of objects, such as chairs, sports equipment, shoes and musical instruments, can all create distress in the musculoskeletal system. The mechanical strains and stresses of misuse lead to a chain reaction of secondary changes, causing pain, tension and trigger points.

Abuse
Injuries, such as whiplash, sporting injuries (torn muscle, broken bone) and surgery can produce scar tissue and changed patterns of use. Over time, such chronic soft-tissue changes, plus joint degeneration and disc narrowing, produce pain and another round of compensation by the rest of the body. Whiplash injuries can apparently sensitise the central nervous system, and set in train the onset of bodywide pain syndromes, such as fibromyalgia.

Disuse
Lack of exercise, immobilisation, protective non-use of an area (as in a fracture, arthritis or a disc problem) and sedentary occupations all lead to underuse of parts of the body and the progressive weakness of disused muscles.

Remedies for overuse, misuse, abuse and disuse
Problems caused by overuse and misuse are clearly avoidable and are often remedied by a simple change of habits. Learning to use the body more efficiently and less stressfully is a matter of re-education and retraining, often accompanied by some form of manual treatment. These include osteopathy, chiropractic, physiotherapy, occupational therapy, massage therapy (including tuina, shiatsu, Ayurvedic massage and Thai massage) and the Alexander technique. Yoga, t'ai chi, Pilates and athletic training can be useful in rehabilitation, too. Conditions that result from abuse may require similar rehabilitation approaches, but are more likely to require more manual and other therapeutic interventions. The after-effects of disuse also require rehabilitation. If muscles have been disused as a result of an injury, surgical operation, stroke or other event, very specialised occupational therapy, physiotherapy or athletic training may be necessary to coax the muscles back into normal working order.

Breathing Pattern Disorders

People with a breathing pattern disorder (BPD) mainly breathe into their upper chest, and do not usually use their diaphragm much. BPDs are extremely common and contribute massively to ill-health. People with a chronic BPD are often persistently fatigued and anxious; many have various musculoskeletal aches, pains and odd sensations. BPDs are not a disease, but a habit, like poor posture. Hyperventilation is an extreme form of a BPD.

When a tendency towards upper-chest breathing becomes more pronounced (usually in stressful situations), biochemical imbalances occur. Excessive amounts of carbon dioxide are exhaled, which makes the blood more alkaline. This in turn produces a sense of apprehension and anxiety, reinforcing the anxious upper-chest breathing pattern. The vicious circle can lead to panic attacks and phobic behaviour as the person begins to avoid situations that trigger these feelings – commonly, queues, crowds and enclosed spaces. Recovery from this cycle may be possible only when breathing is normalised.

This breathing pattern can disturb the normal oxygen supply to the heart in three ways, at times causing it to beat abnormally. First, the smooth muscles that surround the blood vessels constrict, reducing blood supply to the heart muscles. Second, the red blood cells release the oxygen they should be delivering to the heart muscles less efficiently. Finally, the sympathetic nervous system becomes stimulated, which unbalances heart rhythms.

Knock-on effects of increased blood alkalinity include constriction of blood vessels, thereby reducing blood supply to all tissues in general but the brain in particular. At the same time, the alkalinity of the blood discourages the release of oxygen from haemoglobin (Bohr effect), reducing further the oxygenation of tissues and the brain. This can lead to so-called "brain-fog" in which consciousness is blurred and mood swings are more likely. Peripheral nerves become more sensitive and easily irritated, thereby lowering pain thresholds. Muscles tire rapidly and a general feeling of fatigue sets in. When the smooth muscle in the walls of the digestive tract are affected irritable bowel symptoms will get worse. Allergies and food intolerances can get worse too, due to increased circulating histamines triggered by other chemical changes.

Additionally, purely "overuse" stresses occur in the breathing muscles themselves, with increased tension and trigger-point activity (*see p.55*) that involve the chest, upper back, shoulder and neck. A cascade of new strains follow, as tensions increase in spinal (especially neck) and rib joints, triggering head, neck, shoulder, arm and upper back pain.

Posture and Internal Organs

The organs of the body are supported by soft tissues and the framework of the skeleton. When the body is distorted (except for a short period), there will be an impact on the way the organs function. Some years ago, one of the leading physicians of the time, Joel Goldthwaite, described the effects of poor posture on the body as a whole. "When the human machine is out of balance, physiological function cannot be perfect; muscles and ligaments are in an abnormal state of tension and strain. A well-poised body means a machine working perfectly, with the least amount of muscular effort, and therefore better health and strength for daily life."

Diaphragm and abdominal muscles

Goldthwaite pointed out that the main supporting structures of the abdominal organs are the diaphragm and the abdominal muscles. If they become lax and weak, ceasing to offer support when posture is faulty, circulation to internal organs becomes disturbed. The diaphragm may also stiffen up and be unable to move freely.

Faulty body mechanics are an aspect of many chronic health problems and an important consideration when thinking of health enhancement and disease prevention. As people grow older, the abdomen tends to relax and sag, which disturbs the regular movement of the diaphragm. This can interfere with normal circulation, leading to congestion in the abdominal and pelvic organs. The congested organs put pressure on their nerve supply, which causes functional irregularities. This may contribute to many digestive problems and possibly to organ disease itself. If the abdomen and its contents sag, the chest tends to droop, the shoulders to become round and the head to be thrust forwards with the chin jutting out. Fortunately, the lower abdominal muscles can be trained to contract properly (achieving what is known as core stability), supporting both the organs and the lower back.

As you read through the ailments in Part 2, you will find a number of references to spinal manipulation being able, at times, to influence internal functions to improve health (*see Angina, p.249; and Menstrual Pain, p.328*). This is possible because of the interconnected relationship between overall posture, the functional state of the spine and the nerve supply from the spine and the internal organs.

Mind–Body Connection

In a classic Charlie Brown cartoon, Charlie stands in a slumped position with his chin on his chest. He says to one of his friends, "This is how you have to stand when you are depressed." There is much truth in Charlie's words, because we judge people's body language all the time. If someone carries himself or herself in a dejected, "depressed" way, or in an anxious, apprehensive manner, or with an aggressive, angry posture – our instant judgement picks up on their current emotional state. Emotion changes our posture, even our breathing (*see Breathing pattern disorders, p.57*). If prolonged or repetitive, the adaptation to such changes then leads on to new symptoms.

Long-held psychological states, and repressed, unspoken emotions, such as anger and fear, can become stored (somatised) in the body. This creates a virtual armour of tension in the muscles, with consequent changes in joint and general bodily function.

"Unclenching the fist"

The osteopath Philip Latey offers a perspective on the way emotions become expressed as muscle tension in his metaphor for the different physical responses to emotional distress. He describes three key areas of the body, and the tensions in them, as the "upper fist" (head/neck area), the "middle fist" (chest area) and the "lower fist" (pelvic area). The clenched fist neatly gives an image of the tense, tight muscles of these areas, as well as the effect of release, as the fist slowly unclenches.

A question raised by Latey's work is worth considering: if the most appropriate response an individual makes is to "lock away" emotions into their musculoskeletal system, is it advisable to unlock the body and release the emotions which the tensions and contractions hold? It may well be that psychotherapy or counselling, in conjunction with appropriate bodywork, offers the best solution to "unclenching the fist", so that emotional and structural changes can occur simultaneously.

Stress and different muscle groups

One research study confirmed that specific emotions seem to affect particular muscle groups more than others. For example, the main muscles affected in agitated people are on the back of the arms; depressed individuals showed greatest activity in the sheet of muscle on the forehead (the frontalis). Another study found that careful physical examination failed in many instances to find a cause for patients' pain. There was, however, a correlation between anger and pain in the neck, between fear and abdominal pain and between sorrow or despair and low back pain. In patients with these correlations it was rare for an organic cause to be found, even after extensive investigation.

A skeletal muscle fibre is revealed in this scanning electron micrograph to consist of bundles of myofibrils (green) sheathed in connective tissue (brown strands).

Another study used electromyography to evaluate the effect that stress-inducing mental exercises had on different parts of neck and shoulder muscles. When a person was intellectually stressed and anxious, type 1 muscle fibres (which are prone to shorten when stressed) became over-active. These fibres, when repeatedly activated through stressful emotions, may eventually respond with a "metabolic crisis" that produces trigger points (*see p.55*).

Emotion and psychological well-being, therefore, are key factors that influence how the musculoskeletal system behaves. At the same time, the state and functionality of the musculoskeletal system has an impact on how we experience ourselves and express our emotions.

Diagnosis, Treatments and Therapies

Many conventional and unconventional ways can be used to assess the status of the musculoskeletal system. Some are high-tech, but most use observation and fingertip examination (palpation), requiring considerable knowledge and skill. In most instances, when you visit a bodywork practitioner (whether a physiotherapist, osteopath, chiropractor or other) a full case history will be taken, even if the problem appears localised. This is because many apparently clear-cut conditions, such as a painful shoulder, can sometimes have serious underlying causes – digestive or cardiovascular disease, for example – that could easily be missed if the practitioner or therapist simply started treating the affected area. Questionnaires may help to identify particular features of the condition – for example, the type, nature and degree of pain.

X-rays and scans, such as MRI, may be required to search inside the area for evidence of pathology or tissue change. Chiropractors regularly take X-rays to assess the position and relationship of bones and joints. Osteopaths tend to use X-rays more rarely, and then usually only to confirm, or rule out, the presence of disease processes, such as arthritis.

Practitioner tests and assessments

To make sense of how a body is adapting to the stresses of life, a therapist may turn to one of several frameworks of evaluation or grids of (relative) normality. An osteopath, physiotherapist, chiropractor or other bodywork practitioner might do one or all of the following:
- Observe your posture, looking for imbalances, asymmetries and "crossed patterns".
- Assess your gait. What happens to your body (from the

feet to the head) as you walk? An increasing number of practitioners use computerised imaging to record a patient's posture and gait to compare images before and after treatment.

- Evaluate your respiratory function. Is your breathing unbalanced and, if so, in what ways? Sometimes questionnaires and other tests are used, but evaluating how a person breathes is normally tested through observation and palpation.
- Assess your muscles for strength or weakness – looking particularly at type 2 muscles.
- Test for relative shortness of skeletal muscles – looking particularly at the postural, type 1 muscles.
- Assess the "firing pattern" of skeletal muscles – checking to see whether the "right" muscles perform a normal, functional movement in the correct sequence, or whether some muscles have come to dominate others.
- Test the range of motion of your soft tissues and joints. Are your normal movements free from pain? Patients may be asked to perform a particular movement, or the practitioner may move the patient's tissues and joints to test for range of motion.
- Test for abnormal nerve function by looking for the presence, absence or overactivity of neurological reflexes.
- Look for trigger points and sensitisation in your spine (spinal hyper-reactivity). Are trigger points feeding in to the patient's symptom picture?
- Assess influences on your nutrition and lifestyle.
- Evaluate psychosocial factors.

Aims of manual techniques

The objectives of all forms of manual treatment are similar. First, to eliminate or ease pain, restriction and patterns of dysfunction. Second, to restore flexibility, stability, strength, balance and postural and functional integrity.

Most "conventional" bodywork therapists, for example physiotherapists, rely on the same assessment methods employed in conventional medical settings. However, some complementary bodywork professions have other ways of examining the patient. Osteopaths, for example, use evidence of neurolymphatic reflexes or cranial palpation. Some chiropractors use methods known as applied kinesiology for testing the resistance of muscles. In general, however, one manual approach is usually distinguished from another by the way the practitioner interprets the examination and sets about treatment.

Osteopaths tend to focus on restoring the harmonious integrated function of the whole body, with particular emphasis on the circulation. Chiropractors have a particular interest in the nervous system and in releasing what they term "subluxations" which they believe interfere with nerve function. Subluxations are essentially the same thing as the restricted joints, treated (often differently) by osteopaths and physiotherapists.

Self-help during treatment

When you have a treatment bear in mind that it will make adaptive demands on you. Afterwards you may experience a "reaction" (something "feels different"), and for a day or so your muscles may ache. This is normal and to be expected and is not a cause for alarm. The condition may also temporarily get worse. Improvements may fluctuate, with minor setbacks along the way.

Normal life means having to cope with a number of stressors at any one time. If you have a musculoskeletal condition, you are more likely to make progress when some of this "load" is reduced. Therefore, any self-help measures you can take, such as improving posture and breathing patterns, will speed your recovery. Remember that your body always tries to heal itself, so that removing some of the obstacles to recovery is crucial to restoring good health.

Re-education

Recovery from long-term musculoskeletal pain and dysfunction often requires some self-education as part of the rehabilitation process. The key issues are:

- To become informed about your condition.
- To move from a passive to an active role.
- To develop effective ways of responding to your pain and the emotions associated with the pain. A key phrase to learn early on is "hurt does not necessarily mean harm".
- To develop a positive attitude towards exercise and personal health management.
- To develop a programme of structured activity to reduce the effects of physical deconditioning.

Bodywork Therapies

The following is a summary of the many manipulation therapies and bodywork practices that are recommended throughout this book. Always check that the practitioner is fully trained, qualified and registered, and inform them fully about your health problem and any medications you are taking before treatment starts.

If you are having treatment with one type of therapy (e.g. osteopathy), consult your therapist before embarking on treatment with another. That said, some therapies combine very well, for example the Alexander technique, Pilates and osteopathy for back pain.

Acupressure

Part of Traditional Chinese Medicine (*see p.78*), the practice of acupressure can be summed up as acupuncture without needles. Acupressure techniques are also used in shiatsu, which is practised in Japan. Acupressure practitioners use finger and thumb pressure on specific acupoints along meridians to stimulate the flow of *Qi* energy in order to restore harmony and health.

TREATMENT METHODS

Treatment methods vary from profession to profession (although far less than in earlier times). They include:

TREATMENT NAME	PRACTITIONER	DESCRIPTION
High-velocity, low amplitude, thrust (HVLAT)	Chiropractors Osteopaths Physiotherapists	HVLAT is the main manipulation technique that chiropractors, many osteopaths and some physiotherapists use. It is a rapid "adjustment" of a joint, often accompanied by an audible "crack" or "pop" as the joint surfaces separate. It produce a nerve reflex response that relaxes all attaching muscles, usually making movement much easier afterwards. Performed well, HVLAT is painless and safe. It should be used with great caution on patients with circulatory problems in the neck or on anyone with weak bones or rheumatoid disease.
Mobilisation of restricted joints	Osteopaths Physiotherapists Some massage therapists	Also known as articulation, this method uses rhythmic movement and stretching to relax tense soft tissue. It is used widely by osteopaths, some physiotherapists and, increasingly, by massage therapists with appropriate training.
Muscle energy techniques (MET)	Osteopaths Physiotherapists Massage therapists Self-treatment	MET uses contractions against light resistance to induce relaxation in muscles so that they can then be safely stretched. They were originally osteopathic techniques, but are now also used by massage therapists and physiotherapists, and can also be used on yourself at home.
Proprioceptive neuromuscular facilitation (PNF)	Physiotherapists	PNF is similar to MET, but uses far greater degrees of force and effort. It improves flexibility, induces muscle relaxation and increases range of movement in the joints. PNF is now a feature of sports therapy.
Positional release techniques (PRT)	Osteopaths Physiotherapists Massage therapists Chiropractors	PRT are very gentle osteopathic manipulations, ideal for use in acute conditions and after recent injury or surgery
Myofascial release (MFR)	All manual therapists	MFR is a very slow form of manually stretching muscles and connective tissue (fascia). It helps injuries to heal, increases the range of movement of joints.
Neuromuscular technique (NMT)	All manual therapists	NMT involves a combination of soft-tissue approaches that focus on normalising trigger point activity and the reasons for the development of trigger points. It involves finger and thumb strokes or pressure. NMT has its origins in Ayurvedic (traditional Indian) massage, modified to meet 20th-century British requirements, and in American chiropractic research of the 1940s.
Direct manual pressure	All manual therapists	Direct manual pressure is also known as ischaemic compression, trigger point pressure release, inhibition technique and acupressure.
Massage methods	All manual therapists	Massage strokes such as cross-fibre friction, specific soft-tissue mobilisation and other techniques.
Moderate aerobic exercises	All manual therapists	Moderate aerobic exercises are used in a fairly standard way by all the bodywork professions. Practitioners give patients a programme of appropriate aerobic, stretching, toning, breathing, balance and other exercises.

BREATHING RETRAINING

The process of rehabilitating yourself from a lifetime of habitual breathing pattern disorders (BPDs) can take up to six months. Many research studies show the effectiveness of breathing retraining (rehabilitation) in treating this widespread, often undiagnosed problem. Breathing retraining involves relearning the mechanics of breathing (with particular emphasis on full exhalation). It also involves the release of tense muscles and joints by judicious bodywork and mobilisation of the machinery of breathing.

Practise the following breathing exercise every day and whenever you feel stressed or anxious.

BREATHING EXERCISE

- Sit comfortably in a chair that has arms. Rest your arms on the arms of the chair. Relax.
- Press down on the arms with your elbows. This prevents you from using the neck and shoulder muscles while you are doing the breathing exercise.
- After a normal inhalation purse your lips (as if in an exaggerated kiss) and exhale through your mouth, counting slowly until you sense a need to breathe in.
- Close the lips, pause for a count of "one", and inhale through your nose while counting slowly.
- By exhaling fully, your inhalation will be deeper without trying.
- Your exhalation should always take longer than the inhalation.
- Repeat this sequence 20 times, morning and evening.

Alexander technique

Teachers of the Alexander technique aim to show people how to avoid patterns of misusing their bodies and to relearn everyday postures, such as sitting and standing. By concentrating on moving in a balanced and fluid way, people can improve their posture, achieve a better use of their bodies, and relieve the stresses and strains that contribute to illness. The technique is usually taught on a one-to-one basis and the teacher starts by showing how to stand and sit with optimum body posture. Later, all kinds of movements are examined, to help people conduct the activities of their everyday life with minimum strain.

Chiropractic

Chiropractors use precise hand movements to manipulate the vertebrae of the spine. The therapy is particularly effective in treating low back pain and relieving muscle tension caused by stress. In correcting the alignment of the spine with the head and pelvis, chiropractors help the nervous system to work normally. Treatment may involve standing, or sitting or lying on a chiropractic couch while the practitioner uses her hands to local the source of the pain and then make the necessary adjustments.

Cranial techniques

These very gentle massage techniques focus on normalising the tissues of the cranium (skull) and their fascial linkage with spinal and pelvic structures. Cranial osteopathy claims to balance the pressure on the bones of the cranium, correcting disturbances in the flow of cerebrospinal fluid, boosting the circulation of blood and draining excess lymph and fluids from the head.

Craniosacral therapy is similar to cranial osteopathy, except that the focus of treatment is on the membranes surrounding the brain and spinal cord – from the cranium to the sacrum. The sacro-occipital technique is preferred by chiropractors and is a blend of cranial osteopathy and craniosacral methods.

Feldenkrais

Feldenkrais teachers employ exercises specially devised by Moshe Feldenkrais in the 1940s to re-educate people to use their bodies more efficiently. Although the outcomes are similar to the Alexander technique, the methods and exercises employed are different.

Hydrotherapy

This is an umbrella term for various spa and water therapies. Physiotherapists often use a heated swimming pool where the water supports the patient's body, enabling exercise without weight-bearing. The resistance of the water can help in a strengthening programme for muscle and joint rehabilitation.

Hydrotherapy can also be used as a home treatment to treat pain and inflammation. Hot packs may help to treat muscle injuries and joint stiffness – they stimulate blood flow and relax muscles. Ice or cold packs help to reduce swelling and relieve pain. Balneotherapy is a traditional spa therapy in which bathing improves well-being and helps to heal disorders of the skin, muscles and joints.

Lymphatic pumping and drainage

Practitioners of manual lymphatic drainage use gentle rhythmic massage to stimulate the lymphatic system to remove toxins from the body.

Massage

Massage involves kneading muscles and stroking the body with long, sweeping movements. Its main aim is to stimulate blood flow,, which relieves inflammation and improves the circulation, and to encourage relaxation. There are many forms of massage, including Swedish, Thai, sports massage, shiatsu, tuina (*see next page*) and Indian head massage. Massage is widely available at health and sports clubs and your doctor or bodywork specialist may be able to recommend an experienced therapist. Check that a therapist has attended an accredited college (*see p.486*) and has completed a suitable training in anatomy and physiology.

Occupational therapy

People who struggle with the tasks of everyday living because of a long-term disorder, such as arthritis or multiple sclerosis, or because they are recovering from a serious injury or a stroke, can be helped by an occupational therapist. The main aim is to help people become as independent as possible, either through the use of aids, such as a walking frame, or through practical activities that improve dexterity and co-ordination.

Occupational therapists take a three-year course and work in hospitals or community care alongside other health professionals. A doctor can refer you to a therapist.

Osteopathy

Osteopaths use manipulation, massage and touch to balance tensions and remove stiffness throughout the musculoskeletal system so that the body's internal organs, circulation, digestion and lymphatic system can function properly. Osteopathy improves mobility and is particularly good for relieving pain in the joints and soft tissues. Treatment will involve the osteopath examining the spine and alignment of structures such as the pelvis before making various adjustments.

Physiotherapy

Physiotherapists generally use physical techniques, such as massage, hydrotherapy and exercise, to restore a person's muscle strength and flexibility, or to help rehabilitate their physical mobility after illness, injury or surgery. People with arthritis can also benefit from physiotherapy to help them maintain normal use of their body. Physiotherapy, which can also be used to relieve pain, is often combined with drugs and occupational therapy.

Qualified physiotherapists complete a three-year training. Some work alongside other medical staff in hospitals, but many work independently, outside hospitals. A doctor can refer you for physiotherapy.

Pilates

Practitioners teach a sequence of "thinking and breathing" exercises that focus on improving core stability and toning the abdominal muscles in order to develop a strong and flexible body. You can learn Pilates with apparatus or without, in which case you practise the sequences on a mat. Pilates is very useful for relieving chronic back problems. Make sure the teacher you choose has completed a full course and is fully accredited.

Reflexology

Reflexologists view the feet and hands as mirrors of the whole body and believe pressure placed on specific points can stimulate the body's natural healing powers. With finger and thumb pressure, they massage particular reflex points (usually on the feet) in order to treat the corresponding areas of the body.

Rolfing

This deep-tissue manipulation loosens the connective tissue (fascia) enveloping the muscles. It releases the physical (and sometimes the emotional) stresses that cause the fascia to harden and lose elasticity, the muscles to become restricted and breathing to be impaired.

T'ai chi

T'ai chi is an ancient Chinese practice that aims to achieve inner strength. It involves meditative sequences of slow, flowing movements (*see also p.79*) and is excellent for relieving stress and improving breathing.

Tuina

Tuina is a traditional Chinese massage technique that manipulates soft tissues and joints. The name which means "push and grasp" describes how the practitioner stimulates acupoints in order to improve energy flow round the body.

Ultrasound

Beams of high-frequency soundwaves generate heat in damaged soft tissues (muscles, tendons and ligaments) in order to combat pain and reduce inflammation.

Yoga

This ancient Indian practice has been practised for thousands of years in India as part of Ayurveda. It combines physical postures and breathing to train the mind and body. All forms of yoga, such as hatha and astanga, can help relieve mental stress while increasing suppleness and fitness. Yoga therapists teach specific poses to treat medical complaints.

FINDING A PRACTITIONER

Practitioners of the bodywork and movement therapies listed on these pages can be found by contacting the relevant organisations, associations, guilds and professional bodies (*see p.486*). Your doctor may be able to put you in contact with a practitioner.

Some therapies, such as physiotherapy and osteopathy, are more established than others, such as Pilates and reflexology, and so their courses and training methods are potentially more rigorous. Before making an appointment, always make sure the practitioner is fully qualified and registered as a member with the appropriate organisation.

Safety and reliability are paramount. You must be able to trust the capability of the practitioner or therapist you have chosen for, after all, you are literally placing your body and mind in their hands. If, after an appointment, you do not feel comfortable then do not hesitate to find another practitioner who suits you. This is as true for teachers of yoga, t'ai chi, the Alexander technique and Pilates teachers as it is for massage therapists osteopaths, chiropractors and physiotherapists.

Western Herbal Medicine

MICHAEL MCINTYRE

The use of herbs to treat illness is as ancient as history itself and is common to all peoples of the world. In fact, in all but the last 60 years or so, humans have relied almost exclusively on plants to treat illnesses ranging from colds to malaria. The human body is geared to digesting and absorbing plant-based foods and therefore may be better suited to treatment with herbal remedies rather than with isolated chemical medicines. While conventional medicines are designed to target and reverse specific disease processes in the minimum amount of time, plant medicines provide remedies that encourage the body's capacity to regulate and heal itself by restoring disturbed physiological processes.

Herbal Medicine in History

An estimated 70,000 plants throughout the world have a medicinal use and about 500 or so are used on a regular basis in Western herbal medicine. In the distant past, sensitivity to the properties of herbs must have been vital to human survival, and using plants as medicine may be a development of instinctive herb-seeking that is found in many animals. Researchers studying chimpanzees in Gombe (Tanzania's National Park) observed that animals with lassitude and diarrhoea, which are common signs of parasitic infections, searched out and ate the leaves of two plants – *Aspilia mossambicensis* and *Vernonia amygdalina*. These plants are bitter and unpleasant to eat, but they have antiparasitic, purging and antibiotic actions that the chimpanzees seem to recognise and want to make use of. The same herbal medicines have been used in Tanzanian folk medicine for hundreds of years and Tanzanian farmers also use the leaves of *Vernonia* to treat parasites and other ailments in themselves and in their lifestock. Scientists are now studying these plants for their potential as sources of new medicines.

Herbs in ancient cultures

Ancient peoples valued herbal remedies and recorded their medicinal uses, for example a medical manuscript dating from the 2nd century BC was discovered in 1973 in a tomb at Ma Huang Dui in Hunan Province, China, which listed some 224 herbal medicines, and the Egyptian Ebers Papyrus, dating back to 1500 BC, describes more than 700 herbs, including aloes, caraway seeds, castor oil and squill.

The domestication of the camel in around 1200 BC stimulated the growth of the herb trade between Egypt and Greece and eventually also with Rome. Precious gums, resins and spices, such as turpentine, myrrh, frankincense and cinnamon, came through Arabia along well-established incense routes and were eagerly purchased by Mediterranean merchants. They then sold them on to satisfy the increasing demands of markets throughout Europe. The Greek island of Chios was the source of a prized resin called mastic, used as a sort of chewing gum (and giving us the word "masticate"). Recent research confirms that mastic chewing gum is a useful antiplaque agent that reduces the bacterial growth in saliva and plaque formation on teeth.

Dioscorides, a Greek doctor attached to the Roman armies of Claudius and Nero, compiled ancient and contemporary herbal knowledge in his famous herbal *De Materia Medica*, which contained descriptions of about 600 herbs in all, and remained one of the principal medical textbooks for more than 13 centuries. The Greek herbal achieved its final form in the work of Claudius Galen, physician to the Roman Emperor Marcus Aurelius.

In the Middle Ages, much of this knowledge was brought back to Europe by Crusader doctors, who learned new skills from their Arab adversaries. The Arab doctors were expert pharmacists who had preserved and synthesised the knowledge of the ancient Greeks and Persians.

Decline and resurgence of herbs

For centuries, plant remedies were the main medicines throughout Europe, and famous herbals were published in English in the 16th and 17th centuries. Some, such as those of Culpeper and Gerard, are still well known today. However, with the dawn of the scientific age came the slow decline of herbal medicine. This decline was accelerated in the 18th century by the widespread introduction into medicine of mineral- and metal-based remedies such as arsenic, lead, antimony, mercury, copper, tin and gold. In the 20th century, with the discovery of antibiotics and other major drugs, which brought serious infectious diseases under control, the vast majority of herbal remedies became relegated to being mere footnotes in official pharmacopoeias.

New role for plant medicines

Recent years have seen a resurgence of interest in herbal medicine. The days when it was believed that science could deliver "a pill for every ill", and that it was just a matter of time before cures could be found for common conditions such as arthritis, migraine, coronary artery disease and cancer, have gone. Lately, we have a more realistic understanding of the importance of maintaining health and the prevention of disease. In many people, the realisation is dawning that diet and natural plant medicines have a vital role to play in boosting the body's powers to cope with even the most serious of conditions.

MEDICINALLY ACTIVE PLANT CHEMICALS

Plants do not have an immune system like ours to protect them from attack. Instead they use chemicals to fight bacteria, fungi and insects. Because these chemicals are biologically active, some also have medicinal properties.

PLANT	ACTIVE COMPOUNDS	PLANT USE	MEDICINAL USES
Garlic Allium sativum	Allyl sulphides	Antimicrobials prevent the bulb rotting in wet soil	Antibacterial and antiviral
Ginseng Panax ginseng	Ginsenosides (triterpene saponins)	Protection against fungal diseases	Stimulates the immune system
Oak Quercus robur	Tannins	The tannins coagulate protein, so are an effective insect deterrent	The coagulating properties of bark tannins can be used for diarrhoea
Echinacea Echinacea purpurea, pallida, augustiflora	Complex mix of alkylamides, caffeic acid derivatives, palyalkynes and polysaccharides	Antifungal compounds are a defence against fungal disease	Stimulates the immune system. Used for upper respiratory tract infections
St John's wort Hypericum perforatum	Hypericin and pseudohypericin (naphthodianthrones)	Defence against insects that try to eat the plant	Blocks neurotransmitter re-uptake. Used for depression
Peppermint Mentha x piperita	Monoterpene oils	Deter or prevent insect or slug attack	Provide its antispasmodic action. Used for indigestion

How Herbs Work

Since the 18th century scientists have been isolating the active constituents in plants. Research has given rise to some of the world's most powerful drugs. Even today, modern medicine relies heavily on plant-derived drugs. Not only have some of the more long-standing drugs such as digoxin, opiates and aspirin originated from plants, but many of the newer high-tech drugs such as the cancer drug vincristine and other cytotoxics (chemicals that kill cells) are also chemicals derived from plants.

Herbal medicines, however, are different from plant-derived drugs in that they consist of many chemical components. The mixture works in concert, making active constituents more easily available to the body, or buffering otherwise harmful ingredients. This means that the total therapeutic effect of the whole plant is considerably more than the sum of its chemical parts, since the active constituents' effects will be modified by other substances. What's more, the complex arrays of chemicals found in even the simplest plant medicines can trigger a cascade of biochemical processes in the living body. The way herbal medicines work is unlike the linear cause and effect of a single chemical (drug) acting on a single receptor system – a mechanism that pharmacologists are familiar with.

Understanding how plant medicines work calls for a leap into notions of "complexity" and "chaos" which are more familiar to physicists, than to biochemists or pharmacologists.

The consequences of using the whole plant rather than an isolated component are easily illustrated by clinical studies of garlic (*Allium sativum*). Recent research has shown that because garlic can lower blood pressure and cholesterol, it may be useful to people with coronary artery disease. Yet despite their best efforts, researchers have so far failed to identify which of garlic's many chemical constituents are responsible for these medicinal virtues. Though formerly attributed to allicin, a compound found in garlic oil, it has recently become clear that the cholesterol-lowering effect of garlic results from a concerted action of several chemicals, not all of which are in the oil itself.

Research into St John's wort (*Hypericum perforatum*) illustrates the same point. Trials have demonstrated that this ancient remedy is very effective in a wide range of depressive disorders, including seasonal affective disorder (SAD; *see p.432*). It is as effective as modern antidepressant drugs in treating mild to moderate depression, but provokes virtually none of their side-effects. Researchers, however, cannot as yet assign the plant's antidepressant effects to specific chemical components. Another group of chemicals with huge medicinal potential that is not yet well understood are flavonoids. These are chemical compounds that give many flowers, fruits and vegetables their colour. They display an amazingly broad range of medicinal activity: improving capillary fragility and circulation, protecting the liver and preventing heart attacks and strokes. Some are antioxidant or anti-inflammatory and antiviral, while others have demonstrable anticancer properties.

The rapidly expanding body of research into plant pharmacology is challenging the very basis of drug-based medicine. The realisation that many apparently minor chemical constituents, until recently overlooked, have significant medicinal properties has come as a revelation.

Consulting a Herbalist

Herbal practice relies on the gentle and supportive nature of the remedies it uses. In contrast to conventional medicine, herbal practitioners focus on the person rather than the disease label. The herbal practitioner will explore the background of the illness taking a comprehensive case history, in which family and personal life are carefully evaluated. Questions cover lifestyle, exercise and diet, as well as how the patient feels about his or her circumstances (job, relationships, aspirations and anxieties). Then the practitioner is likely to perform a physical examination and may order clinical tests. All this information is used to assess the vitality of the patient, and establish which systems are sluggish and which are overworked. The practitioner will prescribe a mixture of herbs accordingly.

The herbal prescription is not a simple matter of using herbs in the place of drugs to treat a particular condition. Drugs are standardised, while herbal treatment rarely is. Each prescription is unique to the patient, matching the needs of that person, supporting ailing systems and/or reducing over-activity when it is apparent.

In practice, herbs are not usually used as "simples" (i.e. given singly), but are combined for extra effect to suit the individual. St John's wort, for example, though marketed as a remedy to treat mild to moderate depression, is commonly combined with other herbs. When St John's wort is combined with lemon balm (*Melissa officinalis*), it is used to treat anxiety and depression; with wild oat (*Avena fatua*) and/or ginseng (*Panax ginseng*), it is given for exhaustion; with valerian (*Valeriana officinalis*), it is a treatment for bipolar mood disorder.

Herbs often confer a wide spectrum of benefits. For example, lemon balm can be used for anxiety and insomnia, but it is also traditionally used for calming a nervous stomach and bowel. Recently it has been found to have a significant antiviral effect and may also help in the treatment of hyperthyroidism. Herbal remedies can support and stimulate the body's healing response. The herbalist and the patient are partners in this aim, working together towards the common goal of restoring health.

Safety and Efficacy

It is clear that "natural" does not always equal "safe", and that herbal medicines, like conventional medicines, can cause adverse effects. Such adverse events may also be due to contaminants present in herbs, such as heavy metals or aflatoxins, or even because of misidentification of a herb. There is a possibility of herb–drug interactions too (*see below*), Therefore herbal practitioners must be very well trained and know exactly what other medicines their patients are taking.

How safe are herbs?

Safety concerns should be set in context. The European Herbal Practitioners' Association estimates that in 2003 there were over a million herbal consultations in the UK. According to a BBC poll (August 1999), herbal medicines are the most popular form of self-care.

It would appear that the incidence of herbal adverse effects is rather low. A five-year study into the occurrence of adverse events involving traditional herbal medicines and food supplements was undertaken by the UK National Poisons Unit. Of the 1,297 enquiries received, a medicine was implicated as a probable cause of the adverse events in only 38 cases. The Ministry of Agriculture, Fisheries and Food commented: "The findings overall are reassuring as they do not indicate any significant health problems associated with most types of traditional remedies and dietary supplements." However, there have been a number of important concerns regarding the safety of herbal medicines in the past two decades. Using toxic *Aristolochia* species instead of safer herbs in some traditional Chinese medicines resulted in cases of serious kidney poisoning and cancer in Europe, China, Japan and the US.

VOLATILE OILS

Volatile oils such as menthol and thymol have a pungent aromatic aroma and a range of actions because they penetrate easily through the body's tissues. Their molecules can even affect the brain directly through the nose. Herbalists have long known that the aroma of crushed mint (*Mentha*) or rosemary (*Rosmarinus officinalis*) can increase alertness and improve concentration. Internally, these oils are carminative, relaxing an over-contracted intestinal tract. They also stimulate the heart and lungs, improving circulation and deepening breathing. These oils are excreted through the lungs, kidneys and skin, so they act as expectorants and mild diuretics, causing therapeutic sweating. The traditional germicidal properties of many volatile oils, such as from thyme (*Thymus*), tea tree (*Melaleuca alternifolia*) and garlic (*Allium sativum*), are effective to a surprising degree. Garlic has recently been shown to combat the common cold and the hospital superbug MRSA.

CONVENTIONAL MEDICINES DERIVED FROM PLANTS

As well as being used in their own right as herbal medicines, plants are also the source of many of our conventional medicines.

Pharmaceutical companies screen plants from all over the world for chemicals that may be medicinal.

COMPOUND	CONDITION	ORIGINAL SOURCE	HISTORY
Vinblastine and vincristine	Cancers, including childhood leukaemia	Madagascar periwinkle (*Catharanthus roseus*)	In Madagascar many traditional remedies are made from the plant. This alerted Western scientists to its potential.
Quinine	Malaria	Chinchona tree (*Cinchona officinalis* and others)	Quinine was extracted from cinchona bark. Now chemists can synthesise the drug.
Taxol	Cancers, especially breast cancer	Pacific yew (*Taxus brevifolia*) and common yew (*Taxus baccata*)	The bark from one Pacific yew tree only supplied enough Taxol for one treatment. Now the drug is made from a chemical extracted from clippings from common yew.
Aspirin	Pain and inflammation	Willow bark (*Salix*) and Meadowsweet (*Filipendula ulmaria*)	Willow stems were used to treat pain and fever. The chemical salicylic acid is now manufactured as acetyl salicylic acid (aspirin).
Cocaine and procaine	Local anaesthetic	Coca plant (*Erythroxylum coca*)	Leaves are used by South American Indians as a stimulant and for altitude sickness. Sigmund Freud found that a small amount of the extracted drug (cocaine) placed on the tongue caused numbness. Synthetic cocaine-like substances including procaine (Novocaine) are now used in medicine and dentistry.

Professor Ernst, Chair of Complementary Medicine at the University of Exeter, has recently downplayed the threat of adverse effects from herbal medicines. In an editorial in the *British Medical Journal* he comments that "Even though herbal medicines are not devoid of risk, they could still be safer than synthetic drugs. Between 1968 and 1997, the World Health Organization's monitoring centre collected 8985 reports of adverse events associated with herbal medicines from 55 countries. Although this number may seem impressively high, it amounts to only a tiny fraction of adverse events associated with conventional drugs held in the same database. However, the relative paucity could also be due to a relatively higher level of underreporting.... At present, the relative safety of herbal medicines is undefinable, but many of the existing data indicate that adverse events, particularly serious ones, occur less often than with prescription drugs."

Only a tiny fraction of herbal medicines have been fully researched. In some cases, this has led to doctors doubting their efficacy. However, in the same editorial, Professor Ernst dispels the myth that herbal remedies are ineffective and lack credibility because they have not been researched. He writes, "The efficacy of herbal medicines has been tested in hundreds of clinical trials, and it is wrong to say that they are all of inferior methodological quality. But this volume of data is still small considering the multitude of herbal medicines – worldwide several thousand different plants are being used for medicinal purposes."

Relatively few rigorous clinical trials have been conducted on herbal therapies mainly because, compared with the pharmaceutical sector, the herbal industry can rarely afford the considerable expense of a clinical trial. Not being able to patent plant medicines and recoup the costs as drug companies are able to do, puts the herbal industry at a very real disadvantage. However, most of those clinical trials that have been conducted have shown that herbal medicines do work. In a recent overview of 23 systematic reviews (which are comparative and critical analyses of many research studies) of rigorous trials of herbal medicines, 11 came to a positive conclusion, nine yielded promising but not convincing results, and only three were actually negative.

Regulation of herbal medicines

In most developed countries, herbal medicines are subject to increasing regulation. Most major professional herbal associations are now reporting any side-effects so information may be shared among professionals. Proposed new European Union and UK medicines legislation will ensure medicinal plants are identified correctly. The European Directive on Traditional Herbal Medicinal Products, which became law in 2004, requires that over-the-counter herbal remedies should demonstrate at least 30 years of safe use to qualify for registration. Herbal remedies are now being officially listed for safety and efficacy by the European Medicines Evaluation Agency (EMEA). In 2003, the Herbal Medicine Regulatory Working Group set up by the British government published a report calling for the immediate statutory regulation of all UK herbal practitioners. This means that British herbalists will be regulated and acknowledged by the state and other fellow health professionals, thereby ensuring that herbal medicines, which have been tried and tested over hundreds of years, will continue to play a part in everyday healthcare.

Using herbs safely

Herbal remedies, like all medicines, must be treated with respect. There are certain conditions and combinations of treatments in which herbs may cause problems.

General cautions
During the first three months of pregnancy, avoid all medicines, herbal or otherwise, unless absolutely essential.
- Certain herbs should be avoided throughout pregnancy, so consult a qualified medical herbalist.
- Women who are breast-feeding should consult a medical herbalist before using herbal medicines.
- Do not give babies under 6 months any internal herbal (or other) medicine without professional advice.
- The elderly, because of their slower metabolism, may require less than the full adult dose.
- Do not stop taking prescribed conventional medication without first consulting your doctor.
- Some herbs interact with drugs. If you are taking a prescribed medicine, consult a medical herbalist.

Herb–drug interactions
Herbs can change the way that your body absorbs and breaks down (metabolises) drugs. They can also affect other aspects of your metabolism, e.g. heart rate and blood pressure, which can mask or exacerbate symptoms. If herbs and drugs have similar actions, the combined effect can be too strong. This list of cautions is a guide to some of the potential drug interactions and situations when herbs should be used with care. Consult a medical herbalist about herb–drug interactions and contraindications.

Coltsfoot (*Tussilago farfara*) in excessive doses may interfere with blood pressure treatment. Also avoid long-term use.

Garlic (*Allium sativum*) in medicinal doses can cause a dangerous decrease in blood-sugar levels if taken with diabetes medication. Do not take it with the blood-thinning drug warfarin or other anti-clotting medication. (Culinary amounts of garlic are safe.)

Ginkgo (*Ginkgo biloba*) should not be taken with warfarin or other anti-clotting medication.

Ginseng, Siberian (*Eleutherococcus senticosus*) can increase blood pressure, so it should be avoided by anyone with this condition.

Goldenseal (*Hydrasatis canadensis*) can raise blood pressure. Consult a qualified herbalist if taking beta-blocker or other antihypertensive medications, or medication to control diabetes or kidney disease.

Hawthorn (*Crataegus spp.*) may interact with other medicines, especially those prescribed for heart conditions.

Hops (*Humulus lupulus*) have a mild sedative effect and act as a depressive. Do not take if you have depression, breast cancer, or other oestrogen-responsive cancers. Do not take with alcohol.

Lily of the valley (*Convallaria majalis*) contains cardiac glycosides and may interact with other heart drugs. It should only be taken when prescribed by a qualified medical herbalist.

Liquorice (*Glycyrrhiza glabra*) should not be taken by anyone who is anaemic, or has high blood pressure.

Schisandra (*Schisandra chinensis*) should possibly be avoided by those with epilepsy or hypertension.

St John's wort (*Hypericum perforatum*) increases the rate at which the liver breaks down drugs, so that a drug taken alongside it may not be effective. Drugs that may be affected include indinavir and other drugs used for HIV infection, as well as warfarin, cyclosporin, digoxin, theophylline and possibly oral contraceptives. St John's wort may also cause sensitivity to sunlight, though this is most unusual within normal dosage range.

WHEN TO CONSULT A PRACTITIONER

The UK National Institute of Medical Herbalists and the National Herbalists' Association of Australia (*see p.486*) keep registers of trained medical herbalists. Your doctor may also be able to make a recommendation. You should consult a medical herbalist before taking herbal medicines if you are pregnant or have a serious condition such as diabetes, heart disease or high blood pressure. Do not stop taking prescribed medication without first consulting your doctor. Some herbs and drugs interact – see above before taking a herbal medicine.

HOMEOPATHY

DR PETER FISHER

Homeopathy (also spelled homoeopathy) is a complementary medicine based on the idea of treating "like with like" (often quoted in Latin, *Similia similibus curentur*), which aims to stimulate and direct the body's self-healing abilities. It can be used to treat a wide range of clinical problems, but it is particularly useful if the disease is "internal" – due to an imbalance rather than to a deficiency, infection or injury. For example, it is very effective for eczema and anxiety. Homeopathy can be used on its own but also combines well with other treatments.

Key Principles

The key features of homeopathic medicine include treating "like with like", the use of the minimum dose and the linked concepts of holism, constitution and idiosyncrasy, which together can be summed up as "homeopathy treats people, not diseases".

For example, the homeopathic remedy *Apis mellifica* is made from crushed honey bees. In line with treating like with like, it is used to treat medical problems with similar symptoms to the effects of a bee sting, i.e. those that appear suddenly, with a severe stinging pain and swelling. These conditions are relieved by cold applications (e.g. an ice pack), but are made worse when pressure is applied – by bandaging, for instance. While not all these features need to be present for *Apis* to work, a homeopath would normally look for at least three characteristic symptoms to make a "picture". The disease's name is less important than the resemblance between the process triggered by a bee sting and the symptoms to be treated. In practice, *Apis* is often used for skin problems and arthritis.

Homeopathy is concerned with a substance's ability to cure problems similar to those it causes, not with similarities between its appearance and its medical use. To understand the symptoms that a particular substance can cause, and what kind of person is particularly susceptible, homeopaths conduct "provings", or homeopathic pathogenetic trials. In a proving, healthy people take the substance, usually in very small doses under controlled conditions, and report any symptoms that they develop.

The controversial minimum dose

Although widespread and popular, homeopathy remains the most controversial form of complementary medicine because the medicines are so highly diluted. Starting from an alcoholic tincture or, in the case of insoluble substances, a "triturate", which is made by grinding the substance with lactose, medicines are made in a process of serial dilution and succussion (vigorous shaking). This process is sometimes known as potentisation.

The original tincture or triturate is diluted on the decimal scale (X) with a dilution factor of 1:10 or on the centesimal scale (C) with a dilution factor of 1:100. In other words, a homeopathic medicine in the 6x potency has been diluted 1:10, six times over, giving a final concentration of one part in 10,000,000. There are also other scales of dilution, such as Korsakovian, which are prepared by slightly different methods.

Matter is composed of particles (atoms and molecules). Therefore, if you dilute a substance enough, you will eventually dilute it out altogether. Thanks to the 19th-century Italian aristocrat and scientist Count Amodeo Avogadro, we can calculate the point at which it is likely that every atom or molecule of the starting substance has been diluted out. Dilutions of homeopathic medicines above about 24X or 12C are extremely unlikely to contain a single molecule of the starting substance – such dilutions are said to be "ultramolecular".

The homeopathic medicines that are sold in most pharmacies in the UK are in 6C and 30C dilutions. While the 6C dilution is likely to contain molecules of the starting substance, it is extremely unlikely that a 30C dilution does.

How does homeopathy work?

There is evidence that homeopathy does work, but if a remedy does not contain any of the original substance, how can it work? Recent scientific work has bought us closer to an answer, but the mode of action is currently unknown. Homeopaths think that the medicines contain information, held by the water/alcohol mixture in which they are made (sometimes referred to as the "memory of water").

Chemically, homeopathic medicines consist of just water, alcohol and lactose (from the pills), but there is now growing evidence that the preparation process alters the physical structure of the water and that this persists even after the solute has been completely diluted out.

This might seem bizarre, and it has even been claimed that if it were true physics textbooks would have to be rewritten. But the evidence suggests that the change is physical, not chemical, in nature. It can be compared to a magnetic medium, such as a video tape. Chemically, these consist of vinyl and ferric oxide: one cannot determine by chemical analysis whether a video tape is blank, contains a computer virus or records valuable data. This information is stored in physical form (the alignment of the magnetic dipoles of the ferric oxide). It is thought that water can store information in a similar way, although it is clear that the structure of liquid water is highly dynamic, not fixed like that of a magnetic medium.

Information medicine

This has given rise to the idea of "information medicine". Recently scientists at Queen's University, Belfast showed in test-tube experiments that ultramolecular dilutions of histamine, which chemically consist of pure water, reduce immune response. As well as these laboratory experiments, there are over 200 published clinical trials of homeopathy. Overviews of these agree that homeopathic medicines are not just placebos, despite the lack of understanding of the mechanism by which they work.

The practice of using highly diluted medicines originally arose because they were safer. However, in the process, homeopaths stumbled upon a different type of medical action. The process is not fully understood, but is thought to relate to the information content of homeopathic medicines. In high homeopathic dilutions, the original substance is no longer present, what remains and is transmitted to the body is information relating to it. For example, the medicine *Apis*, made from bee stings, is thought to give a message to the body: "your problem is similar to the effects of a bee sting". Similarly, the medicine *Natrum muriaticum*, which is made from common salt (sodium chloride), transmits a message: "there is an imbalance in your sodium metabolism". The body then responds and corrects itself. This has been described as "holding a mirror up to Nature", stimulating and directing the natural healing force (sometimes referred to in Latin as "*Vis medicatrix naturae*").

Holism, constitution and idiosyncrasy

In prescribing a medicine, homeopaths take these three principles into account. Holism means that in deciding which treatment to use, a homeopath considers every aspect of a person, as well as the ailment the person has. Constitution refers to the type of person as a whole (*see Constitution and constitutional prescribing, below*), which includes factors such as build, personality, general physical features (such as intolerance of cold and heat) and susceptibility to particular illnesses. Idiosyncrasy describes a person's unusual or atypical features or unexpected reactions to a health problem from which they suffer – homeopaths sometimes refer to the latter by the quaint phrase "rare, strange and peculiar" symptoms.

Origins of Homeopathy

Homeopathy originates in the work of the German physician Samuel Hahnemann (1755–1843), who coined the term from the Greek word *homoios*, which means same or similar, and *pathos*, meaning disease or suffering. He became a doctor during a brutal period in medicine when treatments involved blood-letting and giving doses of medicine so large the patient often died. Hahnemann vehemently denounced these practices, accusing his contemporaries of "killing gradually more millions than Napoleon ever slew in battle." He also condemned the chaining and beating of "lunatics", instead advocating "humanity combined with firmness".

Hahnemann grew so disillusioned that, for a while, he abandoned medical practice. The inspiration for homeopathy came as he translated a medical book by the Edinburgh physician William Cullen. He disagreed with what Cullen said about cinchona bark, the source of quinine and an effective treatment for malaria, which at that time was common in parts of Europe. Using himself as a guinea pig, he took regular doses of quinine and developed symptoms very similar to malaria, which inspired him to think of the idea of similarity. In 1796, Hahnemann launched homeopathy by publishing an article entitled "On a new curative principle".

Early homeopaths introduced many new medicines and radically changed the uses of others. Homeopathy grew rapidly through the 19th century, largely because of its success in treating epidemics, particularly of cholera. During the infamous London cholera epidemic of 1854, eventually traced to a water pump in Broad Street in Soho, the overall hospital mortality rate was 52 per cent (over 500 people), but at the London Homeopathic Hospital (which was the hospital nearest the infamous pump) the death rate was only 16 per cent.

In 200 years, homeopathy has become a worldwide practice. It is particularly popular in Latin America and the Indian subcontinent. In Western Europe over 50 per cent of the French have used it, and usage is only slightly lower in Germany. In the UK, homeopathy is currently used by 10 per cent of the population, with annual growth in sales of around 12 per cent.

Homeopathy suffered a sharp decline in many parts of the world in the 20th century, but is now growing again. For example, in the US, it almost died out in the 1970s and 1980s, but sales grew by a staggering 500 per cent in a seven-year period in the 1990s.

Types of Homeopathy

There are four main types of homeopathy: individualised or "classical" homeopathy; clinical homeopathy; complex homeopathy; and isopathy.

Individualised homeopathy
The practitioner builds up a "clinical picture" of the patient, often drawing on "constitutional" (*see p. 73*) and psychological factors in particular (*see box, p. 74*). The homeopath may also consult a "repertory" – a book or, more commonly now, a computer programme, which lists symptoms. The medicine is usually given in high potency at relatively long intervals.

Clinical homeopathy
This is a more pragmatic form of prescribing. It is based on a limited number of "keynote" indications and is more often used for acute problems.

Complex homeopathy

Complex homeopathic medicines are combinations of several substances that are likely to be useful for a particular problem. They tend to target particular conditions rather than a constitutional type or symptom picture. Various brands of complexes are widely available from pharmacies for common problems such as travel sickness or insomnia.

Isopathy

Isopathy means treating the "same with the same". For instance, homeopathic dilutions of grass pollen may be prescribed for hay fever.

Homeopathic Treatment

Although it has a wide range of uses, homeopathy should not be seen as an exclusive system of medicine. It does not necessarily provide the right treatment for every complaint or illness. For many diseases homeopathy is best integrated with other forms of treatment, and it is important that everyone involved in the patient's care communicates with each other and works together.

Is homeopathy safe?

All homeopathic medicines are generally safe, because of the high dilutions in which they are used. A worldwide survey of adverse effects concluded that they were "minor and transient". The main risks associated with homeopathy are "indirect" – not due to the medicine itself, but to other, associated factors. For instance, factors include using homeopathic medicines to treat yourself for the symptoms of a serious disease that requires medical diagnosis. Poor advice given by inadequately trained practitioners also poses a risk.

A common indirect risk is the claim made by some practitioners that homeopathy can immunise against diseases such as whooping cough or measles. There is no evidence that this is so, and it is not recommended.

What can homeopathy treat?

Homeopathy is particularly useful when the disease is "internal" – due to an imbalance within the person rather than to an external agent, such as an infection. For instance, homeopathy is very effective for children with eczema and other allergies, and for people with anxiety, depression, sleep problems, recurrent coughs, colds and flu, arthritis and rheumatism, and for women with PMS and menopausal problems. It can complement other treatments, too – for example, homeopathic medicines are sometimes taken alongside conventional medication to help with the side-effects and symptoms of cancer.

Homeopathic medicines are diluted and vigorously shaken many times in a process called succussion. As a result, the medicines are said to become more potent and more specific in the effect they have on an individual patient.

Constitution and constitutional prescribing

The constitution is the basic and essentially unalterable physical and psychological type of a person. The notion that individuals differ in their physical and psychological make-up, and that the differences predispose them to different illnesses, is found throughout medical history. The concept of constitution was known in classical Greece, where the Hippocratic doctors classified people as being of a choleric, phlegmatic, sanguine or melancholic temperament. These were respectively dominated by one of the four traditional "humours": bile, phlegm, blood or black bile. Similar ideas are found in the five-element theory of Traditional Chinese Medicine (*see p.80*) and in Tibetan medicine in which practitioners believe that all aspects of a person are governed by three humours (phlegm, bile and air).

A "constitutional medicine" is said to be the medicine which best encompasses the sum total of an individual's physical, mental and emotional expression over an extended period of time. Constitutional prescribing is, therefore, one of the central concepts in homeopathy because by considering a patient's constitution, the homeopath treats the person not the disease.

"Constitutional prescribing" can be contrasted with "keynote prescribing" when the prescription is based on a few characteristic symptoms of the disease (for instance, the homeopathic medicine *Magnesia phosphorica* is used for a severe pain with a cramping character, which is relieved by heat). Keynote prescribing is usually used for acute problems, constitutional prescribing for chronic or recurrent problems.

MAJOR HOMEOPATHIC MEDICINES

A homeopathic medicine is referred to as a "constitutional medicine" when it is prescribed more for the person than the illness. It is called a "polychrest" when it can be used for different conditions providing it matches the person's constitution or the symptom picture. In practice there is a lot of overlap between the two.

This list provides details of some of the more important homeopathic medicines.

MEDICINE	MADE FROM	COMMENTS
Argentum nitricum	Silver nitrate	Most patients who respond to this medicine have marked psychological features, including anxiety with restlessness and phobias. They nearly always feel too hot. There are frequently digestive problems, particularly burping and diarrhoea. *Argentum nitricum* may be indicated for headaches, vertigo, conjunctivitis and sore throats.
Arsenicum album	Arsenious trioxide	Those who respond to this medicine tend to be anxious, tidy and meticulous, and feel the cold greatly. They often feel weak, and may indeed be seriously ill. *Arsenicum album* may be used for many problems, including rashes, asthma and neuralgia.
Bryonia	*Bryonia alba* (white bryony)	*Bryonia*'s keynote symptom is pain aggravated by movement. This includes headaches, chest pain due to pleurisy and inflammation of joints and tendons. Symptoms are relieved with firm support – for instance, an elastic bandage. People who respond to it often have a dry mouth and are thirsty.
Calcarea carbonica	Calcium carbonate in oyster shells	*Calcarea carbonica* is frequently indicated for children who get recurrent coughs and colds. Adults who respond to it tend to be solid, both physically and psychologically, but this may conceal anxiety, fear of serious disease or inability to cope. They perspire freely, especially on the head at night. *Calcarea carbonica* may help with a wide range of different illnesses when these constitutional features are present.
Causticum	A potassium compound introduced by Dr Hahnemann	The most important mental feature of people who respond to this medicine is a strong sense of justice and sympathy. Physically, they are very sensitive to changes in the weather – for instance, they can predict when it will rain. *Causticum* may be appropriate for arthritis, hoarseness and facial paralysis.
Graphites	Graphite (a form of carbon)	The characteristic symptom of *Graphites* people is skin eruptions, mostly in skin folds, which crack and exude when bad. The medicine can also be useful for flatulent dyspepsia, colitis and menopausal symptoms.
Kalium bichromicum	Potassium bichromate	The most characteristic indication for this medicine is sinusitis with thick, stringy mucus. *Kalium bichromicum* is also useful for arthritis that moves from joint to joint.
Lachesis	The venom of *Lachesis mutus* (the bushmaster snake)	Some of the most characteristic features of *Lachesis* types are loquacity, aversion to tight clothes and a tendency for the problem to be worse on the left side of the body. It is often helpful for menopausal hot flushes, migraine and rosacea.
Lycopodium	The spores of *Lycopodium clavatum* (a kind of moss)	Individuals who respond to this medicine are often anxious and reserved. They may have stomach trouble, crave sweets and their symptoms are often worse between 4pm and 8pm. *Lycopodium* may help headaches and many other problems.
Mercurius solubilis	An oxide of mercury	This is the most important medicine for coughs and colds if taken after the initial stage when there is a thick, greenish nasal discharge, a sore throat that makes swallowing difficult, a sore tongue with too much saliva, and sweating.

MAJOR HOMEOPATHIC MEDICINES CONTINUED

MEDICINE	MADE FROM	COMMENTS
Natrum muriaticum	Sodium chloride (common salt)	It may seem odd to make a medicine from salt, but this is one of the most commonly indicated of all homeopathic medicines. Masked depression, where depressed feelings are not expressed, is a characteristic feature of people it helps. They cope and care for everybody else, without revealing how they feel themselves. Other symptoms include cold sores and migraine.
Nux vomica	The seeds of *Strychnos nux vomica* (poison nut tree)	*Nux vomica* is the classical "stress" medicine. The stress-related problems may be triggered or made worse by overwork. The patient becomes irritable, sleeps poorly and may develop indigestion. They may seek relief in alcohol or other drugs.
Phosphorus	The element phosphorus	Those who respond to this important polychrest are typically sensitive, both to the physical and psychological environment. They are easily tired, but recover after a short rest. They may also bruise easily. *Phosphorus* may be appropriate in hepatitis, haemhorragic conditions and vertigo in the elderly.
Pulsatilla	*Pulsatilla pratensis* (the pasque flower)	Those who respond to this important polychrest are typically indecisive and "changeable": their moods change swiftly – they weep easily, but quickly cheer up when comforted. *Pulsatilla* may be used for nasal catarrh, menstrual problems, circulatory problems and arthritis in people with *Pulsatilla* characteristics.
Rhus toxicodendron	*Toxicodendron radicans* (poison ivy)	Although this medicine is good for itchy, blistering skin rashes, it is most frequently used for arthritis and rheumatism. Its most characteristic indication is restlessness and rapid stiffening up from immobility – sitting still for as little as half an hour makes *Rhus toxicodendron* patients feel uncomfortable.
Sepia	The ink of *Sepia officinalis* (cuttlefish)	This important medicine is most often indicated in women. Typically, the patient is emotionally flat, fed up and snappy. She resents others asking what the matter is and may hide her feelings. She may lose her sex drive, but may gain a remarkable, if temporary, improvement by doing exercise.
Silicea	Sand (silicon dioxide)	Patients who respond to *Silicea* are run down and susceptible to infections. They seem to "pick up every cold", and their infections are slow to resolve. These individuals feel the cold, and have cold, clammy hands and feet. They are often thin and pale with fine hair and nails that have lengthwise ridges.
Staphysagria	*Delphinium staphysagria* (wild delphinium)	*Staphysagria* is indicated for people who are seething with anger, and who may have outbursts of rage. It is also used for genito-urinary problems and styes.
Sulphur	The element sulphur	People who respond to this polychrest are often extrovert and untidy. They nearly always feel too hot and often have hot feet. They tend to have skin trouble, such as intensely itchy eczema.
Thuja	A coniferous tree, *Thuja occidentalis*	Those who respond to *Thuja* often have warts and moles, and may have strange, fixed ideas. *Thuja* may be useful for chronic nasal catarrh, bladder and prostate problems, and neuralgia.

The homeopathic medicine *Arnica* comes from the flowers of *Arnica montana*, shown highly magnified with pollen grains (grey) on the flower's stigma (yellow).

Constitutional features

In deciding on a constitutional prescription the homeopath looks at the patient's physical type: for instance, patients whose constitutional homeopathic medicine is *Calcarea carbonica* or *Graphites* tend to be of solid build, inclined to be overweight, while those of *Silicea* or *Phosphorus* constitutional type are typically of slight build.

Constitutional features can be positive and adaptive, but when a person comes under strain they have a negative and maladaptive side which determines how he or she will break down. For example, patients whose constitutional medicine is *Calcarea fluorica* are usually very supple and may be "double jointed". Because of this they are often talented gymnasts or dancers when young, but when they strain their joints, and also later in life, they are predisposed to joint pain and arthritis.

The underlying psychological and emotional make-up also has adaptive and maladaptive aspects. For instance, *Lycopodium* constitutional types are typically reserved, intellectual and conscientious. Because of this they often occupy senior and responsible jobs, but when they fall ill, these characteristics become maladaptive and they feel they are failing and become anxious, tyrannical and depressed.

Similarly, *Natrum muriaticum* types are often found in the caring professions – they feel greatly for others, and sometimes seem better at dealing with other people's problems than their own. When stressed beyond the limit of adaptation they can become very depressed and have great difficulty telling anyone how they feel.

The extrovert, garrulous *Sulphur* constitutional types become Nature's politicians and trade unionists. This sort of personality, combined with a tendency to develop itchy skin problems as a feature of almost any illness (even if they are not the main problem), suggest *Sulphur* as the constitutional medicine.

Recent research using psychological questionnaire methods and sophisticated statistical analysis supports the proposition that at least some of these constitutional types can be identified scientifically.

Building the picture

A homeopath will take a detailed case history, asking questions about medical health, lifestyle, moods, likes and dislikes to build the "clinical picture". Traditionally, the clinical picture is divided into three parts:

"Locals"

These are the particular symptoms – for instance, a pain or a rash – of which a person complains. The precise details of the quality of the symptoms are important (whether the rash is itchy or sore, for example). The homeopath will also ask what factors make the symptoms better or worse. These indicate the symptom's "modalities" and can be of great importance in determining the treatment.

"Mentals"

As well as taking account of the patient's medical problem, the homeopath also notes the patient's "mentals": whether he or she is extrovert or introvert, assertive or unassertive, for example. Their emotional reactions to their illness, e.g. depression or anxiety, and the exact form they take, are important, as too are any fears and phobias.

"Generals"

The homeopath takes into account a person's "generals" when building a picture. These are general features, which include their build, what they like and dislike to eat, their reaction to temperature and their quality of sleep.

Prescribing homeopathy

Having built up a picture of the person, a homeopath tries to match it to a "medicine" picture – i.e. the medicine that most resembles the disease and sensitivity of the patient. He or she will also decide on the dilution and frequency.

The dilutions most commonly available in the UK are 6C and 30C. Homeopaths usually advise taking two pills of the 6C strength two or three times daily. Higher dilutions (e.g. 30C) are usually taken less frequently, although in an acute situation they may also be used several times per day. In general, the regime corresponds to the pace of the illness – for acute conditions the treatment is repeated frequently, while for long-standing problems the patient usually takes the medicines less frequently.

Taking Homeopathic Medicines

Homeopathic medicines come in a range of strengths that are sometimes called "potencies". The potency routinely stocked by high-street pharmacies is 6C.

For self-treatment it is usually best to start with a 6C potency. Avoid touching the medicines with your hands and fingers. Instead, tip the pills or tablets into the bottle cap then into your mouth. They should be sucked or chewed, but not swallowed whole. The pills should be taken "on a clean palate", at least ten minutes before or after eating or drinking, cleaning the teeth or smoking.

Homeopathic medicines have an "all or nothing" effect: the number of pills or tablets taken is not critical. Four pills of a 6C medicine have the same effect as two 6C pills, not two 12C pills. A dose of two pills or tablets is usually recommended for safety.

Potencies

A good general-purpose potency is 6C, but others, most often 30C, are also prescribed by homeopaths. A higher potency may be necessary in the following circumstances: when a lower one seems to have stopped working; when the problem is psychological or functional, without structural changes; or when the "fit" between the patient's symptom picture and that of the medicine is very good.

Some medicines, such as *Natrum muriaticum*, work better in higher potencies. However, the main objective is to find the right medicine – the right medicine in any potency will do something, and the potency can always be adjusted later in treatment.

It is sometimes said that higher dilutions are "stronger" than lower ones. This is not true, at least not in a simple sense, although different dilutions do vary in their range and duration of action.

Homeopathy for babies and young children

Homeopathic medicines are safe for babies and young children. Getting a baby to take homeopathic medicines is not difficult. The easiest method is to crush two pills or one tablet between two clean teaspoons, and put a small amount into the baby's mouth on the tip of a spoon. They taste sweet and babies usually take them quite happily. Because the effect is all or nothing, it does not matter if the baby does not swallow the whole dose.

Lactose intolerance

Homeopathic pills and tablets are usually made of lactose (milk sugar), which may contain tiny amounts of cows' milk protein. This means that, theoretically, the tablets might upset people with lactose intolerance (lactase deficiency), a condition that is quite common in people of East Asian descent, or children who are intolerant of cows'

milk. In fact, the amounts of lactose and cows' milk protein are so small that they rarely cause problems. However, if they do then you can buy homeopathic medicines that are made with saccharose (cane sugar) or that come in liquid form (these contain some alcohol).

Precautions

Some people develop an "aggravation", or healing reaction (a temporary flare-up of their symptoms), when they start a course of homeopathic treatment. This is nothing to worry about. In fact, it is a good sign because aggravations are usually associated with a promising long-term response. If you do develop an aggravation, however, stop taking the medicine until it has settled completely.

Coffee has a reputation for being an antidote to homeopathic medicines, but in fact interferes with only a few, such as *Nux vomica*. Very strong, penetrating smells, such as menthol and camphor, seem to interfere with the action of most homeopathic medicines, and so you should avoid preparations such as Vick and Tiger Balm while on homeopathic treatment. You can use mint toothpaste for brushing your teeth, but you should not take homeopathic remedies immediately afterwards.

FINDING A PRACTITIONER

In general, homeopathy can safely be used to treat yourself or your family for minor or acute complaints. For chronic or complex problems, which may require "constitutional" treatment, it is best to consult a practitioner.

If you want to reduce your conventional medication, you should do so under the supervision of a competent practitioner who understands both homeopathy and your conventional medication. But, because there is no legal regulation of who can call him- or herself a homeopath, it is not always easy to identify a reliable homeopath.

Qualifications and registration requirements for homeopaths vary widely between countries, even within the European Union. The UK has no legal regulation of who can practise homeopathy or style themselves a "homeopath", and there are no current plans to establish such regulation. In the UK, there are homeopaths who are also medically qualified. The Faculty of Homeopathy is a legal body which trains only registered health professionals. There are also homeopaths who are not medically qualified. Bodies that register homeopaths include the Society of Homeopaths and the Homeopathic Medical Association. In Australia, the Australian Homoeopathic Association represents professional homeopaths.

When you are looking for a suitable homeopath, take recommendations from friends, colleagues or your family doctor. It is always wise to ask at the first session about their training, registration, experience of treating your condition and insurance. (*For useful websites and addresses, see p.486.*)

TRADITIONAL CHINESE MEDICINE

PROFESSOR GEORGE LEWITH

Traditional Chinese Medicine (TCM) is an ancient healing system that incudes acupuncture (*see p.82*), herbal medicine, dietary therapy, massage (tuina), relaxation and special exercises, such as t'ai chi and qigong. Practitioners view the individual as an integrated whole, whose health or ill-health is determined by the flow of *Qi* (energy), and consider symptoms to be signs of a pattern of disharmony and not the result of a particular named disease.

Chinese Medicine

The *Huang Di Nei Jing* (The Yellow Emperor's Classic of Internal Medicine) is the first record of the teachings that form the foundation of Traditional Chinese Medicine. Written between around 200 BC and 100 AD, the teachings appear to be transcripts of discussions between the Yellow Emperor and his disciple, Ji Buo. The book emphasises three of the ideals of Taoist philosophy – balance, harmony and moderation in all things.

TCM practitioners see the main external causes of disease ("pathogenic factors") as the following environmental factors: Wind, Cold, Summer Heat, Damp, Dryness and Fire. The main internal causes of disease are the "Seven Emotional Factors": Joy, Anger, Sadness, Worry, Grief, Fear and Fright. Each of these, if excessive, can cause disease, and tends to affect a particular organ. Other causes of disease include a weak constitution, incorrect diet, lack of physical exercise, over-exertion, excessive sexual activity, pollution and trauma (accidents).

Traditional Chinese diagnosis

Chinese diagnosis takes note of a broad range of symptoms and signs, many of which would not be considered especially significant in Western conventional medicine. The pattern of the symptoms and signs of an ailment are the outer manifestations of "dis-ease" and are considered to reflect the condition of *Qi* and the Internal Organs. Analysis of the symptoms and signs leads to identification of a "pattern of disharmony", which is quite different from a conventional Western diagnosis. Examining the tongue and making a detailed pulse diagnosis are important procedures. Observation of the colour and shape of the tongue body, as well as the tongue's coating, can reveal the state of the Internal Organs and the presence or absence of various pathogenic factors.

Pulse diagnosis is a complex technique and involves a high degree of subjectivity. The radial pulse is felt with the index, middle and ring fingers at three different regions in the wrist, and the pulse characteristics are noted at three different levels (superficial, middle and deep). The various pulses are said to reflect the state of the *Qi*, blood, *yin* and *yang*, and Internal Organs, as well as the presence of pathogenic factors.

Consulting a practitioner

At first, the TCM practitioner will look at the condition of your tongue and hair, the tone of your skin and the way you move. He or she will notice the sound of your breathing and voice and will note any distinctive odours. You will expected to give details of your family history, habits, bodily functions and symptoms of ill-health. Finally, the practitioner will feel your radial pulse, checking for strength, rhythm and quality, and explore your body for hard or tender areas. Treatment can involve herbal medicines, acupuncture (*see p.82*), dietary regimes and movement therapies, such as t'ai chi.

Herbal remedies

The Chinese herbal practitioner can choose from around 6,000 herbs, a few mineral and animal sources and hundreds of different formulas. Herbal remedies are used to restore the *yin–yang* balance within the body and to

work in specific organs and channels (meridians – *see p.84*) to correct the relationship between the five elements. The herbs are classified under the five elements according to the remedial action of their taste – sweet, sour, bitter, pungent and salty – and their opposing *yin–yang* qualities of hot and cold. For example, skullcap is a bitter, cold herb that can be used to lower a fever.

Herbs are usually prescribed as a formula of 10–15 dried herbs on the basis of their reputation and record for treating a particular pattern of disharmony. For example, a practitioner might decide to treat a case of infected allergic eczema, which he would diagnose as "damp-heat eczema with fire poison" (*see p.170*) with Gentian Drain the Gallbladder Decoction (*Long Dan Xie Gan Tang*).

The practitioner often adapts a basic formula to match the patient's individual pattern of disharmony. Remedies are usually taken as teas that are prepared in daily doses. They may also be taken as pills, powders, ointments, creams and lotions.

T'ai chi

This ancient movement therapy is practised daily by millions of Chinese people. It is sometimes referred to as meditation in motion. T'ai chi is a non-combative martial art that combines breathing techniques with sequences of slow, graceful movements that improve the flow of *Qi*, calm the mind and promote self-healing. T'ai chi is a safe and enjoyable form of exercise and can be learned and practised by people of any age. Research shows that it relaxes the muscles and calms the nervous system, so improving the function of the body. It also benefits

THE FIVE ELEMENTS

Practitioners of Traditional Chinese Medicine have a profound understanding of the relationship between *yin* and *yang* and a practical grasp of the qualities that feature in five element theory. The five elements of TCM are fire, earth, metal, water and wood. These categories represent the qualities of everything in the universe, including the body's Internal Organs, which are more than simply organs as understood by the Western mind. The interplay between these elements gives rise to the unfolding and unceasing changes that are involved in maintaining well-being and restoring balance in our lives. Each element relates to a *yin* organ and a *yang* organ, and is associated with a specific taste, emotion and season (*see below*). In five element theory, one element supports or inhibits the function of another: fire melts metal, water douses fire, wood breaks through earth, metal lets water condense, water nourishes wood, earth dries up water, metal cuts through wood. In the body, the organs share the same relationships: the Heart (fire) controls the Lungs (metal); the Kidneys (water) control the Heart. The TCM practitioner will use the qualities of the five elements to understand the pattern of disharmony in the body and to restore the balance of the fundamental forces.

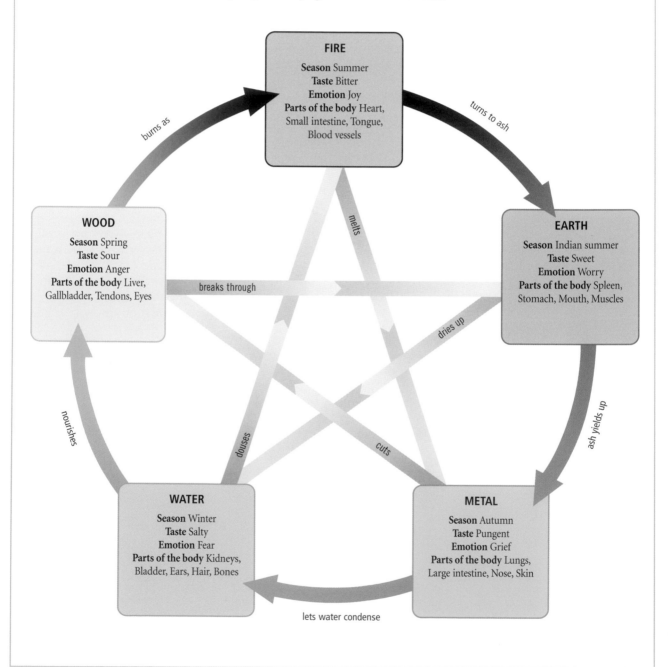

posture, balance and flexibility, thereby helping people who have arthritis and other musculoskeletal disorders.

Many people with arthritis who have practised t'ai chi praise its benefits, saying that it helps to relieve their pain and stiffness, brings relaxation and a lift to their spirits and increases their flexibility and muscle strength. Studies have shown that t'ai chi can not only improve balance but can also prevent falls. In 1996, a trial in Atlanta in the US found that t'ai chi improved the health of elderly people and another American study in 1989 found that it improved breathing without straining the heart.

Key Concepts of TCM

Holism means that a person's mind, body and emotions are seen as a single interacting whole. Ideally, they are in a state of harmony, both internally and in relation to the external environment. Problems in one part of the whole person affect the health of other parts. Holism is one of the key concepts of TCM, which also include *yin* and *yang*, the five elements (*see box, left*), *Qi*, the Internal Organs, the meridians and the acupoints.

Yin and yang
These are the two complementary and fundamental processes of nature of ancient Chinese philosophy. They are qualities that are both opposite and yet at the same time interdependent. Many of the familiar pairs of opposites are described as either *yin* (contraction, cold, water, female, moon, black) or *yang* (expansion, hot, fire, male, sun, white). From the unceasing interplay of *yin* and *yang*, everything grows, develops and changes.

Yin and *yang* are in a state of continual change and influence everything in the universe, from the very large to the very small. This includes a person's health, which is affected by qualities in the external environment and the harmony of internal energy. Disease-causing (pathogenic) factors can disturb the balance between *yin* and *yang*. For example, a disturbed balance might lead to *yin* conditions that involve hardenings, such as osteoarthritis, or to *yang* conditions that involve inflammations. A TCM practitioner will diagnose the imbalance by assessing the flow of *Qi* with various techniques, such as feeling the pulses in the wrist (*see p.79*), and will then direct treatment towards restoring the balance.

Qi
Qi is the "vital energy" or "life force" that exists in every living thing. It is a concept that is very difficult to explain in Western terms. One way of looking at *Qi* is to say there are three kinds. The first is the *Qi* that is given to a child by its parents at conception – this *Qi* is stored in the kidneys and contributes to the child's constitution. The second is the *Qi* which we receive from the digestion of food. The third is the *Qi* which we absorb from the air we breathe.

Qi moves between *yin* and *yang*: it can move inwards to the centre (*yin*) or outwards to the surface (*yang*). It governs the functions of the Internal Organs, and circulates via the meridians to every part of the body. Pain, for instance, results from disturbances in this circulation.

Two main categories of *Qi* can bring disharmony – deficiency and stagnation. When *Qi* becomes deficient it might affect the whole person or a single Internal Organ, such as the Kidneys. When it stagnates, *Qi* ceases to flow smoothly through the meridians, leading to aches and pains or a dysfunction of an Organ.

Internal Organs
The Internal Organs are not the same as the Western equivalent although, confusingly, they have the same names, such as liver, kidneys, heart and spleen. To help avoid this confusion, the Chinese are written as starting with a capital letter – hence, Liver, Kidneys, Heart and Spleen and Internal Organs.

TCM sees each organ as a complex system which includes not only its anatomical entity and physiological functions, but also recognises its corresponding emotional and mental function.

Meridians
The meridians are pathways, or channels, in which *Qi* energy circulates throughout the body (*for a diagram of their locations see p.84*). Each meridian is associated with an Internal Organ.

Acupoints
Acupuncture points, also known as acupoints, are specific sites through which the *Qi* reaches the body's surface. An acupuncturist can manipulate the circulating *Qi* via these points to restore health in the relevant organs or meridians.

FINDING A PRACTITIONER

It is essential to find a suitably qualified Chinese herbalist. The Register of Chinese Herbal Medicine and the Australian Acupuncture and Chinese Medicine Association (AACMA) (*see p.486*) hold lists of practitioners. Expect the first session to last about an hour and subsequent ones about 30 minutes. You may be given a mixture of herbs to prepare as a tea each day, but herbs may also be prescribed as pills, powders and ointments.

Do not treat yourself with Chinese herbs unless they are prescribed by your herbalist. Make sure you give the practitioner full details of any conventional drugs and nutritional supplements you are taking.

If you would like to learn t'ai chi, the T'ai Chi Association (*see p.486*) can help you locate a qualified teacher.

ACUPUNCTURE

PROFESSOR GEORGE LEWITH

Acupuncture is an integral part of Traditional Chinese Medicine (*see p.78*). Traditional Chinese acupuncturists understand patterns of health and illness according to the flow of *Qi* (energy) in the body and apply needles or moxibustion to stimulate acupoints situated along energy channels called meridians. Acupuncture is now becoming an accepted part of modern clinical healthcare, particularly for conditions such as pain management.

History of Acupuncture

"Acupuncture" is a European term that was coined by Willem Ten Rhyne, a Dutch physician, for the practice he observed on his visit to Japan in the 17th century. It literally means "to puncture with a needle", from the Latin *acus* (needle) and *punctura* (puncture). Acupuncture can be defined as a method of stimulating certain points on the body by inserting special needles in order to modify the perception of pain, normalise physiological functions and treat or prevent disease. Its aim, like the other practices in Traditional Chinese Medicine (*see p.78*), is to restore the balance of *yin* and *yang* in the body and to harmonise the flow of the energy known as *Qi*, which is disrupted in illness.

The *Huang Di Nei Jing* (The Yellow Emperor's Classic of Internal Medicine) is the first record of the teachings that form the foundation of Traditional Chinese Medicine. The book emphasises three of the ideals of Taoist philosophy – balance, harmony and moderation in all things.

The Chinese practised acupuncture for several centuries before knowledge of it reached the rest of the world – it was first practised in Korea in about 600 AD and soon after in Japan. The West first learned of acupuncture in the 17th century when Jesuit missionaries brought European medical practice to China. At this time, Western medicine was still based on the four humours and used purges, leeches and herbs. However, Western physicians and surgeons had a good knowledge of anatomy, derived from dissection.

Acupuncture reached its zenith during the Ming dynasty (1368–1644), then declined during the Qing dynasty (1644–1911) under Manchu rule and Western influence. During this period, herbal medicine was emphasised more than acupuncture and, in 1822, the authorities ordered the closure of the acupuncture–moxibustion department of the Imperial Medical College. In Europe, acupuncture came to be widely practised by the medical profession during the first half of the 19th century, and good results were reported in the treatment of pain and rheumatism. In 1823, acupuncture was mentioned in the first issue of *The Lancet*. However, it gradually fell into disrepute when practitioners failed to employ it in a selective and discerning manner. However, now a growing number of Western doctors practise acupuncture to supplement conventional treatment.

Acupuncture Treatment

There are two main types of acupuncture. In traditional Chinese acupuncture, the acupoints are selected in accordance with traditional Chinese theories, such as the individual "pattern of disharmony" (*see p.78*), rather than a Western medical diagnosis. In medical acupuncture, certain trigger points (*see p.55*) are needled to treat pain. Although doctors who use acupuncture make no use of Chinese theories, there is a close correlation between trigger points and acupuncture points for pain.

Modern acupuncture needles are usually made of stainless steel and are single-use, disposable needles. In general, one of the first things a patient will want to know before commencing treatment is "Will it hurt?" In skilled hands, it is not a particularly painful experience. It is much less traumatic than an injection, as it involves the use of a very small-gauge "atraumatic" needle. The Chinese often use moxibustion with acupuncture. This involves burning moxa, the dried leaves of the herb mugwort (*Artemisia vulgaris*), near particular acupoints. The heat is believed to help stimulate the acupoints and flow of *Qi*.

The Chinese believe that for acupuncture to obtain its maximum effect, a patient should feel a "needling sensation", which involves manipulating the needle after insertion into an acupoint. The patient may experience a dull, aching, heavy, numb, sore, distending or warm sensation around the needle. This is known in Chinese as *De Qi*, and signifies the arrival of *Qi* at the needle. Sometimes, sensations may radiate along the path of a channel (meridian) on which the acupoint is situated – the so-called "propagated channel sensation" (PCS). Interestingly, needling trigger points produces the same sort of local sensation.

Generally, only a few needles (perhaps 6–10) are inserted during a treatment. They are usually left in place for about 20 minutes before being removed. It is common for patients to experience a degree of relaxation during and following acupuncture. Some patients may experience drowsiness or go to sleep; others say they feel elated and "high" for a short time. These effects may be due to release of endorphins (opioid, pain-relieving chemicals which are produced by the brain).

In general, acute conditions will respond quickly and need few treatments. Chronic disorders respond more slowly and require a more prolonged course of treatment. However, individuals vary quite considerably in their response to acupuncture. Sometimes, immediate relief may be experienced on insertion of a needle, but in other situations three or four sessions may be required before any benefit is noticed at all. Occasionally, patients may find improvement only some weeks after treatment.

MERIDIANS AND ACUPOINTS

There are 14 meridians in the body. Six are associated with a solid *yin* organ (such as the Liver) and six with a hollow *yang* organ (such as the Lungs). Two more meridians, the Conception and the Governing vessels, control the other 12. *Qi* energy flows along the meridians and is accessible to the acupuncturist via acupoints.

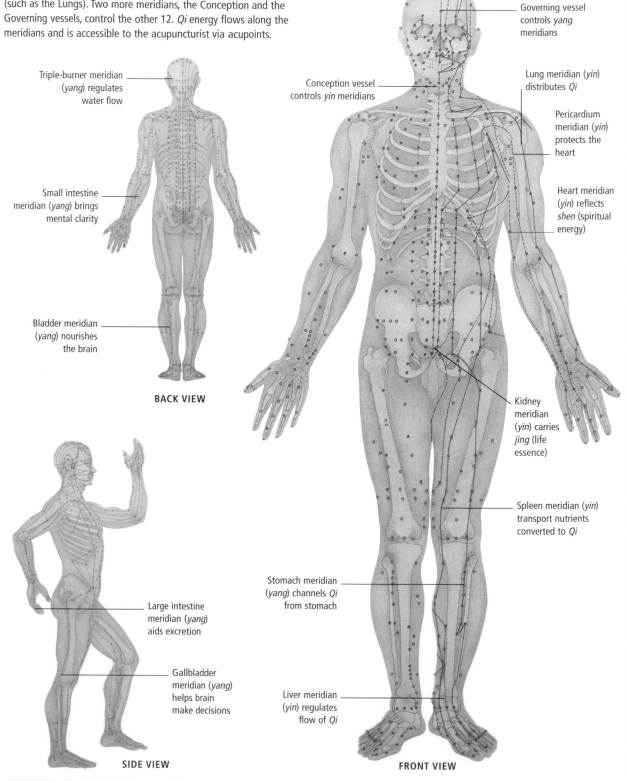

Triple-burner meridian (*yang*) regulates water flow

Small intestine meridian (*yang*) brings mental clarity

Bladder meridian (*yang*) nourishes the brain

BACK VIEW

Large intestine meridian (*yang*) aids excretion

Gallbladder meridian (*yang*) helps brain make decisions

SIDE VIEW

Governing vessel controls *yang* meridians

Conception vessel controls *yin* meridians

Lung meridian (*yin*) distributes *Qi*

Pericardium meridian (*yin*) protects the heart

Heart meridian (*yin*) reflects *shen* (spiritual energy)

Kidney meridian (*yin*) carries *jing* (life essence)

Spleen meridian (*yin*) transport nutrients converted to *Qi*

Stomach meridian (*yang*) channels *Qi* from stomach

Liver meridian (*yin*) regulates flow of *Qi*

FRONT VIEW

Improvement after the first treatment may be only temporary and short-lived, but with each treatment a better and more prolonged effect should occur. Three or four treatments should be adequate to assess whether a patient will respond. If there is no response after four treatments, then it is unlikely whether treatment will work.

Most acupuncturists will continue to treat patients until they are fully recovered or until there is no further improvement in their condition. A typical course of acupuncture might consist of four to twelve sessions.

Western uses of acupuncture

Traditional Chinese acupuncturists treat a wide range of conditions, such as irritable bowel syndrome or asthma. In the West, acupuncture is mainly used for the treatment of pain, particularly neuromuscular pain. The underlying mechanism of how acupuncture works in conventional medical terms is unclear, but in all probability its therapeutic effects are mediated through the autonomic nervous system (the part of the nervous system that controls involuntary functions).

Acupuncture treatment for pain works either locally through release of encephalins (opioid, pain-relieving chemicals produced by the brain) or more centrally through nervous pathways that are mediated by neurotransmitters, such as serotonin (*see p.437*) and noradrenaline. Increasingly detailed research reveals the neurophysiological mechanisms by which acupuncture may bring about its effects.

Effectiveness of Acupuncture

It is difficult to design placebo-controlled trials that test the effectiveness of acupuncture. Researchers involved in clinical trials continue to argue about acupuncture, largely because they tend to look for specific effects compared to a placebo. No appropriate placebo has yet been developed for acupuncture. This adds to the confusion, particularly when comparing so-called "real acupuncture" (acupuncture that needles the correct acupoints) with "sham acupuncture" (acupuncture that does not use acupoints) – the difference in treatment outcome between the two seems to be much less than might be expected. In other words, it may not matter so much exactly where the practitioner places the needles – the benefit may come from the patient experiencing the whole process of having acupuncture.

Evidence for its effectiveness

Positive evidence from clinical trials, based on systematic reviews and meta-analyses of acupuncture trials, supports its use for nausea and vomiting, dental pain and headaches. The efficacy of acupuncture treatment in back pain is less clear, with one positive systematic review, one neutral and one negative review.

Inconclusive evidence exists for the treatment of stroke, asthma and neck pain, and there is clear negative evidence for the use of acupuncture in weight loss and giving up smoking. However, the effect of acupuncture in smoking cessation trials is similar to that of nicotine patches. Acupuncture is currently used in at least 84 per cent of pain clinics in the UK and in primary care for painful and non-painful symptoms.

Needling trigger points

One particularly effective aspect of acupuncture is the practice of needling trigger points (or intramuscular stimulation) in the treatment of pain. Interestingly, the pain referral pattern emanating from a myofascial trigger point often radiates along the pathway of a meridian, and it seems possible that some of the traditional meridian ideas may have developed as a consequence.

Is Acupuncture Safe?

Although serious side-effects may occur with acupuncture, they are rare. They include local infection and local tissue damage, such as bruising. Very rarely, serious damage to superficial nerves or internal organs may cause events such as a punctured lung or kidney. The chances of a needle breaking are extremely small, but if one does there may be problems due to the migration of broken or embedded needle fragments.

Two surveys of acupuncture safety, involving 66,000 consultations, demonstrated a very low incidence of minor side-effects, but warned against some preventable ones. The transmission by acupuncture needles of infections such as hepatitis B and C is a very real possibility. Unsterilised needles probably caused millions of liver disease cases in China and Japan. It is vitally important to use disposable needles. It is also essential to establish a clear diagnosis before initiating acupuncture treatment, particularly for persistent pain. The reason for this is that in theory, at least, acupuncture might mask a disease because it can reduce pain, breathlessness and other troublesome symptoms.

FINDING A PRACTITIONER

The British Medical Acupuncture Society (see p.486) keeps a register of doctors trained in acupuncture techniques and the British Acupuncture Council can also recommend practitioners. In Australia, contact the Australian Acupuncture and Chinese Medicine Association (AACMA). When you receive acupuncture, check the practitioner is using disposable needles. Always tell the practitioner if you are pregnant (certain acupoints should be avoided). Avoid alcohol, large meals, hot baths or showers and strenuous exercise immediately before or after treatment as they may counteract the effect of treatment.

ENVIRONMENTAL HEALTH

DR DAVID KIEFER

Environmental health examines the impact the environment makes on human health and disease. The World Health Organization includes physical, chemical, biological, social and psycho-social factors in their definition of environmental health, and is concerned with both present and future generations of people. For centuries, scientific research has made connections between symptoms of ill health and their possible environmental causes. This knowledge helps doctors to treat existing environmental illnesses, and to encourage changes that will help to prevent them in future.

Environmental Hazards

The physical environment is a very important factor in human health. Clean air, sunlight and clean water are all vital for everyone. Realising that environmental factors can have serious consequences for human health is not new: the detrimental effects of overcrowding, poor sanitation, infectious diseases and breathing or ingesting toxins have long been recognised. Environmental health experts use data from animal tests, ecology studies, laboratory tests and the observation of the effects that substances have on humans to assess the risks that different hazards pose. Following is a summary of some of the most potent threats.

Environmental toxins

Toxins can take the form of chemicals, biological agents, radiation (e.g. X-rays or ultra-violet light) or even tobacco smoke, all of which can have negative effects on health. They may enter the body in several ways, including ingestion, inhalation or from contact with the skin. In some cases toxins can have immediate effects, so the cause of ill health is relatively easy to pinpoint. Some toxins, though, have effects that may only become apparent after many years of low-level exposure.

Many of the chemicals in use in the modern world have not been adequately assessed for their toxicity to humans or the environment.

Air pollution

In the past, a few major episodes of stagnant air pollution in large cities resulted in many deaths among people with lung and heart problems. Subsequent investigations led to the identification of many different air pollutants connected to human illness and disease, such as sulphur dioxide, carbon monoxide, nitrogen oxides, polycyclic aromatic hydrocarbons and ozone. Many of these are produced by the burning of fossil fuels (such as coal, oil and petrol) and they constitute the growing problem of "smog" in major cities across the globe, adversely affecting the health of many people. Other air-borne pollutants, e.g. CFCs (*see p.90*), can create distant health problems.

Indoor air pollution is also a problem that affects people, whether it results from smoke from tobacco, indoor fires or cookers, or the compounds emitted from modern building materials (including carpets, paint and walls) used in modern office buildings and homes.

Water contamination

Water supplies can be contaminated with potentially dangerous microbes and chemicals, either from a specific source ("point pollution", e.g. from a factory) or from many scattered sources (e.g. runoff from agricultural fields). Both types of pollution can contaminate lakes, rivers, reservoirs and other surface waters, and seep into groundwater, contaminating wells and aquifers.

Industrial pollution is responsible for contamination by a wide range of compounds, including volatile organic solvents and heavy metals (especially lead and arsenic).

Lead is a well-researched contaminant. It often enters the water supply from old pipes, which are either made of lead, or lead has been used as a solder, or it leaches from soil contaminated by the fallout from combusted leaded petrol.

Microbes from human and animal waste, such as *Cryptosporidium*, and the common gut bacteria *E. coli*, can contaminate water. These can lead to intestinal disease outbreaks. Nitrates and pesticides can enter drinking water supplies, mainly from farmland run-off. Nitrates can be harmful to very young babies. In the UK, water is treated and pesticide and nitrate levels are usually very low.

Some chemicals are intentionally added to drinking water such as chlorine, which is a common disinfectant, used to kill pathogens such as *E. coli* from sewage. Trihalomethanes (THMs) are produced when chlorine combines with naturally present organic matter. THMs in drinking water have been linked to higher incidences of miscarriage, but evidence is inconsistent and inconclusive. Chlorine and THMs evaporate easily, so leaving tap water in an open container, preferably in the fridge, for a few hours can reduce the chlorine content and improve the taste.

Our bodies need a trace amount of fluoride and it is added to mains water in some areas for dental health. There have been widely publicised health concerns about fluoride, but little good evidence for harm has been published.

Water filters can remove pesticides, nitrates and chlorine, but the filters must be changed regularly or they become ineffective, and they need to be cleaned regularly. Tap water undergoes a series of mandatory test so in most cases it is exceedingly pure. If you are concerned about the quality of your tap water, your local supplier should be able to give you quality control statistics.

Food contamination

Even healthy foods, such as fruit and vegetables can be contaminated with potentially harmful chemicals. In agriculture, chemicals are used to reduce pests (pesticides), diseases (fungicides, anti-microbials and anti-parasitics) or weeds (herbicides). They are also used control the rate of crop growth and ripening (growth regulators). Some crop sprays stay on the surface of the plant, while others (called systemic chemicals) are designed to spread throughout the plant. Chemicals can also be added after harvesting, to improve the appearance or shelf-life of the crop.

Crop chemicals are generally designed to stick to the plant, so that they are not washed off when it rains. This means that a quick rinse under the tap is not enough to remove them: thorough washing with soap or other detergent is required. Some may also be absorbed into the plant's surface layers, so peeling helps to reduce the amount ingested. Other chemicals, described as systemic, permeate the whole plant, so are not removable.

Current pesticide regulations and testing ensure that residues of pesticides in food are extremely low and, in many cases, below the detection limit. However, almost all tests for chemical safety are conducted on individual chemicals, rather than on the cocktail that we are exposed to through our food. There are, however, steps you can take to minimise your exposure to these chemicals. One such step is to buy organic foods. By doing this, as well as reducing your intake of chemical residues, you are also supporting an industry that pollutes the wider environment far less than intensive agriculture does.

Cereal and cereal products

We tend to consume large quantities of cereals (e.g. bread, breakfast cereals and pasta) so the chemicals that are used to cultivate these plants are particularly important. Intensively-grown wheat, barley and other cereals are sprayed with a range of chemicals during their growth, including Chlormequat, Pirimiphos-methyl (an organophosphate), glyphosate and phosphine. The effects of this chemical cocktail on human health has not yet been studied.

On the positive side, chemicals have helped to eliminate problems caused by contamination of cereals with poisonous weed seeds and fungal diseases. A fungus called ergot used to cause major health problems in Western countries, especially in wet years. Symptoms of poisoning included hallucination, manic depression, gangrene and abortion, and could lead to a painful convulsive death.

Fruit and vegetables

Potatoes are another staple food that people tend to consume in large quantities. After harvesting, potatoes are usually sprayed with chemicals to stop them sprouting. Unless you are using organic potatoes, always peel them and avoid eating the skin.

Surface contamination can also be avoided in many fruits. Non-organic oranges and lemons are treated with waxes and other post-harvest chemical sprays to prolong shelf-life and add shine. Try to buy organic, unwaxed lemons, especially if you are using the zest (peel). Alternatively, scrub them thoroughly, using warm soapy water.

Buying organic bananas is another good idea. Non-organic bananas often contain pesticide residues and pesticides have been implicated in thyroid gland disorders in banana plantation workers. Some chemicals are applied before shipping to prevent mould, so are in high quantities at the peel surface.

Strawberries and other soft fruits are highly susceptible to moulds, so fungicides are often used on them. These fruits obviously cannot be scrubbed. Also, high levels of the insecticides acephate and methamidophos have been found in non-organic peaches and nectarines. Because these chemicals are systemic, they spread through the fruit, so washing will not remove them. Fruit and vegetables produced organically have much lower, or negligible, chemical contamination.

Red meat

Animals can be contaminated with potentially harmful chemicals through their food and medication. If their pastures have been sprayed, or their food is contaminated, the chemicals are absorbed into their bodies. Fat-soluble chemicals, such as dieldrin, DDT and dioxins are present in small quantities in plants, but the accumulate in animals that eat those plants. When humans eat the animals in turn, the chemicals accumulate in higher concentrations. Meat reared organically is inherently lower in contaminants as far fewer chemicals are allowed: animals are fed organic foodstuffs and have only minimal medication.

Chicken and eggs

Poultry can be medicated for parasites and disease-causing bacteria, or chemicals can be routinely added to their food. Residues can survive in meat or eggs if the birds are not given enough time to clear the chemicals from their systems.

Low doses of antimicrobial chemicals have been routinely fed to poultry as growth promoters. This has sparked worries that the practice could lead to drug-resistant bacteria evolving and threatening human health.

Birds reared in high-intensity conditions are likely to need the most chemical treatments to keep them healthy, so try to avoid factory-farmed eggs and meat.

Fish

Through the food they eat, fish are able to absorb chemical pollution from the general environment. Farmed salmon can contain 16 times more PCBs (cancer-causing, dioxin-like chemicals) than wild salmon. This mainly comes from the fishmeal (ground, pelleted fish) on which they are fed. Farmed fish are also likely to have been treated with anti-

HARMFUL CHEMICALS AND THEIR EFFECTS

CHEMICAL	SOURCE AND TOXIC LEVELS	PEOPLE AT RISK AND EFFECTS ON HEALTH
Arsenic	**Source:** natural and man-made, such as wood preservatives and pesticides. **Toxic levels** (for adults of normal body weight): between 300 and 30,000 ppb of inorganic arsenic in food or water can cause adverse health effects. Above 60,000 ppb in food or water can be fatal.	**At risk:** people who (a) breathe in air with sawdust or smoke from arsenic-treated wood (b) live near contaminated waste sites (c) live near rocks with high levels of arsenic. **Health effects:** stomach ache, nausea, vomiting and diarrhoea, darkening of skin; small corns/warts on torso, palms or soles.
Benzene	**Source:** natural (volcanoes, forest fires, fossil fuels) and man-made (rubber, pesticides, dyes, drugs, lubricants, etc.). **Toxic levels:** (for adults of normal body weight): between 700 and 3,000 ppm can cause adverse health effects. Exposure to 10,000 to 20,000 ppm for 5 to 10 minutes can be fatal.	**At risk:** people who breathe tobacco smoke, exhausts, industrial emissions, vapour from glues, paints. **Health effects:** high levels cause dizziness, drowsiness, increased heart rate, vomiting, irritated stomach. Persistent exposure damages bone marrow, disturbs immune system and may cause leukaemia.
Lead	**Source:** natural and man-made (industrial). **Toxic levels:** (for adults of normal body weight): more than 1.5 µg/m3 inhaled on average over 3 months and more than 0.015 mg/L in drinking water may cause adverse health effects.	**At risk:** people who (a) drink water from lead plumbing (b) work with lead (c) eat food from lead-contaminated soils. **Health effects:** damage to the central nervous system (especially children's), kidneys. High levels may slow reaction times, weaken joints, cause anaemia, lead to miscarriages and damage sperm production. May be carcinogenic.
Nitrates	**Source:** fertiliser, manure, sewage. **Toxic levels:** (for adults of normal body weight): more than 10 mg/L of nitrate-nitrogen or 45 mg of nitrate in drinking water may have adverse effects.	**At risk:** babies who drink water with high levels of nitrate. **Health effects:** high levels in drinking water can reduce the haemoglobin's ability to carry oxygen, especially in babies up to 6 months old (gut bacteria turn nitrates into toxic nitrites).
Phthalates	**Source:** man-made (plastic softeners, plastic and vinyl toys, solvents, insecticides, wood finishes, cosmetics, personal care products). May be absorbed through skin. **Toxic levels** (for adults of normal body weight): more than 6 ppb in drinking water may cause adverse health effects.	**At risk:** people who (a) eat food stored in plastic wrapping (b) eat fatty foods, fish, meat, vegetable oils (c) breathe in certain perfumes, nail polishes, deodorants, hair sprays (d) drink contaminated water (e) have excessive mouth contact with plastic (plastic tubing, plastic toys). **Health effects:** gastrointestinal problems, nausea, vertigo. Long term, potential damage to developing testes and liver, and to developing foetus. May be carcinogenic.
Polycyclic aromatic hydrocarbons (PAHs)	**Source:** natural (volcanoes, forest fires) and man-made (pesticides, dyes, plastics, medicines). **Toxic levels** (for adults of normal body weight): more than a level of 0.3 to 0.06 mg (depending on the PAH) per kg of body weight per day may cause adverse health effects.	**At risk:** people who (a) breathe air from incomplete burning of fossil fuels, waste or other organic substances (b) breathe soot, exhaust fumes, contaminated dust (c) drink contaminated water or milk. **Health effects:** not proven, but animal research suggests PAHs may affect reproductive system, skin, body fluids and immune system, and may cause cancer.
Polychlorinated biphenyls (PCBs)	**Source:** man-made (pre-1977 manufacture of electrical insulation equipment). **Toxic levels** (for adults of normal body weight) causing adverse health effects vary from 0.5 ppb (drinking water) to 3 ppm (fat of poultry and red meat), and consistently breathing air with more than 0.5 to 1 mg/m3.	**At risk:** people who (a) breathe air from spills and leaks from hazardous waste sites, or from combustion of PCB-containing products (b) drink contaminated water (c) eat fish and aquatic mammals in which PCBs accumulate. **Health effects:** animal research suggests large amounts of PCBs may damage the liver, stomach, blood, immune system and skin (causing acne and rashes). Probably carcinogenic.

(ppm= parts per million; ppb=parts per billion)

biotics and pesticides to control infections and infestations. Wild fish, however, can also be contaminated with harmful environmental chemicals. Some substances such as PCBs and DDT (a pesticide), are oil-soluble, so accumulate in fat and oil. Oily fish (e.g. mackerel) and predatory fish (e.g. tuna), which are higher up the food chain, are likely to have accumulated more contaminants.

When there is a choice, opt for wild fish, and, if possible, try to be selective about the source of your fish. Those caught in restricted waters, such as the Baltic, are much more likely to be more polluted than those caught in the open Pacific or Atlantic oceans.

Since contamination levels can be high, women who are pregnant, or may become pregnant, or who are breast-feeding should eat fewer than the one to four portions of oily fish per week that is recommended for others.

Nuclear radiation

Radioactive contamination occurs with nuclear fallout from nuclear reactor accidents, spills at military, research and commercial facilities, and nuclear weapons testing. All these sources have exposed workers and the general public to varying doses of radiation. Although the details are being debated by scientists, radiation seems to be related to an increased incidence of cancer beyond what would normally be expected in a population. Some researchers even point out that "there is no threshold level below which radiation exposure is safe".

Global climate change

Environmental change has many far-reaching effects, including changes in patterns of human health problems. The weather affects health directly (e.g. heatstroke) or indirectly (e.g. warm, wet weather encourages insects to breed that may transmit diseases).

Current climate variations offer clues to how long-term climate change might affect health. Every few years, natural changes in ocean temperature affect convection currents (the mass movements of air that form weather systems) creating warmer, more stormy conditions than usual in various parts of the world. During these "El Niño" years higher temperatures in some areas of Peru have been connected to more gastrointestinal diseases, whereas El Niño-related droughts and fires in Indonesia contributed to a worsening of air pollution and a risk in related health conditions such as asthma in south-east Asia. If climate change proceeds as predicted, health effects will be diverse. Some experts predict, for example, that if global warming increases flooding of major rivers and coastal areas, these may release and distribute toxins from agricultural fields, human septic systems and toxic dumps. Also, some areas of the world may become more susceptible to drought, worsening malnutrition and its resulting health problems.

The ozone hole

It is now widely realised that pollution in one part of the globe can affect people and environments elsewhere. For example, ozone-depleting chlorofluorocarbons (CFCs) produced in industrialised nations may travel thousands of miles and contribute to the "ozone hole" in the southern hemisphere. These chemicals, combined with compounds from natural sources such as volcano eruptions, react in the atmosphere to deplete ozone and permit greater amounts of certain types of ultraviolet radiation (UV-A and UV-B) from the sun to reach the earth's surface. Some of these UV rays are very harmful, increasing the occurrence of skin cancer and eye problems, such as cataracts. It is also possible that UV rays may cause a suppression of the immune system. The global dispersal of CFCs is an example of how environmental problems and resulting health effects have become international as well as regional.

Furthermore, human health may also be indirectly affected by changes to the environment resulting from stratospheric ozone depletion. For example, UVB radiation contributes to photochemical smog: it can increase ozone at ground level and so aggravate respiratory conditions, such as asthma. A potentially more dramatic effect could stem from a decrease in food production due to the effects of stratospheric ozone depletion on certain plants and animals. However, these indirect health effects are less easily measured than direct effects on human health.

Children's health

Children are exposed to a large quantity of different pesticides and toxins through their food, water, at home, in schools and in gardens and parks. The effects of a toxin on children's behaviour, physiology and physique may be different from its effects on adults. Children have a higher caloric and fluid intake relative to their body weight compared to adults, making low-level contamination of food and water a more significant factor for them. Children also favour certain foods and drinks over others, and this too can contribute to toxic exposure. For example, in the US, toddlers are estimated to drink 16.7 times more apple juice than the average for the population. Thus, any pesticide residues in apple juice would be more significant for toddlers than for other age groups. Also, children are growing and developing in many ways and small, seemingly insignificant exposures may not cause obvious symptoms for many years.

Governments are beginning to recognise these factors and establish recommendations that are specific to children. In the US, the 1996 Food Quality Protection Act dictated that the Environmental Protection Agency must assess the pesticide content of foods and their safety for children. The act also made allowable levels of pesticides lower for infants and children.

Workplace exposure

Many workplace risks are related to environmental exposures. By understanding the risks in your particular occupation, you can act to lessen or eliminate possible harm, and stay healthy in your career.

A thorough assessment by an environmental or occupational health expert should help you to pinpoint hazards. These will be specific to each job, but may include exposures to corrosive substances (acids, alkalis), dusts, fibres (asbestos, fibreglass), gases, heavy metals, agricultural chemicals, plastics (di-isocyanates, phthalates), petro-chemicals, physical agents (such as noise, heat, vibration, repetitive lifting), radiation (including electromagnetic, X-rays and ultraviolet), and solvents.

When you have identified relevant exposures, ensure that you are trained to deal with them, and take all necessary safety precautions. For example, if you are a mechanic you may be exposed to fumes from exhaust, petrol, and solvents, so you should ensure that your workplace is well ventilated. Or, if you use agricultural chemicals, follow the manufacturer's instructions when mixing or applying them, and wear appropriate protective clothing.

In the office, the compounds emitted from modern building materials and furnishings create indoor air pollution. Some people feel that low-level exposure to these compounds causes sick building syndrome: headache, fatigue, inflammation, and respiratory symptoms. Low-emitting building materials, continuous ventilation and non-toxic office supplies will reduce these exposures.

HEALTHY HOUSE

Most homes contain potential environmental health hazards. Here are some ways you can minimise your exposure risks.

Choose wood preservatives of low toxicity

Use natural loft insulation, e.g. sheep's wool

Water tanks, where bacteria may breed, usually supply the bathroom taps. Only drink from direct mains-supplied taps (usually the kitchen cold water tap)

Avoid using air fresheners as these often contain chemicals that have not been adequately tested for health effects

Older houses may contain asbestos insulation. If you expose any during structural modifications, arrange specialist removal

Keep bathrooms free of mould

Wash bedding in hot water, and air mattresses regularly

Make sure your kitchen is well ventilated to prevent condensation and mould growth

If re-decorating, use low emission paint

Try to garden as naturally as possible. Collect rainwater for watering, and minimise your chemical use

If you have an old house, check that pipes are not made of lead

Noise pollution can affect the well-being of those around you. Use CD players and TVs considerately

Ensure that cookers and other gas appliances are adequately ventilated and serviced

Ensure that desk environments are comfortable and safe. Reduce screen glare, adjust seating to the correct height for good posture and avoid trailing cables

If you live with anyone with a dustmite sensitivity, replace carpets with wood floors and vacuum with a hepa-filtered vacuum cleaner

Environmental Health and Cancer Risk

Many factors in the environment are potentially carcinogenic, i.e. are capable of causing changes in body cells that can lead to cancer. Often though, the links have been difficult to study. Epidemiologists (scientists who study the causes and patterns of disease in populations) need large numbers of cases before they can untangle the issues involved. As well as environmental factors, people's diet, lifestyle and genetic susceptibility all play a role. This means that environmental factors are rarely the "cause" of cancer. Instead, they can only be described as "risk factors", i.e. things that increase the chance of a cancer forming.

Scientists continue to work on current cancer concerns. It is worth noting that research has not shown, to date, that artificial sweeteners and using mobile phones are carcinogenic. There is also no good evidence to link antiperspirant use to breast cancer.

Risk factors

Cancer is essentially a condition where cells keep dividing, out of control. Anything that affects cell division, or that damages the cells' DNA (molecular instructions), is likely to be a risk factor.

Ionising radiation, of the type given off by X-rays, cosmic radiation from the solar system and radioactive particles, is known to damage DNA. Many individual chemicals are toxic and directly interfere with cell division. Free radical compounds also increase cancer risk. These are short-lived but very destructive compounds that can damage DNA. One of the main sources of free radicals in the body is oxidation of certain types of fats. Antioxidants such as vitamin C and beta carotene "mop up" these free radicals, so a diet high in the antioxidant vitamins is especially important (*see p.36*).

Organs and susceptibility

Different parts of the body interact with the environment in different ways. The lungs are vulnerable to airborne contaminants. The link between cigarette smoke and lung caner is well established. Other breathable carcinogens include asbestos and radioactive particles (dust).

The skin is relatively impermeable to chemicals because of its protective, waterproofing layer. However, skin is exposed to sunlight, and the damaging effects of its UV rays. The risk of developing skin cancer is higher for people living or holidaying regularly in an area with strong sunlight. People with fair skin are particularly at risk, since their skin contains less melanin, the pigment that gives skin its colour and helps protect it from the sun's rays. Over-use of tanning booths may also contribute to skin cancer.

The ozone layer of the upper atmosphere filters the sun's damaging UV rays, but it has thinned over the last few decades. This may be a factor in the rise in skin cancer cases. The thinnest region – the "ozone hole" – is over the Antarctic.

Female breast tissue is naturally very responsive to certain hormones. The hormone oestrogen appears to play an important role in the development and progress of breast cancer. Oestrogen "mimics" taken either as contraceptive or HRT drugs may in long term use slightly increase the risk of breast cancer. Many pesticides and other environmental contaminants also mimic natural hormones, and so can potentially affect cell reproduction.

The digestive system is also exposed to environmental contaminants, through the food we eat. Some foods are known to be carcinogenic. These include salted, pickled and smoked foods, charred meat and meats treated with nitrites, all of which should be eaten in only small amounts or avoided altogether. A very salty diet has been linked to stomach cancer, and a diet low in fibre is thought to be a risk factor for colorectal cancer. Long-term exposure to aflatoxins, chemicals produced by a fungus that can contaminate peanuts and grains, increases the risk of developing liver cancer.

Cancer and genetics

Genes control how our cells deal with toxins and other contaminants, and how well our DNA is repaired when it does get damaged. Each of us has a unique combination of genes, which partly explains why some people get cancer when others do not, even if they have been exposed to the same environment. About 10 per cent of breast cancer cases, for example, are linked to an abnormal gene. Your doctor can advise on screening programmes if you have a relative with cancer and are concerned about genetic links.

Improving Environmental Health

If you suspect that an illness has an environmental health component, an important first step in any diagnosis is to visit an environmental health specialist. He or she will try to discover if you have been exposed to a toxin from food, water, air, building materials or cleaning supplies and then connect any exposures with your clinical symptoms.

Tests

Tests may provide evidence of certain exposures. For example, a blood test can reveal if you have been exposed to dangerous levels of lead. Blood tests can also detect exposure to elemental mercury (found in dental amalgams, thermometers, and gas meters), whereas urine samples collected over 24 hours are the best way to detect chronic or recent exposures to the other two forms of mercury, methylmercury (found in fish) and inorganic mercury (found in a variety of substances, including industrial pollutants). In many other cases, laboratory tests may be inaccurate, have technical limitations or otherwise fail to help to establish a diagnosis.

Treatment strategies

There are many possible treatment strategies for environmental health problems. In general, environmental health experts recommend decreasing exposure to toxins that may be related to health problems and encouraging the excretion or release of toxins from the body.

Decreasing exposure involves awareness of the sources of the problem, and then taking steps to minimise exposure. These might include changing the cleaning products used in the home, or eating organic food where possible.

Detoxification

Some experts recommend taking steps to improve the liver's ability to metabolise and dispose of toxins. This detoxification approach is a strategy employed by many other cultures and traditional healing systems, such as Ayurveda, Traditional Chinese Medicine and Native American medicine, where it is used as a preventive and treatment option for "periodic cleansing of the body". Liver detoxification may be improved by using liver-toning

herbs, such as milk thistle (*Silybum marianum*), or specific supplements, such as vitamin C, vitamin E, selenium, green tea and mixed carotenes. To help release toxins from the body, some experts recommend increasing fluid intake to flush certain toxins out through the kidneys. They also recommend increasing fibre intake to facilitate bowel clearance, and sweating by exercising or taking saunas. Other possibilities include bodywork, such as massage, to free toxins from the muscle tissue so that they can then be excreted; homeopathy, to increase the excretion of certain toxins; and colonic irrigation to facilitate bowel excretion of some compounds. However, although these therapies are advocated by some practitioners, they are not yet supported by research or clinical trials.

A strategy example: lead removal

People are exposed to lead in various ways (*see table, p.89*). Most of the adverse effects of lead exposure occur in babies and small children, causing reduced IQ and behavioural difficulties. In adults, low levels of lead exposure may be related to high blood pressure, slow reaction times, anaemia and hearing loss. However in many cases there are no symptoms.

Governmental and individual efforts have reduced lead exposure in recent decades. These measures have included controlling dust and paint chip residues, using cold water (not hot) from the main water supply for drinking and mixing baby formula milk, and switching to unleaded petrol to prevent lead from entering the environment.

Time outdoors

Everyone can benefit from being in and interacting with the natural environment, whether gardening, sitting in a park, taking a walk on a beach or hiking through mountains. Research has demonstrated some of these benefits, such as improved responses to stress when compared to people restricted to man-made environments. People recovering from surgery do better in hospital rooms with windows, and people are also able to concentrate better after surgery if they are engaged in a restorative nature activity, such as sitting in a park or tending plants. A close association with trees can help improve well-being. And, of course, our parks and other open spaces are common grounds that foster social interactions and contribute to our overall social well-being.

FINDING A PRACTITIONER

When looking for an environmental health expert, make sure he or she is a member of the www.bsaenm.org (www.bsaenm.org). See also p.486 for useful addresses. In Australia, contact the Australian Institute of Environmental Health (www.aieh.org.au).

MIND–BODY MEDICINE

DR KENNETH R. PELLETIER

Mind–body therapies not only improve overall health but also have a positive and measurable effect on specific conditions and diseases. Two key principles underpin the various therapies. First, the mind can affect the body in positive or harmful ways. Second, whatever you do physically also has an impact on consciousness. A great deal of research reveals that psychological and spiritual practices, such as meditation, relaxation, guided imagery and biofeedback, can have a useful impact on physical problems, including pain.

The Role of Mind–Body Medicine

Doctors are traditionally sceptical about innovation. When the stethoscope was introduced in 1916, for example, critics were concerned that the unorthodox diagnosis device might distance doctors from their patients. Integrating mind–body medicine fully with other forms of medicine remains a challenge, but of all CAM (complementary and alternative medicine) therapies, mind–body practices are supported by the greatest body of scientific evidence for the greatest number of conditions for the largest number of people. Compared to other CAM therapies, they have also gained the widest acceptance within conventional healthcare systems. In fact, mind–body medicine is so widely used by the public and by the medical profession that it may be considered to belong more to conventional than to complementary medicine.

According to the National Center for Complementary and Alternative Medicine (NCCAM) in the US, "Only a subset of mind–body interventions are considered CAM. Many that have a well-documented theoretical basis – for example, patient education and cognitive behavioural approaches are now considered mainstream." On the other hand, meditation, dance, music and art therapy, and prayer and mental healing are categorised as alternative. NCCAM states that "Many CAM therapies are called holistic, which generally means they consider the whole person, including physical, mental, emotional, and spiritual aspects."

What is mind–body medicine?

In 2001, NCCAM defined mind–body practices as those that employ "a variety of techniques designed to facilitate the mind's capacity to affect bodily function and symptoms." Generally speaking, mind–body practices, which include meditation, relaxation, guided imagery, hypnosis and biofeedback, produce a beneficial, biologically regenerative, relaxed state, in which the body is more able to heal itself and function optimally. Under the direction of a skilled clinician, these therapies can be used to treat a wide array of medical and psychological conditions. However, they can also be safely used by everyone as "self-care practices" to prevent and reverse the harmful effects of stress and to complement conventional treatments.

Generally, the extensive research into the efficacy of mind–body medicine focuses on major chronic diseases, such as general pain syndromes and insomnia (*see below*), where a combination of professional therapy and self-care practice is the most effective way of achieving the maximum improvement in health and well-being.

History of Mind–Body Medicine

Mind–body medicine is an ancient concept. Until about 300 years ago, virtually all philosophy and medicine treated the body and mind as an integral whole. Then, in the 18th century, adherents of the Enlightenment introduced a mechanistic and reductionistic scientific model that meant the study of body and mind were separated. The 18th-century paradigm reached its height in the 20th century when modern scientific medicine helped to end the epidemics of infectious diseases, such as smallpox, cholera and tuberculosis which had formerly been major causes of mortality. (It should be said, though, that these diseases had already declined due to public health measures, such as improved sanitation, safer water, improved housing and better nutrition.)

Currently, the diseases that are killing more people in the developed nations worldwide are no longer these infections, but chronic degenerative conditions, such as coronary artery disease, high blood pressure, cancer and diabetes, for which there are no chemical "magic bullets". These diseases are inextricably related to psychological, environmental and lifestyle factors. Increasingly, stress is recognised as a major causal factor in both the onset of acute diseases and in chronic diseases. Mind–body practices can give people the skills to manage the inevitable stress of life and, therefore, have an increasingly important role in preventing and reversing the effects of stress and disease.

Asian healing systems

The rise in popularity of mind–body medicine has been stimulated by the introduction of Asian healing methods and systems, such as yoga and Traditional Chinese Medicine, into mainstream Western culture. In the 1970s, Western medical researchers discovered that people who practised advanced forms of yoga, for example, were able to regulate physical functions that were once considered beyond the reach of conscious control. These include the electrical activity of the brain, the temperature of the body, the heart rate and blood pressure. Incorporating some of

THE INTRICATE MIND–BODY CONNECTION

Mind–body interactions are not rare events but common occurrences in our everyday lives. Often mediated by the activities of nerves and hormones, the effects that one has on the other indicate that they are integrated and part of the same whole. The table (*right*) lists some of these effects.

EFFECTS OF THE MIND ON THE BODY

Emotions
Emotions such as embarrassment cause physical responses such as blushing.

Stress responses
Stress and anxiety raise the levels of the hormones cortisol and adrenaline in the body. These have a variety of physical effects including:
● changes to the immune system
● increased heart rate
● slowing the digestive system.

Humour
Laughter has been shown to:
● lower blood pressure
● reduce levels of stress hormones
● boost immunity (increasing T-cells and B-cells)
● release endorphins that are natural painkillers and produce a general sense of well-being.

Imagery
We can affect the way our body behaves just by using our imagination. For example, imagine unwrapping a chocolate. Feel the paper crinkling under your fingers, smell the aroma that is released, then imagine the taste and feel of it melting on your tongue. This imagery will no doubt have activated your salivary glands!

Placebo response
Placebos (dummy treatments, such as sugar pills) can be effective in around 30 per cent of patients. In other words, believing that the treatment will work can produce positive physiological responses.

EFFECTS OF THE BODY ON THE MIND

Exercise
Exercise has a variety of effects on the brain including:
● improved blood flow to the brain
● release of endorphins, mood enhancers and painkillers similar to morphine
● alteration of serotonin levels in the brain
● increased production of a chemical called BDNF (Brain-Derived Neurotrophic Factor). This chemical helps neurons (brain cells) to grow and connect.

Massage and physical contact
Physical contact with another human (or an animal) can induce feelings of relaxation and well-being.

Massage is a recognised destressing agent.

Sex hormones
Sex hormones (testosterone and oestrogen) alter thoughts and behaviour.

Posture
Studies have established that if we stand upright, head erect, smile and breathe deeply, it is impossible to "feel" depressed.

Immune system
Immune molecules known as cytokines can initiate brain actions. Some cytokines help the body recuperate by sending messages to the brain that set off a series of sickness responses, such as fever. The immune molecules also can trigger feelings of sluggishness, sleepiness and loss of appetite – behaviours that encourage people to rest while they are ill.

Listening
Music can enhance mood and even have a painkilling effect through encouraging endorphin release.

Biological sounds, such as a mother's heartbeat, have been used to de-stress infants. Conversely, noise can increase heart rate, blood pressure, respiration rate and blood cholesterol levels.

Breathing
By controlling breathing patterns, it is possible to reduce anxiety and stress responses (*see pp. 408 and 414*).

these Asian healing systems, researchers have discovered new ways to forestall and heal diseases that have long been considered inevitable consequences of ageing.

Reclaiming wholeness

Mind–body medicine recognises that healing does not necessarily stop when all the physical symptoms of an illness or condition disappear. Healing literally means "to make whole". From this perspective, treating illness can be viewed as an opportunity to reclaim wholeness and restore completeness, even in the face of ongoing disease. However, this can occur only when the mind and body are integrated into a whole, dynamic healing system. It is not simply a question of "mind over matter", but rather that mind matters. The Asian healing systems, such as Traditional Chinese Medicine, have affirmed the power of techniques such as relaxation and meditation and made it clear that a person's inner well-being is crucial to health.

Benefits of Mind–Body Medicine

Essential to all complementary and alternative therapies, but often overlooked, is the notion that the healing process does not work independently of the individual. Rather, it relies on internal changes in an individual's consciousness and behaviour – their attitude, lifestyle, self-orientation and environmental awareness are all important. Such a holistic approach demands continuous change from an individual – he or she has to transform their psychology and actively engage in the well-being of their mind and body. Since mind–body approaches necessitate such an orientation, they constitute an integral and vital part of all complementary and alternative therapies.

From the perspective of mind–body medicine, the mind, body and spirit are interrelated, not only with each other but also with the larger social and physical environment. Physical interventions are not solely physical in their effect, but also have an impact on consciousness.

Exercise, yoga, meditation, dance, relaxation therapies, visualisation, imagery and manipulative therapies can not only resolve problems in the physical organism, but can also create an enhanced psychological and spiritual sense of well being. Psychological treatments, such as meditation, psychotherapy or imagery work, can have a demonstrable impact on physical problems, such as pain and high blood pressure, as well as their extensive psychological benefits.

Relieving stress and depression

An ever-growing body of evidence has demonstrated that psychosocial stress is an important factor in many medical conditions, ranging from coronary artery disease and chronic pain to immune problems. Within the confines of our modern environment, mental cues such as anxious thoughts, crowds, work pressures and traffic jams, are often perceived as threatening and can trigger the fight-or-flight response, even though no physical threat is involved. Moreover, psychological stressors may linger and allow the alarm response to persist far beyond its useful time. Powerful hormones released during this stress response have a specific physical impact on the body and can contribute to disease (*see Coping with Stress, p.408*).

Other negative emotions and personality traits have also been found to be associated with the risk of chronic disease. It was once thought that the "Type A" personality, which is marked by highly stressed, time-pressurised and aggressive behaviour, was a reliable predictor of mortality from coronary artery disease. Actually, "hostility" is the Type A factor that seems to be predictive of heart attacks. In 1995, Dr Murray Mittleman and other researchers at Harvard Medical School in the US reported their analysis of interviews with patients after they had had a heart attack. They reported that the likelihood of having a heart attack was 2.3 times greater within two hours of having an angry outburst than at other times.

Depression is also common in patients with coronary artery disease and is associated with a higher incidence of heart disease as well as an increased mortality rate following heart attacks. In 1996, a team of researchers led by Dr Barefoot at Duke University in the US studied mortality statistics for people who had a documented history of heart disease. They discovered that the mortality rate was 78 per cent higher in those individuals with moderate to severe depression compared to those who were not depressed. Of course, this depression could have been the result rather than the cause of the physical illness, but clearly the entanglement of mind and body influenced the outcome of the illness.

Among their other benefits, most mind–body therapies create a relaxed state which is the opposite of the arousal characteristic of the stress response. Practising meditation, relaxation techniques, imagery work, hypnosis and movement therapies, such as yoga and qi gong, can all produce a beneficial relaxed state.

Techniques from cognitive behavioural therapies (*see also Psychology Therapy, p.104*) are also employed in teaching stress management. Individuals learn to recognise stress triggers and respond to them in a different, healthier way by learning a technique called reframing, which allows them to think more positively about the stress-inducing situations they encounter. Through practising a wide variety of CBT techniques, people learn to master symptoms that had previously been overwhelming. This allows them to build up self-confidence which then spills over into other aspects of their professional and personal life and enables them to make positive lifestyle changes which go well beyond the alleviation of specific symptoms.

Self-care for good health

Eighty per cent of all medical symptoms are self-diagnosed, self-treated and self-limiting, which means they resolve without the need for formal medical care. Nevertheless, people often need help in learning how to take care of their health (self-care) in order to avoid more serious conditions. Mind–body therapies address the kind of psychosocial issues that need to change before people can successfully implement effective self-care. The therapies provide simple structured steps for individuals to take to benefit their health and well-being. Meditation, for example, helps people to relax and become more focused. Consequently, they find it easier to give up smoking, which in turn sets up an upward spiral of health improvement.

In 1993, Dr McGinnis and Dr Foege published an article in the *Journal of the American Medical Association* citing a dire yet familiar litany of mortality – in other words, the ten leading causes of death. Their contention was that this list, which included cancer, heart disease and HIV, belied a more fundamental issue. These are the terminal diseases cited in a pathologist's report or upon autopsy, but the actual causes of death include factors such as tobacco, alcohol, poor diet and inactivity patterns, stress, certain infections, drug use, deadly drug interactions from prescription medications, and so on.

Many of these "causes of death" can be avoided with better self-care practices. Mind–body therapies provide the behavioural basis for individuals to make healthy changes and so are the foundation for helpful self-care strategies, such as exercise, good nutritional habits and more appropriate use of conventional medicines.

Mind–Body Approaches

There are four main mind–body approaches in Western medicine: meditation and relaxation, guided imagery, clinical biofeedback and hypnosis. In addition, there are a number of other therapies recommended throughout the ailment section of this book. Some therapies overlap. Relaxation and stress-management techniques, in particular, are essential components of all of the therapies. Physiological benefits of relaxing include:

- Decreased levels of adrenaline, sugar and cholesterol in the blood.
- Reduced blood pressure and less stress on the cardiovascular system.
- Slower breathing with improved lung function and metabolic rate.
- Relaxed muscles, which contain less lactic acid.
- Improved digestion.
- Skin cools down with less activity from the sweat glands.

Meditation and relaxation

Meditation is a long-standing feature of various spiritual and religious traditions. In the secular context, it is a self-directed practice that quietens the mind and relaxes the body, bringing benefits for health and a sense of well-being. The heightened awareness and inner peace that meditation brings can combat stress and anxiety, relieve headaches and fatigue, and help people to cope with long-term pain.

During the 1960s, reports reached the West about yogis and practitioners of meditation in India and elsewhere who were able to achieve an extraordinary degree of

An electroencephalogram (EEG) involves fixing electrodes to the scalp and measuring brain activity. Blue is the lowest activity, then green and yellow to red, which is the highest. Delta waves on the left screen are dominant in adult sleep. Next come theta waves, typical of a young child. Alpha waves feature in relaxed adults with closed eyes. Beta waves on the right are typical when we focus on something.

control over supposedly involuntary bodily functions such as breathing, pulse rates and blood pressure. Studies by myself and my colleagues at medical research centres, including Harvard Medical School, UCLA, Menninger Foundation and the University of California School of Medicine in San Francisco, substantiated the reports of these remarkable abilities of self-regulation.

While there are major philosophical differences under-pinning the hundreds of forms of meditation, at a biological level they have very similar effects on human biochemistry and on the nervous and immune systems. The benefits that research has discovered are based mainly on studies into transcendental meditation, but they can be attributed equally to other types of meditative practice.

Transcendental meditation

One of the most prominent meditation movements in the US in the 1960s was Transcendental Meditation (TM), developed by the Maharashi Mahesh Yogi and popularised by the Beatles. This practice consists of sitting and silently repeating a mantra (a word or a sound) twice a day for 20 minutes, for the stated purpose of achieving "restful alertness" and a state of "unifying capacity".

Studies by Professor Herbert Benson (of the Mind/Body Medical Institute of Harvard Medical School in the US) and others in the late 1960s showed that TM brings about a healthy state of relaxation. An individual in this relaxed state exhibits a decreased responsiveness of the autonomic nervous system, a reduced heart and respiration rate, a decreased output of cortisol released by the adrenal glands and an increased occurrence of alpha waves, the brainwave frequency associated with a relaxed state. Eventually, Benson developed a generic relaxation method which he termed the "relaxation response" (*see box, right*).

Mindfulness meditation

Among the most commonly used and well-documented forms of meditation in clinical research is "mindfulness" meditation. The art of this Buddhist-based practice is to maintain awareness, in the present moment, of the bodily sensations and flow of thoughts but without passing judgment on them. It differs from concentrative meditation, such as TM, which maintains passive attention on a word, a bodily process (such as breathing) or other stimulus.

Guided imagery

Imagery is a flow of thoughts the embody sensory qualities. It has been used for millennia in every indigenous culture and country of the world as part of shamanic healing practices. As a mind–body therapy, it enlists an individual's imagination in evoking one or more of the senses, usually sound, vision, warmth and movement. In modern clinical settings the therapist generally guides the individual's creation of images. Individuals may also employ imagery

RELAXATION

Practise the following steps for 10–20 minutes every day (but not within two hours of eating a meal) to help ease tension and relieve stress.
- Find a comfortable position, sit quietly and close your eyes.
- Starting at your feet, relax your muscles. Work your way up your legs, torso, hands, arms, neck, face and head, relaxing the muscles as you go. Keep all the muscles relaxed.
- Inhale through your nose and focus on your breathing. As you exhale, silently say "ONE" in your mind. Continue breathing consciously but naturally for 10–20 minutes. Thoughts will try to distract you – just repeat "ONE" as you exhale and continue your breathing.
- To finish, sit quietly for a few minutes – at first with closed eyes and then with them open.

on their own without any instruction or supervision from health practitioners. Sometimes spontaneous imagery in sleep or daydreaming episodes can provide profound personal insights and can be the basis for creativity and scientific discoveries.

Imagery is often incorrectly referred to as visualisation, but it can equally entail imagining smell, touch, hearing, taste, proprioception (the unconscious perception of movement and spatial orientation) and motion.

Many mind–body therapies contain a spontaneous and/or a "guided" imagery component. Guided imagery is purely psychological and can occur with or without a physically quiet state. Biofeedback, desensitisation and aversion techniques, hypnosis, autogenic training, gestalt therapy, Jacobson's progressive relaxation, neurolinguistic programming (NLP) and rational emotive behaviour therapy (REBT) include guided imagery in their approach.

Meditation that involves focusing on a mantra, imagined sound, or object of contemplation also uses imagery, as do relaxation techniques that include sensory instructions. Imagery is also related to hypnosis in that they both elicit similar states of consciousness and have similar uses in practice. In fact, research has discovered that there is a correlation between the ability to imagine and the capacity to enter into an altered or hypnotic state.

Imagery for better health

Imagery may be used early on in a therapy session to help the practitioner with diagnosis. A person may be asked to describe his or her condition or problem in sensory terms. Often, the resulting description can provide a basis for the kinds of therapeutic treatments that are chosen and give a significant insight into the person's subjective experience of their condition. Imagery is also a powerful aid in achieving insight and perspective into a person's health and in making contact with emotions.

EXERCISES FOR IMAGERY AND AUTOSUGGESTION

Imagery can help you to relax and deal with pain or other problems by imagining positive images and desired outcomes. Here are some suggestions for images:

- Imagine your symptoms as a slowly melting block of ice.
- Picture the affected part of your body working perfectly.
- To induce serenity, try a "focused daydream". Imagine walking up a sunlit path alongside a waterfall, or picture a stormy sea that slowly quietens down as you sail into port.

Practise the following up to three times a day:

- Choose an image or desired outcome that you wish to visualise.
- Find a quiet place and either lie down or sit comfortably so that your whole body can relax and you can let your mind go.
- Inhale and exhale slowly through your nose until you relax.
- Concentrate on your chosen image for as long as you can. Focus on every detail. What can you hear? How do you feel?

You can learn to hypnotise yourself safely and effectively with the following autosuggestion technique. Make sure you are clear about the purpose of the self-hypnosis – for example, to ease your asthma, be less anxious or become more confident – and be prepared to practise it every day.

- Sit or lie in a comfortable position, close your eyes and relax your whole body.
- Count from ten to zero and imagine yourself walking down a flight of stairs or along a clearly defined woodland path.
- Repeat words that positively summarise what you want to achieve, such as "the pain is getting less". Alternatively, listen to a recording of the words.
- When you have finished, count from zero to ten as you walk up the flight of stairs or return along the path.
- Rest for a minute with your eyes closed.

One way of doing this is to use imagery in a receptive mode, in which the person has an imaginary dialogue with an image that represents his or her symptoms or illness, and the image communicates information about the meaning of sensations and symptoms.

Imagery work can also be used by therapists to put patients in touch with an "inner advisor" who helps them to achieve insight into their medical problems.

Mental rehearsal

In a technique called mental or psychological rehearsal, imagery is used to help the person prepare for medical procedures, such as invasive diagnostics or surgery. The technique can help to relieve pain and anxiety, and prevent side-effects from procedures, such as chemotherapy, which may be aggravated by intense emotional reactions. When imagery is used in this way, the patient is generally guided by a therapist into a relaxed state and then led through a series of images in which the treatment and the recovery process are described in sensory terms, along with the desired outcome.

Patients may be encouraged to create their own system of images involving the healing process, or they may be guided through a series of images to relax, divert their attention or diminish sympathetic nervous system arousal. Preparatory imagery work can help patients to experience less pain following surgery. It can encourage them to relax the muscles around the incision site as well as hasten the return of bowel function and prevent excessive blood loss by redirecting blood flow to other parts of the body. Mental rehearsal imagery also helps patients deal with anxiety-producing diagnostic procedures, such as CAT scans, which can make some people feel claustrophobic because they have to spend time inside a scanner.

Research with mental rehearsal has yielded highly positive and often dramatic results, which include: reduced pain and anxiety, shorter hospital stays, less need for medication and a reduction in the number and intensity of side-effects from treatment. Mental rehearsal is also used regularly to help prepare mothers-to-be for natural childbirth.

Clinical biofeedback

Clinical biofeedback is a training technique in which people learn to consciously regulate bodily functions, such as heart rate or blood pressure, that are not normally accessible to voluntary control. It applies to any process that measures and reports back information about the system that the individual is attempting to control, with the goal of improving or eliminating a symptom or illness.

Biofeedback dates back to the late 1930s, when Dr O. Hobart Mowrer invented an alarm that could be triggered by urine as a way to train children to stop bedwetting. In 1961, noted psychologist Dr Neal Miller from Yale University in the US explored the unorthodox hypothesis that responses of the autonomic nervous system, such as heart rate and bowel movement, could be conditioned. He conducted a series of groundbreaking experiments that demonstrated how control of autonomic processes could be learned through biofeedback techniques.

In the early 1960s, Dr Joe Kaniya of the University of California School of Medicine in San Francisco, Dr Barbara Brown at the Veterans Administration Hospital in Sepulveda, California, and Dr Elmer and Dr Alyce Green at the Menninger Foundation, Kansas, used biofeedback devices to monitor and record self-regulatory feats of yogis. It was through these remarkable experiments that biofeedback began to attract wider attention.

Measurements and devices

Most commonly, clinical biofeedback is a feature of several measurements and devices. Electrocardiographs (ECGs), for example, reveal the electrical activity of the heartbeat (*see Angina, p.249*) and echocardiographs provide ultrasound scans of the heart muscle. Electroencephalographs (EEGs) provide feedback on electrical brainwave activity and electromyographs (EMGs) monitor muscle tension via visual or auditory signals. Skin temperature gauges measure the heat generated at the surface of the skin and galvanic skin response (GSR) sensors detect the electrical conductivity of the skin which increases when the skin sweats because of stress.

In a typical biofeedback session, people are wired up to biofeedback devices and then use breathing, muscle relaxation and other techniques to help them relax. The machines transmit signals when this is achieved. In this way, people learn to relax at will and and so achieve their desired outcome, such as reducing blood pressure, relieving headaches and coping with asthma. It takes practice, but soon people can attain a slow but even heartbeat, plenty of alpha brainwaves, low-level muscle activity and a warm skin with little activity in the sweat glands.

With the development of increasingly sophisticated monitoring devices and computerised, multiple-channel instrumentation, new possibilities have been opened up for clinical biofeedback training. For example, sensors can monitor and feed back the activity of the rectal sphincter and the muscles controlling the bladder to help people who are incontinent. Oesophageal motility can be monitored to provide feedback on the muscles of the oesophagus since oesophageal spasms are very painful and can be self-regulated through hypnosis and/or clinical biofeedback. Other instruments can monitor gastrointestinal functions and stomach acidity.

Hypnosis and hypnotherapy

In the late 18th century, the practice of the power of suggestion was introduced to medicine by the French physician Dr Franz Anton Mesmer under the name of Mesmerism. He attributed the effects of hypnosis to the presence of a universal fluid that produced disease when it was out of balance in the body. After his ideas were discredited, the name was changed to hypnosis (from the Greek word *hypnos*, meaning sleep). Dr James Esdaile, an English surgeon stationed in India, performed surgery using hypnotic anaesthesia. In the late 19th century, hypnosis became popular when Sigmund Freud used it in his early psychiatric practice.

A hypnotherapist guides an individual from ordinary consciousnesses into a state of focused concentration, in which the individual is highly responsive to suggestion. Hypnotherapy, as the practice of hypnosis has come to be called, was recognised as a valid medical treatment by the British Medical Association in 1955 and by the American Medical Association in 1958.

Today, the American Society of Clinical Hypnosis (ASCH) is the main professional organisation in the US, with more than 4,000 members who must be licensed health professionals and have achieved a minimum of 20 hours of training in hypnotherapy. There are between 3,000–6,000 other practitioners of hypnotherapy, including nurses, social workers and lay therapists.

In the UK, there are about 300 qualified hypnotherapists registered with the UK Council for Psychotherapy (UKCP), with a larger number registered with other organisations, such as the General Hypnotherapy Register and the National Council for Hypnotherapy (NCH).

Benefits of hypnosis

Physiologically, the hypnotic state, which does not necessarily involve a trance, is similar to other forms of deep relaxation, with reduced sympathetic nervous system activity, decreased blood pressure, slowed heart rate and increased activity of the alpha and theta brainwaves. Compared to guided imagery, self-hypnosis is much more purely physical and can occur without the use of any imagery – guided or otherwise.

Hypnosis has come to be viewed as a way of gaining access to deep levels of the mind in order to bring about changes in behaviour or alterations in psychological states. Hypnotherapy often uses imagery to modify feelings of pain, anxiety and fear, or to introduce suggestions regarding the behaviour required to achieve therapeutic goals. Once out of the hypnotic state, the subject is expected to practise these new behaviours.

How hypnosis works

Doctors, psychotherapists, dentists and other healthcare providers use hypnotherapy to treat a wide variety of medical and psychological problems. Methods of hypnotic induction and specific suggestions and imagery are tailored to meet the needs of the individual client. It can be used as a form of analgesia in surgery, to control allergies, reduce stress and produce changes in behaviour for better health, for example it can help people to quit smoking.

Hypnotherapy can be employed either by itself or in conjunction with other forms of treatment. When used in the treatment of chronic illness, hypnosis can help to alleviate anxiety, decrease the need for medication and make medical procedures more comfortable. In 1989, one study showed that hypnosis could increase pain tolerance by 113 per cent among highly hypnotisable subjects when compared to a control group.

When employed by qualified practitioners (*see above*), hypnosis is very safe, but it is a powerful technique that must be used with caution. Consequently, individuals who have a history of serious psychiatric problems are not appropriate candidates for hypnotherapy.

Hypnotisability

Individuals vary greatly in their "hypnotisability" – their susceptibility to hypnosis. According to a 1983 World Health Organisation estimate, 90 per cent of people can be hypnotised and 20–30 per cent are susceptible enough to enter the deep state that makes them ideally responsive to hypnotic suggestion. Most people can learn to hypnotise themselves, either from a book with audio tapes or from a hypnotherapist, with a technique called autosuggestion. You may be able to use this self-hypnosis to relieve pain, boost self-confidence and ease an attack of asthma.

Experimental evidence suggests that elderly people are less susceptible to hypnosis, and hence they may not make such good candidates for hypnotherapy as younger subjects. A 1972 study tested susceptibility to hypnosis among different age groups and produced evidence that confirmed hypnotisability decreases with age. Other factors that may influence hypnotisability include a compromised autonomic nervous system, which is also characteristic of some elderly people. Many studies of hypnosis have been based on research with students and other young people, which may mean the results are inapplicable to the elderly.

Other mind–body techniques

As well as the four main approaches described above, a number of other mind–body therapies are suggested in this book. In addition, yoga, t'ai chi and other movement therapies (*see p.62*) have mind–body components and there is also an overlap between mind–body therapies and psychological techniques (*see p.104*).

Autogenic training (AT)

This is a series of six mental exercises that switch off the body's stress responses and encourage calmness in the mind and relaxation in both involuntary and voluntary muscles. The name is derived from Greek and means "generated from within". Devised by German neurologist and psychiatrist Dr Johannes Schultz in Berlin in the 1920s, AT is normally taught by a practitioner in eight weekly sessions that last for 90 minutes each. AT can help various ailments, from stress and anxiety to high blood pressure and eczema. The length of treatment does not seem to affect clinical outcome.

Gestalt therapy

In this technique, which is also used in humanistic psychotherapy (*see Psychological Therapy, p.104*), a practitioner helps the client to gain self-awareness of habitual thoughts, feelings and actions, and express any thoughts and emotions that may be repressed. The name derives from German and means "organised whole". Developed by German psychoanalyst Fritz Perls in the 1960s, gestalt therapy sessions are held weekly, either on a one-to-one basis or in groups, and may involve recalling a dream and role playing.

Eye-movement desensitisation and reprocessing (EMDR)

This information-processing therapy is a technique that integrates elements of various psychotherapies, such as cognitive behavioural therapy, psychodynamic therapy, experiential therapy and interpersonal psychotherapy (*see p.107, and Post-Traumatic Stress disorder, p.422*). EMDR was discovered by US psychologist Francine Shapiro in 1987 and has proved useful in treating traumatic disorders, such as PTSD, phobias and anxiety.

Meditation helps to bring thoughts under control and to relieve any stress you may be feeling. Regular practice can lower the breathing and heart rate, and induce a sense of calm.

During treatment, patients move their eyes from side to side while simultaneously discussing their anxieties with the therapist. The eye movement is thought to help the brain process painful thoughts. Sessions are held on a one-to-one basis and vary according to an individual's needs.

Jacobson's progressive relaxation

US physiologist Edmund Jacobson developed his relaxation method in the 1930s. It involves systematically tensing and relaxing every major muscle group in their body (*see box on Relaxation, p.99*).

Neurolinguistic programming (NLP)

Developed in the 1970s by US psychotherapists John Grinder and Richard Bandler, this technique combines cognitive behavioural therapy with elements of humanistic psychotherapy (*see Psychological Therapy, p.104*) and hypnotherapy. An NLP practitioner helps a person to consciously reprogramme their patterns of speech and body language with the aim of improving their communication skills and bringing about personal change. Sessions may be held weekly on a one-to-one basis and vary according to an individual's needs.

Psychoeducation

By using books, brochures, illustrations, videos and/or audio tapes the patient can literally be educated on the specific nature of their condition to give them a sense of greater mastery and control through better understanding. This can be an important method of providing advice and information about a person's psychological or behavioural problems. Psychoeducation benefits the person and their families so that they are better informed about the kinds of treatment that are required and better prepared for the treatment itself. The technique has proved useful for people with cancer, eating disorders, ADHD and depression.

Rational emotive behaviour therapy (REBT)

This cognitive behavioural technique aims to replace the irrational thinking behind negative emotions with more positive and flexible patterns of thought to help people to attain their goals and objectives. It was developed by US psychoanalyst Albert Ellis in 1955 and is useful for anxiety, stammering, depression and addictions. Generally, REBT sessions lasting up to an hour may take place once a week, with homework assignments designed to help patients learn skills faster.

Visualisation

More correctly known as imagery (*see Guided Imagery, p.99*), visualisation encourages people to imagine positive images and desired outcomes in order to help them change negative attitudes and overcome various ailments, such as stress, pain, anxieties and phobias, and to cope with chronic illnesses, such as cancer.

Summary of Research Evidence

Dr John A. Astin of the Complementary Medicine Program at the California Pacific Medical Center, San Francisco, has conducted one of the best designed overviews of the applications of mind–body medicine. He writes "There is now considerable evidence that an array of mind–body therapies can be used as effective adjuncts to conventional medical treatment for a number of common clinical conditions". Astin's 2002 review underscores the fact that mind–body therapies can be readily integrated into the treatment of many conditions, often combining self-care practice with clinical care.

Moderate to strong evidence

Extensive randomised controlled trials (*see p.21*) and/or systematic reviews (critical statistical analysis of previously published research) reveal that there is moderate to strong evidence of the clinical efficacy of mind–body therapies for the following 11 conditions: coronary artery disease (*see p.252*); high blood pressure (*see p.244*); insomnia (*see p.448*); general pain syndromes (*see Persistent Pain, p.144*); low back pain (*see p.268*); headaches (*see p.114*); fibromyalgia (*see p.298*); arthritis self-care (*see p.289 and p.293*); living with cancer (*see p.464*); incontinence; and recovery from surgery.

Mind–body therapies are at least as good as, if not better than, many common conventional treatments. Given their relative simplicity, low cost and absence of side-effects, the findings are particularly significant.

Positive efficacy

Most current randomised controlled trials indicate that mind–body therapies are useful for the following conditions: allergies (*see p.456*); asthma (*see p.205*); chronic obstructive pulmonary disease; dermatological disorders (*see Skin Ailments, p.156*); diabetes (*see p.314*); living with HIV (*see p.470*); irritable bowel syndrome (*see p.222*); peptic ulcers (*see p.219*); post-stroke rehabilitation (*see p.148*); pregnancy and labour (*see p.358*); and tinnitus (*see p.188*).

FINDING A PRACTITIONER

Many practitioners work in the field of mind–body medicine so before arranging a consultation make sure they are qualified and registered. Contact the relevant professional organisation for details and lists of practitioners in your area (*see Useful Addresses, p.486*). Some psychologists working within the NHS practise hypnosis – your doctor may be able to refer you. Classes for meditation and other self-help mind–body skills are widely available – check your local listings for details.

PSYCHOLOGICAL THERAPY

DR ADRIAN HEMMINGS

Psychological therapy focuses on the talking therapies, which are grouped together into five general approaches. Qualified practitioners provide a formal and professional relationship within which a person can usefully explore difficult, and often painful, emotions and experiences. These may include feelings of anxiety, depression, trauma or perhaps the loss of meaning in life. It is a process which seeks to help the person gain an increased capacity for choice, thereby becoming more autonomous and self-determined.

Psychological health

The health of the human mind (*psyche*) is much more difficult to establish than the well-being of the body. How we deal with people and the world around us says a lot about our ability to cope with the ups and downs of life, but whether it exposes the secret world of unconscious motivations is another matter.

In general, a healthy mind implies being content with yourself. For healthy people, on the whole, life has meaning and fulfilment. They have friends and family to whom they can express thoughts and emotions. They do not fear change and are always ready to learn. Amid the stresses and strains of everyday life they are able to enjoy themselves. A healthy mind is one that can deal with both positive and negative events, from getting married to a death in the family. It is normal to feel frustration as well as happiness, or anger as well as joy. It is how people deal with the stresses and the intensity of feelings that is important. This depends on an innate ability (nature) as well as the psychological responses learned during the growing up process (nurture).

Psychological problems and their causes

There are many signs of psychological problems. There may be a marked personality change or simply an inability to cope. Some people may have strange, grandiose or obsessive ideas. A prolonged period of depression and apathy, as well as marked changes in eating or sleeping patterns may also be indications of psychological problems.

Thinking or talking about suicide, extreme emotional highs and lows and the abuse of alcohol or drugs are signs of psychological difficulties, as are excessive outbursts of anger, hostility or violent behaviour.

Psychological problems have various origins, which can be placed in a number of categories. An individual's life history is an important factor in the development of psychological problems. It is when people are young that they develop their basic assumptions of others and themselves, as well as their strategies for coping with life. These strategies need continual updating – a strategy that may have been appropriate at the age of five is no longer useful at the age of 40. Sometimes people cling to outmoded and detrimental strategies that then lead to difficulties in current relationships and eventually to psychological and emotional distress.

Some people have a genetic propensity to psychological problems. This could be due to the way in which their brain is formed or because they easily produce excess stress hormones, making them more likely to be susceptible to stressful life events. Physical ill-health can affect a person's psychological well-being, too. Seriously ill people may become depressed or anxious. This in turn can affect their physical health, slowing their recovery and possibly making them more depressed – and so the cycle continues.

Situational factors can negatively influence psychological well-being – for example, living in a socially deprived area with frequent vandalism and drug abuse. Trauma, such as a car accident or physical attack, or even the witnessing of a traumatic event, can produce adverse reactions that can lead to post-traumatic stress. Loss and bereavement, while a natural part of life, can also affect people's psychological health and while all societies have rituals in place to facilitate the grieving process some people find it very difficult to come to terms with their loss.

Cultural factors can affect the person's sense of identity and belonging and can have a direct effect on individual's sense of psychological well-being. For example, people from immigrant populations encounter more psychosocial problems than those in the dominant culture.

Each category can produce psychological problems on its own, but it is usually when there are two or more factors that psychological "dis-ease" takes hold. For instance, if someone has had a very difficult early life, he or she may respond more negatively to a traumatic event than someone who has had stable, loving childhood. However, people's reactions are unpredictable. Someone with a difficult early life, for example, may have learned at an early age to cope with trauma and so manage better than the person with a stable background who has not encountered any traumatic events.

The beginnings of psychoanalysis

Many identify the birth of talking therapies as we know them with Sigmund Freud and his mentor Josef Bruer. When Bruer hypnotised a woman with symptoms that included paralysis, blackouts and an aversion to water, she revisited her childhood memories and became distressed. The experience had a profound cathartic effect, causing many of her symptoms to disappear. Such cases inspired Freud to introduce the concept of the unconscious where, he believed, the motives for our emotions, thoughts and actions lie buried. He developed psychoanalysis to allow his

THE FIVE APPROACHES OF PSYCHOLOGICAL THERAPIES

Talking therapies can broadly be grouped into five categories, depending on the approach adopted.

APPROACH	DESCRIPTION	EXAMPLES	CONDITIONS
Psychoanalytical and psychodynamic	A therapist listens to your experiences and explores links between present emotions and actions and past events, particularly those in childhood.	Jungian analytic therapy Psychodynamic therapy	Personality disorders Depression Eating disorders
Cognitive behavioural	This combines concepts and techniques from cognitive (thinking) and behaviour therapies. The therapist listens to your experiences and offers insights into your negative thoughts, beliefs and behaviours, and then encourages you to explore and practise a new way of thinking or behaving.	Cognitive-behavioural therapy (CBT) Systemic desensitisation Behavioural therapy 12-step programme for addiction	Post-traumatic stress disorder Depressive disorders Anxiety disorders and phobias Eating disorders Schizophrenia Addiction Chronic fatigue
Systemic	A systemic therapist explores relationships by treating them as systems,. For example, in a family system one person's behaviour provokes reactions in others. Systemic approaches are most often used with couples and families or other groups, but can be used by individuals.	Family therapy	Eating disorders in adolescents (involving a whole family)
Humanistic	Counsellors often use a humanistic approach. By exploring and understanding your experiences in an accepting and non-judgmental atmosphere the therapist can help to increase your awareness of your problems and your potential for finding solutions.	Client-centred therapy (a form of counselling, though counsellors can use many different approaches)	Help adjusting to life events, illnesses, disabilities or losses
Interpersonal	In-depth exploration of how people relate to others, and ways of changing the pattern of those relationships.	Interpersonal group therapy	Relationship difficulties Depressive disorders Eating disorders Addiction

patients to talk freely so they could reveal their buried motives and be released from their psychological crisis. One of his pupils, Carl Jung, believed that people share a collective unconscious and that individuals had a "shadow" side, which they repressed. He evolved his own version of psychoanalysis to help individuals integrate this shadow side into their lives and so find their true self.

The five approaches

Since the time of Freud and Jung, the talking therapies have developed considerably. Around 400 recognisable types can be grouped into five approaches that differ mainly in their emphasis rather than in fundamental assumptions.

Psychoanalytic and psychodynamic approach
These therapies originate in the ideas of Freud and include Jungian analytic therapy and psychodynamic therapy, which is used for depression, post-traumatic stress disorder and eating disorders. The therapist listens to the person's account of their experiences and explores the connections between what the person is thinking, doing and feeling in

their present life and their past experiences, particularly in childhood. Thoughts, emotions and feelings that were repressed earlier in life emerge into consciousness and may cause problems, such as conflicts, anguish or anxiety.

Analysing the person's dreams, creative experiences and relationships with others is crucial. The key to the process of psychoanalysis is "transference", by which the person transfers their feelings on to the therapist as a means of exposing, identifying and resolving them.

This approach often takes a long time (several sessions a week for one to seven years). However, adapted techniques can shorten this to about 10 weeks when there is a specific problem such as a bereavement. Psychoanalysis can be carried out individually or in groups.

Cognitive behavioural approach
Clinical psychologists developed this approach in the 1960s by combining features from behavioural and cognitive therapy. Behaviour therapy, which is based on the work of Ivan Pavlov and B. F. Skinner, uses reward and punishment as a way of "reconditioning" behaviour. Cognitive therapy, developed by psychotherapist Aaron T. Beck, relies on the

power of a person's mind to identify and transform their negative mental processes (cognition) into more positive powers of self-perception.

Cognitive behavioural therapies (CBTs) focus on the "how" rather than the "why" of problems. At first, the therapist helps people become more aware of problematic thoughts and habits, and then initiates a plan whereby the person is encouraged to think of new ways of behaving and to records the thoughts and feelings inspired by them.

CBTs can prove particularly useful for depression and anxiety. Individual therapies include gradual exposure therapy for phobias and obsessive–compulsive disorder (OCD); systematic desensitisation for phobias; behavioural therapy for insomnia; ritual prevention for OCD; and brief therapy for depression. CBTs for post-traumatic stress disorder include anxiety management, stress inoculation therapy, systematic desensitisation and eye movement desensitisation and reprocessing (*see p.424*).

Systemic approach

In the 1940s systems theory was developed to explain the way phenomena were organised, by focusing on the arrangement and relationship of the parts as they belonged to the whole. Systemic psychological therapies developed when systems theory was considered in tandem with the feedback mechanisms of cybernetics and the family studies of social anthropology. The systemic approach focuses on a human system, such as a family, team or community, in which people live or work together. The family therapist examines how members of a family relate to and communicate with each other, and how the family as a whole maintains itself and what, for them, constitutes "normality". If, for instance, a family member behaves uncharacteristically, the other members are likely to change their behaviour in order to keep things as "normal" as possible (known as maintaining homeostasis). Therapists may then actively help the family resolve their problems. Systemic approaches are usually short term and carried out with groups, such as families or couples, but they can also be used as a way of understanding an individual.

Experiential or humanistic approaches

These approaches from the 1950s and 1960s are rooted in the work of Abraham Maslow and others, and in the philosophies of humanism, existentialism and phenomenology. Humanists believe moral values come from human nature and experience. Existentialists believe that, because of our desire to be rational in an irrational universe, the individual defines everything in his or her own world. Phenomenologists believe in the primacy of perception and consider that the human mind needs to re-learn the way it engages with immediate experience.

These approaches include gestalt therapy, client-centred therapy, person-centred psychosynthesis, transactional analysis, psychodrama, primal therapy and re-birthing.

Their emphasis is on the experience of the person living in an environment that is often hostile and dehumanising. The therapist encourages the person to become more aware of their immediate experience and to notice how they have adapted to their environment. They may then be facilitated to risk becoming more authentic and "real". Experiental and humanistic therapies are carried out with individuals, couples and groups.

Interpersonal approach (ITP)

ITP was developed in the 1980s by Gerald Kerman and Myrna Weissman from the ideas of Harry Sullivan, as a way of treating depression. The approaches have been adapted for use with various problems, such as bulimia and substance abuse. ITP is highly structured and focuses on the problems that arise between people in a work, social, family or marital environment. The therapist encourages people to examine how they relate to others and to look at ways of changing their "relational style". It involves identifying why breakdowns in communication and unreasonable expectations take place. ITP is short term: individuals attend 12–16 sessions that last an hour and take place weekly.

Do psychological therapies work?

Talking therapies can help people to cope better with depression, anxieties, eating disorders, relationship problems, substance abuse and behavioural dependency, psychotic illness, sexual dysfunction, sexual abuse, bereavement, IBS, asthma, chronic pain and long-term illnesses such as cancer and HIV. Thousands of research studies support the use of talking therapies. Meta-analyses (statistical overviews of independent studies) have shown that people who have participated in a talking therapy are 80 per cent more likely to recover than those who did not participate. Some studies have compared the effectiveness of different pyschological approaches but not enough research has been done in this area. When reading about diseases in this book, bear in mind that where one particular talking therapy is suggested as effective for an ailment, it may simply mean that others have not yet been researched for that condition.

FINDING A PRACTITIONER

Membership of a recognised organisation and a list of qualifications may not be a guarantee of good practice, but it does provide some safeguards. Check if a therapist is an accredited member of an organisation such as the British Association of Counselling and Psychotherapy (*see p.486*). At the first session, ask the therapist to explain about confidentiality, payment, and how many sessions you are likely to need.

Diseases &

Disorders

GENERAL ADVICE & PRECAUTIONS

The 110 conditions that appear in this book have been selected because they respond best to an integrated, holistic approach to treatment that combines complementary therapies with conventional medical practice. The objective of the book is to provide readers with an overview of each condition – what it is, why it occurs, who is most likely to be affected – and a unique summary of the best treatments for these conditions. The text for each treatment has been written by a leading practitioner in the field (*see Contributors, p.5*). The juxtaposition of these varied approaches demonstrate how, in many cases, complementary and conventional medicine can work in tandem to alleviate symptoms, improve well-being and, in some cases, provide a cure.

Essential Components

Information is organised for each condition in a standard way. Each ailment has a number of essential components. These include lists, boxes and bulleted compilations of practical advice to which you can turn for help or immediate relief.

Symptoms, factors and triggers The symptoms of a condition, and the reasons it may have arisen, are listed on the left-hand side of each opening page. Predisposing factors make the condition more likely. Triggers are known to cause the condition.

Caution boxes warn you of side-effects, alert you to potential interactions between treatments, provide advice on when some treatments are not appropriate and tell when you should consult a practitioner.

WHAT ARE THE SYMPTOMS?

Symptoms usually begin 1–3 weeks following infection and may include:
- A mild fever, headache or flu-like symptoms
- Rash that appears as crops of small red spots. The spots become itchy and fluid-filled, then dry out and form scabs
- Discomfort in the mouth if spots develop there
- Possible complications include bacterial infections of the rash

WHY MIGHT MY CHILD HAVE THIS?

PREDISPOSING FACTOR
- Weakened immune system

TREATMENT PLAN

PRIMARY TREATMENTS
- Fluids, paracetamol, etc. (*see Helping your child*)
- Antiviral drugs (in some cases, e.g. when immunity is compromised by other illnesses or drugs)

BACK-UP TREATMENTS
- Antibiotics (if a secondary infection occurs)
- Nutritional therapy
- *Rhus toxicodendron* and other homeopathic medicines

For an explanation of how treatments are rated, see p.111.

CHICKENPOX

Chickenpox, also known as varicella, is a contagious viral illness that is common in children. It is caused by the varicella zoster virus and results in a characteristic rash of fluid-filled spots which are usually widespread over the body. Chickenpox is usually mild in children, but symptoms tend to be more severe in young babies, adolescents and adults. The main aim of treatment is to fight the virus and to enhance the function of the immune system.

WHY DOES IT OCCUR?

The varicella zoster virus, which causes chickenpox, is transmitted through air-borne droplets contained in the coughs and sneezes of infected people. It can also be transmitted by direct contact with the rash of spots and blisters.

Once the rash appears, the tiny red spots quickly turn into itchy, fluid-filled blisters These dry out within 24 hours and form scabs. Several crops of spots can appear.

Someone with chickenpox is infectious from about two days before the rash appears until the last spots have formed scabs, usually 10–14 days after the onset of the rash.

COMPLICATIONS Bacterial infection of the blisters caused by scratching the sometimes unbearably itchy rash is the most common complication of chickenpox. Newborn babies and people with weakened immune systems (such as those who are undergoing chemotherapy) are more likely to have a more serious chickenpox infection and may also develop other complications, such as pneumonia.

THE RELATIONSHIP OF CHICKENPOX WITH SHINGLES People who have had chickenpox are then immune to the disease and cannot catch it again. However, the virus remains dormant in nerve cells and may be reactivated later in life, causing shingles (*see p.165*). People who have not had chickenpox can catch it from someone with shingles, but only via direct contact with the shingles rash and not via coughs and sneezes. However, it is not possible to develop shingles without having first had chickenpox, even if it was only a very mild episode a long time ago.

The chickenpox rash first affects the skin on the body, then spreads to the face and limbs. The spots become itchy, fluid-filled blisters that dry out and then form scabs.

HELPING YOUR CHILD

PRIMARY TREATMENT For a child with a mild infection who does not need to see a doctor, try the following measures:
- Let him rest.
- Help to reduce the fever by stroking his skin with a cool flannel.
- Encourage him to drink plenty of cool fluids to prevent dehydration. Thirst is

IMPORTANT

Pregnant women who develop chickenpox, or who are exposed to the infection and think they may never have had the infection, should see their doctor.

often absent and dehydration is a real danger, especially for babies. Offering lots of small sips is usually best, especially when nausea is a problem. A plastic medicine dropper that holds a few fluid ounces is useful.
- Follow your child's cues about whether to bundle up or throw off the covers: fevers can go up and down.
- Don't force food on a child with a fever. Offer tasty, favourite foods, but avoid giving too much sugar, which may slow immune responses.
- To relieve the discomfort of chickenpox, give liquid paracetamol to children over three months (but do not use aspirin as there is a risk of Reye's syndrome).
- A bath with plenty of warm water that contains either a handful of bicarbonate of soda or two cups of powdered oat-meal can be soothing.
- Use cotton wool to gently dab calamine lotion on to the spots to relieve the itching. Alternatively, you can apply a gel of chickweed (*Stellaria media*) and/or a paste made from slippery elm (*Ulmus rubra*) powder, baking soda and water to the spots.
- Keep your child's fingernails short and try to prevent him from scratching the spots and blisters, which could lead to skin infections. Babies may need to wear mittens to stop the scratching.

TREATMENTS IN DETAIL

Conventional Medicine

If your child is otherwise healthy, the infection is likely to be mild and will not need treatment. The child will normally recover fully between 10 and 14 days after the onset of the first crop of the chickenpox rash. Simply focus on relieving the itching and preventing your child from scratching the blisters (*see Helping your child*). Permanent scars may result from blisters that have been scratched and become infected.

PRIMARY TREATMENT Babies or individuals with reduced immunity, such as those who are undergoing chemotherapy or who are HIV positive, should see a doctor at once regarding possible treatment with antiviral drugs.

Chickenpox does not usually require any treatment, although antiviral drugs, such

as aciclovir, may be considered for adults. Antiviral drugs may limit the effects of the varicella infection but they need to be administered in the early stages of the disease if they are to be of help.

Antibiotics are needed if a secondary bacterial infection of the rash occurs.

IMMUNISATION A vaccination against varicella has been developed. However, it is not recommended for immunising healthy children in the UK. The health services in some other countries, such as the US and Australia, have introduced a programme of varicella immunisation as a routine measure for children who are aged between 12 and 18 months.

CAUTION
Antiviral drugs have potential side-effects: ask your doctor to explain these to you.

Nutritional Therapy

PRIMARY TREATMENT **VITAMIN C SUPPLEMENTS** Although no conclusive clinical trials have been performed, vitamin C supplements may be able to boost the immune system of children with chickenpox. They may help to fight the infection, encourage healing and speed recovery. The recommended dose is 500–1,000mg of vitamin C supplements per day, divided into three or four doses.

VITAMIN A SUPPLEMENTS Studies show that the chickenpox infection causes a lowering of vitamin A levels in children. Consequently, giving 3,000–5,000 IU of vitamin A every day for 10 days from the start of infection seems to help children with chickenpox.

If they are given at the very start of the chickenpox infection, vitamin A supplements may be effective in shortening the duration of the illness. Moreover, the supplements may also help to protect against complications, such as pneumonia, conjunctivitis and gastroenteritis.

CAUTION
Consult your doctor before giving vitamin C with antibiotics (*see p.46*).

Homeopathy

Chickenpox is usually a mild disease in young children, settling without complications. However, it can be a severe illness in people with a suppressed immune system (which occurs, for example, as a side-effect of certain drugs).

RHUS TOXICODENDRON The classical homeopathic treatment for chickenpox is *Rhus tox.* This medicine is frequently helpful, particularly if the rash is very itchy and is accompanied by small blisters. Give your child two pills of the 6C strength, 4 times a day until the rash heals (*see p.77*).

> Chickenpox during pregnancy, especially the second half, can endanger the baby

OTHER MEDICINES *Belladonna* or *Aconite* are two homeopathic medicines that may help in the early stages of the infection, where there is fever and the child is generally unwell. *Aconite* is likely to help if the child feels both chilly and frightened. *Belladonna* is appropriate if the child feels hot and flushed.

Pulsatilla may help with children who are miserable, clingy and tearful with the illness. They may have a fever, but strangely are not thirsty. *Antimonium tartaricum* has a reputation for helping when the skin rash is slow to settle.

PREVENTION PLAN

The following may help to prevent your child from catching chickenpox:
- Avoid people infected with either chickenpox or shingles.
- Give a daily multivitamin and mineral supplement, as well as a diet rich in fruit and vegetables.
- An immunisation against varicella.

Treatment Plan lists treatments in order of priority, helping you to make more informed choices. Primary treatments should be the first line of treatment in all cases. For an explanation of ratings, see p.111.

Important boxes highlight safety information regarding a condition, including special situations when it is essential that you see your doctor or go to hospital.

Prevention Plan appears at the end of ailments for which preventive measures may be effective. It lists simple things you can do yourself to help prevent a condition.

General Precautions

- Always consult your doctor for a diagnosis – do not try to diagnose an illness or condition yourself.
- See a doctor immediately if you have any of the red flag symptoms listed below.
- See your doctor if there is no improvement in a condition within two weeks (48 hours for children under five years old).
- Do not stop taking prescribed medicine without consulting your doctor first.
- Tell your doctor about any complementary therapies you are using, and tell a complementary practitioner about any conventional treatment you are receiving.
- If you have a diagnosed medical condition, check with your doctor before using any complementary treatments.
- If you do not exercise regularly, check with your doctor before starting a new exercise programme. This is especially important if you have heart disease, back pain or you are pregnant.
- If you pregnant, breast-feeding or trying to conceive, do not take any over-the-counter medicines or any herbal medicines without consulting your doctor.

Specific Precautions

Conventional Medicine
- Tell your doctor (or pharmacist if you are buying over-the-counter medicines) of all the other medicines and complementary remedies you are taking.
- Only take medicines that are prescribed for you and complete the full course.
- Seek medical help if you develop unexpected side-effects.
- Do not keep medicines beyond their expiry dates.

Nutritional Therapy
- Do not take more than the recommended dose. Excessive doses of vitamins and minerals may have toxic side-effects.
- Some nutritional supplements interact with conventional drugs See p.46 before taking a nutritional supplement.
- Check with a doctor before taking high-dose nutritional supplements of any kind.
- Check with your doctor before giving supplements to children under 12.
- During pregnancy, limit your intake of supplements that contain vitamin A. If you are in doubt, consult with your doctor.

Western and Chinese Herbal Medicine
- See p.69 before taking a herb. Some interact with drugs and supplements.
- Do not take herbal medicines along with conventional medicines (whether they are prescribed or bought over the counter) without first consulting your doctor or a qualified medical herbalist.
- Do not give herbal remedies to children under 12 years of age without consulting a qualified herbalist.
- Do not take herbs during pregnancy, while breast-feeding or while trying to conceive without the advice of your doctor or a qualified medical herbalist.
- Seek medical advice before taking herbal medicines if you have ever had hepatitis or another liver disease.
- Always seek professional advice if you do not recover as soon as expected when taking a herbal remedy.

Bodywork Therapies and Massage
- Inform your practitioner of your medical condition. This is especially important if you are pregnant or have osteoporosis, a fracture, cancer, or circulatory problems.

Acupuncture
- Ensure your practitioner is qualified and uses disposable needles.
- Tell your practitioner if you are pregnant or if you have hepatitis B or C or HIV/AIDs.

Mind–Body Therapies
- If you have severe depression, psychosis or epilepsy, you may be disturbed by hypnosis or hypnotherapy. Ask your doctor or psychiatrist before using these therapies.

How Treatments are Rated

Throughout this section, treatments are divided into three categories to help readers decide on their treatment path. Primary treatments are those that a reader should definitely try first. In many cases there is good scientific evidence from randomised controlled trials and meta-analyses (*see* p.480) to support their use. In all cases they are recommended by the authors of this book, who are doctors and complementary practitioners with extensive knowledge of treatments for these conditions.

Back-up treatments have some positive evidence to support their use. Treatments in the third category are worth considering because they have a history of traditional use or there is some practitioner experience to suggest they may work.

This is an evidence-based book and the authors have cited references for all the treatments described. The scientific evidence for the primary treatments is listed on p.494. All the other references for treatments are listed on the Dorling Kindersley website. Go to www.dk.com/newmedicine.

RED FLAG SYMPTOMS

You should see a doctor immediately if you experience any of the following symptoms:

- Chest pain or shortness of breath. If you have pain in the chest, arms, jaw or throat, call an ambulance.
- Unexplained dizziness
- Persistent hoarseness, cough, sore throat
- Difficulty swallowing
- Persistent abdominal pain or indigestion
- Coughing up blood
- Persistent weight loss or fatigue
- A mole that has changed shape, size or colour, or itches or bleeds
- Change in bowel or bladder habits
- Passing blood in the stools or urine

- Vaginal bleeding between periods, after sex or following the menopause, or any unusual vaginal discharge
- Thickening or lump in a breast; discharge or bleeding from a nipple; change in shape or size of a breast
- Swelling or lump in a testicle; change in shape or size of a testicle; total and persistent failure to get an erection
- Severe headaches; persistent one-sided headaches; visual disturbance
- A sore that does not heal, or unexplained swellings under the skin
- Frequent and persistent back pain
- Unexplained leg pain and swelling

Brain & Nervous System

The mysterious brain and the nerves that network through the body co-ordinate the way we think, feel and sense. Integrated medicine treats the whole person – body and mind. Nutritional and herbal medicines support the nervous system and drugs and complementary therapies work well in tandem for disorders ranging from stroke to migraine.

HEADACHES

Most people have at least one headache every year, making this a very common complaint. The majority of headaches last only a few hours, but some can last for days or even weeks. They have a variety of causes, most of which are not serious. As well as painkillers for immediate relief, treatment might involve other drugs, adopting a regular eating pattern and making other dietary changes. Depending on the cause, postural rehabilitation, manipulation techniques, dental treatment, biofeedback training and relaxation therapy could also be appropriate.

WHAT ARE THE SYMPTOMS?

- Pain that may involve the entire head or only one area, such as the temples or the area above the eyes

WHY MIGHT I HAVE THIS?

PREDISPOSING FACTORS

- Tense neck muscles
- Depression
- Food sensitivities
- Low magnesium levels
- Prolonged use of painkillers
- Noisy, stuffy environment
- Poor posture
- Trigger points and joint restrictions
- Polluted environments

TRIGGERS

- Stress
- Caffeine withdrawal
- Too much caffeine
- Low blood-sugar levels
- Dehydration

WHY DOES IT OCCUR?

TENSION A variety of factors may cause headaches, but the majority are brought on by tension in the neck or scalp muscles. The trapezius muscle, which runs from the middle of the back to the shoulders and base of the neck, is one of the strongest and most responsive muscles in the body. When it contracts, it causes the muscles of the neck to contract as well, and the resulting "pull" or tension at the base of the skull generates a tension headache, along with constriction of other muscles of the head and face. Recurrent tension headaches often affect people with depression or those under prolonged stress. Noise and stuffy rooms make tension headaches worse.

OTHER CAUSES There may be various other triggers for headaches. Low blood-sugar levels, mild dehydration, food sensitivities, too much caffeine and low levels of magnesium in the diet are thought by many nutritional experts to contribute to headaches. Headaches may also result from stuffy environments or from prolonged use of strong painkillers. Caffeine withdrawal can be another cause.

Poor posture, trigger points (sensitive areas in muscles), joint restrictions in the neck and upper back and stress can contribute to headaches. Similarly, problems with the temporomandibular joint that connects the jaw to the skull, as well as dental problems or whiplash injuries, can also result in headaches (*see p.280*).

Headaches may occasionally have a serious cause, such as temporal arteritis (*see right*), meningitis or subarachnoid haemorrhage, in which the pain is usually felt at the back of the head.

IMPORTANT

If you have an unusual, severe, one-sided or persistent headache, see a doctor. This is very important if the headache is accompanied by scalp tenderness, a stiff neck, nausea, fever, sensitivity to light, a rash that does not fade when pressed or drowsiness.

TREATMENT PLAN

PRIMARY TREATMENTS

- Rest, painkillers and other self-help measures (*see Immediate Relief, right*)
- Blood-sugar stabilising diet
- Food elimination diet
- Increased water intake
- Avoid caffeine
- Magnesium supplements
- Relaxation training and biofeedback

BACK-UP TREATMENTS

- Fish oil supplements
- Homeopathy
- Western and Chinese herbalism
- Alexander technique (if poor posture is a factor)
- Environmental health measures
- Chiropractic and osteopathy
- Acupuncture
- Mind–body therapies

For an explanation of how treatments are rated, see p.111.

CLUSTER HEADACHES A cluster headache is similar to a migraine in that it often affects one side of the head only and the pain is usually severe. However, cluster headaches last for only an hour or so, and attacks tend to come in groups, with headache-free periods in between.

TEMPORAL ARTERITIS A headache and tenderness over the scalp or temple may occur as a result of temporal arteritis, a serious condition that particularly affects older people and is caused by inflammation of blood vessels in the head. The cause is unknown. Temporal arteritis requires immediate treatment with corticosteroids because it can cause sudden blindness.

IMMEDIATE RELIEF

PRIMARY TREATMENT The following measures can help to relieve a headache:
- Take a painkiller such as ibuprofen or paracetamol and drink plenty of water.
- Splash your face with cold water and lie down for 30 minutes. Applying an ice pack to the back of the neck may help.
- Practise deep breathing and try to rest.
- With your fingertips, massage around the neck, the base of the skull and over the scalp, focusing on any particular areas of tenderness.

TREATMENTS IN DETAIL

Conventional Medicine

PRIMARY TREATMENT The doctor may arrange investigations, such as an MRI scan, to exclude an underlying cause for headaches. However, in most cases no tests will be needed. He or she may recommend ways of dealing with underlying stress and may prescribe painkillers such as paracetamol or ibuprofen. These strategies are largely based on clinical experience. In some cases it may be helpful to stop taking painkillers because overuse of these drugs can contribute to persistent headaches. Antidepressants may be helpful; their use for headache is supported by clinical trials.

CAUTION

Drugs for headaches can cause a range of possible side-effects: ask your doctor to explain these to you.

Nutritional Therapy

PRIMARY TREATMENT **BLOOD-SUGAR STABILISING DIET** One factor that can be common in non-migrainous headaches is low blood-sugar levels. People who are prone to headaches when they skip a meal are most at risk of this condition. Taking steps to stabilise blood-sugar levels and reduce the effects of stress are often very effective in combating headaches associated with low blood-sugar levels (*for more details, see p.42*).

PRIMARY TREATMENT **FOOD ELIMINATION DIET** Food sensitivity is a common cause of migraine headaches. The foods most commonly reported as headache triggers in one study were alcoholic drinks, chocolate and cheese. Citrus fruits and citrus juices can also trigger migraines in some people. (*For more information about food sensitivity, see p.39.*)

PRIMARY TREATMENT **INCREASE WATER INTAKE** A common and often overlooked cause of headaches is dehydration. The tissues that surround the brain are mostly composed of water. When these tissues lose fluid, they shrink, and this can give rise to pain and irritation. Low levels of fluid in the body may also encourage the accumulation of toxins, which have been implicated in headaches. Many people find that just drinking about two litres of water a day can lead to a substantial reduction in the frequency and/or severity of their headaches.

PRIMARY TREATMENT **AVOID CAFFEINE** People who regularly drink coffee, tea or other caffeinated drink normally find that stopping caffeine can lead to a headache for a day or two, after which headaches are very much reduced or stop altogether. For the best results, you should eliminate all forms of caffeine-containing foodstuffs from your diet, including coffee, tea, chocolate, cocoa and caffeinated soft drinks. Naturally caffeine-free beverages, such as herb and fruit teas and coffee substitutes based on barley or chicory, make good alternatives to caffeinated drinks.

PRIMARY TREATMENT **MAGNESIUM SUPPLEMENTS** There is some evidence that magnesium deficiency may play a part in the development of headaches. Clinical experience supports the advice to people with chronic headaches to take 200mg of magnesium once or twice a day.

FISH OILS Taking fish oils at a dose of approximately 800mg EPA and 500mg DHA per day may help both to prevent and treat headaches. A study showed that teenagers who took fish-oil supplements for two months had an 83 per cent reduction in the number of headaches they experienced. Those who did have headaches found that did they were 74 per cent shorter in duration.

CAUTION

Consult your doctor before taking magnesium and fish oils because they can interfere with other medication (*for more information, see p.46*).

The majority of people who experience recurrent cluster headaches are male

Homeopathy

Homeopathic treatment of headaches is controversial, and some clinical trials have been negative. However, a non-clinical study into the effects of homeopathic treatment of headache by Gennaro Muscari-Tomaioli and colleagues in Italy showed that 60 per cent of patients receiving homeopathic treatment for headaches were much improved after about five months. It is difficult to generalise about homeopathic treatment of headaches and which remedy is best because it very much depends on the individual. For best results always visit a reliable practitioner rather than try to self-treat.

NATRUM MURIATICUM, a remedy made from salt, is probably the most commonly used homeopathic medicine for chronic headaches, although many others may be appropriate. It is usually prescribed on "constitutional" grounds (treating the person, not the disease, *see p.73*), for people who are conscientious and controlled. They may be quite depressed, but hide it well, and do not like to discuss their own feelings, although they may be very sympathetic to the problems of others. They may also crave salty, savoury food. If it is indicated, take two 30C pills of *Natrum mur.* once or twice a week.

NUX VOMICA, which is derived from the southeast Asian poison-nut tree, is a homeopathic remedy that is used to treat "sick headaches". It is therefore suitable for treating headaches that are accompanied by feelings of nausea or by actual vomiting. These headaches are normally at their worst first thing in the morning and may be triggered by overindulgence in food or alcohol the night before.

Western Herbalism

Calming herbs, such as chamomile (*Matricaria recutita*), valerian (*Valeriana officinalis*), lavender (*Lavandula officinalis*) and lemon balm (*Melissa officinalis*), help to reduce the stress that contributes to tension headaches. Applying diluted essential oils of rosemary (*Rosemarinus officinalis*), lavender or mint (*Mentha spp.*) to the temples when a headache threatens can be very helpful. Follow this by sipping a cup of chamomile or lemon balm tea.

> **CAUTION**
>
> See p.69 before taking a herbal remedy.

Chinese Herbal Medicine

In Traditional Chinese Medicine, headaches are treated according to the individual's pattern of symptoms. Headaches in this medical system are viewed as a sign of imbalances in *Qi* (energy), deficiencies of

some kind, or caused by disruptive influences on the patient's health. One common type that particularly affects women is a "blood-deficient" headache, which is treated with the Four Substances decoction. This remedy also treats another type: the "blood stasis" headache, which is marked by chronic unremitting episodes and may be associated with injury to the head. There are many other types of headache and a diagnosis by a qualified practitioner is essential.

> **CAUTION**
>
> Self-medication with Chinese herbal medicine is inadvisable for headaches. Consult a qualified Chinese herbalist.

Environmental Health

It is thought that environmental chemicals may injure the nervous system, resulting in symptoms such as headaches. For example, some claim that the myriad symptoms

---

TRIGGER POINTS AND HEADACHE

Tension headaches may be partly due to areas of sensitised tissue in the muscles of the jaw, neck and shoulders, known as trigger points (*see p.55*). These sensitive areas often develop from habitual tightening of the muscles when a person is under stress. Trigger points may be responsible for causing pain not only at the site where they have developed, but also in tissue some distance away ("referred pain"). It is possible to release the trigger points (*see Osteopathy and Chiropractic, p.118*). This, together with regular relaxation exercises, can help to reduce both the duration and frequency of tension headaches.

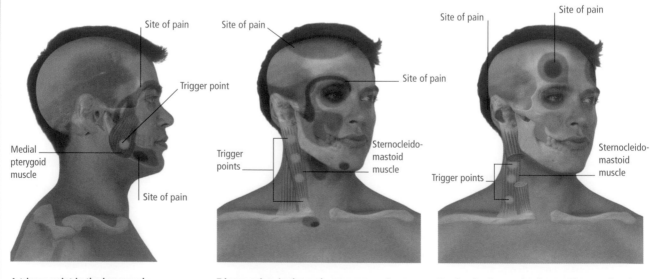

A trigger point in the jaw muscle can cause pain in both the jaw and above the eye.

Trigger points in the neck may cause pain at the back of the head and around the eyes.

Forehead pain may be due to trigger points in the sternocleidomastoid muscle.

(including headaches) in Gulf War syndrome may represent injury to the nervous system. There are many possible causes for this, including exposure to chemical warfare agents, pesticides, extremes of heat and cold, dust and smoke from oil-well fires. However, other studies have found no association between such exposures or combat experience in the Persian Gulf and resulting symptoms.

EVERYDAY HAZARDS Loud noises, strong light and altitude changes can give some people headaches. The weather can also be a culprit: some people may experience a worsening of their headaches during thunderstorms or humid conditions, a phenomenon that has been borne out in scientific studies. Other individuals may develop symptoms from the use of hand-held mobile phones, with symptoms worsening with longer use.

SPECIFIC POLLUTANTS Sometimes acute contamination with a single chemical can be the cause of a cluster of headache cases.

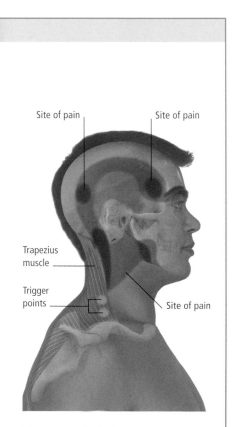

Site of pain

Site of pain

Trapezius muscle

Trigger points

Site of pain

Trigger points in the trapezius muscle may cause pain in both the neck and temple.

In one community, for example, well-water contamination with trichloroethylene may have contributed to the development of moderate to severe headaches in the people using water from the well.

Similarly, there was a case in 1993, when affected individuals complained of various symptoms, including headaches, following an accidental spraying of paraquat over a residential community.

Headaches may be distressing, but they only rarely have a dangerous cause

LEAD AND PETROL High blood-lead levels, such as those found in people living close to and downwind from lead smelters, are related to increased incidence of headaches. Headaches may also arise from exposure to petrol fumes and other environmental toxic substances (such as benzene, sulphur dioxide and photoionisable dust) in the air at petrol stations. Exposure to these substances is a particular problem for workers at these sites.

MERCURY Leaching of mercury from dental amalgam fillings is often mentioned as a cause for a variety of health problems, including headaches, but this claim is doubted by many researchers. Part of the problem is that some forms of mercury-level testing, such as hair analysis and certain urine tests, are not reliable. Also, there does not appear to be evidence for the efficacy of chelation therapy (a technique for washing mercury out of body tissues) or dental amalgam removal in ridding the body of chronic, low-dose mercury. However, most mercury toxicity arises as a result of occupational exposure (mining, ore smelting and in dental clinics) or from eating tainted fish.

The best advice is to avoid suspect fish, especially shark and swordfish, and occupational exposures. You can see an environmental health expert for assistance in reviewing possible mercury exposures in your work and home, and for advice about appropriate screening tests.

SICK BUILDING SYNDROME It is thought that a group of symptoms, including

headaches, fatigue, inflammation and respiratory symptoms, could be the result of low-level exposure to compounds such as chemicals in new carpets in inadequately ventilated buildings .

Also, carbon monoxide, a by-product of combustion of fossil fuels, can build up in poorly ventilated rooms near cars, furnaces, air-conditioning systems and gas stoves. Carbon monoxide can be very dangerous because it is odourless and is therefore not easily detected. It can build up to the point where it can cause symptoms that are much more severe than headaches, including serious central nervous system toxicity and, eventually, death. You can reduce your exposure to these by using low-emitting building materials, continuous ventilation, non-toxic office supplies and by carefully storing all chemicals.

AVOIDING FOOD ADDITIVES Monosodium glutamate (MSG), a flavour-enhancing substance often found in Chinese food, crisps and many types of processed foods and seasonings, is known to cause headaches in some people. Also, in some people headaches may be caused by sodium nitrate or sodium nitrite, which are ingredients used to preserve cured meats. If you think you may be sensitive to these compounds, you should carefully read the ingredient labels on foods, and make a point of avoiding anything that contains MSG.

Acupuncture

It may be well be worth trying acupuncture for headaches. There have been a number of studies of it as a treatment for tension headaches, which all point to it being an effective treatment. The most recent large study involved over 400 people and showed that acupuncture offered substantial benefits compared to routine conventional treatment, both in the short and long term, with the study's authors noting significant improvement in the frequency, severity and duration of individuals' symptoms.

In the study, researchers found that compared to the control group, patients receiving acupuncture treatment took 14 per cent less medication, made 30 per cent fewer visits to their GPs and took 25 per cent fewer days off sick due to ill health.

To treat headaches successfully, a series of treatments is usually needed. Treatment and its duration depends on the symptoms.

Pressing the L7 point in the hollow between the thumb and index finger may provide temporary relief.

Bodywork and Movement Therapies

The many different causes of headaches require different approaches to treatment. Some approaches focus on posture, some on neck restrictions, some on trigger points (sensitive areas in muscles; *see p.55*), and others on imbalances affecting the jaw (*see also p.280*).

ALEXANDER TECHNIQUE Spending a great deal of time standing or sitting with your head poked forward, in a slouched posture, puts a great deal of stress on the muscles and joints of the upper back and neck, which can lead to formation of trig-

Cranial osteopaths and dentists apply techniques to ease the stresses in the jaw area that may cause headaches, either by working on correcting possible misalignment of the upper and lower teeth or by encouraging better function of the jaw itself.

OSTEOPATHY AND CHIROPRACTIC Some injuries to the neck, particularly whiplash (which is caused by a sudden, extreme "whipping" movement of the head and neck; *see p.268*), can cause long-term irritations to the nerves that lead to chronic headaches. Chiropractors and osteopaths manipulate restricted joints of the neck or use soft-tissue techniques to encourage greater freedom of movement and ease possible nerve irritations. Research has shown that this approach can help to reduce the incidence of chronic headaches in many cases.

A review of randomised controlled trials found that spinal adjustment was as effective as antidepressants in preventing tension headaches or migraines.

Many (but not all) headaches may result from activation of trigger points in muscles, and there is evidence that deactivating these sensitive points in muscles reduces the incidence of headaches. The headaches

A review of psychological treatments found that relaxation and cognitive behavioural therapy can reduce the severity and duration of headaches in both children and adolescents.

Another study found that stress associated with negative life events, such as divorce, was related to how frequently people experienced headaches. Finally, a national survey of Taiwanese people found a strong link between job stress and the incidence of a number of health-related problems, including both headaches and musculoskeletal discomfort.

PRIMARY TREATMENT **BIOFEEDBACK, RELAXATION TRAINING** and other specific psychological skills can help to relax tense muscles that lead to headaches and counteract the negative effects of pain caused by excessive muscle tension. Electromyographic (EMG) biofeedback, in which electrodes are attached to muscles in the forehead and temple region, is often used. The electrodes monitor tension in the muscles, which is translated to an audio or visual signal. Patients learn to relax the muscles contributing to tension headaches by learning to slow down the signal.

A comprehensive review of studies that examined non-drug approaches to recurrent tension headaches found that relaxation training and biofeedback, as well as a combination of the two, produced nearly a 50 per cent reduction in the frequency of headaches.

Evidence has also shown that home-based psychological approaches, such as relaxation exercises or meditation, are as effective as clinic-based treatments given by professionals. They are worth trying if you have headaches on a regular basis.

> ## About 3 per cent of people experience a tension-type headache on most days

ger points, nerve irritation and headaches. The Alexander technique aims to correct such "patterns of misuse". It takes time and you need an Alexander teacher to guide you through the procedure. What feels uncomfortable at first (such as holding the head in its correct position) gradually becomes comfortable and eventually starts to "feel right". Teachers of the Alexander technique have perfected a gradual rehabilitation programme, which should ideally be accompanied by treatment (and self-treatment) aimed at stretching and releasing tight muscles and joints and at toning and balancing the body as a whole.

CRANIAL OSTEOPATHY AND DENTISTRY Talk to your dentist to see if jaw misalignment could be a cause of your headaches.

that are most improved by trigger-point treatment are those where there is also tenderness of the muscles attaching to the head. Trigger points can be eliminated by practitioners with a neuro-muscular training. *See also Migraine, p.119.*

Mind–Body Therapies

STRESS AND HEADACHES Numerous scientific studies have shown a strong link between stress and both tension and migraine headaches (*see p.119*). A study of young adults who experienced regular tension headaches found that feeling under stress and not functioning well emotionally were both predictive of greater frequency, intensity and longer duration of headache symptoms.

PREVENTION PLAN

If you are prone to headaches, the following may help:

- Eat regular meals to ensure stable blood-sugar levels.
- Drink plenty of fluids, especially water.
- Avoid caffeine and alcohol.
- Do daily relaxation exercises.
- Try to have some free time each day.

MIGRAINE

Migraine is characterised by recurrent headaches which are often accompanied by visual disturbances, nausea and vomiting. Migraines can last for several days and may be preceded by a period of feeling off-colour and irritable, known as the prodrome. A tendency to migraines sometimes runs in families, suggesting that genetic factors may play a role. Treatment involves a range of measures, such as dietary changes, massage and relaxation, as well as medication to treat an attack and prevent further attacks from occurring.

WHAT ARE THE SYMPTOMS?

- Throbbing or pounding pain on one or both sides of the head
- Nausea and vomiting
- Dislike of bright lights, noise and movement

WHY MIGHT I HAVE THIS?

PREDISPOSING FACTORS

- Genetic factors
- Pre-menstrual hormones
- Taking the combined oral contraceptive pill
- Low magnesium levels
- Trigger-point activity in muscles

TRIGGERS

- Certain foods, especially cheese, chocolate, red wine and wheat
- Food additives, such as monosodium glutamate and nitrates
- Strenuous exercise
- Low blood-sugar levels
- Stress

WHY DOES IT OCCUR?

Migraines are thought to be caused by a sudden widening of blood vessels that supply the brain, which in turn irritates the nerves surrounding the blood vessels. The reason for this is unknown, but various factors may be involved. Certain foods, for example, play a role in triggering migraines in many people. Low blood-sugar levels, low levels of magnesium in the diet, female hormones and stress also seem to be contributory factors. Some people develop migraine-type headaches in response to vigorous exercise, possibly because it causes an increase in blood pressure and blood flow. Trigger points (sensitive points in the muscles, *see p.55*) and nerve irritation in the head and neck are also thought by some to trigger severe headaches that are either true migraines or very similar.

IMPORTANT

See your doctor if a headache comes on after vigorous exercise; is accompanied by fever, stiff neck, drowsiness or a rash; if the headache follows a head injury; or if self-help remedies do not bring relief after three days.

TYPES OF MIGRAINE There are two main types of migraine. The first is "classical" migraine, in which the headache and nausea are preceded or accompanied by an event known as an aura. This may involve a range of phenomena, including visual disturbances, tingling and/or numbness in various parts of the body and feelings of restlessness or depression. What causes the aura is not fully understood. The second type is common migraine, in which there is no aura preceding the headache. Some

TREATMENT PLAN

PRIMARY TREATMENTS

- Rest and other self-help measures (*see Immediate Relief*)
- Over-the-counter painkillers and antinausea drugs
- Triptan and other drugs (for severe attacks)
- Feverfew and other Western herbs
- Magnesium supplements
- Food elimination diet
- Blood-sugar stabilising diet
- Neck manipulation and massage

BACK-UP TREATMENTS

- Nutritional therapy
- Bodywork therapies
- Relaxation training
- Acupuncture

WORTH CONSIDERING

- Homeopathy
- Chinese herbal medicine
- Environmental health measures

For an explanation of how treatments are rated, see p111.

people experience "visual" migraine, in which they have visual disturbances but no headache. Others, especially children, have "abdominal" migraine, in which the pain is experienced as a stomach ache or stomach upset rather than a headache. Migraine is a significant cause of headache in children.

IMMEDIATE RELIEF

PRIMARY TREATMENT The following can help relieve a migraine:

- Take painkillers and other medication as prescribed by your doctor.
- Splash your face with cold water or put a cold compress or an ice pack on your forehead and the back of your neck.
- Rest in a darkened, quiet room.
- Drink plenty of water.
- Massage your temples and neck with a few drops of lavender, rosemary or peppermint essential oil.
- Sip a cup of peppermint tea or a glass of ginger beer to help relieve any nausea associated with migraine.

TREATMENTS IN DETAIL

Conventional Medicine

Your doctor will diagnose the condition from a description of the symptoms. He or she will be able to give you advice about lifestyle changes and prescribe drugs if necessary. He or she will also be able to help you to identify and avoid migraine triggers, with the aim of reducing the number and severity of attacks.

PRIMARY TREATMENT **OVER-THE-COUNTER DRUGS** Painkillers and anti-nausea medications, such as aspirin and metoclopramide, may be helpful when an attack occurs. It may be necessary to experiment to see which one works best. Ibuprofen and other non-steroidal anti-inflammatory drugs (NSAIDs), may also be useful.

PRIMARY TREATMENT **PRESCRIPTION DRUGS** Your doctor may prescribe triptans such as sumatriptan, which are often helpful in relieving more severe migraine attacks. They work by narrowing the blood vessels that supply the brain. As well as being available as tablets, these drugs may be given by injection or nasal spray. In addition, if your migraines occur fre-

quently, there are various drugs available that may be prescribed for use on a daily basis, for example the beta-blocker propranolol and the antidepressant amitriptyline.

CAUTION

Drugs for migraine can cause a range of possible side-effects: ask your doctor to explain these to you.

Nutritional Therapy

PRIMARY TREATMENT **FOOD ELIMINATION DIET** Food sensitivity is a major cause of migraine according to a number of research studies. Certain foods known to trigger migraine are sometimes referred to as "the five Cs": chocolate, cheese, claret (and other red wines), caffeine and citrus fruits. However, research suggests that the most common food trigger of migraine is actually wheat. The same research also found milk and eggs to be common migraine-trigger foods.

People with such sensitivities can be treated with elimination diets. In one study of 60 people on a five-day elimination diet, which was limited to pears, spring water and lamb, participants reported a very significant improvement in their symptoms after eliminating on average 10 foods to which they were sensitive. (*For more details about food elimination diets, see p.39.*)

PRIMARY TREATMENT **BLOOD-SUGAR STABILISING DIET** Migraine can sometimes be triggered if the level of sugar in the blood becomes too low – a condition known as hypoglycaemia. This may explain why some people are prone to a migraine attack if they miss a meal. To ensure a stable blood-sugar level, avoid long periods without food: eat regular meals with healthy snacks, such as fresh fruit and nuts, in between. In general, base your diet on unprocessed foods, such as fresh fruits and vegetables and meat and fish. Choose wholegrain starches, such as

wholemeal bread and brown rice, which are broken down more slowly by the body than their white counterparts. This type of wholefood diet gives the body a steady release of glucose and helps to prevent blood-sugar levels from fluctuating (*for more information, see p.42*).

PRIMARY TREATMENT **MAGNESIUM SUPPLEMENTS** Migraine has also been related to low magnesium levels and magnesium deficiency, which increases the risk of spasm in the arteries. This mineral may be particularly helpful for women who suffer from premenstrual migraines. Research has found that 360mg of magnesium a day decreases menstrual migraine. If you have migraines regularly, try taking 200mg of magnesium twice a day. This seems to help with many migraines, even those unrelated to menstruation.

ESSENTIAL FATTY ACIDS Certain healthy fats known as the essential fatty acids (particularly omega-3 fatty acids) have been found to be helpful in migraine, probably because they reduce the amount of inflammatory substances that are implicated in headaches. One study found that gamma-linolenic acid (found in evening primrose oil) and alpha-linolenic acid (found in flaxseed oil) supplements reduced the frequency, severity and total duration of migraine attacks by 86 per cent. During the sixth month of the study, 22 per cent of the patients became free of migraine and more than 90 per cent experienced less nausea and vomiting.

FISH OILS Studies also show that fish oils (756mg per day of EPA and 498mg of DHA per day) may be beneficial in the treatment of recurrent migraines. If you have migraines, you may benefit from eating a diet rich in omega-3 fatty acids (found in oily fish such as salmon, sardines, mackerel and trout, as well as in flaxseeds and walnuts). You could also try taking 15ml of flaxseed oil, or 2–3g of fish oil supplements each day.

> Around 20 per cent of people have migraines, in both developed and undeveloped countries

AVOIDING FOOD ADDITIVES Certain chemicals and food additives can cause migraines. Some of the most common are nitrates (preservatives added to preserved meats), and monosodium glutamate, which is naturally present in mushrooms, kelp and scallops, but is also added to Chinese restaurant food and snack foods. Aspartame, an artificial sweetener found in many products from soft drinks to chewing gum may cause migraines. Interestingly, aspartame may have been involved in continuing headaches as there is anti-migraine medication with aspartame added to it. If you are prone to migraines it is worth checking the ingredients listed on packaging and trying to avoid aspartame.

CAUTION

Consult your doctor before taking magnesium and fish oils because they can interfere with other medication (*for more information see p.46*).

Homeopathy

The evidence on homeopathy as a treatment for migraine is rather confusing – there are some positive results, some negative results and some equivocal results. The differences may be accounted for by different types of patients, different types of homeopathic prescribing and different ways of measuring outcomes. However, an Italian research group led by Gennaro Muscari-Tomaioli found that homeopathy had very positive results on the quality of life of people with migraines. The usual medicines given were *Natrum muriaticum*, *Staphysagria*, *Lycopodium*, *Lachesis* and *Nux vomica*. All were prescribed at least partly on a "whole person" basis (*see p.73*).

NATRUM MURIATICUM is suggested by homeopaths for severe headaches with visual problems that tend to be worse in the sun. The affected person may also have streaming eyes. It is one of the medicines for "weekend migraine", which typically comes on when the patient relaxes.

STAPHYSAGRIA may be used for headaches brought on by anger or indignation, especially if these feelings are not expressed. Affected people may also have styes.

LYCOPODIUM is often appropriate when the headache is right-sided or moves from right to left. These migraines tend to be worse in late afternoon and are often associated with bloating and wind.

LACHESIS is given for headaches that are usually left-sided and worse in the morning. In women they occur before periods or as menopause approaches.

OTHER REMEDIES *Kalium bichromicum* is suggested if there is an aura preceding the headache by several hours. Affected people may also experience sinusitis. The remedy *Spigelia* is often recommended to treat left-sided headaches that also affect the eye. This type of headache is also sometimes accompanied by palpitations.

Western Herbal Medicine

Herbalists see migraine as a sign of disrupted normal physiology rather than focusing on pain as the essential problem. The fundamental message is to improve lifestyle and diet. People who suffer from frequent migraines tend to be perfectionists, who are often addicted to their own internally generated stress hormones and find it hard to relax. Regular food and fluid intake, as well as sufficient sleep and relaxation, are essential to prevent migraines. Without this, herbal treatment is unlikely to be anything more than a short-term palliative. For best results, visit a medical herbalist, who can assess your symptoms and prescribe an appropriate mixture of herbs to take.

IMPROVING CIRCULATION Herbal treatment aims to restore healthy circulation of nutrients to the brain by improving blood supply and supporting an overstressed nervous system. A mixture of wild oats (*Avena fatua*), skullcap (*Scutellaria laterifolia*), celery seed (*Apium graveolens*), wood betony (*Stachys officinalis*), vervain (*Verbena officinalis*) and mistletoe (*Viscum album*) may be suggested. Ginkgo biloba, hawthorn (*Crataegus spp.*), rosemary (*Rosmarinus officinalis*), sage (*Salvia officinalis*) and peppermint (*Mentha x piperita*) are also useful for migraines because they help to increase blood flow to the brain.

RELAXING HERBS Chamomile (*Matricaria recutita*), rose (*Rosa gallica*), lavender (*Lavandula officinalis*), lemon balm (*Melissa officinalis*), limeflower (*Tilea cordata*) and valerian (*Valeriana officinalis*) have relaxing properties, while ginseng (*Panax ginseng*), Siberian ginseng (*Eleutheroccus senticosus*) and astragalus (*Astragalus membranaceus*) help relieve migraines by combating any underlying chronic fatigue.

If during a migraine the person has a ruddy face, the herbalist may also suggest bitter, cooling remedies, including such herbs as feverfew (*Tanacetum parthenium*), gentian (*Gentiana lutea*), wormwood (*Artemisia absinthium*) and centaury (*Erythraea centurium*).

Very tense, tight shoulder and neck muscles can be eased by taking cramp bark (*Viburnum opulus*) and chamomile and by gentle massage of tense areas with essential oils such as lavender, rosemary, cinnamon (*Cinnamomum verum*) and orange (*Citrus aurantium*), diluted in almond oil. Massaging the neck and temples with a few drops of diluted essential oils of rosemary, lavender or mint (*Mentha spp.*) as soon as a migraine threatens can also help.

The visions of medieval mystic Hildegard of Bingen may have been due to migraines

---

PRIMARY TREATMENT

FEVERFEW AND OTHER HERBS The substances salicylates and parthenolide, which are the active constituents in meadowsweet (*Filipendula ulmaria*) and feverfew, can be effective pain-relievers. Feverfew is well known as a remedy for migraine and a number of scientific trials have demonstrated the herb's effectiveness. Extracts of the fresh herb inhibit the painful contraction of smooth muscle caused by serotonin and phenylephrine. The herb is available in tablets or tinctures and a folk remedy for preventing migraine is to eat a leaf daily.

During a migraine, blood flow to the body's extremities is reduced. This thermogram reveals decreased heat in the hands and fingers, which show up as green and blue.

After the person has used thermal biofeedback, the hands are much warmer. This technique can help relieve migraine by encouraging blood to flow to the hands and away from the head.

to increased carbon monoxide levels). Keeping track of these factors may help you identify problems and make changes that could lead to fewer migraines.

OTHER FACTORS Other environmental factors for migraine headaches include exposure to strong light, changes in the weather, and being at a high altitude.

There is some mention by "alternative" researchers of a gastrointestinal cause for migraines. This stems from what is called "leaky gut" syndrome, a phenomenon by which toxins supposedly penetrate the wall of the intestines and enter the bloodstream. However, despite a possible mechanism, some supportive testimonials and some relevant treatments, most of the leaky gut hypothesis still remains to be definitively studied and proven.

Acupuncture

Migraine has frequently been treated with acupuncture and there are a number of quality studies in this area. However, many look simply at headache in general and do not necessarily differentiate "classical" migraine from regular headaches alone.

Studies have looked at using a traditional Chinese approach to the diagnosis and treatment of migraine, as well as more Westernised techniques involving the use of tender trigger points in the head and neck. A number of these studies, particularly those published in the early 1980s, have been of poor quality, but on balance there is much more evidence to show that acupuncture is beneficial in treating the condition than reports that it has no effect.

A large study recently showed that acupuncture (up to 12 treatments over a period of three months) for chronic headaches, most of which were migraines, offered substantial benefits compared to conventional treatments. Frequency of headaches was reduced immediately after the study and remained reduced a year later. Medication use was reduced as well.

Acupuncture treatment for migraine can be based on either a traditional Chinese or a Western approach and usually needs to be given initially on a weekly basis. Usually, at least six to eight treatments are required for lasting relief, with the frequency of treatment related to the frequency of migraine attacks.

PREMENSTRUAL MIGRAINES can respond to chasteberry (*Vitex agnus-castus*), motherwort (*Leonuus cardiaca*), *Dang Gui* (*Angelica sinensis*) and black cohosh (*Cimicifuga racemosa*).

> **CAUTION**
>
> See page 69 before taking a herbal remedy and, if you are already taking prescribed medication, consult a medical herbalist first.

Chinese Herbal Medicine

Traditional Chinese Medicine (TCM) decides the treatment of migraine on an individual basis according to the pattern of symptoms. In TCM, headache can be externally or internally generated.

WIND INVASION If you feel under the weather, practitioners believe you may indeed have been invaded by adverse climatic factors. Wind is seen as a particularly disrupting influence, unsettling *Qi* (vital force) and blood flow to the head. Wind may invade together with cold, damp or heat. "Wind-cold" headaches are often treated with Ligusticum-Tea Blended Powder, a formula containing green tea, while "wind-heat" headache is treated with Chrysanthemum Tea Adjusted Powder. Chrysanthemum, *Ju hua* (*Chrysanthemum morifolium*), a key Chinese remedy for headache, is a relative of feverfew used by Western herbalists for the same purpose.

ENERGY IMBALANCES In TCM, the liver provides *Qi* (vital force) to enable the smooth flow of blood and nutrients to the brain. Its function is easily disrupted by stress, anger, worry and tension.

This disordered flow of *Qi*, which is described as "liver *yang* and internal wind rising", brings on a painful, throbbing headache, typically affecting one side of the head only – this is a characteristic migraine presentation. The classical prescription in TCM for this condition is Gastrodia Uncaria Decoction.

> **CAUTION**
>
> Self-medication with Chinese herbal medicine is not advisable for migraine. Consult a qualified Chinese herbalist.

Environmental Health

ENVIRONMENTAL TOXINS can be a trigger for migraines. An important first step is to thoroughly assess your workplace and home, perhaps with the help of an environmental health expert, looking for exposures to chemcials in building materials, cleaning supplies, paints or foods that may be causing your symptoms.

You may notice that you have more migraine headaches after working with solvents (for example those used in some hobbies), after spraying with pesticides or herbicides around the house or garden, or when the gas heater is turned on (leading

Bodywork Therapies

Despite having many of the same symptoms as true migraine (such as nausea), many one-sided headaches may not in fact be migraines at all but may arise instead from nerve irritation, or trigger-point activity, in the neck.

It is also not uncommon for people to experience both migraines and severe headaches that derive from the nerve irritation in the neck. A recent study of patients with neck injuries reported that 35 per cent of participants experienced headaches deriving from their necks, while another 11 per cent had both neck-related headaches and migraines.

> ## Peak prevalence for migraine is from 30 to 39. After the age of 50 they are less common

PRIMARY TREATMENT **NECK MANIPULATION AND MASSAGE** Your headache, whether diagnosed as migraine or not, may be helped by treatment of the neck muscles and joints. This might involve mobilisation or manipulation of restricted joints, release of excessive tension in muscles of the region, or deactivation of trigger points. However, not all the evidence is positive: one study showed that chiropractic manipulation did not help migraine.

Massage releases muscle tension and helps to restore normal blood flow to the blood vessels in the neck, scalp and face. It also has a wider therapeutic effect, helping to relieve stress and tension, which are often factors in migraine.

A 1998 study evaluated the potential benefits of massage in the treatment of migraine. After five weeks, the group of participants receiving massage therapy for their migraines reported a greater number of headache-free days, a reduced need for migraine medication when migraines did arise, more hours of sleep per night and better quality, less interrupted sleep.

THE DEACTIVATION OF TRIGGER POINTS Migraines in particular are often associated with trigger points (sensitive areas in the muscles, see p.55) in the neck and facial muscles. It is very simple to prove the connection between trigger points and headaches for yourself. If you have a particular pattern of headache, gently feel around in the muscles of the neck and face for tender areas (trigger points). Once you locate them, press them firmly, one at a time for 10 seconds or so, until you identify points that reproduce or exaggerate the headache pain pattern you usually have.

If you do find such points (there may well be more than one), you will have identified active trigger points, which should be treated and thus deactivated by a suitable practitioner. This might be an osteopath, chiropractor, physiotherapist, massage therapist, neuromuscular therapist or acupuncturist.

Mind–Body Therapies

Many scientific studies have shown a strong link between psychological stress and the onset of both tension and migraine headaches. Emotional factors, such as stress or anxiety, seem to be able to influence physiological factors that can act as triggers for migraine headaches.

RELAXATION TRAINING AND BIOFEEDBACK, as well as a combination of the two, yielded nearly a 50 per cent reduction in headaches in a review of the literature examining non-drug treatments for recurrent migraines. Moreover, home-based relaxation techniques were as effective at reducing headaches as treatment that was given in a clinic. The consensus panel of the United States Headache Consortium concluded there is strong evidence for the effectiveness of psychological therapies, including relaxation, biofeedback and cognitive behavioural therapy (CBT), in the prevention of migraines.

If you experience migraine headaches on a regular basis, it may be a sign that you need to make relaxation a higher priority. Experiment with a programme of relaxation exercises or try to meditate for 20 minutes each day (*for relaxation and meditation sequences, see p.99 and 100*).

THERMAL BIOFEEDBACK is a technique that has been shown to be particularly valuable in preventing migraine. Visualisation is used to get blood to flow to the body's periphery and away from the brain, an action which seems to prevent the full onset of a migraine (*see p.100*).

The best time to do thermal biofeedback is during the early onset or "aura". The technique, which must be learned in a clinic, involves placing a temperature sensor, called a thermistor, on the fingers. When a migraine begins, temperatures in the fingers can fall from their usual range of the mid-30's C (90's F to the low 30's C (80's F) or even lower. When a patient can see these lowered temperatures on the thermistor, he or she uses general relaxation and/or visual imagery (such as imagining the warm sun shining on the hands) to help the hands warm up. By watching the tiny changes registered on the thermistor, the patient can learn which relaxation techniques and/or visual images are most useful for making the temperature of the hands go up.

As well as being a preventive technique, even during a migraine attack the use of thermal biofeedback can occasionally alleviate the severity and/or duration of the migraine. However, it must be said that medications that act quickly to constrict excessive blood flow to the brain are still the first line of treatment once the headache has started.

PREVENTION PLAN

If you experience migraines on a regular basis, the following may help:

- Keep a diary of when migraines occur and likely triggers. Make a note of factors such as foods eaten, changes in the weather, sleep patterns and stress levels.

- Try to avoid any foods or situations that seem to bring on attacks.

- Take propranolol or other medication prescribed for prevention.

- Eat regular meals and try to get enough sleep at night.

- If stress is a trigger, do relaxation exercises every day (*see p.99*).

WHAT ARE THE SYMPTOMS?

- Pain that may involve any part of the body, depending on the cause
- In postherpetic neuralgia, burning and continuous pain in the area previously affected by shingles
- In trigeminal and suboccipital neuralgia, intense, stabbing pain in attacks lasting from a few seconds to a few minutes

WHY MIGHT I HAVE THIS?

PREDISPOSING FACTORS

- Shingles
- Heavy dental work
- Head or back injury
- Aspartame (an artificial sweetner), in trigeminal neuralgia
- Caffeine, in trigeminal neuralgia

TRIGGERS

For trigeminal neuralgia

- Eating, talking, brushing the teeth and washing the face
- Touching certain areas on the face (known as trigger points)
- Exposure to cold

NEURALGIA

Episodes of severe pain in the area supplied by a nerve is known as neuralgia. In one common type, trigeminal neuralgia, a severe, stabbing pain is felt around the side of the face and the cheek – areas supplied by the trigeminal nerve. Postherpetic neuralgia is persistent pain in an area previously affected by shingles (*see p.165*). Neuralgia may also occur in the suboccipital region, which is at the back of the head, or in an arm or a leg if a nerve is affected by a prolapsed disc. A variety of treatments bring relief, including drugs and bodywork therapy.

WHY DOES IT OCCUR?

The pain of neuralgia is caused by damage to a nerve. Various factors can cause it, including prolonged pressure on or injury to the nerve, as may happen due to a prolapsed disc (*see p.274*). Infection, such as with the herpes zoster virus in shingles (*see p.165*), may also cause postherpetic neuralgia in the area that is affected. Facial surgery or heavy dental work, such as having a tooth extracted or root canal treatment, may also cause neuralgia.

However, in many cases the cause of neuralgia is not known. For example, doctors are not usually able to identify a cause for trigeminal neuralgia or glossopharyngeal neuralgia (in which there is severe, stabbing pain at the back of the tongue and in the back of the throat).

Trigeminal neuralgia is more common in women and in people with multiple sclerosis (*see p.140*). In rare cases, trigeminal neuralgia may be found to be caused by compression of the trigeminal nerve by a tumour or an enlarged blood vessel.

WHAT SETS OFF THE PAIN? Some people with established neuralgia find exposure to cold triggers attacks. In some instances, only very slight disturbance to an affected area is enough to bring on stabbing pain. In trigeminal neuralgia, for example, facial movements such as smiling or frowning may be enough to set off an attack. In postherpetic neuralgia, merely touching the skin may be enough to bring on the pain, while sometimes attacks can occur spontaneously, without a trigger.

IMPORTANT

See your doctor if you experience symptoms of neuralgia. In rare cases there may be a serious underlying cause.

TREATMENT PLAN

PRIMARY TREATMENTS

For postherpetic neuralgia:

- Drugs and anaesthetic creams for pain relief

For trigeminal neuralgia:

- Carbamazepine (and other antiepileptics) for pain relief
- Acupuncture

BACK-UP TREATMENTS

- Avoiding aspartame and caffeine

- Vitamin B supplements
- Capsaicin cream

WORTH CONSIDERING

- Homeopathy
- Osteopathy, chiropractic and cranial manipulation
- Relaxation and biofeedback
- Surgery (if trigeminal neuralgia persists)

For an explanation of how treatments are rated, see p.111.

TRIGEMINAL NEURALGIA

One of the most common types of neuralgia affects the trigeminal nerve. This transmits sensation from some areas of the face to the brain. It is also involved in controlling the muscles that move the jaw to chew. Damage to the trigeminal nerve may cause bursts of stabbing pain that are felt anywhere along the path of the three branches of the nerve on a single side of the face. The cause is often not known. Attacks of trigeminal neuralgia may be brought on by chewing or certain facial movements, or by touching the face.

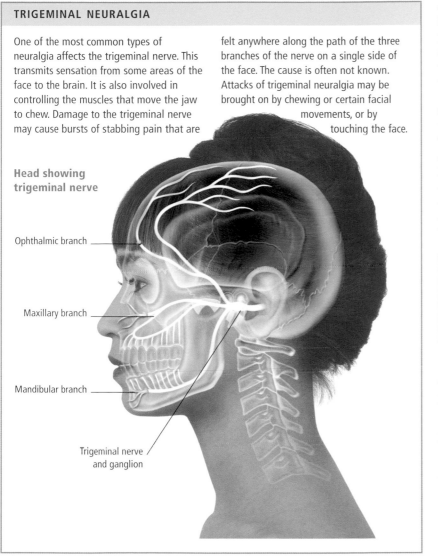

Head showing trigeminal nerve

Ophthalmic branch

Maxillary branch

Mandibular branch

Trigeminal nerve and ganglion

TREATMENTS IN DETAIL

Conventional Medicine

The doctor will probably be able to diagnose neuralgia from a description of the symptoms. He or she may also evaluate other possible causes of the pain, such as injury to the area. In some cases, neuralgia may resolve spontaneously. In other cases, the doctor will aim to treat any underlying cause (such as a prolapsed disc) in order to relieve the pain.

PRIMARY TREATMENT **ANTIVIRAL DRUGS** (such as aciclovir) reduce the likelihood of persistent postherpetic neuralgia developing if they are started early in attacks of shingles (*see p.165*). Starting a course of antiviral drugs early enough in an attack of shingles can also shorten the duration of the attack itself.

PRIMARY TREATMENT **ANAESTHETIC CREAMS** for postherpetic neuralgia can be applied directly to the affected area to help bring relief from pain.

PRIMARY TREATMENT **AMITRIPTYLINE**, an antidepressant, may reduce the likelihood of persistent neuralgia lasting six months or more. It is not known why this drug should be effective in shortening the course of neuralgia.

PRIMARY TREATMENT **CARBAMAZEPINE** is an antiepileptic drug which can help relieve the pain of trigeminal neuralgia. Other antiepileptic drugs, such as clonazepam, may be effective in some cases. As with antidepressant drugs, it is not known why antiepileptic drugs relieve neuralgia. It may be that both drugs alter the nerve impulse transmission, but this has not been shown.

SURGERY may be considered if the symptoms of trigeminal neuralgia are persistent. The options include heat treatment to destroy the nerve or microsurgery to cut it. Both procedures will result in numbness on the affected side of the face. If a tumour or enlarged blood vessel is found to be the cause of trigeminal neuralgia, surgery may be recommended to remove it.

> **CAUTION**
>
> Drugs for neuralgia can cause a range of possible side-effects: ask your doctor to explain these to you.

Nutritional Therapy

ELIMINATING ASPARTAME, an artificial sweetener widely found in soft drinks and processed food, from your diet may help if you have trigeminal neuralgia. A component of aspartame, the alcohol methanol, is known to be toxic to the nerves. Check all packaging for this carefully.

CAFFEINE Avoiding caffeine, which is found in cola, chocolate and even in some painkillers – as well as in coffee and tea – may help if you have trigeminal neuralgia. In a case study, a woman had complete relief from trigeminal neuralgia after adopting a caffeine-free diet. Caffeine may trigger trigeminal neuralgia because it has a nerve-stimulating action.

VITAMIN B SUPPLEMENTS A German study showed that neuralgia symptoms improved with a B-vitamin preparation. If you have neuralgia, try taking a daily multi-B vitamin supplement containing at least 25mg of each major B vitamin.

> **CAUTION**
>
> Ask your doctor before taking vitamin B supplements. These may interfere with the action of certain drugs. See p.46.

Homeopathy

ACONITUM NAPELLUS AND ARSENICUM ALBUM People who respond to *Aconitum napellus* and *Arsenicum album* are anxious and restless during the attack, and the pain is made worse by cold.

Aconitum napellus often helps with acute attacks of neuralgia, especially if it has been triggered by exposure to cold and particularly to cold wind. In people who respond to it, the pain may alternate with tingling or swelling and the person is usually anxious and restless during the attack.

Arsen. alb. is deeper acting and more likely to help with the underlying condition. People who respond to it are often very organised and "uptight"; they feel the cold greatly and often have dry, flaky skin. The pain is usually of burning character, relieved by heat.

OTHER REMEDIES *Agaricus muscarus* (made from the fly agaric toadstool) may help when the pain is described as being like "icy needles". People who respond to it may have twitching or a facial tic, sometimes with very itchy chilblains. *Spigelia antihelmia* is one of the most important medicines for trigeminal neuralgia, especially when it is left-sided. The pain affects the eye and there may be palpitations.

Kalmia latifolia is associated with rather similar symptoms to those of *Spigelia antihelmia*, but usually on the right side. *Hypericum perforatum* may be helpful if the neuralgia came on following an injury.

Western Herbal Medicine

CAPSAICIN CREAM This cream, which is made from a derivative of the chilli pepper, can be applied to the skin to treat the pain of neuralgia (see also p.129).

Acupuncture

PRIMARY TREATMENT Acupuncture, as well as related techniques such as transcutaneous electrical nerve stimulation (TENS), are frequently used in pain clinics to treat a variety of chronic pain syndromes. Acupuncture has a bearing on a number of pain processes. It can affect the nerve transmission of pain and stimulate the production of chemicals in the body that act naturally to relieve pain (for example, endorphins and encephalins). (*See also Persistent Pain, p.144.*) Acupuncture is commonly used and appears to be an effective treatment for many neuralgias, although it does not appear to be effective in postherpetic neuralgia. The evidence for its wide use is unfortunately lacking, largely because there are so few clinical trials in this area.

TREATMENT The acupuncturist should, in general, try to avoid placing needles in the painful area. Usually needles will need to be placed in other parts of the body, possibly the ear. Treatment should be given once or twice a week initially, but if after six to eight treatments there is no obvious benefit, then acupuncture is unlikely to be helpful. Frequently, neuralgia is an indication of some underlying imbalance that may be amenable to acupuncture. If initial treatment with acupuncture is successful, regular treatment, on a monthly basis is likely to be recommended.

Bodywork Therapies

OSTEOPATHY OR CHIROPRACTIC may be able to relieve the frequency and intensity of trigeminal or suboccipital neuralgia when it is associated with restrictions of the facial or cranial joints.

Research at the University of Florida College of Dentistry suggests that 5 to 10 per cent of patients may experience secondary trigeminal neuralgia after facial surgery, and that between 1 and 5 per cent of patients may experience secondary trigeminal neuralgia after dental extractions. If the area was injured or subjected to heavy dental work before the onset of symptoms, there may be a mechanical feature involved in the nerve irritation that manipulation might relieve.

Research has also shown that trigeminal neuralgia can originate from damage not only to the nerve itself, but also from damage to the upper spinal cord and neck area. Trauma to the head and neck, such as concussion or whiplash, may result in injury to nerve pathways. Following the trauma, facial pain may be triggered immediately or may take months or years to develop.

CRANIAL MANIPULATION (also known as cranial osteopathy, craniosacral technique or sacro-occipital technique) is the specialised application of very mild forces to areas of the head and is designed to restore normal freedom of the extremely small degrees of movement that are possible at the various sutures (fixed joints in the skull) and other joints of the skull and between the facial bones. Cranial manipulation may help to relieve the pain of neuralgia when it affects the face and back of the head.

TRIGGER POINTS (tender points in the muscles; *see p.55*) either in the face itself or in the muscles at the front and side of the neck can produce pain that is so similar to that of trigeminal neuralgia that it can be easily confused with it.

Researchers into trigger points report, "The pain from sternocleidomastoid trigger points can mimic true trigeminal neuralgia in distribution." Trigger points can be deactivated by acupuncture, as well as by manual pressure and stretching techniques, as used by osteopaths, massage therapists (particularly those with a neuromuscular therapy training) and some physiotherapists and chiropractors.

Mind–Body Therapies

RELAXATION EXERCISES AND BIOFEEDBACK may be worth considering, using either electromyographic (EMG) or muscle tension biofeedback techniques. (*See also Persistent Pain, p.144.*) For some people, psychological stress may be a factor in their neuralgia, and reducing the incidence of stress and finding time for relaxation may help. (*For meditation and relaxation sequences, see pp. 99.*)

PREVENTION PLAN

To reduce the likelihood of neuralgia:

- If you develop shingles, see your doctor promptly so a course of antiviral drugs can be started.

- Get plenty of rest after shingles in order to recuperate fully.

- Try to avoid triggers such as exposure to cold weather.

- Give up caffeinated beverages and aspartame if you are prone to trigeminal neuralgia.

NEUROPATHY

The peripheral nerves originate from the spinal cord and branch out to supply the body. Any disorder of these nerves is known as neuropathy. The cranial nerves, which extend from the brain to supply the head and neck, may be affected and cause facial palsy. Nerves supplying internal organs may also be affected. Neuropathies cause a range of symptoms and may be acute and short-lived or long term. Drugs, dietary supplements, creams, acupuncture and bodywork therapies may be used to treat the underlying cause and/or to relieve symptoms.

WHAT ARE THE SYMPTOMS?

SENSORY NEUROPATHIES

- Tingling, pain (which may feel like an electric shock) or burning and numbness in the hands, feet and limbs

MOTOR NERVE NEUROPATHIES

- Muscle weakness and wasting, and eventually impaired mobility in some cases

AUTONOMIC NEUROPATHIES

- Fainting, diarrhoea or occasionally constipation, inability to pass urine, impotence and an irregular heartbeat

WHY MIGHT I HAVE THIS?

PREDISPOSING FACTORS

- Exposure to toxic substances
- Alcohol abuse
- Some cancers
- Overuse of power tools that cause vibration

TRIGGERS

- Diabetes mellitus
- Vitamin deficiencies
- Infection
- Certain drugs
- Cancer
- Injury or compression of a nerve
- Inflammation of blood vessels supplying a nerve

IMPORTANT

See a doctor if you develop the symptoms of neuropathy. In some cases neuropathy may have a serious underlying cause.

WHY DOES IT OCCUR?

While some causes seem to damage the nerve cells directly, others harm the outer layer (the myelin sheath) of the nerves. Sometimes both are damaged. In all cases, the normal passage of signals along the peripheral nerves is disrupted, leading to symptoms of neuropathy. Areas on the skin supplied by spinal nerves, called dermatomes, may be the sites of neuropathies affecting those nerves (*see diagram, p.128*).

Depending on the particular nerve or nerves affected, neuropathy may affect sensation (sensory neuropathy), movement (motor neuropathy) or autonomic functions, such as bladder control (autonomic neuropathy). Neuropathy affecting the neck is known as cervical radiculopathy; if it affects the low back it is known as lumbar radiculopathy. If the facial nerve is affected, facial palsy may result. Bell's palsy is a type of facial palsy that causes weakness or paralysis on one side of the face.

In a mononeuropathy, one nerve is affected and the symptoms are restricted to the area supplied by that nerve. Damage to a single nerve may be due to injury or compression. For instance, carpal tunnel syndrome (*see p.152*) is caused by compression of the median nerve that supplies the hand. If many nerves are affected, symptoms are more widespread.

COMMON CAUSES The most common cause of neuropathy in developed countries is diabetes mellitus (*see p.314*). If diabetes is poorly controlled, high glucose levels may damage the peripheral nerves and blood vessels supplying them. Deficiencies in certain B vitamins and other nutrients may cause neuropathy. The most common cause worldwide is Hansen's disease (leprosy); infection with other viruses, such as HIV (*see p.470*), may also cause neuropathy.

Neuropathy may develop if the blood vessels that supply the nerves become inflamed, as occurs in polyarteritis nodosa. Some cancers can cause neuropathy. Certain drugs and toxic substances can damage nerves, as can vibration from overuse of power tools. Sometimes the cause of a neuropathy is unknown.

TREATMENT PLAN

PRIMARY TREATMENTS

- Treatment of underlying cause

BACK-UP TREATMENTS

- Vitamin B12 injections and vitamin B6
- Capsaicin (for diabetic neuropathy)
- Environmental health measures
- Acupuncture

WORTH CONSIDERING

- Bodywork therapies and yoga
- Evening primrose oil (for diabetic neuropathy)

For an explanation of how treatments are rated, see p.111.

SELF-HELP

The following measures can help you to manage diabetic neuropathy:

- Check your feet every day for signs of injury, which you may not be able to feel due to nerve damage. See your

doctor at the first sign of injury.
- Make sure that nothing in your shoes can injure or irritate your feet, such as ill-fitting linings or soles.
- Use a moisturiser if the skin on your feet is dry and/or thin.
- Limit your caffeine intake. Caffeine may make the pain of neuropathy worse.
- Take regular exercise.
- Massage your hands and feet every day.

TREATMENTS IN DETAIL

Conventional Medicine

Your doctor will probably diagnose neuropathy from your symptoms. He or she may do a physical examination and arrange other tests, such as electromyography and nerve conduction tests, to find out more. Further tests may be arranged to look for an underlying cause for example, a blood test to measure blood-sugar levels.

PRIMARY TREATMENT **TREATING AN UNDERLYING CAUSE** where possible is the first approach. If alcohol abuse is a cause, vitamin B1 supplements will be recommended. Corticosteroids may be given for polyarteritis nodosa.

Nutritional Therapy

VITAMIN B12 (the methylcobalamin form of this nutrient) may accelerate recovery from Bell's palsy. In one study, 60 people with Bell's palsy were given standard steroid therapy, standard steroid therapy plus methylcobalamin or methylcobalamin alone. The group given methylcobalamin alone recovered the quickest. The time required for complete recovery of facial nerve function was significantly shorter in the methylcobalamin and methylcobalamin plus steroid groups (average of about two weeks) than in the steroid group (average of about nine weeks). The dose of methylcobalamin used in the study was 500mcg. It was injected into the muscle three times a week for at least eight weeks, or until recovery was complete. People considering vitamin B12 injections for facial palsy should consult their doctor.

Vitamin B12 treatment may also be useful in treating other forms of neuropathy. Vitamin B12 (cobalamin) deficiency can produce a number of neurologic problems, including neuropathy in the nerves in the limbs and in the optic nerve, and these always need thorough investigation. If you have a neuropathy and vitamin B12 deficiency is suspected, medical investigation is always needed.

VITAMIN B6 (pyroxidine) may also be useful. People with diabetic neuropathy may have an underlying vitamin B6 deficiency. In one study, a group of people with diabetic neuropathy took supplements of 150mg of pyridoxine per day. Most of those in the study experienced some initial relief of pain and also from abnormal sensation within approximately 10 days. Improvement continued throughout the experimental period with lessening or resolution of symptoms.

After the experimental period, 70 per cent of patients asked to continue taking B6 supplements. Within three weeks of stopping pyridoxine therapy, the remaining 30 per cent of patients had a recurrence of their diabetic neuropathy symptoms. If you have diabetic neuropathy, try taking 50mg of B6, two or three times a day.

GAMMA-LINOLENIC ACID (GLA) is an essential fatty acid in the omega-6 series. It is formed in the body from linoleic acid (provided by vegetable oils). People with diabetes generally have a reduced ability to convert dietary linoleic acid to GLA. The lack of GLA and the molecules it converts to in the body may play a role in the development of neuropathy.

GLA supplements have been noted to bring about improvements in diabetic neuropathy. In one trial, GLA at a dose of 480mg per day for a year was shown to reverse existing diabetic neuropathy.

Evening primrose oil contains GLA and has been found to help alleviate the symptoms of diabetic neuropathy. If you have diabetic neuropathy, try taking 4–6g of evening primrose oil a day.

CAUTION

Vitamin B may reduce the effectiveness of certain drugs: ask your doctor for advice (see also p.46). High doses of vitamin B6 (over 500mg per day, or 150mg per day for some people) can cause neuropathy.

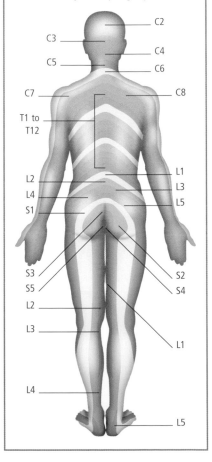

NERVES AND DERMATOMES

The spinal nerves branch out from the spinal cord and supply different areas of the body. The areas of the surface of the skin supplied by specific spinal nerves are known as dermatomes. The dermatomes in the trunk are all horizontal, while the dermatomes in the limbs are vertical. Dermatomes are named according to the spinal nerves that supply them – "C" stands for cervical (neck region), "T" indicates the thoracic (chest region), "L" stands for lumbar (low back and parts of thighs and legs) and "S" refers to the sacral (parts of thighs and legs, buttocks, genital areas and feet). Areas of sensation may overlap slightly.

Western Herbal Medicine

CAPSAICIN CREAM Capsaicin is the active ingredient in chilli peppers, making them irritating to the tongue and skin. When used in a cream to treat diabetic neuropathy, capsaicin appears to deplete the chemical messengers that send signals through the peripheral nerves, lessening the sensation of pain despite the fact that the cause is still present. Several trials suggest that capsaicin cream is an effective and safe way to treat diabetic neuropathy.

Creams and gels containing capsaicin are available in strengths ranging from 0.025 per cent to 0.075 per cent. It is probably best to begin using capsaicin cream at the lowest strength and progress to stronger concentrations if necessary. Some people experience a burning sensation and redness at the site where the cream is applied, but this generally lessens with repeated applications. Capsaicin cream should not be applied more than four times a day, and it may take up to four weeks for maximum benefit to be seen.

> **CAUTION**
>
> Keep all medications containing capsaicin away from the eyes and the mucous membranes. Do not apply the cream immediately after bathing or showering. Wash your hands very carefully after each application.

Acupuncture

Acupuncture does appear to provide pain relief in some cases of neuropathy. It affects some of the pain mechanisms, for example it affects the nerve transmission of pain, and encourages production of certain chemicals, such as endorphins and encephalins, that act to inhibit pain. Acupuncture can also deactivate trigger points (tender areas in muscles) that may arise due to a neuropathy. The evidence for acupuncture to treat neuropathy is limited and few clinical trials are available. The main disadvantage of using acupuncture in degenerative neurological conditions is that treatment may need to be repeated very frequently. Acupuncture treatment for neuropathy should be given on a weekly basis and abandoned if no positive effect is seen after six to eight sessions.

Environmental Health

An environmental health expert may be able to help in detecting the cause of a neuropathy. Environmental causes include compounds that are toxic to the nerves, certain medications (including some of the chemotherapeutic agent used to treat cancer) and mechanical injury resulting in compression of a nerve. Even simple pressure on nerves, such as prolonged use of crutches or sitting in the same position for a long time, can cause it, as can therapeutic drugs, workplace chemicals and environmental pollutants.

Exposure to heavy metals such as mercury, arsenic and lead has well-documented neurological effects. Recreational drugs can induce neurological or psychiatric impairments: nerve degeneration, for instance, can be associated with chronic cocaine or stimulant abuse.

EXTREME COLD AND VIRUSES There are two possible environmental causes of the specific neuropathy known as Bell's palsy, which affects the facial nerve. In some people, exposure to extreme cold temperatures can lead to symptoms consistent with Bell's palsy. Also, there is some evidence to suggest that a viral cause for some cases of Bell's palsy occurs with exposure to anything that lowers activity or effectiveness of our immune systems. This immune system weakening allows latent viruses to become activated and infect certain nerve cells, as with the case of trichloroethylene and the herpes simplex virus.

Bodywork Therapies

TRIGGER POINT DEACTIVATION Some forms of neuropathy, such as cervical radiculopathy or lumbar radiculopathy, can activate trigger points that perpetuate and aggravate the symptoms caused by the neuropathy itself. If you have a neuropathy, it may be useful to consult an acupuncturist or an osteopath, physiotherapist, massage therapist or chiropractor in order to deactivate any trigger points. This can be helpful in addition to whatever else is done regarding the neuropathy itself.

CRANIAL MANIPULATION When neuropathy causes Bell's palsy, gentle cranial manipulation aimed at restoring normal movement to the joints of the face and skull is sometimes effective.

Neuropathic symptoms elsewhere in the body that are specifically caused by nerve entrapment or compression can often be eased or relieved by specialised physical therapy methods involving very precise, carefully performed stretching and mobilisation techniques. Among the commonest neuropathies that are capable of improvement using these methods are carpal tunnel syndrome (*see p.152*) and the ulnar tunnel neuropathy (affecting the elbow).

OSTEOPATHY AND CHIROPRACTIC When neuropathy results from spinal nerve compression, possibly involving disc damage, osteopathic and chiropractic manipulation may effectively ease the pain that can result from the nerve compression or irritation. However, manipulation in the presence of a prolapsed disc requires expert skills and you should be certain that your practitioner has experience in dealing with prolapsed discs.

MASSAGE Regular massage of the hands and feet can help to maintain circulation in diabetic neuropathy and so help to prevent complications, such as ulceration, that result from poor blood flow to the extremities. Massage appears to be effective whether it is self-administered or done by another person.

Yoga

Certain neuropathic conditions where nerve entrapment is involved, such as carpal tunnel syndrome (*see p.152*) have been successfully treated using yoga stretching techniques. For peripheral neuropathy, yoga may help to relax tense muscles, lessen pain and make it easier for individuals to cope with their condition. Yoga is also a good form of exercise for people with diabetic retinopathy because it tends to be gentle and is unlikely to cause damage to tissues.

> **PREVENTION PLAN**
>
> The following may help to prevent the development of neuropathy:
> - Avoid environmental hazards.
> - Take a vitamin B-complex supplement.
> - If you have diabetes mellitus, keep your blood-sugar levels well controlled.

MEMORY IMPAIRMENT

A certain degree of memory impairment is a normal consequence of ageing. The decline may begin as early as the mid-30s and be noticeable by the mid-40s. It usually has a gradual onset and mainly affects short-term memory. Lack of regular mental stimulation, which can occur when a person retires, may contribute to the condition. Treatment for poor memory might involve drugs if there is an underlying cause, dietary changes, vitamin supplements, homeopathy, exercise and psychological techniques to improve memory recall.

WHAT ARE THE SYMPTOMS?

- Inability to recall short-term events
- Inability to remember short-term information
- Difficulty finding the right word or name for something or someone

WHY MIGHT I HAVE THIS?

PREDISPOSING FACTORS

- Age and lack of mental stimulation
- Free radical damage
- Raised homocysteine levels
- Underlying physical or psychological disorder
- Certain drugs, such as antiepileptic drugs and mood stabilisers

TRIGGERS

- Rapid upper-chest breathing
- Low blood-sugar levels

TREATMENT PLAN

PRIMARY TREATMENTS

- Drugs to treat any underlying condition
- Ginkgo biloba
- Memory tasks

BACK-UP TREATMENTS

- Oily fish
- Antioxidants and B vitamins

WORTH CONSIDERING

- Homeopathy
- Acupuncture
- Exercise
- Breathing techniques

For an explanation of how treatments are rated, see p.111.

WHY DOES IT OCCUR?

NORMAL AGEING Some degree of memory impairment can be expected as the brain ages. As a person grows older, the ability to learn gradually declines, although life experience becomes greater and the intellectual faculties continue to develop. By 50 to 70 years of age, short-term memory and the ability to concentrate tend to become reduced. By the age of 90, the brain has lost up to 10 per cent of its tissue.

BRAIN DISORDERS Memory impairment may occur as a result of various brain disorders. It may be caused by dementia (*see p.133*), or it may follow a head injury. An underlying physical illness, such as hypothyroidism (*see p.319*), or a psychological condition, such as depression (*see p.436*) or anxiety (*see p.414*) may also be contributory factors to poor memory. Some drugs, including antiepileptic drugs and mood stabilisers, can affect memory.

OTHER FACTORS Low levels of essential fatty acids and vitamin E in the diet have been linked with poor memory, as have raised levels of the amino acid homocysteine in the body. A condition known as respiratory alkalosis, in which the blood becomes too alkaline as a result of habitual shallow breathing, may also contribute to poor short-term memory by creating an oxygen deficit in the brain. Lack of mental stimulation can be a factor.

IMPORTANT

See your doctor if memory impairment is causing concern or interfering with daily life.

TREATMENTS IN DETAIL

Conventional Medicine

The doctor will assess memory and brain functions. If memory impairment is considered to be worse than expected for a person's age, tests (such as thyroid function tests and CT or MRI scanning of the brain) may be arranged to rule out any underlying conditions.

PRIMARY TREATMENT **UNDERLYING CAUSE** A doctor will aim to treat the underlying cause wherever possible. For example, hypothyroidism is treated with thyroid hormone supplements and depression may be relieved with antidepressant drugs.

Nutritional Therapy

Brain tissue is rich in healthy essential fats known as long-chain polyunsaturated fatty acids (PUFAs). In recent years, a lot of scientific attention has been focused on the role in brain function of the omega-3 PUFAs, such as eicosapentaenoic acid (EPA) and docosahexaenoic acid (DHA).

Some people have a tendency to low blood sugar. Their concentration and memory may deteriorate whenever blood-sugar levels dip too low. (*For information on stabilising blood sugar, see p.42.*)

OILY FISH EPA and DHA are found in abundance in oily fish (such as salmon, trout, tuna, mackerel, herring and sardines), and studies suggest that high fish consumption helps to reduce the risk of brain function decline. In one study, men who ate a lot of fish were found to have half the rate of mental decline compared

MIND MAPPING

Mind mapping brings the creative thinking and visual areas of the brain into play to help jog memory recall. To start a mind map, write down in the centre of some paper a main theme, for example "holiday". From the central word, draw a line or arrow and jot down items to be remembered such as "passport". Use another line for tasks to be done before you leave, such as "empty fridge". Your map can be as elaborate or simple as you like. Below are some tips to guide you.

DRAW YOUR MAP

- Write the map's theme in the centre and work outwards.
- Group related items together.
- Use coloured pens for different sections.
- Look for relationships and use arrows or lines to link related ideas.
- Leave some space to add more ideas later.
- Try capital letters to make key words stand out clearly.

KEEP IT SIMPLE

- Just have key words or images – not sentences.
- Write down words as they occur.
- Allow ideas to flow.
- If you can't think what to add in one area, move on to another.

THINK VISUALLY

- Illustrate with doodles, shapes or little pictures. They create a visual relationship with the idea that helps you remember things later.
- Try an image at the centre of the map – this is particularly effective.
- Use colours to highlight key tasks or to group related items.
- Enjoy the task – creativity aids memory.

to men who only ate fish occasionally. No clinical studies have been done in humans, but supplements of EPA and DHA have been shown to improve memory in animals. Aiming to eat at least two portions of oily fish per week might help to maintain memory. Taking daily supplements of concentrated fish oils at a dose of 2g may also help preserve memory in the long term.

ANTIOXIDANTS The mental decline that occurs with ageing may be related to damaging molecules known as free radicals. Free radicals are quenched in the body by antioxidant substances, such as beta-carotene and vitamins C and E. There is some evidence that increasing intakes of antioxidant nutrients might help to maintain mental sharpness. One study found that people who consumed 2.1mg (3,500IU) of beta-carotene per day were half as likely to experience cognitive impairment, disorientation or have difficulty solving problems compared to those taking 0.9mg (1,500IU) or less per day. Another study found that higher levels of vitamin C and beta-carotene in the body were associated with better memory. Citrus and kiwi fruits, strawberries, broccoli and Brussels sprouts are especially rich in vitamin C, while deep green and yellow-orange vegetables (e.g. carrots, spinach and sweet potato) are all good sources of beta-carotene. It would be reasonable to supplement the diet with 5000– 10,000IU of beta-carotene and 1g of vitamin C daily to see if it helps memory.

The antioxidant vitamin E has also been related to memory. In one study, people with the lowest vitamin E levels were almost three times worse at remembering than those with the highest levels. Other studies also show that high vitamin E levels are associated with good brain function. Good sources of vitamin E include nuts and seeds. In addition, supplementing with vitamin E at a dose of 400–800IU per day may be helpful.

FOLIC ACID AND OTHER B VITAMINS Another link between nutrition and brain function concerns the amino acid homocysteine. Raised levels of homocysteine have been linked to chronic diseases such as heart disease and osteoporosis. Research also shows a relationship between raised homocysteine levels and reduced mental performance. Folic acid (which is a B vitamin), vitamin B12 and vitamin B6 have all been found to help reduce homocysteine levels in the body.

Interestingly, studies have found people with low folic acid levels have impaired memory function compared to people with normal folic acid levels. Folic acid is found in green leafy vegetables, while liver, avocado, bananas and fish are rich in vitamin B6. Foods that contain vitamin B12 include meat, fish and eggs.

You may also want to take a supplement. A study into the effects of supplements on women found that taking 750mcg of folic acid, 15mcg of vitamin B12 and 75mg of vitamin B6 each day for 35 days had a significant positive effect on some measures of memory performance in comparison to a placebo, which had no effect. Taking a vitamin B-complex supplement each day may help to improve memory.

CAUTION

Consult your doctor before taking fish oils or omega-3 supplements, which can enhance the action of warfarin; vitamin B6, which can cause neuropathy in high doses; and folic acid (*see p.46*).

Herbal Medicine

PRIMARY TREATMENT | **GINKGO BILOBA** Herbs for dementia (*see p.133*), especially ginkgo biloba, may also be useful in treating memory impairment. Recent research has shown that the herb rosemary (*Rosmarinus officinalis*) can improve memory, and sage (*Salvia officinalis*) and lemon balm (*Melissa officinalis*) are both thought to help in improving memory as well.

CAUTION

See p.69 before taking a herbal remedy and, if you are already taking prescribed medication, consult a medical herbalist first.

Homeopathy

A number of homeopathic medicines may help with memory. For dosages, see p.77.

BARYTA CARBONICA AND LYCOPODIUM are the most important for age-related memory problems. *Baryta carbonica* is effective where there are arteriosclerosis (hardening of the arteries), memory problems and mental slowness. The person affected may become timid and childish and have offensive foot sweat. Symptoms may be worse in cold, damp weather and affected people may get recurrent colds, with neck glands that become very hard and swollen. *Baryta carbonica* may also be helpful for younger people who experience memory problems after illnesses, especially glandular fever.

People who respond to *Lycopodium* are often serious intellectual people who may have held responsible jobs. They tend to become depressed and reclusive because they lose self-confidence over their memory problems. These people also often have stomach trouble, with wind and bloating, and a sweet tooth.

PHOSPHORIC ACID is another medicine that may be helpful for younger people, especially when they experience the effects of intellectual and emotional stress combined, for instance the stress of exams combined with relationship difficulties.

ANACARDIUM ORIENTALE is sometimes helpful if there is sudden loss of memory, as happens when a name or idea suddenly goes out of someone's head. Affected people may also have sudden, violent tempers.

Acupuncture

If memory impairment is considered as part of a traditional Chinese diagnosis, then regular acupuncture treatment may improve overall balance and function including memory, either through a traditional Chinese approach or through the more Westernised explanation of improved cerebral circulation. While there are no controlled trials suggesting that acupuncture does improve memory, there are a number of anecdotal suggestions that it may help. Usually, repeated treatments are required to obtain a sustained effect. If the underlying cause of memory impairment is a disease such as Alzheimer's, acupuncture might slow down the development of dementia. However, there is no research to guide us and acupuncture is not effective at treating the underlying cause of the condition. The individual's memory capacity should be tested at the beginning of treatment and after six to eight weekly sessions have been completed. If no progress is being made, acupuncture should probably be abandoned.

Exercise and Breathing

Respiratory alkalosis (*see p.57*) may cause short-term memory loss and an inability to "stay focused". The condition also prevents the red blood cells that transport oxygen around the body from releasing their oxygen efficiently, which adds to the oxygen deficit in the brain. This consequence of respiratory alkalosis is known as the Bohr effect. The solution is to increase the efficiency of delivery of oxygenated blood to the brain and to aid the release of oxygen to body tissues.

EXERCISE is one of the most obvious and beneficial ways to improve delivery of oxygenated blood to the brain. Researchers have also found that there is a clear link between high blood-sugar levels and reduced volume of the hippocampus, a structure within the brain concerned with memory and learning. People with impaired blood-sugar regulation commonly perform more poorly than normal in memory tests. Since weight loss and exercise can both normalise blood-sugar levels, it seems obvious that a healthy lifestyle that includes regular exercise can help to improve your memory.

In important research it was found that immediately after 20 minutes of riding a stationary bicycle, at a rate that reached their peak performance level, people with the respiratory condition chronic obstructive pulmonary disease (COPD) showed instant improvement in their thinking processes and memory. The assessment after exercise evaluated verbal processing, attention span, short-term memory and motor skills. The results "indicate that they were able to process and retain information better than they could prior to exercising." These people, because of their diseased lungs, in their normal lives were forced to adopt a breathing pattern that led to excessive carbon dioxide exhalation and an oxygen deficit in the brain, which the exercise helped to reverse. The research results clearly show the potential for improving short-term memory loss by stimulating circulation through even modest amounts of exercise.

BREATHING TECHNIQUES Learning to slow down the breathing rate and improve abdominal breathing is another good way to improve the efficiency of delivery of oxygenated blood around the body. (*For details, see p.62.*)

Mind–Body Therapies

Memory impairment is a common aspect of ageing. However, along with physical trauma, it can be associated with a number of other psychological problems, such as anxiety (*see p.414*) and depression (*see p.436*). Post-traumatic stress (*see p.422*) may also affect memory in that traumatic memories intrude into everyday life.

PRIMARY TREATMENT | **MEMORY TASKS** Dementia (*see p.133*) is probably the most common cause of memory impairment and recently some talking therapy techniques have been developed to help address the memory loss aspect of this distressing condition.

Spaced retrieval (SR) is a technique whereby a client is given a memory task at increasingly extended intervals, which helps the person to recall how to remember. A number of studies have supported this method of working.

Cueing hierarchy, in which a correct sequence of words must be remembered, is another method and has been compared directly with SR. In studies both treatments were effective, although more goals were attained using SR.

PREVENTION PLAN

To avoid further memory loss:
- Take ginkgo biloba supplements.
- Practise memory techniques.
- Take plenty of regular exercise.

WHAT ARE THE SYMPTOMS?

- Impaired memory, especially regarding recent events
- Loss of intellect that affects reasoning and understanding
- Difficulty holding a conversation
- Reduced vocabulary
- Emotional outbursts and agitation
- Physical wandering
- Neglect of personal hygiene

WHY MIGHT I HAVE THIS?

PREDISPOSING FACTORS

- Risk factors for stroke, including high blood pressure, smoking and diabetes mellitus
- Long-term alcohol abuse
- Low antioxidant intake
- Raised homocysteine levels
- Advanced age
- Genetic factors
- Possibly aluminium exposure

IMPORTANT

Anyone suspected of having dementia should have a thorough medical assessment. Elderly people with severe depression may seem to have dementia because the conditions share some symptoms, such as forgetfulness.

DEMENTIA

Memory loss, personality changes and a decline in intellectual ability characterise dementia. The condition is more common in people over the age of 65, and genetic factors may play a part in some types. Important first steps are to assess intellectual function and look for an underlying cause. Although the condition cannot usually be cured, a range of treatments might help to control the symptoms, including drugs, dietary methods, massage, music therapy and relaxation training.

WHY DOES IT OCCUR?

The underlying abnormality in dementia is degeneration of the brain tissue, but the exact cause of the condition is often not known. Alzheimer's disease is probably the best-known type of dementia, but there are many others, including multi-infarct dementia (see below), Pick's disease and Lewy body disease. All of these are less common than Alzheimer's disease.

In Alzheimer's disease, cells in some areas of the brain are destroyed, while other cells become less responsive to neurotransmitters (chemicals that transmit messages in the brain). Chemical changes in the brain are thought to play a role in the condition, with a decline in levels of acetylcholine and other neurotransmitters. Abnormal tissues and deposits of abnormal protein also appear in the brains of people with Alzheimer's disease.

Dementia sometimes results from an underlying cause, such as damage to the brain from interruption to its blood supply by recurrent small strokes (known as multi-infarct dementia). Alzheimer's disease usually develops gradually, while multi-infarct dementia tends to develop more rapidly. Other possible causes of dementia include long-term alcohol abuse, hypothyroidism (see p.319) and HIV infection (see p.470). Dementia may also develop after a heart attack or a brain injury. Some types of dementia may have genetic factors.

Recent research has shown that people who have had a stroke (see p.148) are at a high risk of developing dementia. Dementia that develops after a stroke begins as an Alzheimer's-type condition, but later takes on the characteristics of vascular dementia.

People with dementia often do not realise that anything is wrong, which can make the condition even more distressing for friends and family. Initially, however, they may realise what is happening, which can cause depression. Caregivers often need support themselves.

TREATMENT PLAN

PRIMARY TREATMENTS

- Treatment of any underlying cause
- Donepezil and galantamine (for mild to moderate Alzheimer's disease)
- Emotional and practical support

BACK-UP TREATMENTS

- Drugs for symptoms (such as agitation)
- Dietary changes
- Antioxidant vitamins
- Western herbal medicine

WORTH CONSIDERING

- Environmental health measures
- Contact with nature (for its calming effect)
- Exercise
- Bodywork therapies
- Acupuncture
- Mind–body therapies

For an explanation of how treatments are rated, see p.111.

This coloured scan of an Alzheimer's disease brain (left) and a normal brain (right) shows how the Alzheimer's brain is considerably shrunken and the surface is more deeply folded than the normal brain.

TREATMENTS IN DETAIL

Conventional Medicine

PRIMARY TREATMENT The doctor will take a careful history from the person affected and often from a close relative or friend as well. He may also refer the person affected for cognitive testing to assess intellectual function, and may arrange other tests, such as blood tests to check thyroid gland function. Where possible, the doctor will aim to treat the underlying cause.

PRIMARY TREATMENT **DRUGS** are now available for treating some people with mild to moderate Alzheimer's disease. Examples include donepezil and galantamine. These have been shown to improve intellectual ability in some cases. Regular assessments are performed to monitor any change. A drug is likely to be stopped if there is no response. Drugs such as sedatives may also be prescribed to treat other features of dementia, such as agitation.

PRIMARY TREATMENT **SUPPORT** People with dementia usually need assistance with day-to-day living and may at some point require full-time care in a nursing home. People who care for someone with dementia in the home usually find the task very demanding and stressful and are often in need of support themselves. The doctor can put carers in touch with organisations and support groups who can offer them both practical and emotional support. (*See also Useful Addresses, p.486.*) Respite care, where the carer is able to have some time off at home or go away on holiday, can often be arranged.

> **CAUTION**
>
> Drugs for dementia have a range of possible side-effects; ask your doctor to explain these to you.

Nutritional Therapy

ALUMINIUM Although the precise cause of Alzheimer's disease is not known, there is at least some evidence that a proportion of cases are linked to the toxic effects of aluminium. More than one study has found accumulations of aluminium in the part of the brain affected by the disease. However, there have also been studies that have not found a link between aluminium and Alzheimer's disease.

Whether aluminium in the diet can cause Alzheimer's disease remains controversial, but it seems prudent for healthy people to minimise their exposure to aluminium. You can do this by reducing intake of foods cooked in aluminium pans, drinks from aluminium cans and foods that have been stored in aluminium foil (*see also Environmental Health, right*).

DIETARY CHANGES Oily fish (e.g. salmon, trout, tuna, mackerel, herring) and foods such as flaxseed oil contain omega-3 fatty acids. A diet rich in these seems to help protect against Alzheimer's disease. In one study, people with Alzheimer's were treated for six months with fish oil capsules containing 1400mg of DHA (an omega-3 fatty acid found in oily fish) per day experienced an improvement in brain function.

In addition, studies show that the levels of DHA are generally lower in the brains and blood plasma of Alzheimer's patients than in those of normal elderly individuals. Individuals wishing to stave off Alzheimer's disease and dementia may do well to consume a diet high in omega-3 fatty acids, for example by eating two portions of oily fish a week.

Monounsaturated fats, which are found in extra-virgin olive oil, avocados and nuts, have also been found to slow brain function decline. Including plenty of these foods in the diet may help to maintain brain function in the long term.

Excessive intake of meat and eggs may increase the risk of Alzheimer's disease. These are rich in arachidonic acid, which encourages inflammation in the body. Inflammation is possibly a risk factor for Alzheimer's disease and reducing the amount of arachidonic acid in the body (by limiting foods such as meat and eggs) may help to prevent Alzheimer's disease.

ANTIOXIDANTS Some scientists have been looking at the role that damaging molecules called free radicals play in Alzheimer's disease. Free radicals damage cell membranes (including nerve cells) and are quenched in the body by antioxidants. It is thought that brain function may be protected if antioxidant intake is increased. Vitamin E (an important antioxidant nutrient) at a dose of 2,000 IU per day has been shown to help protect against Alzheimer's disease, and to extend the time that people with Alzheimer's disease are able to care for themselves. Studies have also found that supplements of vitamins C and E and high dietary intakes of these nutrients are associated with a reduced risk of dementia and Alzheimer's disease.

An estimated 18 million people worldwide have dementia. By 2025 that number will double

Another antioxidant, beta-carotene, may also be helpful in preventing cognitive decline. In a study of more than 5,000 individuals aged between 55 and 95, it was found that those consuming 2.1mg (3,500 IU) of the antioxidant beta-carotene per day were half as likely to suffer cognitive impairment, disorientation and have difficulty in problem-solving compared to those who took 0.9mg (1,500 IU) or more per day. Taking 5000–10,000 IU of beta-carotene per day, along with 600–800 IU of vitamin E and 1–2g of vitamin C each day, may afford some protection from the onset of dementia in the long term.

VITAMIN B High levels of the blood chemical homocysteine have also been found in people with Alzheimer's disease. One study concluded that an increased plasma homocysteine level is a strong, independent risk factor for the development of dementia and Alzheimer's disease. A raised homocysteine level can often be successfully treated with supplements of vitamin B6 (at least 10mg per day), vitamin B12 (at least 50mcg per day) and folic acid (at least 400mcg per day). Taking a daily B-complex supplement may help to preserve brain function in the long term.

CAUTION

Consult your doctor before taking vitamin C and vitamin E with anticoagulant drugs, such as warfarin; and vitamin B, which in high doses can cause neuropathy (*see also p.46*).

ACETYL-L-CARNITINE can increase the production of the important brain neurotransmitter acetylcholine. Examinations of the brains of Alzheimer's disease patients have revealed decreases in the amount of acetylcholine, and acetyl-L-carnitine supplementation has been shown to improve memory and slow the progression of Alzheimer's disease. Nutritional experts normally recommend taking 500–1,000mg, three times a day.

Western Herbal Medicine

Several herbal medicines have direct use in the prevention and treatment of dementia, in particular Alzheimer's disease. People seeking to treat dementia with herbal medicine should consult a professional medical herbalist who will prescribe herbs to enhance cerebral blood flow, promote anti-inflammatory and antioxidant activity within the brain and support elimination of toxins via the liver and kidneys.

Anxiety and depression are common features of dementia, so uplifting herbs such as lemon balm (*Melissa officinalis*) and St John's wort (*Hypericum perforatum*) may well be suggested. Massage of tense neck and shoulder muscles with lavender oil may be greatly appreciated.

GINKGO BILOBA and members of the mint family, such as sage (*Salvia officinalis*) and rosemary (*Rosmarinus officinalis*), are among the best-known herbal treatments for dementia. Ginkgo is the herb of choice in treating dementia, having been the subject of extensive laboratory and clinical research. It improves circulation to the brain and inhibits inflammation there, the net effect being to stabilise and strengthen nervous system function. Cognitive activity, including memory and recall, is stimulated. Clinical research shows that ginkgo is most effective in mitigating mild to moderate dementia, although there are indications that it also slows deterioration in severe dementia. A review of clinical trials using ginkgo extract concluded that it

was at least as effective as the currently available conventional treatments in treating Alzheimer's disease. Side-effects at recommended dosages are rare.

SAGE (*Salvia officinalis*) has been investigated by researchers at Newcastle University to determine its potential to maintain brain acetylcholine levels. As Alzheimer's is marked by low levels of acetylcholine, herbs that inhibit its breakdown within the brain may prove useful. The research indicated that sage acts to strengthen mental function and memory.

CHOTO-SAN is a Japanese formula of which the main ingredient is the herb *Uncaria sinensis*. This herb has traditionally been used to treat stroke in China and is known to lower blood pressure.

Two different studies were done on the efficacy of Choto-san on patients with vascular dementia. Both showed that it was effective in improving dementia symptoms, including psychiatric symptoms and the ability to cope with the daily living.

CAUTION

See p.69 before taking a herbal remedy and, if you are already taking prescribed medication, consult a medical herbalist first.

Environmental Health

There are many chemicals that potentially could damage neurons and lead to dementia, but definitive proof is often lacking.

ALUMINIUM One well-studied agent associated with Alzheimer's disease is aluminium. Elevated levels of aluminium in drinking water, for example, are associated with an increased risk of Alzheimer's disease and dementia. You can check with your local water supplier for details about the content of specific substances in your water. Government agencies also have information about drinking water; in the UK, check with the Department for Environment, Food and Rural Affairs. (*See also Nutritional Therapy, left.*)

ENVIRONMENTAL HAZARDS People in occupations that could expose them to electromagnetic fields (such as in airports, radio and television stations, power plants, electrical plants or those who work in telephone repair) could be at greater risk of developing dementia than others.

Chronic solvent exposure may lead to memory problems. However, one study did not find an association between Alzheimer's disease and exposure to solvents, although this may be due to the difficulty in characterising and measuring exposure to solvents. The true nature of many of these exposures and the risk that they pose for the development of dementia in the general population are still speculative, and need further research.

CONTACT WITH NATURE may have a beneficial influence on people with dementia. A study has shown that people with progressive Alzheimer's disease who live in care homes without gardens tend to become more aggressive than people with the condition who have access to the outdoors.

PROTECTION There may be a significant amount of individual variation with respect to susceptibility to environmental chemicals that may lead to dementia. It is possible that the mechanism for damage from these compounds is through free-radical formation (*see Nutritional Therapy, p.134*). If further research shows that is indeed the case, then free-radical scavengers (antioxidants) such as vitamin E may be useful in both prevention and treatment of dementia.

Bodywork Therapies

Dementia is often accompanied by outbursts of agitated behaviour, sometimes verbal and sometimes involving violent activity. This behaviour can be extremely upsetting and disturbing to others. Research studies have shown that body massage, hand massage and/or peaceful background music can play an important role in reducing the incidence of agitated behaviour in people with dementia.

MASSAGE AND MUSIC In a study comparing the effects of ten minutes of soothing music with ten minutes of calming hand massage, it was found that both methods reduced non-aggressive agitated behaviour for at least an hour afterwards, but had no effect on aggressive behaviour. The music used in this type of research had a slow tempo, soft dynamic levels, and repetitive themes; care was taken to avoid recognisable melodies that might evoke unwanted emotional responses.

Back massage too can be a soothing influence: in one study people with dementia in a care home were given back massage and displays of agitated behaviour reduced in frequency, athough verbal agitation was unaffected.

Exercise

Physical activity may help to prevent dementia. One study found that men and women over the age of 65 who exercised regularly had about half the risk of developing Alzhemer's disease or other types of dementia. Exercise may also help relieve depression in patients with Alzheimer's disease. Intellectual stimulation is another factor that may protect against dementia.

Mind–Body Therapies

RELAXATION TRAINING A relaxation session may temporarily help relieve symptoms. A study of the effects of relaxation on dementia investigated the effectiveness of intensive relaxation training in people ranging in age from 52 to 93 years old who had been diagnosed with either Alzheimer's disease or multi-infarct dementia. Results showed that relaxation training may be an effective aid in the management of behavioural problems such as forgetfulness and disorientation in elderly patients who have dementia. Music may also aid relaxation (*see Bodywork Therapies, left*).

COGNITIVE STIMULATION THERAPY A recent study showed that cognitive stimulation therapy (CST) appears to improve both cognitive function and quality of life in people with dementia. This technique involves having people with dementia do various cognitive "tasks" that are related to real-world events and people. In the randomised controlled study, 115 older people with dementia took part in a CST programme that ran twice weekly for 45 minutes at a time. Sessions began with a physical warm-up activity, followed by activities that encouraged the processing of information rather than simple recall of facts. The topics that were included involved money, present-day events, famous faces and word play. None of the participants in the programme took medication for their dementia.

At the end of the 14-week trial period, the group who had attended the CST sessions showed significant improvement in cognitive skills and quality of life over the control group, who had no treatment. However, the authors concluded that CST

Only a small number of dementia cases are thought to be due to genetic factors

sessions would need to be ongoing and done on at least a weekly basis for improvements to be maintained.

REMINISCENCE THERAPY is a psychological technique that helps people with dementia to recall events in their lives, using videos, objects and music from the past. Reminiscence therapy is valuable because it may help dementia patients to regain a sense of self.

PREVENTION PLAN

The following may help protect against the advance of dementia:

- Eat oily fish twice a week and eat foods high in antioxidants.

- Take ginkgo biloba and vitamin E supplements daily.

- Have blood pressure and homocysteine levels checked regularly (these may be risk factors for dementia).

- Avoid environmental hazards.

- Learn new skills and maintain social networks and existing hobbies to keep the mind active.

- Take regular exercise and avoid factors that provoke stress as far as possible.

DIZZINESS AND VERTIGO

The term dizziness is commonly used to describe various symptoms, from mild light-headedness to vertigo, a more specific term that describes a false sensation of moving or rotating. Both may be accompanied by nausea and vomiting. Dizziness may result from various causes, including panic attacks or anaemia. Vertigo may result from disturbance to the organs of balance in the inner ear, or from other causes. There are no well-established natural treatments for vertigo, but dietary changes, breathing exercises and chiropractic might bring relief.

WHAT ARE THE SYMPTOMS?

- A sensation of moving or rotating
- Nausea
- Vomiting

WHY MIGHT I HAVE THIS?

PREDISPOSING FACTORS

- Labyrinthitis
- Benign positional vertigo
- Ménière's disease
- Head or neck injury
- Fluctuations in blood-sugar levels
- Anaemia and fatigue
- Autonomic dysfunction
- Standing motionless for long periods
- Arthritis in neck joints
- Multiple sclerosis
- Tumour

TRIGGERS

- Inner ear infection
- Hyperventilation
- Excessive alcohol consumption
- Stroke

TREATMENT PLAN

PRIMARY TREATMENTS

- Immediate Relief measures *(see left)*
- Antihistamines; adjusting medication

BACK-UP TREATMENTS

- Blood-sugar stabilising diet
- Epley procedure (for benign positional vertigo)
- Chiropractic or osteopathy

WORTH CONSIDERING

- Homeopathy
- Craniosacral therapy/cranial osteopathy
- Breathing retraining
- Mind–body therapies

For an explanation of how treatments are rated, see p.111.

WHY DOES IT OCCUR?

Mild dizziness may be caused by various factors, including panic attacks, anaemia, fatigue, shallow breathing, low blood-sugar levels or drinking too much alcohol. It may also occur after long periods of standing still. Often no cause can be found.

Vertigo is due to problems with the nerve that connects the inner ear to the brain, or to problems in the areas of the brain that are concerned with balance. Another cause of vertigo is an infection of the inner ear that affects the organs of balance (labyrinthitis). This type of vertigo usually comes on rapidly. It may last for up to two weeks but tends to resolve on its own.

Benign positional vertigo, which is due to a build-up of calcium debris in the semicircular canals in the inner ear, is a common cause of episodes of vertigo that are triggered by moving the head. These episodes are normally short-lived, typically lasting for less than one minute.

Recurrent vertigo may result from the inner ear disorder Ménière's disease, in which the pressure in the inner ear is intermittently raised. If vertigo is due to Ménière's disease, it may be accompanied by nausea and vomiting.

Arthritis in the joints of the neck can sometimes cause recurrent episodes of vertigo and, in rare cases, vertigo may be a feature of multiple sclerosis (*see p.140*). Other rare causes of dizziness and vertigo include a tumour affecting the nerve that connects the inner ear to the brain, a stroke or a head or neck injury. These serious conditions may cause other symptoms affecting speech, vision or movement and require immediate medical attention.

IMMEDIATE RELIEF

PRIMARY TREATMENT — During an attack, lie still and avoid sudden movements.

- Press the pericardium 6 (P6) point for 5 to 10 minutes. It lies about two thumb-widths above the front wrist crease, in line with your ring finger.
- You can also buy special wrist straps ("sea-bands") designed to help motion and morning sickness; they put pressure on these points. Ask for them at your local pharmacy.

IMPORTANT

If your dizziness or vertigo is accompanied by problems with your speech, vision or mobility, seek medical help immediately.

TREATMENTS IN DETAIL

Conventional Medicine

Your doctor will do an examination focusing on the ears, eyes and the functioning of the nervous system, and may also arrange tests to check the vestibular apparatus (structures of the inner ear). Investigations, such as blood tests and CT scanning, may be done to look for underlying disorders, which will be treated where possible.

EPLEY PROCEDURE If you have benign positional vertigo, your doctor may recommend that you try doing the Epley procedure. This is a series of head movements that help to reposition any calcium debris that has become loose in the semicircular canals in the inner ear, helping the vertigo to resolve (*see box, overleaf*).

PRIMARY TREATMENT **ANTIHISTAMINES**, such as cinnarizine, may help to reduce vertigo and any associated nausea. Antihistamines can cause drowsiness.

Nutritional Therapy

BLOOD-SUGAR STABILISING DIET Dizziness or vertigo can be symptoms of blood-sugar fluctuation; dizziness is associated with low blood-sugar levels (*see p.42*).

Homeopathy

Many remedies may be suitable for dizziness and vertigo. You will need to visit a homeopath as the choice of remedy is dictated by your constitution and symptoms (*see p.73*). Some of the more commonly prescribed remedies are as follows:

VERTIGO HEEL is a complex homeopathic medicine that has been shown to be equally effective as one of the leading conventional treatments for treating Ménières disease – Betahistine (Serc®). *Vertigo Heel* contains *Conium*, *Cocculus maculatum*, *Petroleum* and *Ambra*.

MENIERE'S DISEASE AND LABYRINTHITIS *Chininum sulphuricum* is among the medicines most frequently prescribed and is often helpful for symptoms of Ménières disease, such as dizziness with ringing in the ears and deafness. *Tabacum* may be helpful for labyrinthitis, symptoms of which include severe dizziness, nausea, vomiting and cold sweats. *Gelsemium* may also be useful in treating this condition when the nausea is less severe but the patient feels weak and tremulous. *Theridion* is rarely used in general but is helpful for vertigo, associated with the rare symptom of extreme sensitivity to noise, which seems to go right through the patient.

VERTIGO IN OLDER PEOPLE *Conium*, *Baryta carbonicum* and *Phosphorus* are medicines often indicated for older people who have vertigo associated with circulatory problems. *Conium* is appropriate when people find that their vertigo is worse while lying down or from any movement of the head. *Baryta carbonicum* is suggested when vertigo is associated with difficulty in thinking and poor memory. There may also be hard, swollen glands, particularly in the neck, and cold feet.

Phosphorus will generally be prescribed on "whole person" grounds, when symptoms include great tiredness that is temporarily improved by rest, along with easy bruising and generally easy bleeding (for example nosebleeds). *Phosphorus* may also be indicated where there is anxiety with phobias and excessive sensitivity both to the physical and human environment. It is associated with emotional changeability.

Acupuncture

Acupuncture has been used quite consistently as a treatment for dizziness and vertigo, particularly if the dizziness is associated with problems in the neck. There are case reports, but unfortunately no good-quality clinical trials which attest to the fact that acupuncture may be of real value in this condition.

Bodywork Therapies

EASING SPINAL RESTRICTIONS A chiropractor or osteopath may be able to ease underlying spinal restrictions. Dizziness that derives from neck problems is characterised by feelings of unsteadiness when walking or standing, and is usually made worse by turning the neck. Causes include restriction of circulation, nerve irritation, or the brain receiving contradictory messages from the tiny nerve structures about the position different parts of the body are in and the movements taking place.

Ménière's disease, which involves dizziness, may sometimes be the result of irritation of nerves in the neck. One research study examined 235 people with symptoms of dizziness following neck injuries. In early 50 per cent symptoms could be brought on by keeping their head still, while they turned their body, so producing rotation of the neck. Almost all 112

THE EPLEY PROCEDURE

The Epley procedure, which is used to treat benign positional vertigo, was developed by Dr John Epley to reposition calcium debris in the inner ear, which can cause vertigo. Tiny calcium crystals, known as canaliths, are usually attached to the base of the semicircular canals in the inner ear. These crystals may become detached, for unknown reasons, and move through the canals, causing a sensation of dizziness when the head moves. The Epley procedure repositions the canaliths back to the base of the canals. Shown here is a modified version for self-help use.

1. Sit on the edge of a bed. Turn your head to the side on which nystagmus (involuntary eye movement) has occurred.

2. Keeping your head turned, lower yourself backwards until you are lying on the bed. This can sometimes trigger the nystagmus.

patients were found to have specific restrictions between the vertebrae of the neck, mainly the part just underneath the skull where it joins the upper neck. After an average of 18 treatments, 101 of these people were symptom-free and a further six had much reduced levels of dizziness. Out of the original group, only five had symptoms that had not improved.

CHIROPRACTIC If dizziness begins after a neck injury (such as a fall or a road accident), try consulting an osteopath or chiropractor. Good results have been achieved using chiropractic manipulation with large groups of people whose vertigo started after a neck injury such as whiplash. Chiropractic can also help dizziness caused by chronic tension in the neck.

CRANIOSACRAL THERAPY AND CRANIAL OSTEOPATHY practitioners maintain that their gentle manipulation of the head and neck achieves good results in many cases of vertigo; however, there are no research studies to back these claims.

Breathing Retraining

A typical effect of rapid and shallow upper-chest breathing (hyperventilation), commonly triggered by stress or anxiety, is elimination of too much carbon dioxide from the body. This can cause the blood to become too alkaline, which in turn makes the smooth muscle layer around the blood vessels contract, causing dizziness.

Another effect of increased alkalinity is the Bohr effect, in which the red blood cells that carry oxygen to the brain (and to other body tissues) release oxygen less readily than usual. This combination of reduced blood supply and poor oxygen release can starve the brain of oxygen, leading to dizziness and other symptoms.

Breathing-pattern disorders that lead to this situation can usually be improved or corrected by breathing rehabilitation, involving slow, diaphragmatic (yoga-type) breathing methods (see p.62), as well as by correction of restrictions that may have developed in overused and stressed muscles and joints. These restrictions tend to reinforce any abnormal breathing pattern that has developed, and, in order to resolve the problem, it is important to treat both.

Mind–Body Therapies

Vertigo can be difficult to treat due to the often subjective nature of dizziness, the frequent failure of drugs to alleviate the condition and the complicating psychological factors. However, relaxation techniques can be useful in combating underlying stress and may also help people who are prone to panic attacks, of which dizziness is a common component.

Dizziness is not uncommon after a road accident, especially if the incident was frightening or involved loss of consciousness. If your dizziness began with a traumatic experience, consider trying psychological treatments as well as bodywork, because the mind as well as the body needs treatment after sudden, shocking events.

RELAXATION and other psychological therapies were used to treat a 26-year-old woman who had debilitating dizzy spells after a mild head injury sustained in a car accident. A nine-week behavioural treatment included biofeedback-assisted relaxation training, psychological counselling, gaze-fixation practice, desensitisation exercises, and generalisation training. Following treatment, the woman reported a 90 per cent reduction in dizzy spells and was fully able to resume independent activities.

PREVENTION PLAN

If you are prone to dizziness:

- Avoid triggers as much as possible.
- Eat regular meals.
- Do regular yoga or diaphragmatic breathing exercises.
- Avoid standing still for long periods.

---

3. After waiting for 30 seconds, turn your head carefully and slowly to the opposite side (your "good" side). Wait another 30 seconds.

4. Keeping your head very still, use your arms to lever yourself up slowly from the bed into a sitting position.

5. Sit for a minute on the edge of the bed looking downwards. This helps the crystals in the ear to settle.

MULTIPLE SCLEROSIS

In multiple sclerosis (MS), nerves in the brain and the spinal cord are progressively damaged, causing a range of symptoms that can affect feeling, movement, bodily functions and balance. Symptoms and their severity differ from person to person. Multiple sclerosis is more common in the northern hemisphere and tends to develop between early adulthood and middle age. Although there is no cure, treatment might include drugs to ease symptoms and improve functioning, as well as dietary changes, chiropractic, acupuncture and homeopathy.

WHAT ARE THE SYMPTOMS?

The symptoms of MS vary according to which parts of the brain and spinal cord are affected and may include:

- Blurred vision
- Numbness or tingling anywhere in the body
- Fatigue, which may be persistent
- Weakness and a feeling of heaviness in the limbs
- Coordination and balance problems, including vertigo (a sensation of moving or rotating)
- Slurred speech
- Stiff movement of the limbs (spasticity)
- Tremor

WHY MIGHT I HAVE THIS?

PREDISPOSING FACTORS

- Living in the northern hemisphere
- Having a close relative with MS
- Diet high in saturated fat
- Smoking
- Exposure to organic solvents
- Exposure to heavy metals
- Exposure to pesticides and herbicides

WHY DOES IT OCCUR?

Many nerves in the brain and spinal cord have a sheath of fatty material called myelin, which acts as insulation. In MS, small areas of myelin are damaged, leaving holes in the sheath (demyelination). Nerve impulses are not conducted normally, causing a wide range of symptoms that affect sensation, movement, body functions and balance. Eventually, the damaged areas of myelin are replaced by scar tissue. Evidence suggests that MS is an autoimmune disorder, in which the body's immune system produces antibodies (substances that normally only attack foreign bodies) against its own tissues.

It is thought that MS may be triggered by factors such as a viral infection in childhood in genetically susceptible people. There is also some evidence that the development of the disease may be related to an intake of certain dietary fats, but no definite trigger has been identified.

There are two types of MS. In the first type, symptoms may be intermittent, alternating with long periods with no symptoms (remission). This type of MS is "relapsing–remitting". Other people have chronic symptoms that become progressively worse. This type is known as "chronic–progressive". Relapsing–remitting MS may become chronic–progressive over time.

Symptoms may occur singly early on in the disorder and together as it progresses. Depression is common and memory may be affected. Eventually, there may be muscle spasms and poor mobility.

IMPORTANT

If you think you may have MS, consult a doctor without delay.

TREATMENT PLAN

PRIMARY TREATMENTS

- Corticosteroids, interferon-beta, immunosuppressants (*see Drugs to treat relapses*)
- The Swank diet

BACK-UP TREATMENTS

- Drugs for fatigue, depression and other symptoms
- Physiotherapy
- Emotional support
- Omega-3 fatty acids
- Nutritional supplements

WORTH CONSIDERING

- Homeopathy
- Environmental health measures
- Acupuncture
- T'ai chi
- Bodywork therapies
- Cognitive behavioural therapy

For an explanation of how treatments are rated, see p.111.

DAMAGE TO NERVES IN MULTIPLE SCLEROSIS

Nerve cells, or neurons, transmit and receive nerve impulses. As well as having nuclei and other features common to all cells, neurons have long projections. Some are called dendrites, and others are known as nerve fibres (or axons). These fibres link the neuron to other neurons or cells and carry nerve signals, often forming long communication chains in the body. Some nerve fibres are covered in a fatty substance called myelin, which helps to speed up the transmission of nerve impulses. If this myelin sheath is damaged, as occurs in MS, nerve impulses along the fibre are slowed or stopped.

In MS areas of demyelination develop. Nerve impulses are not conducted normally across nerve fibres, leading to symptoms such as blurred vision and poor balance.

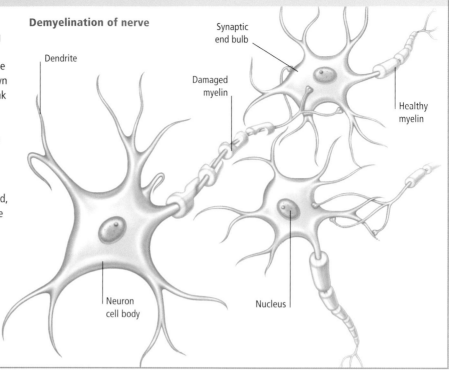

Demyelination of nerve

Dendrite

Synaptic end bulb

Damaged myelin

Healthy myelin

Neuron cell body

Nucleus

TREATMENTS IN DETAIL

Conventional Medicine

The doctor will arrange for tests, such as magnetic resonance imaging (MRI) of the brain and spinal cord to look for areas of demyelination. Drug treatments for MS can be divided into two main groups: those that aim to reduce the severity or frequency of relapses in relapsing–remitting MS and those that aim to relieve specific symptoms. Research is in progress into the use of cannabinoids to relieve some MS symptoms, such as spasticity and tremor.

PRIMARY TREATMENT **DRUGS TO TREAT RELAPSES** Intravenous or oral corticosteroids may be given as short courses to reduce the severity of symptoms during relapses. These drugs reduce inflammation, which has a role in demyelination. Short courses of corticosteroids should not cause any significant or long-term side-effects. Interferon-beta given by injection may be prescribed in some cases and may reduce the number of relapses, as may immunosuppressants drugs, such as azathioprine, and other medications including glatiramer acetate.

DRUGS FOR SYMPTOMS Many types of medication are available to treat symptoms. For example, the drug amantadine may help with fatigue and antidepressants may be recommended for depression. Drugs that act on the muscles of the bladder, such as oxybutinin, may be given to relieve bladder symptoms. Treatments for impotence include sildenafil. Muscle spasms may be relieved by muscle-relaxant drugs, such as baclofen.

PHYSIOTHERAPY may be recommended, to improve mobility and help relieve muscle spasms if they occur. If movement is affected, occupational health practitioners can offer advice on the many aids available. They can also advise on other measures to help with everyday living, for example, cooking, sleeping and bathing facilities can be adapted so that a high degree of independence can be maintained.

EMOTIONAL SUPPORT is extremely important for people with MS and their families in the long term. An affected individual's healthcare team will help to provide this, and there are support groups and organisations that can also offer both practical and emotional assistance (*see p.486*).

CAUTION

Drugs for multiple sclerosis can cause a range of possible side-effects: ask your doctor to explain these to you.

Nutritional Therapy

OMEGA-3 FATTY ACIDS, such as those found in oily fish, appear to be protective. This type of fat may be important through its modulation of the inflammatory and immune processes. Inflammation in the blood vessels of the brain may be an underlying feature of multiple sclerosis. The omega-3 fatty acids EPA and DHA, which are found in abundance in oily fish, can be made into anti-inflammatory chemicals in the body. By contrast, arachidonic acid, which is an omega-6 fatty acid found in foods such as red meat, eggs, liver and kidneys, can be made into chemicals that have an inflammatory effect. One study found that people who eat more red meat, which is rich in arachidonic acid, have higher rates of MS. If you have MS, you may wish to eat more oily fish and less red meat. Some people with MS have been found to be deficient in the omega-3 fatty acids EPA and DHA. Fish oil supplements, which are rich in EPA and DHA, may be useful for people with MS. If you have MS, you may wish to take about 350mg per day of EPA and 250mg per day of DHA. Taking 1–2g concentrated fish oils each day will provide good levels of EPA and DHA.

PRIMARY TREATMENT **THE SWANK DIET** There is some evidence that the sooner the Swank diet is started in MS, the less risk there is of significant disability. Dr Roy Swank studied the effect of a low-fat diet in 150 patients with MS between 1949 and 1984. The diet restricted saturated fat to

The further you live from the equator (in either direction), the greater your risk of having MS

20g per day and eliminated partially hydrogenated fats, such as margarine and many processed fats. People were given healthy fats in the form of cod-liver oil (5g per day) and vegetable oils (10–40g per day). Compared to untreated individuals, those who kept strictly to this regime deteriorated less. The treated group also had better survival rates, with about 70 per cent surviving over the study period compared to only 20 per cent in the untreated group.

NUTRITIONAL SUPPLEMENTS Taking a high-potency multivitamin and mineral supplement each day may help those with MS. There is evidence to suggest that calcium, magnesium, selenium, vitamin D, vitamin E, vitamin B12 and other B vitamins may be important in MS.

> **CAUTION**
>
> Consult your doctor before taking fish oil supplements, magnesium or calcium because they can interfere with certain medications. (*For more information, see p.46.*)

Homeopathy

There has not been any scientific research into the homeopathic treatment of MS, but a number of case reports show that it can create an improvement in symptoms or,

apparently, even in the underlying disease itself. Because the condition can be so variable, individualised treatment from a trained homeopathic practitioner is required (*see p.73*) and the condition is not suitable for self-help.

PHOSPHORUS may be helpful in MS, particularly if blurred vision or vertigo are problems. People who respond to this homeopathic remedy usually feel very tired and may catnap. They may also have numbness or altered sensation, particularly burning sensations in the hands, feet and elsewhere. They are often thirsty, especially for cold, refreshing drinks, and may also crave salty foods. They tend to be nervous and oversensitive.

SILICEA AND NATRUM MURIATICUM are other constitutional medicines (i.e. they match the person' constitutional type, *see p.73*) that may help.

People who respond to the remedy *Silicea* typically are thin, pale and chilly but have sweaty, cold hands and feet. A very characteristic feature of these people is weak nails, often with lengthwise ridging. Affected people often say that their nails became weak and their hair thinner and finer around the time they fell ill. They seem to pick up infections easily and are slow to recover. Mentally, they are timid, although they may be stubborn and push themselves to exhaustion if they have decided to do something.

In people who respond to *Nat. mur.* it is not uncommon to find that the problem seems to have been triggered by mental stress, for instance an unhappy relationship or bereavement, but it is very typical of these patients that they try to avoid discussing their inner feelings.

MEDICINES TO RELIEVE SYMPTOMS *Nux vomica* or *Ignatia* may be useful for the painful spasms, usually in the legs, which may occur in MS and are sometimes triggered by quite trivial stimuli or even have

no apparent stimulus. The person who responds to *Nux vomica* tends to be bad-tempered and often has indigestion. The *Ignatia* patient is nervous, sometimes to the point of being hysterical. *Equisetum* may help with bladder control, *Gelsemium* with double vision and tremor and *Conium* with vertigo.

> **CAUTION**
>
> Coffee may interfere with the action of *Ignatia*, avoid it if you are using this remedy.

Environmental Health

GEOGRAPHICAL DISTRIBUTION The view that the environment has a bearing on MS is supported by population studies showing that the disease occurs in clusters. The geographical distribution of MS is not random. Cases of the disease increase as latitude increases (in both directions), even in ethnically homogeneous countries. The northern portion of the US, northern and central Europe, and New Zealand are among the high-risk regions for the development of the disease. When people move from an area of low MS risk to an area of high risk, they automatically become at high risk of MS. It is likely that something in the environment, perhaps combined with a genetic predisposition, causes MS.

Environmental triggers proposed for MS are many and include viral infections, smoking, injuries, lack of sunshine, heavy metals, anaesthesia, psychological stress, organic solvents and artificial sweeteners. However, it has so far been impossible to assign specific causes to a disease that has so many different presentations and has a genetic component as well. In the absence of carefully controlled studies, we are left with epidemiological studies and some specific avoidance advice.

INFECTIONS There is strong evidence that viral infections act as triggers for MS flare-ups. People with MS are twice as likely to experience an acute flare-up following an upper respiratory infection, and this risk is more than threefold in people who have a high level of antibodies to viruses in their bloodstream. Bacterial infections may also play a role in causing relapses in MS. If you have MS you should avoid such exposure as much as possible. This means avoiding crowded, confined places during outbreaks of flu and respiratory disease. Most importantly, wash your hands frequently and avoid touching your face.

SMOKING Smoking has been associated with a transient worsening of MS symptoms, and if you have MS you should not smoke. Many studies show a strong association between smoking and the development of MS as well. There are no studies examining the role of second-hand smoke, but if you have MS, it would be wise to avoid all exposure to smoke.

CHEMICAL SOLVENTS Exposure to certain chemical solvents has been proposed as a trigger for MS, but the evidence is controversial. There have been over a dozen studies in the past decade that have suggested a relationship between solvents and the development of MS, but many occupational exposure studies have not shown any MS clusters in people such as painters, printers and carpenters whose jobs involve high exposure to organic solvents. However, if you have MS you should avoid exposure to all toxic solvents, including household cleaning chemicals, paints, petrol, and other solvents.

contain lead), and some calcium supplements (which, like gelatin, may contain lead from bones).

PESTICIDES AND HERBICIDES Many compounds used in pesticides and herbicides sold for domestic gardens can be toxic to the nervous system. Do not use these chemicals in your garden or walk where they have recently been applied.

SUN EXPOSURE Exposure to sunlight has been examined in relation to MS ever since the geographical distribution was noticed. In people with MS, it seems that higher sun exposure is linked to a decreased risk of death. Some researchers feel that this protective effect of sunlight is due to increases in vitamin D production, since sunlight is necessary for the body to make vitamin D. People with MS who have higher levels of vitamin D have fewer MS lesions on MRI scans. Studies on animals with MS-like diseases also show improvements with vitamin D treatments.

If you have MS, try taking a daily vitamin D supplement and make sure you go outside in the sunshine every day. However, limit your sun exposure to 15–20 minutes daily (without sunscreen) to protect against skin cancer.

Practitioners attempt to restore the normal curves of the spine, especially those of the neck area, to prevent mechanical stresses to the spinal cord from aggravating the symptoms of MS. However, research evidence is so far limited to a few case studies.

MASSAGE has been shown in several small research studies to be helpful in treating various aspects of MS. In one study, patients who were massaged had significantly improved levels of self-esteem, better body-image and enhanced social functioning, although there did not appear to be any improvement in neurological symptoms. In another study, massage appeared to improve well-being and mood in people with MS, while helping to reduce tension and fatigue.

REFLEXOLOGY is recommended on the basis of some randomised controlled trials. In one study, over 70 people with MS were divided into two groups, one receiving reflexology and the other just massage of the calf. The reflexology group showed significant improvement in the amount of control they had over their muscles as well as increased bladder control. In another study, 14 people with MS received a one-hour reflexology treatment every week, while 12 acted as a control group. After 18 weeks those patients in the treatment group experienced some improvements in 45 per cent of their symptoms.

T'AI CHI The gentle flowing movements of t'ai chi can help to control MS symptoms. When a group of people with MS did t'ai chi, symptoms such as depression, problems with balance and walking, muscle spasms and bladder control all improved.

Mind–Body Therapies

COGNITIVE BEHAVIOURAL THERAPY shows promise in the treatment of MS. Stress is known to be a factor that makes MS symptoms worse. Relaxation or meditation exercises may help (*see p.99*), but cognitive behavioural methods may be even more effective. In a small 2002 study, MS patients using a cognitive behavioural programme to improve their coping skills developed fewer MS-related brain lesions. Ask your caregiver about these methods and their suitability for you.

> Sclerosis means scars. In MS, scars in the brain and on nerve fibres interrupt nerve transmission

HEAVY METALS Exposure to heavy metals, such as mercury, seems to play a role in the development of the disease, according to studies into MS clusters. Some researchers believe that exposure to heavy metals in the soil is responsible for the geographic variation in MS cases. This has been used as an argument to link mercury in amalgam dental fillings with MS, a theory that has not been supported by any meaningful research. It is not neccesary to remove fillings, but it may help to have your drinking water tested and install a purifying system if the heavy metal content is high (this is especially important if you use water from a well). Limit or avoid tuna, shark and swordfish (which often contain high levels of methylmercury), gelatin (which may

Acupuncture

There is no evidence that acupuncture will alter the course or severity of MS. However, neuralgia-like pain (*see p.124*) is common in MS, and acupuncture can be used to provide pain relief, although no clinical trials have been done to study its use in this specific condition. Acupuncture may only work for a short time, and treatment may need to be repeated frequently.

Bodywork and Movement Therapies

CHIROPRACTIC Chiropractors claim that spinal restrictions can play a part in aggravating many of the symptoms of MS.

- Long-term pain anywhere in the body

WHY MIGHT I HAVE THIS?

PREDISPOSING FACTORS

- An infection, injury or other cause, even if it has healed
- Being depressed (states of mind and other mind–body issues can affect perception of pain)

PERSISTENT PAIN

Acute (sudden) pain is the body's warning signal that something specific is wrong. Persistent (chronic) pain is defined as pain lasting for six months or longer. It may be the result of chronic inflammation, as occurs in some kinds of arthritis, or nerve damage. However, persistent pain may also derive from a complex problem involving both mind and body, when the nervous system begins to generate pain signals even though no underlying physical cause is involved. Mind–body therapies are important to treatment, along with painkillers and acupuncture.

WHY DOES IT OCCUR?

The sensation of pain can stem from injury, infection and many other causes. Some of the most common causes of pain include injuries, rheumatoid arthritis (*see p.293*), osteoarthritis (*see p.289*), back problems (*see p.268*) and neuralgia (*see p.124*). Sometimes pain is perceived in the wrong area of the body. In angina, for example, pain signals from the heart travel up the sensory nerves of the spinal cord together with signals from the left arm. The brain becomes confused and senses pain in an unexpected part of the body (the left arm, neck or jaw).

PERSISTENT PAIN AND "GATE CONTROL"
In some cases it is not possible to identify an underlying cause for chronic pain and

there is often no clear explanation for why some pain persists even after the disease or condition that triggered it has healed. However, persistent pain syndromes are very real and incapacitating to those who develop them, having a devastating effect on work and relationships. Persistent pain is increasingly viewed as a disorder in its own right instead of a symptom of an underlying cause.

According to the "gate control" theory, nerve impulses travelling from the body via the spinal cord to pain receptors in the brain can be influenced by nerve cells in the spinal cord that behave like gates. By shutting or opening these "gates", the brain is able either to magnify or to reduce pain signals. Chemicals called endorphins are the body's natural painkillers. They work by slotting into receptors located in the

TREATMENT PLAN

PRIMARY TREATMENTS

- Treatment of underlying cause where possible
- Painkillers (for short-term use)
- Other drugs to relieve pain, such as NSAIDs
- Physical treatments, e.g. TENS
- Psychological treatments, e.g. counselling

BACK-UP TREATMENTS

- Corticosteroid injections for joint pain
- Opioid drugs for intractable pain
- Nerve blocks for severe pain
- Antidepressants

WORTH CONSIDERING

- Fish oil supplements
- Tryptophan
- Acupuncture
- Bodywork and movement therapies
- Exercise
- Meditation
- Cognitive behavioural therapy

For an explanation of how treatments are rated, see p.111.

IMPORTANT

If you experience persistent pain, see your doctor to determine any underlying cause and for help with managing the pain.

brain, spinal cord and nerve endings, where they block pain impulses. How wide the pain gates open and how much pain information reaches the brain depends partly on the quantity of endorphins that are circulating in the body.

The spinal cord's pain gates can be shut by nerve impulses travelling down from the brain, or conversely, they can be opened by messages from the brain. A wide-open pain gate results in pain even if nerves coming to the spinal cord are not sending in any pain messages.

TOLERANCE of pain varies, partly due to an individual's psychological state. This is because emotional states modify the levels of endorphins in the body. The effect of psychological state on perception of pain explains why athletes who are injured in competition are often able to carry on regardless or how soldiers are sometimes able to fight on in the heat of battle despite devastating injury. Pain is perceived as being worse when people are depressed, and better when they are distracted by something enjoyable.

How someone interprets pain and any ideas they may have about it and its consequences affect pain tolerance. Past experiences and associations with pain, along with general life stresses, also play a part in perception and tolerance of pain.

VICIOUS CIRCLE People with chronic pain often tend to become sedentary. This is unfortunate because the painkilling endorphins released by exercise would reduce their fear and depression. Lack of activity also weakens and shortens muscles and causes them to become tense, creating muscle spasms and more pain. This pain–tension cycle can cause deepening depression, helplessness and lower pain tolerance. People in pain also tend to overbreathe, which makes the muscles prone to spasm and alters the way nerve impulses are transmitted to the brain.

HYPERSENSITIVITY Continual pain can make a pain pathway more sensitive to pain impulses, long after the original cause of the pain has been healed. Psychological states are known to directly affect the body: in one experiment, just thinking about painful experiences caused the back muscles of people who complained of

---

USING TENS FOR PAIN RELIEF

Transcutaneous electrical nerve stimulation (TENS) is a technique that is used to help relieve pain. The TENS unit produces minute electrical impulses that pass into the body via electrode pads that are attached to the skin. The pulses are supposed to interrupt the pathways along which pain signals travel and prevent them from reaching the brain, where they are registered as pain. Here a TENS unit is being used on the knee. TENS is frequently used to relieve pain during labour.

---

chronic back pain to become tense. By expecting the worst when a migraine begins, people who have regular migraines may tighten muscles and restrict blood flow, thereby making the attack longer and more severe.

SELF-HELP

The following measures may help to reduce pain and improve well-being:

- Keep a diary to record episodes of pain in order to be able to better identify factors that make it better or worse.
- Avoid becoming tired and take plenty of rest each day.
- Take regular aerobic exercise such as walking, swimming or tennis, as well as yoga or stretching to prevent muscles from becoming stiff.
- Do meditation or relaxation exercises (*see p.98*) every day.
- Take fish-oil supplements (*see below*).
- Make time for friends and family as well as for enjoyable hobbies and activities that distract you and lift your mood.
- Have regular relaxing massages.

TREATMENTS IN DETAIL

Conventional Medicine

PRIMARY TREATMENT **TREATING THE UNDERLYING CAUSE** Your doctor will arrange various investigations to look for an underlying cause of persistent pain, which will be treated if possible. Various measures may be helpful in treating persistent pain, and there is ongoing research into potential new treatments. For example, research shows that cannabis may relieve muscle pain in multiple sclerosis, although prescribing it remains a controversial issue in most countries. You may also be referred to a local pain specialist or to a multidisciplinary pain clinic, if there is one available in your area, where experts in pain management can help to reduce pain levels and restore your normal function and well-being.

PRIMARY TREATMENT **PAIN-RELIEVING DRUGS** Various pain-relieving drugs are available, ranging from mild analgesics to some powerful opiate drugs. Non-steroidal anti-inflammatory drugs (NSAIDs) are also helpful in some cases, for example in joint pain caused by inflammation.

Even though they are not primarily prescribed for pain, some drugs relieve certain types of pain in addition to their primary action. Such drugs include the antidepressant amitriptyline and the anticonvulsant carbamazepine, both of which may be used to treat the pain of neuralgia.

INJECTIONS AND NERVE BLOCKS Corticosteroid injections into joints may help relieve pain in certain joint diseases, such as osteoarthritis. Nerve blocks are another option for certain types of chronic pain. For example, epidurals, in which a local anaesthetic is injected into the space around the membranes enveloping the spinal cord, may offer temporary relief for back pain. Very severe pain arising from surgery or serious injury may be treated with opioid injections. These drugs are not prescribed for long-term use due to their addictive properties, but the opiods morphine and diamorphine (heroin) may be prescribed lfor the intractable pain of some cancers and other conditions.

PRIMARY TREATMENT **PHYSICAL TREAMENTS** Various physical treatments are available to help relieve pain, including acupuncture, massage and ultrasound therapy. In transcutaneous electrical nerve stimulation (TENS), electrical impulses are relayed from a portable impulse generator to electrodes stuck to the skin in the painful area. They are left in place usually for about 30 minutes. TENS treatment may relieve persistent pain, such as chronic back pain, for several hours.

PRIMARY TREATMENT **PSYCHOLOGICAL HELP** Pain is stressful, and your doctor may suggest counselling to help you cope. Cognitive behavioural therapy may be especially helpful. In addition there are organisations (*see p.486*) that can offer emotional support and advice. Antidepressants may be prescribed for the depression that often accompanies persistent pain.

> **CAUTION**
>
> Drugs for persistent pain can cause a range of possible side-effects: ask your doctor to explain them to you.

Nutritional Therapy

FISH OIL SUPPLEMENTS Pain associated with inflammation may be helped by supplementation with omega-3 fatty acids. A diet rich in omega-6 polyunsaturated fatty acids (found in vegetable oils and fast foods) and relatively lacking in omega-3 fatty acids (found in oily fish such as trout, sardines and salmon) seems to promote inflammation and pain.

Supplementation with omega-3 fatty acids has been shown in studies to reduce inflammatory processes and pain in the body. The omega-3 fatty acids EPA and DHA at doses of 378mg per day of EPA and 259mg per day of DHA for at least two months have been used in other studies to reduce inflammation. Omega-3 fatty acids can be found in some nuts and seeds and in oily fish such as salmon, mackerel, trout and sardines. Including these foods in the diet may help to control pain. Taking 1–3g of fish oil each day is likely to help persistent pain also.

TRYPTOPHAN The amino acid tryptophan is required for the release of the substance beta-endorphin, which is one of the body's natural pain-relieving compounds. Tryptophan is also needed for the production of serotonin, a brain chemical that may reduce a tendency to sense pain. Supple-

mentation with tryptophan may be able to change the body's pain threshold so that pain is not sensed so readily. Tryptophan exists naturally in foods such as meat, tofu, almonds, peanuts and pumpkin and sesame seeds. Tryptophan supplements are not available over the counter in many countries, including the UK and the US. However, 5-hydroxytryptophan (5-HTP), which is a substance that tryptophan is converted into before it is made into serotonin, is a good alternative. If you want to see if 5-HTP will benefit you, take 50mg two or three times a day.

> **CAUTION**
>
> Consult your doctor befor taking fish oil supplements because they can interfere with certain medications (*see p.46*).

Acupuncture

Acupuncture is often used by multidisciplinary pain teams to treat unexplained pain and appears to be an effective treatment. It is said to work by stimulating the release of endorphins and "closing pain gates" by stimulating nerve fibres that block pain. It may also be helpful in relieving the anxiety and depression that accompanies long-term pain. It is very

Acupuncture has a good track record for treating unexplained persistent pain. Fine needles are inserted (here on the Kidney meridian). The needles stimulate nerve fibres and block pain impulses from reaching the brain.

possible to manage persistent pain using acupuncture, but since persistent pain is not in itself a diagnosis, it is almost impossible for clinical trials to provide evidence in this area.

Almost all acupuncture techniques have been used at some point to treat persistent pain and there is no real evidence to suggest which approaches are best, but it is

local anaesthetic injection and acupuncture. Releasing trigger points allows the circulation to be restored to tense muscles.

HYDROTHERAPY can be both relaxing and invigorating, helping to improve the circulation. There are a number of forms of hydrotherapy, from exercising in heated swimming pools to applying cold com-

level of pain you will tend to experience. These and a body of other findings provide very strong support for using psychological approaches to control chronic pain that is not cancer-related.

MINDFULNESS MEDITATION One of the most innovative studies of the therapy of "mindfulness" meditation was undertaken by Dr Jon Kabat-Zinn and his colleagues at the University of Massachusetts School of Medicine in the US. Patients with chronic pain were trained in this form of meditation as part of a 10-week stress-reduction and relaxation programme. The people in the study found that, using this technique, they could ignore "present-moment pain". They also found that their other symptoms, such as depression and negative body image, improved. At the same time, use of pain-relieving drugs decreased and activity levels and feelings of self-esteem increased. Improvements were mostly maintained for up to 15 months after the initial mediation training and many of the participants continued the meditation practice as part of their daily lives.

Five out of six people with chronic pain take painkillers, but 70 per cent still have pain

clear that it is worth persisting with treatment over a month or two to see if pain relief can be obtained. Further treatment may be required if some, but not complete, pain relief is achieved.

Bodywork and Movement Therapies

MANIPULATION THERAPIES Easing pain that arises from the central nervous system may require surgical or other interventions, such as nerve blocks (injections, *see Conventional Medicine, left*), that aim to interrupt the transmission of pain signals. This is especially true if pain is extreme and/or long-standing.

However, if pain stems from a peripheral source, such as nerves in an arm or leg, some manual therapies (such as neuromuscular therapy, osteopathic soft-tissue manipulation, and so forth) may be able to alter the mechanism that is giving rise to the pain either through manipulation or soft-tissue treatment or a combination of both. Practitioners, through teaching certain breathing rehabilitiation and relaxation methods, can also help patients to reduce their general sensitivity to pain.

DEACTIVATION OF TRIGGER POINTS The researchers Wall and Melzack have shown that, whatever other factors are involved, all chronic pain involves trigger points in muscles. They are a factor in the continuing painful state and may even be the primary cause of the pain. Trigger points (particularly sensitive areas in the muscles, *see p.55*) can be eliminated by various means, including soft-tissue manipulation,

presses to the painful area. There have been various studies of therapies using water, particularly involving supervised exercises in seawater known as balneotherapy, as a means of relieving general chronic pain. The hydrostatic force of the water is considered to help bring about pain relief. Balneotherapy is often prescribed for people with psoriatic or rheumatoid arthritis, and can significantly help to relieve pain and improve general functioning.

Exercise

Pain can make people reluctant to exercise, but this should be resisted since lack of activity weakens, tenses and shortens muscles, which can in turn create more pain. It is easy to fall into a vicious circle. Taking gentle exercise each day, such as walking, cycling or swimming, as your condition allows, helps to promote the release of endorphins, improve sleep, relieve depression and reduce the perception of pain. Start slowly and remember to work within your limitations. A doctor or physiotherapist may be able to advise on suitable activities. As well as aerobic forms of exercise, gentle yoga or stretching at home may be therapeutic.

Mind–Body Therapies

A 1994 study showed that there is a strong link between someone's "control belief" and their experience of pain. This means the more you believe you can influence or control your symptoms, the less pain you are likely to experience. Specifically, the higher your control belief, the lower the

COGNITIVE BEHAVIOURAL THERAPY A major 1999 review looked at the effectiveness of certain psychological therapies for persistent chronic pain. Psychological treatments, such as cognitive behavioural therapy (CBT), were associated with significant physical and psychological improvement in people who participated in the studies. The review concluded that active psychological treatments based on the principle of behavioural therapy are very effective in managing persistent chronic pain. If you have chronic pain (whatever the cause), try talking to your doctor about the possibility of having CBT. Also try spending 20 minutes each day doing relaxation exercises or meditation (*see p.98*). In addition, you could also learn biofeedback techniques (*see p.100*) which are another useful technique for pain relief.

PREVENTION PLAN

See your doctor if you begin to experience persistent pain. Many people put off having treatment for their condition, and delay can make the problem worse.

WHAT ARE THE SYMPTOMS?

Symptoms often develop rapidly over seconds or minutes. The exact symptoms depend on the area of the brain affected, but may include:

- Weakness or inability to move on one side of the body
- Numbness on one side of the body
- Tremor and clumsiness
- Blurred vision or loss of vision in one eye
- Very severe headache, possibly at the back of the head
- Difficulty in speaking or understanding what is said
- Vomiting, loss of balance and vertigo (feeling of dizziness)
- Unconsciousness

WHY MIGHT I HAVE THIS?

PREDISPOSING FACTORS

- High blood pressure
- Smoking
- Being over 70
- Sedentary lifestyle
- Obesity
- Diet high in saturated fat
- Raised homocysteine levels
- Atrial fibrillation (an abnormal heart rhythm)
- Diabetes mellitus

STROKE

Damage to the brain caused by an interruption of its blood supply is known as a stroke. It may occur due to a blockage or a leak in one of the arteries that supply the brain. Stroke is more common over in those over 70 and affects more men than women. Smoking and a diet high in saturated fat are risk factors for stroke, as is having high blood pressure. Rehabilitation and prevention of further strokes might incorporate various approaches, including dietary and lifestyle changes, drugs, and speech, occupational and physiotherapy.

WHY DOES IT OCCUR?

Most strokes are due either to cerebral thrombosis, in which a blood clot forms in an artery in the brain, or to cerebral embolism, when a fragment of a blood clot that has formed elsewhere travels to the brain. Blood clots are more likely to form in arteries damaged by atherosclerosis, a condition in which fatty deposits build up in the lining of the arteries. In this sense, the disease is generally similar in cause to coronary artery disease (*see p.252*).

About 10 per cent of strokes result from cerebral haemorrhage, which occurs when an artery in the brain ruptures, leaking blood into the brain tissue. In some cases, the underlying cause is an aneurysm, a tiny bulge in the blood vessel.

Strokes caused by a cerebral haemorrhage tend to be more serious and are often accompanied by a very severe headache. In the type known as subarachnoid haemorrhage, the first symptom is usually a headache, which comes on sud-

IMPORTANT

If someone develops any of the symptoms of a stroke (*see left*), call an ambulance immediately.

denly and is often felt at the back of the head. Haemorrhagic strokes are more likely than other types to result in loss of consciousness and to be life-threatening.

If the symptoms of a stroke disappear in 24 hours, the condition is known as a transient ischaemic attack (TIA), which may be a warning sign of susceptibility to a future stroke. However, in most cases strokes come on without warning. TIAs usually result from tiny emboli (blood clot framents) that block narrowed blood vessels. Other causes include reduced blood flow through carotid arteries (in the neck) that have been narrowed by atherosclerosis.

The after-effects of a stroke vary greatly in their severity (*see box, p.151*). They range from mild, temporary symptoms,

TREATMENT PLAN

PRIMARY TREATMENTS

- Giving up smoking (*see Self-help right*)
- Treatment of underlying cause, e.g. high blood pressure
- Aspirin, anticoagulants and other drugs
- Carotid endarterectomy and other surgery
- Rehabilitation
- Treadmill walking

BACK-UP TREATMENTS

- Nutritional therapy
- Physiotherapy

WORTH CONSIDERING

- Acupuncture
- EMG biofeedback

For an explanation of how treatments are rated, see p.111.

This X-ray shows an aneurysm (balloon-like swelling) in the carotid artery. If an aneurysm in the brain ruptures, cerebral haemorrhage and stroke result.

such as localised muscle weakness, to permanent disability, loss of speech and cognition and even death. In some cases, people who have had a stroke develop dementia (*see p.133*). Most treatment aims to prevent further strokes.

SELF-HELP

If you have had a stroke:
- Do not smoke.
- Eat a diet rich in fruit, vegetables and oily fish and low in fat (*see p.44*).
- Take exercise on a regular basis.
- Watch your weight.
- If you have high blood pressure, follow your doctor's advice on how to reduce it and take any medication correctly.

TREATMENTS IN DETAIL

Conventional Medicine

ASSESSMENT Anyone suspected of having a stroke should be taken to hospital as soon as possible. A doctor will carry out a thorough examination to assess the symptoms, identify any risk factors (such as high blood pressure) and look for possible sources of emboli (fragments of blood clots) that may have caused the stroke.

The doctor may arrange various tests, which may include CT scanning or MRI, which will show the site and extent of the damage, as well as revealing whether the stroke resulted from a blockage or a haemorrhage. Carotid doppler scanning, in which ultrasound is used to assess blood flow, may be used to look for narrowing of the carotid arteries. Other tests may be done to evaluate the heart's rhythm and the motion of the heart muscle.

TREATMENT will involve identifying and treating any underlying conditions, such as high blood pressure. Other possible measures depend on whether the stroke was caused by a blockage or a haemorrhage. If you smoke, your doctor will advise you to stop. You will also be advised to change your diet to include less fat and more fresh fruit and vegetables (*see p.44*).

PRIMARY TREATMENT **ASPIRIN AND OTHER DRUGS** If the stroke resulted from a artery blockage, you may be prescribed a high dose of aspirin for several days. This has been shown to improve chances of recovery and reduce the risk of death. High-dose aspirin treatment will be followed by a regime of low-dose aspirin to take every day. Long-term, low-dose aspirin has been shown to reduce the risk of a further stroke because it makes the platelets in the blood less likely to clump together, a process that happens when clots form. Other drugs that aim to reduce the risk of a further stroke include dipyridamole. Anticoagulant drugs, which reduce the clotting tendency of the blood, may be prescribed, also. For people who have had a subarachnoid haemorrhage, the drug nimodipine may be prescribed, since

CAUTION

Drugs for stroke can cause a range of possible side-effects: ask your doctor to explain these to you.

it improves the prognosis. Drugs that lower cholesterol are important if high cholesterol levels are a factor.

PRIMARY TREATMENT **CAROTID ENDARTERECTOMY** If the carotid arteries in the neck are found to be greatly narrowed, carotid endarterectomy may be performed. In this procedure, material that is causing the narrowing is removed from the lining of the arteries. Risks include the small possibility of causing a further stroke.

PRIMARY TREATMENT **SURGERY** If the stroke resulted from a haemorrhage, urgent surgery may be performed to remove the clot formed by the leaked blood. In certain cases, where aneurysms are present, it may be possible to clip off the aneurysm to prevent further leakage of blood.

PRIMARY TREATMENT **REHABILITATION** is a key part of treatment for stroke. It may involve physiotherapy (*see also p.150*) and speech and language therapy, depending on the disability experienced. If disability is ongoing, occupational therapists can advise on special utensils, walking aids and other items that help with everyday living. There are also a number of organisations that can provide both practical and emotional support for people who have had a stroke and their carers. Talk to your care-provider or see p.486.

Nutritional Therapy

DIET In general, the best diet for stroke prevention is one rich in fruits, vegetables, nuts, seeds and oily fish, and low in fast and processed foods and other sources of salt and saturated fat. Fruit and vegetables seem to be particularly important because they are rich in potassium, which helps to lower blood pressure in the body and may help to reduce stroke risk. Interestingly, low potassium levels (hypokalaemia) have been found to be common after a stroke, and may be associated with a poorer recovery.

Flavonoids, which are also found in fruit and vegetables, are associated with a lower risk of stroke. In one study, people with the highest levels of quercetin, a flavonoid, had a 71 per cent lower risk of stroke. If you want to protect yourself from stroke, try to eat at least five portions of fruit and vegetables each day.

Studies have found that people who eat fish regularly tend to be at less risk of stroke than those who do not eat fish. The protective effect seems to be due to the

omega-3 fatty acids that fish contains. To reduce your risk of stroke, eat at least two portions of fish a week, especially oily fish (such as salmon, mackerel, trout and sardines), which are especially high in omega-3 fatty acids.

SUPPLEMENTS There is some evidence that supplementation with vitamins, minerals, protein and energy may improve general nutrition and health and reduce mortality in stroke patients. Along with a healthy diet, a multivitamin and mineral supplement may help to improve outcome in

individuals who have had a stroke. One study found that people with high blood levels of vitamin C had a 41 per cent lower risk of having a stroke. Taking 1g of vitamin C per day, in addition to a multivitamin supplement, may help to prevent stroke.

Some studies show that moderately raised homocysteine levels may be a risk factor for stroke. Raised homocysteine levels are associated with a low dietary intake of folic acid, vitamin B6 and vitamin B12. Taking a vitamin B-complex supplement, in addition to a daily multivitamin, may help you to reduce your risk of stroke.

See p.44 for more information on nutritional approaches that may help in the prevention and treatment of stroke.

> **CAUTION**
>
> Consult your doctor before taking vitamin B and vitamin C supplements because they may interfere with other medication and high doses of vitamin B can cause neuropathy. *(For more information see p.46.)*

Acupuncture

The Chinese tend to use acupuncture for stroke and head injury on a daily basis. There are some quite specific techniques that are claimed to help accelerate the

> ## Catherine the Great, Empress of Russia, died in 1796 of a sudden stroke

recovery from stroke. The accepted wisdom is that the quicker one intervenes with acupuncture, the more likely it is to be effective and help damaged areas of the brain recover, but because acupuncture is said to work by enhancing the local blood circulation around the injured area of brain, treatment should not be started for a week or two after the stroke occurred in order to avoid further bleeding.

RESULTS OF TRIALS There have been a number of very rigorous clinical trials looking at the use of specific acupuncture

points in the treatment of stroke, in particular the use of scalp acupuncture, which involves prolonged electrical stimulation of needles inserted just into the skin of the scalp overlying the damaged area of brain.

These trials show that acupuncture does not appear to have a specific effect in aiding stroke recovery. The original clinical trials, which suggested that it might be very effective, were small and not well designed. The more recent clinical trials leave no doubt and suggest that while acupuncture may have some effect on improving spasticity and enhancing individual independence, it does not accelerate stroke recovery.

If acupuncture is to be considered following stroke, at least 10–15 treatments are needed, and they should be given over a month or so before deciding whether this treatment is effective.

Bodywork and Movement Therapies

It is well established that early treatment of a stroke, using tactics such as exercise and movement to ensure an optimal supply of oxygen to the brain and other body tissues, reduces the risk of long-term neurological damage and also serves to decisively improve survival chances.

PRIMARY TREATMENT **PHYSIOTHERAPY AND OTHER TECHNIQUES** Recovery from the effects of a stroke depends, to a large extent, on efficient rehabilitation strategies, based on physiotherapy, occupational therapy, and possibly speech therapy. A recent review concluded therapy-based rehabilitation services (physiotherapy, occupational therapy and speech therapy), targeted at stroke patients living at home, appeared to improve independence in personal activities of daily living. A study looked at patients who still had difficulty with normal functions such as walking a year after a stroke. The results showed that in such cases rehabilitation treatment leads to significant, but clinically small, improvements in mobility and walking. However, these improvements were not usually sustained after treatment ended, and the treatment was found to have no lasting effect on the patients' daily activity, social activity, anxiety, depression and number of falls, or on the emotional well-being of their carers.

AFTER-EFFECTS OF STROKE

The after-effects of stroke depend on what caused the stroke, its severity and the location in the brain where it occurred. Different areas of the brain are responsible for different functions and abilities in the body. The right side (or hemisphere) of the brain is responsible for controlling the left side of the body, and vice versa. A stroke may also affect the brain stem, which is located at the base of the brain and is responsible for the control of many of the body's vital functions, such as breathing and heart beat.

STROKES IN THE RIGHT SIDE OF THE BRAIN MAY CAUSE:	STROKES IN THE LEFT SIDE OF THE BRAIN MAY CAUSE:	STROKES AFFECTING THE BRAIN STEM MAY CAUSE:
• Weakness or paralysis in the left side of the body • Denial that weakness or paralysis has occurred ("left neglect") • Visual problems, especially with the left visual field • Problems with spatial awareness, such as depth perception • Difficulty recognising or locating body parts • Difficulty reading maps or finding clothing or other items • Problems with memory • Changes in behaviour, including lack of concern about problems, impulsiveness, inappropriate actions and depression	• Weakness or paralysis in the right side of the body • Difficulties with speech and comprehension • Visual problems, especially with the right visual field • Problems with mathematics and with organising and reasoning • Behavioural changes, including cautiousness, inability to make decisions and depression • Problems with reading and writing • Difficulty in assimilating new information • Problems with memory	• Problems with breathing and heart functions • Trouble controlling body temperature • Problems with balance and coordination • Weakness or paralysis affecting the entire body • Difficulties with chewing, speaking and swallowing • Problems with vision • Coma

PRIMARY TREATMENT **TREADMILL WALKING** Recent studies have shown that walking on a treadmill, with the body weight partially supported on the arms of the equipment, is among the most effective ways of regaining the ability to walk independently after a stroke. This method gives patients who cannot walk unaided the chance for repetitive practice, encouraging them to walk more symmetrically, with less muscular spasm and better cardiovascular efficiency, when compared to walking on the floor. Several controlled trials looking at survivors of acute strokes have shown treadmill training is at least as effective as other physiotherapy approaches.

ROBOT-ASSISTED MOVEMENT Results of trials showed that using a robot to assist the shoulder and elbow movements of people who had had a stroke helped them to recover faster and more fully compared with those who had had conventional rehabilitation that involved exercising and physiotherapy. By six months after the stroke, however, there was no effective difference between patients who had had conventional treatment and those who had had robotic assistance.

CHINESE TECHNIQUES In China, acupressure, acupuncture (*see left*) and Tuina (TCM manipulation and massage), are commonly used to treat the after-effects of strokes and to encourage rehabilitation. Cases have been described showing the effectiveness of these methods when they are used as part of an intensive rehabilitation programme.

Mind–Body Therapies

EMG BIOFEEDBACK can be an effective way to regain control of weakened muscles. You may be taught electromyographic (EMG), or muscle activity, biofeedback. This involves using special instruments to measure the electrical activity of the muscles, and then learning to increase this activity through various techniques. EMG biofeedback treatment has also been used specifically for walking rehabilitation, but the results of trials are controversial. However, a recent study concluded that EMG biofeedback increases muscle strength and improves walking in people with impaired function on one side and foot-drop after a stroke. Another study showed that it is superior to physiotherapy alone for improving ankle muscle strength in people having rehabilitation after a stroke.

PREVENTION PLAN

To prevent another stroke:
• Give up smoking.
• Eat a healthy diet low in saturated fat.
• Take regular gentle exercise.
• Lose excess weight.
• Have treatment for high blood pressure if necessary (*see p.244*).

CARPAL TUNNEL SYNDROME

In carpal tunnel syndrome, the median nerve, which supplies certain parts of the hand, is compressed where it passes through the narrow space (the carpal tunnel) formed by the bones of the wrist and the strong band of tissue that overlies them. The compression causes painful tingling in the hand, wrist and forearm, which is often worse at night and first thing in the morning, or after strenuous exercise. A combination of yoga stretches, anti-inflammatory drugs, nutritional supplements and other therapies all help to bring relief.

WHAT ARE THE SYMPTOMS?

Initial symptoms may include:
- Burning or tingling sensation in the hand
- Pain in the hand that may extend up the forearm

As the condition progresses, further symptoms may develop, including:
- Numbness of the hand
- Weakening of the grip
- Wasting and weakness in some muscles in the hand, especially at the base of the thumb

WHY MIGHT I HAVE THIS?

PREDISPOSING FACTORS
- Repetitive hand movements, e.g. using a keyboard
- Pregnancy
- Obesity
- Low thyroid function (hypothyroidism)
- Diabetes mellitus (*see p.314*)
- Oral contraceptives

TREATMENT PLAN

PRIMARY TREATMENTS
- Splinting the wrist at night
- Corticosteroids
- Osteopathic manipulation
- *Namaste* pose and other yoga exercises

BACK-UP TREATMENTS
- Vitamins and bromelain
- Surgery (in severe cases)

WORTH CONSIDERING
- Homeopathy
- Acupuncture

For an explanation of how treatments are rated, see p.111.

WHY DOES IT OCCUR?

The underlying cause of the nerve compression that causes carpal tunnel syndrome may not be identifiable. However, in some cases the soft tissues inside the carpal tunnel swell, putting pressure on the median nerve. This swelling may be associated with fluid retention in pregnancy or with obesity.

Sometimes the carpal tunnel becomes narrowed because of a joint disorder, such as rheumatoid arthritis, or a wrist fracture. Repetitive hand movements, such as typing on a keyboard or playing a musical instrument, may cause inflammation of the tendons in the wrist, which may in turn affect the median nerve.

In women, taking the contraceptive pill may sometimes be a factor in developing the condition. Carpal tunnel syndrome is more common in people between the ages of 40 and 60 and tends to affect people who have diabetes mellitus (*see p.314*) or hypothyroidism (*see p.319*).

Symptoms typically affect the area supplied by the median nerve: the thumb, the first and middle fingers, the inside of the third finger and the palm of the hand. Both hands are often affected. Symptoms may be worse at night, and pain may be severe enough to disturb sleep.

IMPORTANT

Consult a doctor if you think you may have carpal tunnel syndrome..

TREATMENTS IN DETAIL

Conventional Medicine

The doctor will usually be able to diagnose carpal tunnel syndrome from your symptoms alone. He will examine your hands and wrists and may tap the inside of your wrists to check whether you experience a tingling sensation. Nerve conduction tests may be done to confirm the diagnosis.

If the condition develops in pregnancy, there is a good chance that it will resolve after the birth. In other cases, treating the cause, if it can be identified, usually relieves symptoms. If carpal tunnel syndrome is linked to repetitive hand movements, it is important to try to avoid the repetitive actions that cause the symptoms.

PRIMARY TREATMENT **SPLINTING** Your doctor may advise splinting the wrist at night to give you some relief.

PRIMARY TREATMENT **CORTICOSTEROIDS** An injection in the affected wrist or a short course of oral corticosteroids may be prescribed. These drugs, which work by reducing inflammation, have been found to bring a period of relief.

SURGERY may be necessary to relieve the pressure on the nerve if symptoms are persistent and severe. This may either involve traditional ("open") surgery or endoscopic ("keyhole") surgery, in which smaller incisions are made. Both procedures carry a small risk of complications, such as temporary numbness and wound infections.

YOGA STRETCH FOR THE WRIST

The yoga pose known as *namaste*, or the prayer position, has been shown to help in treating carpal tunnel syndrome. Bring the hands together with the palms flat against each other at the centre of the chest. The elbows should be pushed out at the sides and you should feel a slight stretch in each hand. Relax your shoulders and hold the position for a few seconds. Do several times each day.

Flexor tendons

Ligament (forms the carpal tunnel)

Sinovial sheath

Median nerve

The median nerve controls some hand muscles and conveys nerve impulses from parts of the hand. It runs through the carpal tunnel, which is formed by the bones of the wrist and the ligament that stretches across them. Stretching this area in the *namaste* pose (*see left*) can help to relieve the pain of carpal tunnel syndrome.

Nutritional Therapy

VITAMIN SUPPLEMENTS One nutrient that seems to be very effective in treating carpal tunnel syndrome is vitamin B6. It helps by reducing inflammatory reactions in soft tissues. There is good evidence that vitamin B6 gives significant relief to a large proportion of people with carpal tunnel syndrome. Vitamin B2 can also be effective for carpal tunnel syndrome and the effectiveness is further improved when vitamins B2 and B6 are taken together. Try taking 100mg each day for three months. Thereafter take a good B-complex supplement.

BROMELAIN The pineapple extract bromelain is naturally anti-inflammatory and may be useful in treating carpal tunnel syndrome, especially when taken with vitamin B6. Try taking 500mg of bromelain three times a day on an empty stomach.

CAUTION

Consult your doctor before taking vitamin B6 which can interacts with certain drugs; high doses may cause neuropathy. (*See also p.46*.)

Homeopathy

Ruta graveolens and *Hypericum perforatum* may be used to treat carpal tunnel syndrome. People who respond to *Ruta* have wrists that feel weak, stiff and achey in the morning, but symptoms ease as the day goes on. There may also be bony arthritic nodes on the fingers. People who respond to *Hypericum* have severe, usually shooting pain. The problem may be brought on by injury to the median nerve.

Acupuncture

The pain and discomfort of carpal tunnel syndrome can often be helped by a few treatments of local acupuncture and it is always worth trying prior to surgery. Sometimes electrical stimulation is required around the wrist, but frequently acupuncture needles alone will provide fairly immediate and sustained relief. This is particularly likely if the condition is triggered by a transitory event, such as pregnancy.

You will know whether acupuncture is likely to be effective for this condition after four or five weekly sessions.

Bodywork Therapies

PRIMARY TREATMENT **OSTEOPATHIC MANIPULATION** methods have been used successfully to treat carpal tunnel syndrome. Myofascial release (a type of stretching) improved carpal tunnel symptoms in a small preliminary trial. Participants' pain, numbness and weakness decreased.

Yoga

PRIMARY TREATMENT **NAMASTE POSE** In one study, people with carpal tunnel syndrome did 11 yoga poses for the arms daily, holding each one for 30 seconds. Researchers noted that the *namaste* pose was particularly helpful (*see above*). After eight weeks, participants reported less pain and said their grip was significantly better.

PREVENTION PLAN

If you work in a job that involves repetitive hand movements, use a wrist support and take regular breaks.

MOTION SICKNESS

Almost everyone experiences motion sickness at some time, but the condition is especially common in children. The condition may be caused by road, sea or air travel or by amusement park rides. Once the motion stops, the symptoms usually subside soon afterwards. Motion sickness can be treated with antihistamine and other drugs, but acupressure, acupuncture, avoiding certain foods before travel, and autogenic training exercises can also bring relief.

WHAT ARE THE SYMPTOMS?

- Nausea
- Vomiting
- Headache
- Sweating
- Pallor
- Fatigue and lethargy

WHY MIGHT I HAVE THIS?

PREDISPOSING FACTORS

- Eating salty or high-protein foods before travelling
- Trigger point activity in neck muscles
- Anxiety

TRIGGERS

- Fumes from traffic
- Reading or doing close work while travelling, especially in cars or buses

TREATMENT PLAN

PRIMARY TREATMENTS

- Pressing pericardium 6 point on wrist and other self-help measures
- Motion sickness drugs or patches

BACK-UP TREATMENTS

- Avoiding certain foods
- Ginger and peppermint
- Homeopathy

WORTH CONSIDERING

- Trigger-point deactivation
- Breathing retraining
- Autogenic training
- Relaxation exercises

For an explanation of how treatments are rated, see p.111.

WHY DOES IT OCCUR?

Motion sickness occurs because of a conflict between the messages the brain receives from the eyes and the messages it receives from the organs of balance (the vestibular apparatus), which are located in the inner ear. For example, if you are travelling in a car, the inner ear senses the motion, but if you are looking at the interior of the car or are focusing on a book in front of you, your eyes may perceive the car as stationary. The conflicting messages the brain receives may bring on nausea or vomiting. The same conflict causes motion sickness from travelling in a plane or boat.

Some practitioners also think that the body's sense of balance can be disturbed by sensitive areas known as "trigger points" (*see p.55*) in the neck muscles, as well as by restrictions in the joints of the neck, and this can contribute to motion sickness. Psychological factors, such as anxiety about the journey or stress, can also contribute to motion sickness. Some people are sensitive to engine fumes and this can also bring on feelings of nausea.

SELF-HELP

PRIMARY TREATMENT
If you are feeling nauseous, try the following:

- Firmly press the pericardium 6 (P6) point for 5 to 10 minutes (*see below*). You can buy wrist straps ("sea-bands") from your pharmacy that put pressure on these points for you.
- Look at the horizon while travelling.
- Open a window, if possible, and breathe deeply and slowly.
- Take ginger or peppermint before and during travel.

THE PERICARDIUM 6 POINT

Feelings of nausea can often be relieved by pressing the pericardium 6 point on the wrist. This point is used in acupuncture, but can also be effective when pressed. To find this point, measure two of your own thumb-widths above the first crease in your wrist as you go up your arm. Then find a point in line with your ring finger on that hand. Press this point firmly, until it hurts just slightly, for five to 10 minutes. You can repeat the procedure on the other wrist. This method can be used as often as necessary to relieve nausea, and is also safe for children to use.

Pressing the pericardium 6 point for nausea

Conventional Medicine

PRIMARY TREATMENT **MOTION SICKNESS MEDICINES** Various treatments are available that may help to relieve motion sickness, some of which can be bought over the counter. Antihistamines, such as cyclizine, taken before the journey, may help to prevent nausea. These drugs are usually used to treat allergic conditions, but they also reduce the vomiting reflex in the brain. Some oral antihistamines, such as hyoscine, can safely be given to children aged four years and over.

Skin patches containing hyoscine are helpful in preventing nausea in some people. These patches have a prolonged action but need to be applied several hours before travel. They should not be used on children under the age of 10 years.

> **CAUTION**
>
> Be aware that drugs for motion sickness may cause drowsiness and blurred vision; do not take them if you will be driving or operating machinery.

Nutritional Therapy

FOODS TO AVOID Eating foods that are high in sodium, such as preserved meats, corn chips, potato crisps and salted nuts, correlates significantly with increased airsickness (a form of motion sickness). Consumption of foods high in protein, such as milk products, cheese and preserved meat, has also been related to an increased risk of airsickness. Avoiding these foods for several hours before travelling may help to combat airsickness and other forms of motion sickness.

GINGER AND PEPPERMINT These traditional nausea remedies can also be effective in preventing and treating motion sickness. They have a warming and soothing action on the stomach and do not cause side-effects, as many drugs for motion sickness do. Try eating crystallised ginger or peppermint drops before and during a journey; alternatively, you can make a tea from ginger or peppermint and drink it before you travel.

Homeopathy

Homeopathic treatments are frequently used for motion sickness. Clinical trials conducted in France by Dexpert and by Ponti show that they are effective.

COCCULUS, which is made from the plant *Anamirta cocculus* – the Indian cockle – is among the several homeopathic medicines that may be appropriate for the condition. A number of other homeopathic medicines may be used as well. In practice, it is best to use a homeopathic complex, which contains several different homeopathic medicines. A number of such complexes are available, all of which include *Cocculus*. These include Travella (containing homeopathic *Apomorph*, *Staphysagria*, *Cocculus*, *Theridion*, *Petroleum*, *Tabacum* and *Nux vomica*) available in the UK and Cocculine, available in France, USA, Canada and elsewhere, which has a similar composition.

It is best to start treatment the day before travel, with two tablets, three times on the day before, and an additional dose just before leaving.

Acupressure

Needling acupuncture points on the front of each forearm, just above the wrists (the P6 points), has been shown by some researchers to have an anti-nausea and anti-dizziness effect. Similar benefits are claimed for acupressure, whether the nausea is caused by motion, medication (such as chemotherapy or an anaesthetic) or pregnancy. Treatment should be given ideally just before the journey and, if necessary, some acupressure should be applied during the journey if symptoms persist (*see box, opposite*).

Bodywork Therapies

TRIGGER-POINT DEACTIVATION Trigger points are sensitive areas in muscles that usually cause pain or discomfort not only where they are situated but also in areas some distance away. Trigger points, particularly in the muscles that run from just behind the ear to the breastbone, can produce symptoms of dizziness and/or motion sickness. Trigger points can be deactivated by acupuncture as well as by manual pressure and stretching techniques

as used by osteopaths, massage therapists (particularly those with neuromuscular therapy training) and some physiotherapists and chiropractors.

Breathing Retraining

It may be that motion sickness is made worse by the anxiety and tension that accompany it. Therefore symptoms may be reduced if the body is relaxed and the breathing pattern is allowed to calm down. Clinical experience suggests that people who learn to relax their neck and shoulders and breathe deeply with the diaphragm rather than using the upper chest can tolerate motion better. See mind–body therapies (*below*), and p.62 for more information.

Mind–Body Therapies

AUTOGENIC TRAINING is a series of six silent verbal exercises for the mind that help people to relax at will. It may be possible to control symptoms of motion sickness using autogenic relaxation techniques, especially if anxiety and tension contribute to the condition.

A study compared the effectiveness of intramuscular injections of promethazine and a training method known as autogenic-feedback training exercise (AFTE) as treatments for motion sickness. People prone to the condition underwent a test in which they were spun round in a rotating chair. Motion-sickness tolerance was significantly increased after four hours of AFTE when compared to either 25mg or 50mg doses of promethazine. The AFTE group reported fewer or no symptoms at higher rotational speeds than people in the control or promethazine groups. Although it was a small study, the positive results suggest that psychological techniques may indeed be helpful in overcoming motion sickness. Try practising relaxation techniques (*see p.99*) before your journey, and use them as you travel.

> **PREVENTION PLAN**
>
> Do breathing and relaxation exercises before you travel, and avoid salty, high-fat and dairy-based foods.

Skin

The skin is the body's largest organ and its first line of defence. Skin ailments are often a visible symptom of internal imbalances, so integrated treatment can be very effective. While treatments usually rely on creams, ointments and oral drugs, nutritional supplements, homeopathy, herbal remedies and mind–body therapies can all help.

ACNE

Acne is a rash that usually appears on the face but may also affect other areas, especially the upper back, the middle of the chest, the shoulders and the neck. The most common form is acne vulgaris, which is the familiar rash that afflicts many teenagers. Regular washing with acne soaps may help to prevent bacterial build-up. Depending on the severity, acne may be treated with topical creams or oral antibiotics. Acne may also respond to special diets, supplements, homeopathic and herbal remedies and deactivation of trigger points.

WHAT ARE THE SYMPTOMS?

- Small blackheads
- Small, firm whiteheads
- Red pimples, sometimes with pus-filled tips
- Painful, large, firm, red lumps
- Tender lumps without obvious heads (cysts)

WHY MIGHT I HAVE THIS?

PREDISPOSING FACTORS

- Hormonal changes associated with puberty
- Exposure to certain oils, such as cooking oils
- Certain drugs, such as corticosteroids
- Excess of toxins in the body
- Overgrowth of yeast organisms
- Food sensitivity
- Irritated areas in muscles (trigger points)
- Genetic factors

WHY DOES IT OCCUR?

Acne vulgaris is more common and more severe in males than in females. The skin condition is triggered by changes in hormones, such as testosterone and other androgens, associated with puberty. The rash usually subsides after adolescence, but can occasionally persist after the age of 30 and scars may form on the skin.

Various factors may predispose an individual to develop acne (*see left*), including genetic factors, since acne vulgaris sometimes runs in families. Stress can make the acne worse. The condition can cause great psychological distress, and often arises during the period when teenagers are most self-conscious about their appearance.

OVERACTIVITY OF SEBACEOUS GLANDS Acne vulgaris is caused by the overproduction of an oily substance called sebum, which is secreted by the sebaceous glands in the skin (*see illustration, right*). Sebum normally drains into the hair follicles and flows out through the follicle openings on the skin surface, lubricating the skin and keeping it supple. However, excess sebum blocks the follicles and hardens into tiny plugs. Bacteria multiply in the blocked follicles, releasing fatty acids from the sebum, inflaming the surrounding tissue.

In some cases, the follicles may become blocked with keratin, a tough protein that is produced by skin cells to strengthen the epidermis. Keratin is also a constituent of hair and nails.

OTHER TYPES OF ACNE Less common forms of acne include occupational acne, which may result from exposure to certain industrial oils; and drug-induced acne, which may be due to prescribed drugs, such as corticosteroids.

TREATMENT PLAN

PRIMARY TREATMENTS

- Benzoyl peroxide cream (*see Self-Help*)
- Topical keratolytics
- Topical antibiotics and retinoids

BACK-UP TREATMENTS

- Oral antibiotics and retinoids (severe acne)
- Oral contraceptives (for some women)
- Wholefood diet
- Antioxidants
- Fish-oil supplements
- Detoxifying and other diets

- Zinc
- Vitamin B6 (for acne before a period)
- Western and Chinese herbal medicine

WORTH CONSIDERING

- Homeopathy
- Trigger-point deactivation
- Hydrotherapy
- Mind–body therapies

For an explanation of how treatments are rated, see p.111.

PRIMARY TREATMENT If you have acne, the following steps may help you:

- Wash twice a day with warm water and a mild cleanser, but do not scrub your skin too vigorously.
- Do not pick your spots and pimples, as this may make them worse and even result in scarring.
- Apply benzoyl peroxide cream to your acne every day.

TREATMENTS IN DETAIL

Conventional Medicine

After making a diagnosis, and depending on the severity of your symptoms, your doctor may recommend antibiotics and other drugs in the form of creams as well as preparations to be taken orally. You may also be referred to a dermatologist.

PRIMARY TREATMENT **TOPICAL KERATOLYTICS,** such as salicylic acid, help to relieve mild acne. Your doctor may prescribe a cream containing these. They help to break down the oily plugs that block the opening to the hair follicle and loosen the dead or hardened cells on the surface of the skin. As a result, the trapped sebum can flow out and air can enter the follicle, reducing the chances of bacterial infection.

PRIMARY TREATMENT **TOPICAL ANTIBIOTICS AND RETINOIDS** can help acne that is mild to moderately severe. Your doctor may prescribe creams or ointments containing these. Retinoids work by reducing sebum production.

ORAL ANTIBIOTICS AND RETOINOIDS If your acne is moderate to severe, your doctor may prescribe oral antibiotics, such as tetracycline, which you need to take for at least 3–4 months. For severe acne, dermatologists may prescribe a course of retinoids, such as isotretinoin, which is usually taken for four months. Over 90 per cent of patients respond to this therapy. Many people are cured by a single course of retinoids, but in some cases a second course may be prescribed.

CERTAIN COMBINED ORAL CONTRACEPTIVES reduce male hormone (androgen) levels and have been shown to reduce the

DEVELOPMENT OF ACNE VULGARIS

Sebaceous glands around the hair follicles produce sebum (an oily substance) to lubricate hair growth and waterproof the surface of the skin. Sometimes too much sebum is produced during puberty in both sexes due to male hormones (androgens). The excess sebum becomes mixed with dead skin cells, clogging the follicle opening and encouraging bacteria to breed. The result is inflammation and acne.

Four stages of acne

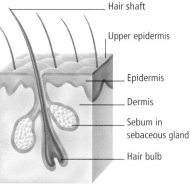

Hair shaft
Upper epidermis
Epidermis
Dermis
Sebum in sebaceous gland
Hair bulb

1 HEALTHY SKIN
The sebaceous glands sit in the dermis layer of the skin, where they produce the right amount of sebum to lubricate the hair shaft and waterproof the epidermis.

Plug of sebum (blackhead)
Excess sebum in sebaceous gland
Hair follicle

2 BLACKHEAD
A surge in production of sebum blocks the pore. The plug of sebum, bacteria and skin debris reacts with oxygen in the air and turns black (blackhead or "open comedo").

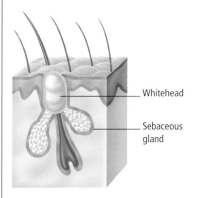

Whitehead
Sebaceous gland

3 WHITEHEAD
Sometimes the plug of sebum does not break through the skin, when it is known as a whitehead or "closed comedo". As it grows larger, it presses on the hair follicle.

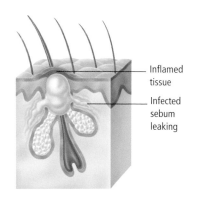

Inflamed tissue
Infected sebum leaking

4 INFECTED FOLLICLE AND ACNE
Sebum and the bacteria that feed on it leak from the growing whitehead into the dermis. The surrounding skin tissue and the hair follicle become inflamed (acne).

severity of acne in some women. These combined pills may need to be taken for at least six months.

CAUTION

Oral and topical acne drugs can have side-effects, particularly if you are pregnant. Ask your doctor to explain these to you.

Nutritional Therapy

WHOLEFOOD DIET Evidence is emerging that the prevalence of acne in developed countries is related to a glut of foods high in refined sugars and starches. These tend to cause the body to secrete copious quantities of insulin, which seem to increase the levels of the male hormones that may be at the root of many acne cases. Cutting back on refined and processed carbohydrates is an important step in clearing acne.

DETOXIFICATION AND OTHER DIETS In natural medicine, acne is viewed as a problem of excess toxicity. Clinical experience shows that detoxification can be effective in reducing acne and in improving the

primrose (*Oenothera biennis*), borage (*Borage officinalis*) or blackcurrant (*Ribes nigrum*) oil, as well as from fish oil.

ZINC from food sources, such as pumpkin seeds, or supplements can be effective for people with acne. One study found that zinc therapy worked as well as antibiotic

Acne that responds to *Silicea* features pustules that never seem to discharge: they sit under the skin for weeks without bursting, but often forming cysts. *Silicea* people are usually chilly and feel cold, even in a warm room. They tend to be pale and thin, with fine hair and weak, ridged nails. Their hands and feet are cold yet clammy.

The sebaceous glands in your skin are active even before you are born

condition of the skin. A common factor in acne is an overgrowth of yeast organisms and food sensitivity also appears to be a common underlying theme in acne. (*See p.40 for diets to address these problems.*)

ANTIOXIDANTS There is evidence to suggest acne is an inflammatory condition in which free radicals play a role. Antioxidants can help to reduce the inflammation by neutralising the damaging free radicals. Eating plenty of antioxidant fruit and vegetables is important.

Regular intake of carrot juice, for example, can provide you with beta-carotene, an antioxidant and a precursor to vitamin A, which helps to control acne. Supplements can help, too: in one study, taking 200mcg of the mineral selenium together with 20IU of vitamin E each day helped to reduce acne symptoms.

FISH OIL SUPPLEMENTS can also help to reduce the inflammation that may be associated with acne. This inflammation may be linked to excessive amounts of omega-6 fatty acids (found in vegetable oils), accompanied by a relative lack of omega-3 fatty acids (found in oily fish). There is some evidence that many people with acne are generally deficient in the essential fatty acids they need.

You may be able to control your acne by cutting down on both margarine and vegetable oils and by eating more oily fish (such as salmon, mackerel and trout), walnuts and flaxseeds.

You may also reduce the inflammation associated with acne by taking essential fatty acids, such as gamma linolenic acid (GLA). These are derived from evening

treatment. Take 30mg of zinc supplements three times a day for 3–4 months and then reduce the dose to 25mg once a day. Taking zinc for a long period can deplete the body of copper, so take 1mg of copper for each 15mg of zinc.

VITAMIN B6 can help some women whose acne flares up before a period. A significant proportion of female acne sufferers have high levels of male hormones (androgens). Women with pre-menstrual acne may benefit from taking a 50mg vitamin B6 supplement a day.

> **CAUTION**
>
> Consult your doctor before taking zinc with antibiotics, or fish oils or omega-3 oils with warfarin (*see p.46*).

Homeopathy

The evidence suggests acne responds well to homeopathy. Treatment needs to be tailored to a particular individual by a skilled homeopath, but if one is not available, try a homeopathic complex consisting of several of the medicines indicated below.

SULPHUR AND SILICEA Two of the most commonly indicated medicines are *Sulphur* and *Silicea*. Rashes that respond to *Sulphur* are typically very itchy, particularly in the heat. *Sulphur* constitutional types are usually extroverted, untidy and may be opinionated or garrulous. They tend to be hot-blooded, needing fewer clothes than most people. In particular, their feet may be hot and smelly.

OTHER REMEDIES *Kalium bromatum* is recommended when the spots are often itchy. Individuals complain of poor sleep, frequently disturbed by bad dreams. They may be mentally slow, finding it hard to remember and think.

Calcarea sulphurica is suitable when there are large yellow pustules that are slow to heal. They may also be itchy. Acne spots which respond to *Hepar sulphuris calcareum* are very sensitive to touch or are painful as they develop.

Pulsatilla is particularly (but by no means exclusively) helpful for girls when crops of spots develop in the week before a period. It is prescribed mostly on constitutional grounds (*see p.73*). *Pulsatilla* types are mild-tempered or sweet-natured. They lack assertion and are indecisive. Although they easily feel cold, they like fresh air (provided they are well wrapped up) and hate stuffy atmospheres.

Western Herbal Medicine

Herbs are highly effective in controlling excess sebum production and combating the bacteria that proliferate in the follicles. A combination of internal and external treatment brings the best results. However, no clinical trials support this claim.

INTERNAL TREATMENTS A daily dose of chasteberry (*Vitex agnus-castus*) may help to control surges of the hormones (especially at puberty) that increase the size of sebaceous glands and the production of sebum. Sage (*Salvia officinalis*), motherwort (*Leonarus cardiaca*) and red clover (*Trifolium pratense*) may also help to reduce surplus sebum by modulating hormone levels. Regular cups of green tea (*Camellia sinensis*) may adjust the overproduction of male and other hormones.

Extracts of poke root (*Phytolacca decandra*), a herb restricted to professional use, seem to cut down the flow of sebum and restrict bacterial proliferation. Burdock

(*Arctium lappa*) root and leaf also combats bacteria and reduces inflammation.

An overloaded bowel is a frequent cause of acne. Rhubarb (*Rheum palmatum*) root eliminates toxic wastes and reduces bacterial inflammation. It is laxative, so take it only for a short time. Oregon grape root (*Mahonia aquifolium*) can significantly reduce acne eruptions, while the bitters in artichoke (*Cynara scolymus*) leaf stimulate the liver and production of bile.

EXTERNAL TREATMENTS help to unblock sebaceous glands and kill off bacteria that lead to inflammation of the skin. Try the gel of tea tree (*Melaleuca alternifolia*) oil, which in clinical trials was as effective as conventional treatments.

Washes of astringent herbs, such as rose (*Rosa gallica*), witch hazel (*Hamamelis virginiana*), burnet (*Sanguisorba officinalis*) root, elderflower (*Sambucus nigra*) or cold Earl Grey tea, can clear impacted sebum. Applying fresh lemon juice and/or live yoghurt to your skin can also help, especially after a chamomile (*Matricaria recutita*) steam bath has opened up the sebaceous glands. Allow the steam made from chamomile tea to rise over your face.

An Ancient Egyptian remedy for acne featured ostrich egg, olive oil, bile, flour and milk

You can clear your skin with a paste of oatmeal, green tea (*Camellia sinensis*), chamomile (*Matricaria recutita*) and calendula (*Calendula officinalis*). Pounded burdock (*Arctium lappa*) leaves mixed with an aqueous cream can calm inflamation and fresh aloe vera gel is good for oily skin.

A topical remedy that is also effective in clearing the skin is an equal mixture of cucumber and beetroot juice – the only drawback is that this can stain the skin.

> **CAUTION**
>
> See p. 69 before taking a herbal remedy and, if you are already taking a prescribed medication, consult a herbalist first. It is unwise for someone taking oral isotretinoin (Roaccutane) to have herbal treatment at the same time.

Chinese Herbal Medicine

In Traditional Chinese Medicine (TCM), herbalists classify acne into four types based on the infection, toxicity, inflammation and stress that contribute to them. The research evidence is not yet available to back up the TCM approach. If you are considering using TCM herbs for relieving your acne, you should consult a trained practitioner (*see p.81*). Self-medication is definitely not recommended.

> **CAUTION**
>
> See p. 69 before taking a herbal remedy. Always consult a practitioner for a diagnosis and do not self-treat.

Bodywork Therapies

TRIGGER-POINT DEACTIVATION When trigger points (*see p.55*) are activated in your muscles, the skin may increase the production of sebum, which encourages bacterial activity and acne symptoms.

Trigger points are local, "irritable" areas that are sensitive to pressure. They usually cause pain or discomfort, not only where they are situated but also some distance away. For example, points in the sternomastoid muscles on the front and sides of the neck can trigger skin symptoms in the face. If you have acne on the face or forehead and have a tendency to sweat in these areas, trigger points in the neck may be part of the problem.

Acupuncture, osteopathy, physiotherapy, massage and chiropractic are all bodywork therapies that can help to deactivate trigger points by massaging and stretching the area. Of the various kinds of massage therapist, those who have training in neuromuscular techniques (*see p.61*) are likely to be the most effective.

HYDROTHERAPY, such as the regular use of a facial sauna, can act as a preventive measure. It helps to reduce the chances of the skin follicles becoming blocked. A facial sauna made from fresh peppermint (*Mentha piperita*), parsley (*Petroselinum crispum*) and lemon (*Citrus limonum*) is especially good for deep cleansing and invigorating the skin.

A refreshing facial sauna for particularly oily skin combines peppermint (*Mentha piperita*), lavender (*Lavandula angustifolia*), yarrow (*Achillea millefolium*) and rosemary (*Rosmarinus officinalis*).

A hydrotherapist may recommend that you cleanse your system by taking a hot bath with Epsom salts. Alternatively, you could try thalassotherapy, which makes use of seawater jets and baths to cleanse and tone your skin.

> **CAUTION**
>
> Do not take an Epsom salts bath if you are elderly or frail.

Mind–Body Therapies

Acne can have a major emotional impact, especially on self-conscious teenagers, and some healthcare practitioners believe that stress can make it worse. In one study, researchers employed a combination of biofeedback, visualisation, relaxation and breathing and found they were effective in reducing stress.

If you are prone to acne, try diaphragmatic breathing (*see p.00*) for 10 minutes a day. If your acne is making you depressed or causing you difficulties in your relationships and emotional life, your doctor may recommend psychotherapy to help restore your self-confidence. By discussing your feelings with a counsellor, you may recapture your self-esteem.

> **PREVENTION PLAN**
>
> **The following may help to prevent acne in the long term:**
> - Eat a wholefood diet.
> - Take zinc supplements.
> - Practise relaxation.
> - Use cleansing hydrotherapy.

HERPES SIMPLEX

Herpes simplex is a highly contagious skin infection, which especially affects the mucous membranes of the mouth and genitals. The viruses responsible cause lesions (blisters and ulcers), which frequently are very uncomfortable. Although there is no outright cure, antiviral creams and pills reduce the severity and duration of attacks. Eating a high-lysine, low-arginine diet may restrict the virus's ability to reproduce. Boosting the immune system and keeping stress to a minimum with relaxation may reduce the chances of a further outbreak.

WHAT ARE THE SYMPTOMS?

For herpes simplex type 1 (HSV-1):

- At first, either no symptoms or painful mouth ulcers
- Cold sores may develop, preceded by tingling in the affected area

For herpes simplex type 2 (HSV-2):

- Painful blisters and ulcers in the genital area – the first episode may be accompanied by a fever and painful urination
- Recurrences may be accompanied by tingling in the affected area

WHY MIGHT I HAVE THIS?

PREDISPOSING FACTORS

- Other infections
- Lowered immunity
- Excessive amounts of foods containing arginine
- Stress
- Depressed mood

TRIGGER

- For HSV-2, unprotected sex with an infected person

TREATMENT PLAN

PRIMARY TREATMENTS

- Topical antiviral creams
- Oral antiviral drugs
- Lysine supplements

BACK-UP TREATMENTS

- Low-arginine diet
- Homeopathy
- Western and Chinese herbal medicine
- Mind–body therapies

WORTH CONSIDERING

- Various supplements
- Zinc sulphate solution

For an explanation of how treatments are rated, see p.111.

WHY DOES IT OCCUR?

Two viruses, herpes simplex types 1 and 2, primarily cause cold sores and genital herpes respectively. You can catch the viruses by direct contact with the lesions (the ulcers and blisters). You are infectious until they have healed. Avoid contact from when symptoms are first experienced until lesions are no longer present.

Both types of the herpes virus remain dormant in the nerves for life, during which time a healthy immune system will normally keep them in check. When the immune system is weakened, the viruses can be reactivated, causing ulcers and blisters to recur and viruses to be shed. The predisposing factors (*see left*) can all cause the viruses to reactivate.

HERPES SIMPLEX TYPE 1 (HSV-1) Most people have been infected with HSV-1 by the time they reach adulthood. The initial infection is often symptomless, although painful mouth ulcers occur in some cases. Afterwards, the virus lies dormant, most commonly in the trigeminal nerve ganglia near the temple region of the head. If it is reactivated, it migrates down the nerve, causing a fresh outbreak of cold sores, mainly on the lips. The face and, rarely, the eyes may also be affected.

HERPES SIMPLEX TYPE 2 (HSV-2) The genital herpes caused by HSV-2 affects 1 in 5 adults and adolescents. The virus can be caught via unprotected sex with an infected person. After the initial attack, this virus retreats to the sacral ganglion, a nerve structure near the base of the spine, from where it may later be reactivated, causing a recurrence of lesions in the genital region.

IMPORTANT

See your doctor immediately if you develop a cold sore in or near the eye.

Occasionally, HSV-1 is transmitted to the genital area during oral sex and HSV-2 may affect the throat. People who have developed antibodies to HSV-1 may have some immunity to HSV-2, and vice versa.

IMMEDIATE RELIEF

- Place a cold, wet, used, Earl Grey tea bag over the affected area as soon as the tingling or painful sensation begins.
- For genital herpes, try sitting in a salt-water or warm bath.

TREATMENTS IN DETAIL

Conventional Medicine

PRIMARY TREATMENT **TOPICAL ANTIVIRAL CREAMS** may be prescribed by a doctor to shorten a cold sore attack. They are also available over the counter. These topical creams contain antiviral drugs, such as aciclovir. To be effective, they must be started very early – as soon as you feel the tingling sensation and often before the ulcers or blisters develop.

PRIMARY TREATMENT **ORAL ANTIVIRAL DRUGS** may be prescribed by your doctor to treat attacks of both types of herpes simplex. A five-day course of oral antivirals, such as aciclovir, famciclovir and valaciclovir, needs to start as early as possible – often when you feel the first tingling sensation. If you have impaired immunity and develop a herpes simplex infection, your doctor may prescribe oral antiviral drugs, such as aciclovir, as the infection may become severe.

> **CAUTION**
>
> Antiviral drugs may cause side-effects: ask your doctor to explain them to you.

Nutritional Therapy

PRIMARY TREATMENT **LYSINE** is an amino acid that inhibits the growth of the viruses and, according to some research, should reduce the frequency and severity of herpes attacks. Clinical trials of lysine supplements have not shown them to be a consistently helpful treatment or preventive measure. However, if you are prone to herpes attacks, it may be worth trying. Take 500mg of lysine supplements every day for three months. Increase the dose to 1g, 2–3 times a day during an acute attack.

A LOW-ARGININE DIET may help to fight the herpes viruses because they need the amino acid arginine to reproduce. Argi-

A human cell is under attack from a number of herpes viruses. After each virus enters the cell, its genetic material (yellow) emerges from the protein coat (blue) and reproduces itself.

nine is found in high concentration in nuts, especially peanuts and cashews, chocolate and grains. Many individuals report that eating these foods can bring on the symptoms of herpes. If this happens to you, following a low-arginine diet, especially at the first sign of an attack, can help you to prevent problems.

A COMBINATION OF VITAMIN C AND BIOFLAVONOIDS Research shows that vitamin C and bioflavonoids can help to reduce the duration of symptoms by more than half. Take 200mg of vitamin C and 200mg of bioflavonoids 3–5 times every day at the first sign of a herpes attack. Applying vitamin C cream 3 times a day may also help to reduce symptoms and heal herpes blisters.

SELENIUM can inhibit the growth of several viruses and so the mineral may also help to reduce herpes attacks. Try taking 300–400mcg of selenium a day as a preventive measure for three months.

VITAMIN E spread on to the skin from a soft gelatine capsule can provide topical relief for herpes blisters. Soak a small piece of tissue in the contents of a vitamin E capsule and apply to the lesions. Studies show that if you do this for 15 minutes,

twice a day, the cold sore will often resolve within a day or two.

ZINC SULPHATE A solution of zinc sulphate (0.2 per cent zinc), applied 8–10 times per day within 24 hours of the appearance of the sores, may also help. The blisters should clear in 4–5 days, with itching, burning and pain often subsiding within a few hours.

> **CAUTION**
>
> Consult your doctor before taking vitamin E or vitamin C with warfarin, or before taking vitamin C with antibiotics (*see p.46*).

Homeopathy

RHUS TOXICODENDRON is the most commonly prescribed homeopathic medicine for acute attacks of both types of herpes. It is specifically suggested for patients whose itching and pain are relieved by the application of heat. For dosages, *see p.77*.

OTHER REMEDIES *Croton tiglium* is helpful for people who have severe genital herpes that is very sensitive to touch.

Natrum muriaticum is the main homeopathic medicine prescribed for people with cold sores of the lips, both for the acute attack and to prevent recurrences.

Causticum is sometimes very effective for people who develop the relatively uncommon but irritating problem of cold sores in the nose.

Sepia is probably the most effective homeopathic medicine for recurrent herpes, wherever it occurs, but particularly on the female genitalia. In women, the attacks often come before a period.

AGARICUS MUSCARIUS AND ARSENICUM ALBUM are two homeopathic medicines that may be used to treat post-herpetic neuralgia. The people who respond to *Agaricus muscarius* describe the pain as being like "icy needles". The patient may also suffer from tics or twitching.

If *Arsen. alb.* is appropriate, the person is likely to be experiencing a burning pain, which is relieved by heat. Their skin is dry and flaky, and the patient in general is characteristically extremely anxious, tense and chilly.

Western Herbal Medicine

RHUBARB ROOT One Chinese study has demonstrated that, even in low doses, an ethanol extract of rhubarb (*Rheum officinale*) root can inhibit the spread of the herpes simplex virus that causes cold sores. In addition, the research discovered that it also helps to prevent infection.

Rhubarb root was one of four herbs identified by Chinese researchers as having significant inhibitory effect on the herpes virus. The others were the tree peony (*Paeonia suffruticosa*), chinaberry (*Melia toosendan*), and yellow mountain laurel (*Sophora flavescens*). The researchers used a variety of extraction mediums that made a difference to the potency of the remedy in each case and their data indicated that these four herbs possess a potential value as a source of new powerful anti-herpes simplex virus compounds.

Other research has confirmed that a sage (*Salvia officinalis*) and rhubarb root cream, applied to the lips, proved as effective as topical aciclovir cream.

PROPOLIS Israeli researchers have revealed the remarkable anti-HSV effect of propolis, a resinous material from poplar (*Populus tremuloides*) and conifer buds that bees use to maintain their hives. Applying an aqueous extract of propolis to cold sores before or at the time of infection gave best effect, but even after infection had occurred it appeared that propolis still gave 80 per cent protection.

OTHER HERBS Other well-known herbs have shown anti-HSV activity. In clinical studies, topical glycyrrhetinic acid (found in liquorice) encouraged herpes blisters to heal and reduced the pain associated with a cold-sore outbreak.

Tea tree (*Melaleuca alternifolia*) oil and eucalyptus (*Eucalyptus globulus*) oil individually show antiviral activity against HSV in the laboratory. Regular use of creams containing concentrated and dried leaf extract of lemon balm (*Melissa officinalis*) has proved highly effective against HSV. Siberian ginseng (*Eleutheroccus senticosus*) is also useful.

Soothing herbs, such as chickweed (*Stellaria media*) and chamomile (*Matricaria recutita*), applied as creams or gels or cold chamomile tea bags may provide relief.

TRADITIONAL TREATMENTS Some traditional treatments have yet to be researched. One is the Earl Grey tea bag (*see Self-Help*), which may be effective because of its bergamot oil and tannin content. Applying either golden seal (*Hydrastis canadensis*) powder mixed into live yoghurt or fresh grapefruit juice to an outbreak is also said to be effective. Some herbalists advocate aloe vera (*Aloe vera*) gel, while others recommend taking flaxseed oil because the omega-3 oils it contains can boost the body's immune defence against the virus.

> **CAUTION**
>
> See p.69 before taking a herbal remedy. Always consult a herbalist for a diagnosis and never self-treat.

Chinese Herbal Medicine

TCM doctors see HSV-1 and HSV-2 infections as typical "damp–heat" toxins. An acute attack is treated with Gentian Drain the Gallbladder Decoction (*Long Dan Xie Gan Tang*), with changes made for legal and safety reasons. For example, akebia (*Akebia trifoliata*) is replaced with phellodendron (*Phellodendron amurense*) bark, yellow mountain laurel (*Sophora flavescens*) root, dyer's woad (*Isatis tinctoria*) leaf and rhubarb (*Rheum officinale*) root.

A paste prepared from natural indigo (*Indigofera suffructicosa* or *Isatis tinctoria*) powder can be applied to the cold sores.

> **CAUTION**
>
> See p.69 before taking a Chinese herbal remedy and if you are taking a prescribed medication consult a Chinese herbalist first.

Mind–Body Therapies

The regular practice of a mind–body technique, along with lifestyle changes, such as stress reduction and regular exercise, may be effective in controlling the severity and/or the frequency of herpes recurrence.

RELAXATION TECHNIQUES Studies suggest that stress, anxiety, worry and depression can all make a recurrence of oral or genital

> ## Approximately 1 in 5 people infected with genital herpes have only one attack

herpes more likely. The social stigma of genital herpes enhances a sense of isolation and guilt. If you have herpes, regularly practising techniques such as progressive muscle relaxation, hypnosis, abdominal breathing and meditation can all help to counter stress by slowing the heart and respiration rates. In a 2002 study, participants who were prone to genital herpes were taught self-hypnosis over six weeks. Results showed their herpes attacks almost halved. Another study suggested cognitive restructuring, a form of cognitive behaviour therapy that focuses on changing attitudes toward a chronic illness, may also help.

STRESS MANAGEMENT In 1997, research showed that when men with genital herpes practised stress-management techniques, the frequency of their herpes attacks significantly reduced. The men also reported less depression and anxiety. Those who practised relaxation most consistently had greater improvement in mood. In 2000, another study revealed a 10-week period of stress management lowered stress levels, decreased the negative impact on the immune system and improved symptoms.

> **PREVENTION PLAN**
>
> **The following may help to prevent further attacks of herpes:**
>
> - Take a long course of an oral antiviral drug.
> - Take a daily multivitamin and mineral supplement.
> - Eat a low-arginine, high-lysine diet.
> - Practise relaxation and take exercise.

SHINGLES

The herpes zoster virus causes chickenpox (*see p.400*) and may later cause shingles, a blistering rash along the path of a nerve. Like herpes simplex, the herpes zoster virus remains dormant in the body and can then be reactivated later. Pain or discomfort, known as post-herpetic neuralgia, may persist in the affected area for many months after the rash has disappeared. Treatment involves painkillers and antiviral drugs, with additional measures to treat the post-herpetic neuralgia.

WHAT ARE THE SYMPTOMS?

- Initial tingling or pain in the affected area
- Tiny, painful blisters appear like a rash in one area of the body – usually on one side of the chest, abdomen or face – and later crust over
- Tiredness
- Fever
- Headache
- Pain and discomfort, known as post-herpetic neuralgia, may continue for several months

WHY MIGHT I HAVE THIS?

PREDISPOSING FACTORS

- Stress
- Illness

TREATMENT PLAN

PRIMARY TREATMENTS

- Oral drugs (antivirals and/or antibiotics)
- Pain relief

BACK-UP TREATMENTS

- Proteolytic enzymes
- Vitamin E
- Acupuncture
- Homeopathy
- Capsaicin cream
- Mind–body therapies

For an explanation of how treatments are rated, see p.111.

WHY DOES IT OCCUR?

Herpes zoster initially causes chickenpox and then remains dormant for the whole of the individual's life in the dorsal root ganglia, which is a nerve structure near the spine (*see next page*). Stress or an illness may reactivate the virus to cause shingles. The herpes zoster virus can be spread by direct contact with a blister. A person who has not had chickenpox can catch the virus from someone with shingles.

Chickenpox rarely recurs, but shingles tends to be a recurrent condition that mainly affects people aged between 50 and 70 years. People who have weakened or depleted immune systems, such as those with HIV/AIDS or cancer patients undergoing chemotherapy, are particularly susceptible to shingles. In older people, there may be prolonged pain (post-herpetic neuralgia, *see p.124*).

TREATMENTS IN DETAIL

Conventional Medicine

Your doctor will be able to diagnose shingles from the appearance of the rash and from other symptoms.

IMPORTANT

- Consult your doctor at once if you suspect you have the symptoms of shingles.
- Consult your doctor if you are pregnant and have been exposed to chickenpox.
- See your doctor immediately if the rash of shingles affects your face. If a nerve that supplies the eye is affected, it may cause inflammation and scarring of the cornea.

PRIMARY TREATMENT **ORAL DRUGS**, such as the antiviral drug aciclovir, may be given for a week and may help shorten attacks if they are started early enough. You will need antibiotics if the blisters become infected. Studies have shown that antiviral drugs and the antidepressant amitriptyline can reduce the likelihood of persistent post-herpetic neuralgia occurring.

PRIMARY TREATMENT **PAIN RELIEF** You can take painkillers, to help relieve the pain and discomfort of post-herpetic neuralgia. Alternatively, your doctor may prescribe a topical preparation containing anaesthetic drugs, which can be applied to the affected area.

A treatment known as transcutaneous electrical nerve stimulation (TENS) may also bring relief from the pain. A small device which you can use at home relays tiny electrical impulses (usually for about 30 minutes) to electrodes stuck to the skin in the painful area. The impulses stop the pain signals reaching the brain.

CAUTION

Antiviral drugs can cause side-effects: ask your doctor to explain these to you.

Do not use a TENS device if you have a pacemaker or if you are in the first trimester of pregnancy. Do not place the electrodes near your eyes or the front of your neck.

Nutritional Therapy

PROTEOLYTIC ENZYMES There is some evidence to suggest that taking a combination of the proteolytic (protein-digesting) enzymes chymotrypsin, papain and trypsin (administered orally) may help to

SHINGLES RASH

The shingles rash caused by the herpes zoster virus usually affects the skin of the chest, abdomen or face. More rarely, the rash may appear on a shoulder or on the scalp. It is common for the rash to occur on only one side of the body, because the virus becomes activated on one of the branches of the 12 pairs of dorsal nerves. After lying dormant in the dorsal root ganglion of a spinal nerve, the virus may be activated by stress or an illness. In a shingles attack, blisters appear on the skin along the path of the nerve. The rash may follow a line from the back to the front of the ribs.

The highlighted areas show the potential path of the shingles rash on the skin of the back as if the two nerves were infected.

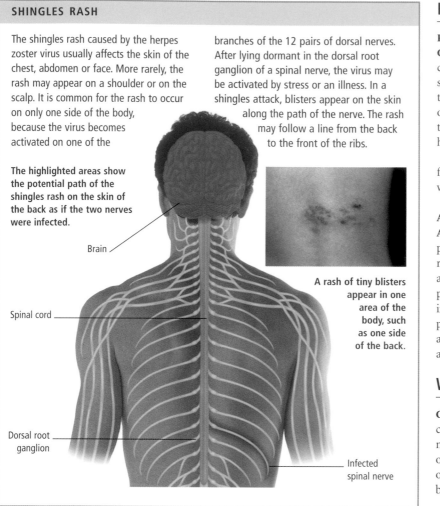

Brain

Spinal cord

Dorsal root ganglion

Infected spinal nerve

A rash of tiny blisters appear in one area of the body, such as one side of the back.

Homeopathy

RHUS TOXICODENDRON OR RANUNCULUS BULBOSUS *Rhus tox.* is the most commonly indicated medicine for acute shingles attacks. It is particularly suitable if there are small, intensely itchy blisters, often on a dusky-red background, and if the itching and pain are often relieved by hot applications.

Ranunculus bulbosus can be very helpful for shingles, especially if it affects the chest, with severe burning or shooting pain.

AGARICUS MUSCARIUS OR ARSENICUM ALBUM may sometimes help people with post-herpetic neuralgia. In those who respond to *Agaricus muscarius*, the pains are reported to be like "icy needles"; the patient may also suffer from tics or twitching. *Arsen. alb.* is associated with a burning pain that is relieved by heat. The skin is dry and flaky, while the patient is extremely anxious, tense and chilly.

Western Herbal Medicine

CAPSAICIN CREAM Post-herpetic neuralgia can be treated with capsaicin, which is made from chilli seeds. It may be available over the counter in creams. You can rub it on to the affected area several times a day, but it may cause a burning sensation.

Mind–Body Therapies

You can combat the psychological factors associated with post-herpetic neuralgia, such as stress and anxiety, with techniques, including progressive muscle relaxation, biofeedback, meditation or abdominal breathing. These techniques lower your heart and respiration rates, and calm your body and mind. Reducing stress appears to boost your immune response to the virus and helps to prevent reactivation.

accelerate the process of healing the shingles rash. The enzymes are thought to be involved in decreasing the body's inflammatory response to the virus. Research also shows that these enzymes may help to reduce the likelihood of having post-herpetic neuralgia.

In one study, the effect of administering 120mg of trypsin, 40mg of chymotrypsin and 320mg of papain five times a day reduced both the blisters and the pain. The effect was as good as aciclovir. The recommended dose is 500mg of a proteolytic enzyme preparation, taken several times a day while symptoms persist.

VITAMIN E A study in 1976 showed that taking vitamin E in a dose of 1,200–1,600 IU per day helped in some cases to alleviate the post-herpetic neuralgia associated with shingles. However, it can take six months or more before real benefit is seen.

> **CAUTION**
>
> Consult your doctor before taking vitamin E with aspirin or warfarin (*see p.46*).

Acupuncture

In Traditional Chinese Medicine, acupuncture is widely used to treat acute shingles: it is usually provided within 48–72 hours of the illness developing. No trials compare acupuncture with antiviral drugs, but circumstantial evidence suggests that it may help to prevent post-herpetic neuralgia if it is given during the acute phase. However, good evidence suggests that acupuncture does not help once the neuralgia has become established. Treatment for shingles should be provided in the first few days, on a daily or every other day basis, and gradually discontinued as the rash settles.

> **PREVENTION PLAN**
>
> **The following may help to prevent further attacks of shingles:**
>
> - Eat a good diet, possibly with multivitamin supplements.
> - Practise relaxation regularly to keep stress to a minimum.

ECZEMA AND CONTACT DERMATITIS

Eczema, also known as dermatitis, is a condition in which patches of skin become red, inflamed and itchy. Affected areas may also be covered in small, fluid-filled blisters. Of the several types, atopic eczema is the most common. The rash of contact dermatitis may result from irritation or from an allergic reaction. With no complete cure for eczema, the aim is to control symptoms with topical creams, special diets, probiotics, avoiding environmental triggers and taking herbal remedies. Relaxation and breathing retraining may also help.

WHAT ARE THE SYMPTOMS?

- Redness and swelling of the skin
- Small, fluid-filled blisters
- Itching, especially at night
- Dry, scaly and cracked skin
- Thickened skin in long-standing eczema

WHY MIGHT I HAVE THIS?

PREDISPOSING FACTORS

For atopic eczema:

- Genetic tendency
- Fatty acid deficiency
- Stress and anxiety
- Depression
- Biotin deficiency
- Vitamin B12 deficiency
- Zinc deficiency
- High histamine levels in the blood

TRIGGERS

For atopic eczema:

- Strong detergents, soaps, dog and cat fur, wearing wool, house-dust mites
- Food sensitivities

For contact dermatitis:

- Exposure to sensitising agents, such as nickel, rubber, plants (e.g. primulas)

For seborrhoeic dermatitis:

- Yeast overgrowth may be a factor

WHY DOES IT OCCUR?

We are witnessing a significant increase in atopic eczema and environmental factors certainly play a part. Centrally heated houses, house-dust mites in pillows and carpets, as well as animal dander from household pets, may all trigger or worsen eczema in susceptible individuals. However, there are also many other factors (*see left*) – some, such as detergents, are actually irritants rather than triggers. Eczema tends to recur intermittently throughout life. Each type of eczema may be triggered by different factors.

TYPES OF ECZEMA Atopic eczema may first appear in infancy and continue to flare up throughout adolescence and adulthood.

The cause is unknown, but this type of eczema often appears in people with an inherited disposition to other allergic conditions, including asthma and hay fever.

The mechanism underlying eczema is not fully understood. In people with atopic eczema, it seems as though the immune system reacts to an otherwise harmless substance, such as dust, as if it were dangerous. It is thought that inflammatory cells are stimulated to destroy the "allergen", and if too many are activated, the skin becomes red, swollen and itchy.

In contact dermatitis and other types of eczema, the skin is irritated and there may be an allergic response. Contact dermatitis can occur at any age and develops after touching something to which you are sensitive – for example, an object made of

TREATMENT PLAN

PRIMARY TREATMENTS

- Emollient creams and topical treatments
- Food-exclusion diet
- Essential fatty acids
- Homeopathy
- Avoidance of environmental irritants

BACK-UP TREATMENTS

- Oral corticosteroids and immunosuppressants (for severe eczema)
- Ultraviolet phototherapy

- Probiotics (particularly for children)
- Western and Chinese herbal medicine
- Mind–body therapies

WORTH CONSIDERING

- Breathing retraining
- Zinc, biotin and vitamin B
- Anti-*Candida* diet

For an explanation of how treatments are rated, see p.111.

nickel or rubber, or the leaves of a plant, such as a primula.

Seborrhoeic dermatitis usually affects the face and scalp, but also the armpits, groin and middle of the chest. The skin tends to become red, scaly and flaky. In babies, it affects the scalp (when it is called cradle cap) and sometimes the nappy area. The cause is unknown, but the condition is sometimes associated with an overgrowth of a type of yeast (not *Candida albicans*) on the skin. It can occur both in infancy and in adulthood.

Nummular, or discoid, eczema, causes itchy, coin-shaped patches on the arms and legs. Affected areas may ooze and become scaly or blistered. It is more common in men. The cause is not known, nor is it clear if there is an immune response.

IMPORTANT

If you have eczema symptoms, consult your doctor for a diagnosis.

SELF-HELP

- Avoid contact with known irritants and keep notes in a diary to find out which factors, whether foods, dust, or stress, could be triggering your attacks.
- Use emollient soothing creams frequently and liberally.
- Do not scratch the affected areas.
- Expose the affected area to sunlight for ten minutes several times weekly.
- Spread *Calendula* cream on the eczema patches. (Homeopathic *Calendula* cream may contain lanolin – do not use this if you are sensitive to lanolin.)
- Wear gloves when doing housework to protect your hands from detergents and cleaning materials.
- Use hypo-allergenic bathwater oil to help moisturise the skin.
- Place 500g (1lb) of oatmeal in a gauze, cotton or cheesecloth bag. Hang it under a running hot-water tap as you fill a bath. The bathwater should be at body temperature (not too hot). Let the bag float in the bath and use it to gently pat areas of particular irritation. Stay in the water for around 20 minutes and then pat yourself dry afterwards, taking care not to rub.

PATCH TESTING FOR CONTACT DERMATITIS

Patch testing of the skin helps a doctor to determine which substances cause an allergic reaction. Tiny amounts of the substances are placed on small discs, which are stuck to an inert tape and placed on a person's back. After about two days, the discs are removed to reveal either red patches (positive reactions) or no changes (negative reactions). In some cases, the reaction may be delayed.

Positive reaction to test

Negative reaction to test

TREATMENTS IN DETAIL

Conventional Medicine

Your doctor will usually be able to diagnose eczema from the symptoms alone, and may be able to distinguish the type from an examination and a discussion about the possible irritants. The location of your contact dermatitis may help to determine the cause. People with contact dermatitis may need patch testing (*see above*) to look for positive or negative reaction to selected trigger substances.

PRIMARY TREATMENT **EMOLLIENTS AND TOPICAL TREATMENTS** are your doctor's first option for controlling symptoms of eczema. Emollients help to keep the skin moist (hydrated). Topical corticosteroid creams, which reduce inflammation, can help to relieve eczema symptoms. If corticosteroid creams are used intermittently and at the right strength for the body area being treated, they are unlikely to cause thinning of the skin or other side-effects. Soap substitutes, such as aqueous cream, can also be useful.

If you have seborrhoeic eczema, the doctor will suggest a mild topical steroid and an antifungal cream. Antifungal shampoos, emollients and soap substitutes may also be recommended. If you have developed contact dermatitis, your doctor will treat it like atopic eczema and will advise you to avoid the irritant where possible and to take preventive self-help measures, such as protecting your hands with barrier creams or gloves.

ORAL DRUGS may be prescribed for people with very severe atopic eczema. These include corticosteroids, cyclosporin and azathioprine. These drugs work by reducing the immune response. Oral antibiotics may be prescribed if the eczema becomes infected. Some antihistamines may be taken at night for their sedating properties.

ULTRAVIOLET PHOTOTHERAPY (UVA) may also be needed in severe cases of eczema in order to reduce the skin inflammation (*see Psoriasis, p.172*).

CAUTION

Oral drugs and ultraviolet phototherapy have a range of possible side-effects: ask your doctor to explain these to you.

Nutritional Therapy

PRIMARY TREATMENT **A FOOD-EXCLUSION DIET** may be needed for children who develop atopic eczema. Evidence suggests that food sensitivity is a common feature in children with eczema. Identifying the suspect food and following a special diet that eliminates it often leads to a very significant improvement in symptoms (*see p.39*).

PRIMARY TREATMENT **ESSENTIAL FATTY ACIDS** are needed for keeping the skin healthy. Research has suggested that people with eczema may be unable to process these acids normally.

Evening primrose oil, which contains omega-6 fatty acids, used to be recommended, but the most recent research shows that it does not help. Although the largest study of fish oil was negative, some studies seem to show that fish oils can reduce the overall severity of symptoms and the scaling and itching of atopic eczema. Take 1.8g of omega-3 fatty acids each day for 1–3 months as a trial. This dose is the equivalent of 3–4g of fish oil, or a daily portion of oily fish.

leakage of food allergens (food particles that initiate immune reactions) across the gut wall, which can be one element in atopic eczema in early childhood. There is some good news for mothers at risk of having a child with eczema (i.e. women who already have a child with eczema, suffer from eczema themselves or have a first-degree relative with eczema). Evidence suggests that if you take probiotics during pregnancy and then feed your child probiotics after birth, your child is less likely to develop eczema.

ZINC OR BIOTIN SUPPLEMENTS may benefit some people with eczema. The clinical research so far fails to identify precisely who is likely to respond to them, but they could be worth trying for a month.

VITAMIN B SUPPLEMENTS Evidence suggests that eczema and dermatitis may be made worse by a deficiency in vitamin B12. It has been known for over 50 years that vitamin B12 supplements may help to alleviate the symptoms of dermatitis. Since studies suggest that a deficiency of other B vitamins, such as riboflavin, may also be involved in exacerbating eczema, try taking

Homeopathy

Each of the various types of eczema respond well to homeopathic medicines. Although there are only a few clinical trials for evaluating the homeopathic treatment of eczema (the same is also true for the conventional treatments), homeopaths consistently report very good results.

PRIMARY TREATMENT Eczema is an ailment that illustrates one of the principles of homeopathy: three different medicines (*Arsenicum album, Graphites* and *Sulphur*) will help in most cases, but a homeopath must choose the correct remedy for the individual (*see p.73*).

ARSENICUM ALBUM AND SULPHUR People who respond to these two remedies have similar characteristic skin symptoms – they experience intensely itchy rashes that burn after scratching. However, the types of people who respond to these two medicines are markedly different. The typical person who responds to *Arsen. alb.* is tidy, fastidious, tends to be anxious and feels the cold excessively.

On the other hand, people who respond to *Sulphur* are often untidy and tend to be extroverts who relish a good argument. In addition, they are often warm-blooded (they feel heat) and have hot feet.

> Between 40 and 60 per cent of people with eczema also have a respiratory allergy

Hemp and flaxseed oils are rich sources of essential fatty acids. Take 1–2 tablespoons of oil a day for one month (doses should be reduced for children, in proportion to their weight). It can also be used in ointments to control dry, atopic eczema.

PROBIOTICS contain healthy gut bacteria that may help infants and young children with atopic eczema. This is because research shows that the large intestines of atopic infants may have a disturbed balance of beneficial and potentially harmful bacteria. Giving probiotics (*Bifidobacterium lactis Bb-12* and *Lactobacillus GG*) in formula milk to infants during weaning can be beneficial in reducing the extent and severity of atopic eczema. Evidence seems to suggest that probiotics benefit the immune system and may also decrease

a high-potency vitamin B complex each day for a month. In addition, applying vitamin B6 cream can help to control seborrhoeic eczema in some children.

ANTI-CANDIDA DIET Nutritionists find that seborrhoeic dermatitis often seems to be related to an overgrowth of the yeast organisms in the small intestine. If the rash is itchy, and your bowel is also upset, then *Candida* may be an underlying factor and an anti-*Candida* diet may help control the symptoms. (*See p.40 for anti-Candida diet.*)

CAUTION

Consult your doctor before taking fish oil or omega-3 oils with warfarin, or zinc with antibiotics (*see p.46*).

GRAPHITES In *Graphites* cases of eczema, the rash tends to crack and ooze a clear or yellowish, sticky liquid when scratched. It often affects particular areas, such as behind the ears or on the nipples; in women, the eczema may become worse before menstruation. (*See also Locals, mentals and generals, p.76.*)

TAKING REMEDIES Start each of the above treatments by taking two pills of the 6C strength, twice daily. Beware of "aggravations", in which you experience temporary flare-ups of the symptoms, followed by improvement. Aggravations are quite common in the homeopathic treatment of skin conditions and are considered a positive sign because they indicate that you are reacting to the medicine. If you develop an aggravation, stop your treatment and do not take any more of the remedy until the aggravation has fully settled. This may take up to two to three weeks.

Western Herbal Medicine

External treatments play a role in controlling the symptoms of eczema, but effective herbal healing of eczema usually requires internal treatment as well. The best way to take the herbs is in an infusion (brewed like a tea) or a decoction (boiled in water to extract the active ingredients) rather than as a tincture (soaked in alcohol and water to extract the active ingredients).

STARFLOWER OIL, when applied to childrens' seborrhoeic dermatitis (cradle cap), sometimes leads to considerable improvement within 3–4 weeks, according to research. Starflower is also known as borage (*Borago officinalis*). Rub ten drops of starflower oil into the affected region of the skin twice a day for a month. Repeat this treatment as necessary.

OTHER EXTERNAL TREATMENTS When washing yourself, try using oatmeal (*Avena sativa*) sealed in an old stocking instead of soap (*see Self-Help, p.168*). If you are having a bath, run the hot water through a bag

lesions, as can a compress of oak (*Quercus robur*) bark tea, which is rich in tannins. Witch hazel also soothes inflamed skin. Liquorice (*Glycyrrhiza glabra*) paste mixed with a drop or two of chamomile or peppermint (*Mentha piperita*) oil applied externally may also reduce the inflammation and itch. Liquorice has a mild steroidal-like effect and an active principle within the plant, glycyrrhetinic acid, applied in an ointment to eczema rashes displayed an improvement similar to the effect of cortisone.

Studies have documented the anti-inflammatory and soothing effects of creams prepared from chamomile in treating inflamed skin. For the few people who develop reactions to chamomile, hypo-allergenic chamomile preparations may be used instead.

INTERNAL TREATMENTS Western herbalists advise patients to drink infusions and decoctions made with so-called blood-cooling herbs to calm inflamed skin. These include nettle, heartsease (*Viola tricolor*), figwort (*Scrophularia nodosa*), red clover (*Trifolium pratense*), burdock (*Arctium lappa*) root and leaf, and yellow dock (*Rumex crispus*) root.

Teas made from elderflower, limeflower (*Tileia cordata*) and Rooibosch (*Aspalathus linearis*) can help to reduce itching. Weeping eczema may respond to the

Chinese Herbal Medicine

Eczema is known in Traditional Chinese Medicine (TCM) as *Si Wan Feng*, in which "dampness" plays an important part. Clinical control trials in the 1990s of a standard formula of ten herbs for the treatment of dry, atopic eczema showed significant effects in both adults and children. Approximately half the children who took part (at Great Ormond Street Hospital in London) continued to benefit from the formula a year later. The researchers noted, however, that the treatment might provoke liver abnormalities, and later trials of TCM herbs for eczema have not confirmed the original good results.

TYPES OF ECZEMA One of a number of typical presentations is damp–heat eczema with "fire poison" (i.e. a bacterial infection). The skin is very red with raised, red papules, vesicles (small, fluid-filled blisters) and pustules (pus-filled spots) that may weep. Treatment is likely to be based on Gentian Drain the Gallbladder Decoction (*Long Dan Xie Gan Tang*) but omitting *Mu Tong*, which is illegal in the UK.

Acute eczema that corresponds to widespread, dry, atopic eczema is "heat in the blood with resulting wind" (i.e. disrupted *Qi* flow) but little or no dampness. There is no weeping from the inflamed skin. TCM doctors may treat this by modifying a combination of three classical treatments that cool the blood and eliminate wind.

In chronic attacks of eczema that are repeated over a period of months or years, a pattern may develop caused by blood deficiency. Affected skin is dry, rough, thickened and very itchy. The patient is chronically fatigued and suffers from dry, thinning hair and ridged nails that break easily. The correct strategy is to nourish the blood, clear the heat and eliminate the wind (disrupted *Qi* flow). A typical prescription is a variation of Chinese Angelica Decoction (*Dang Gui Yin Zi*).

EXTERNAL TREATMENTS Skullcap (*Scutellaria laterifolia*) root, phellodendron (*Phellodendron amurense*) bark and sophora (*Sophora flavescens*) root can be combined to make a soothing wash for inflamed skin. A paste, wash or ointment that contains burnet (*Sanguisorba officinalis*) root can calm irritated skin.

> The incidence of eczema has increased threefold in the last 30 years

of oatmeal. To control the symptoms of dry, atopic eczema apply an ointment containing hemp oil to your skin.

Try a paste of slippery elm (*Ulmus rubra*) powder and oatmeal mixed with chamomile (*Matricaria recutita*) and elderflower (*Sambucus nigra*) tea and distilled witch hazel (*Hamamelis virginiana*). An ointment prepared from nettle (*Urtica dioica*) juice may bring relief, too.

Compresses of chickweed (*Stellaria media*) or cold cucumber are soothing. The healing astringent action of a compress prepared from the leaves of walnut (*Juglans regia*) can bring relief to weeping

antibacterial action of Oregon grape root (*Mahonia aquifolium*), fumitory (*Fumaria officinalis*), dandelion (*Taraxacum officinale*) root and golden seal (*Hydrastis canadensis*). A substance called inulin in dandelion and burdock root may increase the resistance of the immune system to infection and reduce histamine release.

Environmental Health

Allergic contact dermatitis and irritant contact dermatitis are the most common skin problems caused by exposure to environmental agents.

PRIMARY TREATMENT **AVOIDING IRRITANTS** Common agents known to cause contact dermatitis are acids, alkalis, solvents and other highly irritant chemicals. They are found in everyday products, such as deodorants, hair products, antistatic compounds, antiseptics, disinfectants, alcohols, soaps, cleaners, detergents, softeners, fibreglass, solvents, petrol, paraffin, paint, adhesives, lacquers, degreasing agents, pesticides and latex. Ultraviolet radiation may also cause contact dermatitis.

Skin irritation may result from a specific product or a specific ingredient in a group of products. For example, an irritant contact dermatitis may be caused by compounds in personal hygiene products, the chlorine-containing compounds in cleaning products or the organohalogen substances present in some pesticides.

Most environmental agents can cause dermatitis in one of two ways. They can act as "sensitisers" by dissolving the protective oily layer on the skin, impairing its barrier function and sensitising it to other chemicals and irritants that would otherwise not pose a problem. Or, they can act as "irritants" directly.

PERSONAL HISTORY Ask an environmental health expert to help identify which chemicals you have been exposed to and to match potential exposures to your particular skin problem. This involves analysing your specific circumstances, such as your work and home environment and even the local weather conditions, to determine when your symptoms are better or worse. You will need to answer questions, such as "Do you live or work near any hazardous chemical facilities?" and "Does anyone around you have similar symptoms?".

NON-TOXIC ALTERNATIVES Try to use low-emitting building materials, continuous ventilation and non-toxic office and cleaning supplies. Carefully store the chemicals in your home or office. For a trial period, limit contact with known irritants, such as latex, antiseptics and detergents, and avoid prolonged exposure to the sun without proper protection.

If you find you are sensitive to a particular substance, look for an alternative. For example, replace products made from latex, which are ubiquitous in both industry and healthcare, with those made from nitrile. Many stores stock environmentally friendly, natural, organic or non-toxic versions of common household and garden products, such as pesticides.

Breathing Retraining

Diaphragmatic, yoga-type breathing exercises help to retrain breathing. People who habitually breathe with only their upper chest expire excessive amounts of carbon dioxide. This makes the blood more alkaline and increases allergic responses, which may make the eczema worse.

Breathing retraining is a simple exercise that focuses on the diaphragm and breaks the habit of upper-chest breathing (*see p. 57*). It is based on yoga and, if practised over at least a three-month period, has been shown to change breathing habits, especially when it is coupled with massage and other types of bodywork that release and relax the chest and upper back.

Mind–Body Therapies

People with eczema may become anxious, stressed and, if the condition affects the face or other visible areas of skin, markedly depressed. Stress may precipitate and make eczema worse in vulnerable individuals.

A 1995 study provided evidence that mind–body therapies, such as biofeedback, autogenic training and hypnotherapy, may help to treat the psychological components of atopic dermatitis and to manage the symptoms, especially in tandem with medical treatment. Group psychotherapy, as a supplement to a regular medical regime, can help, too.

BIOFEEDBACK When combined with progressive relaxation at home, biofeedback can help to reduce the severity of atopic eczema and the associated irritation. Research shows that mind–body relaxation

In the UK, eczema affects around 1 in 5 children and 1 in 12 adults

combined with guided imagery may be more effective than relaxation alone in lowering the anxiety levels and itchiness.

AUTOGENIC TRAINING As a way of managing the stress and anxiety associated with eczema, autogenic training compares well with other mind–body therapies, such as biofeedback and techniques focused more exclusively on muscular relaxation. It is a series of six mental exercises that changes body chemistry to encourage relaxation. It regulates unwanted tension in both involuntary muscles (e.g. those in the blood vessels) and voluntary muscles (e.g. those in the back). The length of treatment does not seem to affect the clinical outcome – even a short period of autogenic training can alleviate eczema symptoms.

HYPNOTHERAPY can control itching. After inducing a state of profound relaxation, a practitioner will aim to plant positive suggestions in the subconscious mind to help relieve anxiety and reduce the desire to scratch the skin.

PREVENTION PLAN

The following may help if you are prone to eczema:

- Avoid irritant chemicals.
- Eat a healthy diet.
- Practise relaxation.

WHAT ARE THE SYMPTOMS?

For plaque psoriasis:

- Patches of thickened, red, scaly skin, usually on the knees, elbows, lower back and scalp, and sometimes on old scars
- Intermittent itchiness or soreness of the affected areas
- Discoloured nails with small pits

For guttate psoriasis:

- Coin-shaped, pink patches of scaly skin, about 1cm (2/5in) across, mainly on the back and chest
- Intermittent itchiness of the affected areas

For pustular psoriasis:

- Small fluid-filled blisters on a red base, mainly on the palms of the hands and the soles of the feet
- Gradual replacement of blisters by brown spots or small, scaly patches
- In the severe form, many blisters usually develop quickly, together with a fever

For inverse psoriasis:

- Large, clearly defined, red areas in the folds of skin. The rash often affects the groin, the armpits and the skin under the breasts

WHY MIGHT I HAVE THIS?

PREDISPOSING FACTORS

- Genetic factors
- HIV infection

TRIGGERS

- Excessive alcohol intake
- Drugs, e.g. some antimalarials and, rarely, beta-blockers
- Food sensitivity
- Overgrowth of yeast organisms, such as *Candida albicans*
- Injury
- Infection
- Stress or anxiety

PSORIASIS

Psoriasis is an inflammatory disorder that can affect many areas of the body at once. The most common type is plaque psoriasis, but all forms of psoriasis involve reddening and thickening of the skin. Treatment combines skin preparations with a nutritional regime that eliminates food sensitivities and incorporates foods that are rich in omega-3 fatty acids, fresh fruit and vegetables, and supplements of selenium or vitamin E. Oral drugs, such as immunosuppressants, are reserved for severe cases that do not respond to other treatments.

WHY DOES IT OCCUR?

In psoriasis, new skin cells are produced at a much faster rate than dead cells are shed, so an excess of skin cells accumulate to form thickened patches. The cause of psoriasis is not known, but episodes may be triggered by local trauma, excessive alcohol, food sensitivity, infection, injury, stress and anxiety, and, according to complementary therapists, *Candida* overgrowth.

TREATMENT PLAN

PRIMARY TREATMENTS

- Topical treatments
- Sarsaparilla
- Homeopathic *Calendula* cream (for immediate relief)

BACK-UP TREATMENTS

- UV phototherapy (for severe psoriasis)
- Oral drugs (for severe psoriasis)
- Food-exclusion and anti-*Candida* diets
- Omega-3 fatty acids and dietary changes
- Homeopathy (*see also Self-Help*)
- Western and Chinese herbal medicine
- Mind–body therapies

WORTH CONSIDERING

- Acupuncture

For an explanation of how treatments are rated, see p.111.

Certain drugs, such as antimalarials, can trigger psoriasis. Free radicals may be involved in generating the inflammation. The condition often runs in families, and around 5 per cent of people with psoriasis develop a particular form of arthritis.

TYPES OF PSORIASIS Of the four types, only plaque psoriasis, which may develop at any age and is the most common type, is usually a lifelong disorder.

Guttate psoriasis, which affects mainly children and adolescents, often develops about two weeks after a bacterial throat infection. This type usually resolves spontaneously after one to two months, but it may recur or plaque psoriasis may develop.

A rare type, pustular psoriasis, may become life-threatening if the severe form

The elbow is one of the common locations for the characteristic patches of thickened skin. Other sites where plaque psoriasis develops include the scalp, knees and forearms.

IMPORTANT

See your doctor if you experience symptoms of psoriasis. In rare cases, there may be a serious underlying cause.

occurs, as dehydration, kidney failure and severe infections may develop. Inverse psoriasis, which mainly affects elderly people, usually clears up without treatment. Some people are affected by more than one type of psoriasis.

IMMEDIATE RELIEF

PRIMARY TREATMENT Apply homeopathic *Calendula* (marigold) cream freely to psoriasis patches. If you are allergic to lanolin make sure the cream is lanolin-free.

TREATMENTS IN DETAIL

Conventional Medicine

Your doctor will be able to diagnose the type of psoriasis from the appearance of the skin patches.

Since plaque psoriasis cannot be cured completely, doctors aim to control the symptoms and will usually start by prescribing creams to apply to the skin.

Guttate and plaque psoriasis are usually treated with topical treatments and, sometimes, with ultraviolet light therapies. Pustular psoriasis that is restricted to the hands and feet may be treated with very strong topical steroids or PUVA light therapy (*see right*).

PUVA phototherapy involves regular exposure to ultraviolet light under hospital supervision. It is believed to help people with psoriasis by reducing skin inflammation.

Severe pustular psoriasis requires urgent hospital admission for monitoring, with drugs and supportive measures provided. Inverse psoriasis can often be controlled by mild topical steroids.

PRIMARY TREATMENT **TOPICAL TREATMENTS** Emollient creams and lotions can help bring relief by hydrating (moistening) and softening the skin. There are various other topical treatments, all of which are usually applied to the psoriasis patches once or twice a day. Some are not to be used by pregnant women but your doctor will advise you about this and any other potential side-effects.

Corticosteroid creams of a mild to moderate strength may provide short-term relief by reducing inflammation. Purified coal tar which is widely available in the form of bath products, ointments and pastes, also helps relieve inflammation.

Calcipotriol, which is derived from vitamin D, can be used either as an ointment and cream or as a preparation to be applied to the scalp but not to the face. Its action appears to slow the production of the skin cells involved in the process of skin thickening and patch formation.

Dithranol cream can help; it also slows down the rate at which skin cells divide. Make sure you wash it off within an hour of applying it. Tazarotene, which is a retinoid drug derived from vitamin A, is a gel that you can spread on affected areas. The mechanism by which it works is not yet fully understood.

PUVA AND UVB PHOTOTHERAPY reduce skin inflammation. They involve treatment with the two different types of ultraviolet light (UVA and UVB) and are sometimes combined with topical treatments.

In PUVA (psoralen ultraviolet A) phototherapy, patients take a psoralen drug, such as methoxsalen, that makes the skin more sensitive to the effects of the light. The drug enhances the treatment with long-wave ultraviolet light (UVA), which is delivered by special lamps in hospitals. The use of PUVA is carefully regulated.

UVB phototherapy involves supervised and regulated exposure to the radiation from ultraviolet B lamps.

ORAL DRUGS may be needed if plaque psoriasis is so severe it does not respond adequately to topical treatments. They are prescribed by a hospital doctor. The drugs include: acitretin, which is a retinoid drug that may start to have an effect after 2–4 weeks; cyclosporin, which is an immunosuppressant; and methotrexate, also an immunosuppressant, which is usually taken once a week.

> **CAUTION**
>
> Topical treatments, oral drugs and phototherapy all have potential side-effects: ask your doctor to explain them to you.

Nutritional Therapy

A FOOD-EXCLUSION DIET may help since clinical experience indicates that some psoriasis cases may be linked to food sensitivity (*see p.39*). Evidence from one study suggests that individuals with psoriasis may improve on a diet that excludes food likely to cause sensitivity problems. Another study reported that eliminating gluten – found in wheat, barley and rye – improved psoriasis in some individuals.

AN ANTI-CANDIDA DIET will resolve an overgrowth of yeast organisms, such as *Candida albicans.* Some studies indicate that too much *Candida* in the intestine is common in people with psoriasis, and that this infection is a potential provoking factor in psoriasis. (*For the diagnosis and treatment of* Candida, *and for anti-*Candida *diets, see p.40.*)

OMEGA-3 AND OMEGA-6 FATTY ACIDS Eating less food containing the unhealthy omega-6 fatty acids and more food containing the healthy omega-3 fatty acids (*see p.34*) may help people with psoriasis, who tend to have raised levels of a fat known as arachidonic acid in their blood. This acid seems to encourage inflammation in the body, leading some scientists to believe that it may be an important underlying factor in psoriasis.

In the body, arachidonic acid can be formed from omega-6 fatty acids – found in many margarines, vegetable oils, processed foods, fast foods and baked goods, such as muffins, cakes, biscuits and pastries. Foods that are rich in arachidonic acid include dairy products and red meat. Consequently, if you have psoriasis, avoid foods containing omega-6 fatty acids and arachidonic acid.

In addition, supplementing your diet with omega-3 fatty acids, which have anti-inflammatory effects in the body, may help to relieve psoriasis. In one study, taking 10g of fish oil daily improved the skin patches of psoriasis. Patients had less itching, scaling and redness, and the affected area had diminished in size compared to those of the people taking the placebo.

FRESH FRUIT AND VEGETABLES Clinical experience has demonstrated that people with psoriasis often benefit from eating a diet rich in fruit and vegetables. These foods are full of many different nutrients, especially vitamin C and beta-carotene, which have antioxidant properties that may help to quell inflammation.

SELENIUM is an antioxidant mineral that may also help, since various studies have shown that people with psoriasis often have low selenium levels. Research suggests that taking 100–200mcg of selenium supplements daily, in combination with 10mg of vitamin E supplements, may help to reduce psoriasis symptoms.

> **CAUTION**
>
> Consult your doctor before taking vitamin E with warfarin or aspirin, or fish oils/omega-3 fatty acids with warfarin (*see p.46*).

Homeopathy

Case studies indicate that many patients with psoriasis benefit from homeopathic treatment, although in the majority of

OTHER REMEDIES *Graphites* may be appropriate in inverse psoriasis and in psoriasis that is unusually distributed – for instance, in the fold behind the ears, where the eruption cracks and may ooze clear colourless or yellow fluid.

The psoriasis that responds to *Sulphur* is usually the plaque type: intensely itchy and often the rash is red and raw because of scratching. Heat makes the itching worse (for instance, in bed). The patient is generally hot-blooded, often with hot feet, kicking off shoes at every opportunity, and sticking their feet out of bed at night. *Sulphur* types are hot, scruffy, usually extrovert and untidy or flamboyant.

The psoriasis in people who respond to *Lycopodium* and *Sepia* is not very specific. Homeopaths prescribe these medicines mostly according to the person's mental and general features (*see Constitutional medicines and polychrests, p. 73*).

Western Herbal Medicine

Although psoriasis appears to have a significant genetic basis, there are various plant-based treatments to which herbalists can turn.

PRIMARY TREATMENT **SARSAPARILLA** (*Smilax ornata*) is a detoxification herb that may help to reduce an overload of toxins, which are derived from the intestines and implicated in psoriasis. Sarsaparilla's anti-inflammatory properties make it useful for combating the arthritis that sometimes affects people with psoriasis.

The little research that has been done on sarsaparilla supports its traditional use in treating psoriasis. In one controlled study of 92 patients, the herb significantly improved the psoriasis of 62 per cent and achieved complete clearance of the condition in 18 per cent of subjects.

OTHER DETOXIFICATION HERBS, such as burdock (*Arctium lappa*) and the root of yellow dock (*Rumex crispus*), are used to clean up an overloaded system and maintain a healthy bowel.

Aloe vera (*Aloe vera*) heals the gut, promoting the growth of healthy intestinal bacteria. Linseed (*Linum usitatissimum*) and the seeds of psyllium (*Plantago psyllium*) both have a detoxifying and soothing effect on the bowel.

Psoriasis affects approximately 2 per cent of people in the UK

Omega-3 fatty acids are a constituent of certain nuts and seeds, especially walnuts and flaxseeds, and of oily fish, such as mackerel, salmon and sardines. People with psoriasis may benefit from regular inclusion of these foods in their diet or from taking a daily supplement of 5–10g of concentrated fish oil. For those who do not like the odour of fish oil, a good alternative is flaxseed oil, which has three times as much omega-3 fatty acids as omega-6 fatty acids.

Research shows that applying fish oil to patches of skin affected by psoriasis effectively relieves scaling, but not itching. Other research reports that intravenous infusions of a fish-oil emulsion can help ameliorate the symptoms of chronic plaque psoriasis.

cases, the problem does not clear up completely. Treatment needs to be prescribed on an individual basis. Among the most important medicines are: *Arsenicum album, Arsenicum iodatum, Graphites, Sulphur, Lycopodium* and *Sepia*.

ARSENICUMS The two *Arsenicums* are usually used for guttate psoriasis in which the plaques tend to be small, rounded and flaky. *Arsen. alb.* may also be very helpful in pustular psoriasis. The rash is often very itchy and burns after scratching. The itching of people who respond to *Arsen. alb.* is relieved by heat and they are anxious, tense and meticulous. *Arsen. iod.* has less of these features, but patients often have severe hay fever and other allergies, particularly affecting the eyes.

> Ten per cent of adults with psoriasis may have developed it before they were 10 years old

BERBERINE Incomplete digestion of proteins can bring about raised levels of amino acids and peptides in the bowel. These are then metabolised by bowel bacteria into potentially toxic compounds called polyamines, which can stimulate skin cells to divide at too fast a rate.

Studies show that people with psoriasis have increased levels of polyamines. Berberine, an alkaloid found in Oregon graperoot (*Mahonia aquifolium*) and golden seal (*Hydrastis canadensis*), inhibits the formation of polyamines.

LIVER REMEDIES In treating psoriasis, herbalists also pay particular attention to ensuring that the liver works to its optimum potential. The liver has a vital function of filtering and detoxifying the blood as it returns from the bowel. Any decrease in its ability to detoxify means an increase in the blood level of toxins, derived from the intestines and elsewhere, that aggravate psoriasis.

People with psoriasis should avoid drinking significant amounts of alcohol because it impairs liver function and damages the lining of the bowel, increasing the absorption of toxins from the intestine. Alcohol also dilates the skin capillaries, increasing cell turnover and inflammation.

Liver remedies that may be used to treat psoriasis include dandelion (*Taraxacum officinale*), Oregon graperoot (*Mahonia aquifolium*), the bark of barberry (*Berberis vulgaris*), milk thistle (*Silybum marianum*), blue flag (*Iris versicolor*), golden seal and the leaves of artichoke (*Cynara scolymus*).

A potent liver remedy for short-term use by professionals only is greater celandine (*Cheldonium majus*). It contains the alkaloid sanguinarine, which has been shown to reduce the proliferation of the protein keratin, a major constituent of the epidermal layer of skin.

OTHER HERBAL STRATEGIES are the lymphatic stimulants that aid detoxification. These include cleavers (*Galium aperine*) and figwort (*Scrophularia nodosa*). Red clover (*Trifolium pratense*) also has a cleansing (alterative) effect and is traditionally used for the treatment of psoriasis.

EXTERNAL TREATMENTS Psoriasis is best treated internally, but trials on aloe vera (*Aloe vera*) gel, when applied to psoriasis patches, have shown some success in controlling this skin disease. Herbalists have also used comfrey (*Symphytum officinale*) ointment to treat the patches of psoriasis.

> **CAUTION**
>
> See page 69 before taking a herbal remedy and, if you are already taking a prescribed medication, consult a medical herbalist first.

Chinese Herbal Medicine

Chinese herbal medicine categorises psoriasis in ways that are unfamiliar to Western doctors. For example, acutely progressive psoriasis, marked by widespread, distinct and raised red patches, is seen as caused by heat in the blood. The main prescription for this is based on the Sarsaparilla and Sophora Decoction (*Tu Hai Yin*), which contains herbs for cooling the blood.

The TCM herbalist will also generally advise those with psoriasis to avoid alcohol, spicy food, shellfish and "hot" meats, such as lamb and beef.

> **CAUTION**
>
> See page 69 before taking a herbal remedy. always consult a medical herbalist for a diagnosis and do not self-treat.

Acupuncture

To date, no trials indicate that acupuncture is effective for psoriasis. In one controlled trial, in which 56 patients were treated with traditional diagnosis and therapy over three months, the control group actually fared better than those patients who were receiving acupuncture. If acupuncture is to have an effect, then the treatment will need to be conducted over a prolonged period of time. Weekly treatment for eight to ten weeks would be reasonable.

Mind–Body Therapies

STRESS MANAGEMENT People with psoriasis may experience significant psychological stress and distress, which appear to aggravate the course of the disease process. If you have psoriasis, yoga or a relaxation therapy, such as diaphragmatic breathing (*see p.62*) may be helpful to reduce stress.

Preliminary studies have suggested that psychological therapies may help in managing psoriasis. In one study, a six-week course of an integrated, multi-disciplinary, stress-management approach – the Psoriasis Syndrome Management Programme (PSMP) – helped patients to experience a greater reduction in the clinical severity of psoriasis symptoms as well as a reduced incidence in anxiety, depression, psoriasis-related stress and disability. Moreover, the reductions were sustained for six months.

MINDFULNESS MEDITATION is one of the most innovative approaches to treating psoriasis. Research suggests that a brief session of mindfulness meditation (*see p.99*), delivered by audiotape during UVA photo therapy or photochemotherapy (PUVA) (*see above*), can reduce the stress of people with psoriasis while increasing the rate at which the psoriatic patches heal.

One study combined the mind–body techniques of meditation and guided imagery to help 18 people with psoriasis of the scalp. Results showed that meditating may be clinically effective for some patients in reducing their psoriasis symptoms, but that guided imagery made no significant impact. Overall, meditation can be regarded as a useful treatment for some patients with psoriasis.

> **PREVENTION PLAN**
>
> **The following may help to prevent psoriasis outbreaks:**
>
> - Eat a wholefood diet with plenty of fruit, vegetables and oily fish.
>
> - Practise relaxation and meditation.

HIVES

Hives, also known as urticaria or nettle rash, is an intensely itchy rash that may affect the whole body or just one area. It is often part of an allergic reaction and consists of red, raised areas and, sometimes, white lumps. The swellings develop rapidly over a few minutes and last for several minutes to several hours. Hives may occur with angioedema or anaphylaxis, both of which require urgent medical attention. Hives can be treated with oral antihistamines. Vitamin C or quercetin may also help. So, too, might a diet in which any trigger foods are excluded.

WHAT ARE THE SYMPTOMS?

- Red, itchy rash, sometimes with white lumps

In angioedema:

- Sudden onset of swelling in any part of the body
- Sudden difficulty breathing, speaking or swallowing
- Hives is present in many but not all cases of angioedema

In anaphylaxis:

- Angioedema, nausea and vomiting, wheezing, flushing of the skin and dizziness or loss of consciousness
- Hives is present in many but not all cases of anaphylaxis

WHY MIGHT I HAVE THIS?

PREDISPOSING FACTORS

- Genetic factors

TRIGGERS

- Food sensitivity, e.g. to nuts, strawberries, food additives
- Drug allergy
- Insect bites or stings
- Allergy to a plant
- Sunlight

TREATMENT PLAN

PRIMARY TREATMENTS

- Oral antihistamines
- Food-exclusion diet

BACK-UP TREATMENTS

- Antihistamine supplements
- Homeopathy
- Nettles and other herbal remedies
- Acupuncture

For an explanation of how treatments are rated, see p.111.

WHY DOES IT OCCUR?

Hives may be part of an allergic reaction, when skin cells release histamines and other substances that cause local inflammation. The itchy red rash may affect a small area of skin or it may emerge over the whole body.

The reaction may follow exposure to a particular substance, such as a drug, or to a food, such as nuts or strawberries. Hives can also follow an insect sting or bite, or contact with a plant, such as nettles. In some cases, no cause can be found. A tendency to develop hives may run in families.

"Physical urticaria" results when the skin temperature is raised, as in a hot bath or shower and during exercise, or as an emotional response, such as anger or stress. Even sunlight or contact with water may trigger the rash.

ANGIOEDEMA Hives may occur with angioedema, when a part of the body (often around the eyes, lips and hands) suddenly swells. Occasionally, the mucous lining of the mouth, tongue and throat may suddenly swell, too. This can seriously affect the ability to talk, breathe and swallow and is a medical emergency.

ANAPHYLAXIS Hives may also be a feature of anaphylaxis, a severe and potentially fatal allergic reaction in which the blood pressure falls, causing light-headedness or even loss of consciousness.

IMMEDIATE RELIEF

- Try not to scratch the rash.
- Apply a cooling lotion, such as calamine lotion, to the rash as soon as you can.

Hives is a rash of red and white lumps surrounded by inflamed skin. It is very itchy and can occur anywhere on the body.

IMPORTANT

Call an ambulance immediately if you or someone you are with develop the symptoms of angioedema or anaphylaxis.

TREATMENTS IN DETAIL

Conventional Medicine

If the symptoms of hives persist or recur, see your doctor, who may arrange a skin prick test (*see p.35*) to discover which substances might be the underlying cause. You can help with this by keeping a diary to record the foods you have eaten and to list other potential triggers. Changes in diet may help in some cases (*see below*).

PRIMARY TREATMENT **ORAL ANTIHISTAMINES**, such as loratadine, may bring the fastest relief. They may be prescribed by your doctor to treat and prevent hives.

CAUTION

Some antihistamines have side-effects: ask your doctor to explain these to you.

Nutritional Therapy

PRIMARY TREATMENT **FOOD-EXCLUSION DIET** Evidence suggests that some cases of hives are caused by a food sensitivity or a reaction to additives, such as colourings, flavourings, preservatives and aspartame. Try to identify and eliminate suspect foods from your diet (*see p.39*).

> ## One in five people will develop hives at some time in their life

ANTIHISTAMINE SUPPLEMENTS Hives may be related to the release of histamine, so taking vitamin C, which seems to have antihistamine effects, may help. Take 1g of vitamin C, 2–3 times a day while symptoms persist. Quercetin is a bioflavonoid that appears to reduce the release of histamine from immune cells known as mast cells. Try taking 400mg of quercetin 2–3 times a day while symptoms persist.

> **CAUTION**
>
> Consult your doctor before taking vitamin C with antibiotics or warfarin, or quercetin with the anti-angina drug felodipine (*see p.46*).

Homeopathy

Case studies suggest that hives responds quite well to homeopathic treatment.

URTICA URENS is one of the main medicines for hives. Made from stinging nettles, it is appropriate when the skin is swollen, with raised areas which may be very itchy or sore. *Urtica urens* is specifically helpful when symptoms are made worse by contact with water and cold objects.

APIS MELLIFICA is made from bee stings and is sometimes used, particularly when the hives is associated with angioedema.

ANARCARDIUM ORIENTALE is particularly appropriate for people who are extremely bad tempered, even violent, when their skin is bad. They may also get indigestion. Eating improves their indigestion and skin.

CALCAREA CARBONICA Many people with a tendency to hives have skin that reacts to a blunt point drawn across it so they can "write on their skin", a phenomenon known as dermatographism. *Calc. carb.* is the main medicine used to treat these individuals. Typically, those who respond to *Calc. carb.* are rather stout, solid both physically and mentally; they are calm, hardworking, conscientious and stubborn. Beneath this solid exterior, they may have many fears and anxieties, particularly if they work themselves to the point of exhaustion. They sweat freely on the head and neck, especially at night.

Western Herbal Medicine

TREATMENT AIMS The affected area, the frequency of occurrence and the severity of the symptoms, such as heat, swelling and itchiness, are key clues for the herbalist. Especially in cases with no identifiable external triggers, a herbalist will pay attention to the following: the presence of other allergic symptoms that result from food sensitivity and hay fever; signs of toxicity, poor diet and constipation; chronic infection; signs of impaired digestive function, including a deficiency in the secretion of gastric acid; and the emotional and psychological state of the affected person – in particular, if they suffer from nervous irritability and chronic anxiety.

The symptoms are best treated internally, although lotions and creams can help. In almost all cases, a herbalist prescribes remedies to aid digestion, liver metabolism and detoxification.

NETTLES Remedies known to have antihistamine and anti-allergy actions include nettle (*Urtica dioica* or *Urtica urens*). The ability of nettle leaf to relieve hives (nettle rash) is an example of a herbal medicine curing "like with like". The stinging hairs contain histamine, serotonin and acetylcholine, a combination that provokes a painful inflammatory rash on contact.

Nettle leaf has proven anti-inflammatory activity. Some clinical evidence suggests it has an anti-allergenic action, too. For hives, nettle leaf is best taken as a tea. However, the tea can also be applied as a lotion to relieve irritated skin.

OTHER HERBS Both liquorice (*Glycyrrhiza glabra*) and rehmannia (*Rehmannia glutinosa*) are anti-allergenic and help to relieve inflammatory skin rashes of all types. Liquorice also has a restorative action on the liver and adrenal glands. Four other herbs that herbalists commonly suggest for hives are German chamomile (*Matricaria recutita*), yellow dock (*Rumex crispus*), calendula (*Calendula officinalis*) and echinacea (*Echinacea spp.*).

> **CAUTION**
>
> See p.69 before taking a herbal remedy and, if you are already taking medication, consult a medical herbalist first.

Acupuncture

Traditionally, acupuncture has been used to alleviate both acute and chronic persistent hives. There have been no rigorous and randomised controlled trials, but good-quality case reports indicate that it may be of real value.

After a traditional Chinese diagnosis, treatment may be repeated regularly, depending on the severity and persistence of the rash. Usually, treatment should be provided weekly, in the first instance, for 6–8 weeks to correct imbalances in the flow of energy through the meridians. Afterwards, treatment is recommended every month or every three months to help maintain a good constitutional balance.

> **PREVENTION PLAN**
>
> **The following measures may help to prevent hives:**
>
> - Avoid any substances to which you are sensitive.
> - Take oral antihistamines.
> - Take vitamin C supplements.
> - Take quercetin supplements.

WHAT ARE THE SYMPTOMS?

For ringworm:

- Red, scaly rash that appears in a small circle
- Itchiness of the affected area
- After 1–2 weeks, further circles may appear
- The circles grow larger and form a red, scaly ring, usually surrounding a central area of normal skin
- Ringworm of the scalp may cause scaling like dandruff. Alternatively, there may be round, scaly patches, often with associated hair loss
- Ringworm may cause whitening and thickening of the nails, often accompanied by crumbly white material under the nails

For athlete's foot:

- Cracked, sore and itchy areas of skin on the bottom of the foot, often between the toes
- Flaking, white, soggy skin in the same areas

WHY MIGHT I HAVE THIS?

PREDISPOSING FACTORS

- *Candida* overgrowth in the intestines
- Having reduced immunity (e.g. from diabetes or AIDS)

TRIGGER

- Contact with the fungus

RINGWORM AND ATHLETE'S FOOT

Ringworm is a fungal infection of the skin that causes itchy, red, ring-shaped patches. It is not caused by worms, despite its name. Ringworm may occur in many parts of the body and common forms affect the scalp and groin. When it affects the feet, the infection is known as athlete's foot. Ringworm may also affect the nails. Topical antifungal creams are the treatment of choice, although if your ringworm is persistent, widespread or affects your scalp, then you will need to take oral antifungal drugs and follow a diet to control *Candida*.

WHY DOES IT OCCUR?

RINGWORM is caused by several species of fungus, such as *Microsporium*, *Trichophyton* and *Epidermophyton*, that live on the dead layers of skin of people and animals. These fungi thrive in warm, humid conditions, which is why ringworm is often seen in the groin area (the genitals, buttocks and inner thighs) and on the feet.

Ringworm can affect people of all ages. Scalp ringworm is more common in children, while ringworm affecting the groin area (sometimes called jock itch) is much more common in men. People with conditions, such as diabetes mellitus (*see p.314*) and AIDS (*see p.470*), that reduce their immunity to infection are particularly prone to ringworm.

Ringworm is spread by direct, skin-to-skin contact with an infected person or animal, such as a cat, or by sharing infected towels and hair brushes.

This red circle on the skin of the neck clearly shows the characteristic mark of ringworm. The circle is, in fact, skin that is recovering as the infection spreads outwards.

ATHLETE'S FOOT tends to be more common in adolescents and young adults. The fungus is usually caught through direct contact or from walking barefoot in warm, humid, communal areas, such as swimming pools and changing rooms.

TREATMENT PLAN

PRIMARY TREATMENTS

- Antifungal creams and drugs
- Anti-*Candida* diet

BACK-UP TREATMENTS

- Homeopathic marigold therapy
- Western herbal medicine

For an explanation of how treatments are rated, see p.111.

SELF-HELP

IF YOU HAVE RINGWORM:

- Always keep your skin clean and dry.
- Change your bed linen every day and wear clean nightclothes every night.
- Apply a topical cream (*see right*) and/or powder to the rash every day.

IF YOU HAVE ATHLETE'S FOOT:

- Only use your own towel to thoroughly dry yourself – especially the skin in between your toes – after swimming or a bath or shower.

- Wear socks and shoes made from natural rather than synthetic materials to allow air to circulate around your feet.
- Dust your socks and shoes with athlete's foot powder each morning.
- Change your socks every day.
- Sprinkle an antifungal powder and/or apply a topical cream (*see below*) between your toes twice a day.

TREATMENTS IN DETAIL

Conventional Medicine

Your doctor will probably diagnose ringworm by looking at the patches of skin. If confirmation is needed, laboratory tests on samples of skin, hair or nail will reveal the fungus responsible.

PRIMARY TREATMENT **TOPICAL ANTIFUNGAL CREAMS** are best if the infection is localised and affects just one area. You can buy some of them over the counter, but you will need a prescription for a stronger cream. Patches of ringworm and athlete's foot may be treated for up to two weeks with prescribed topical creams containing antifungal drugs, such as miconazole or terbinafine. These drugs may cause some local irritation.

PRIMARY TREATMENT **ORAL ANTIFUNGAL DRUGS**, such as itraconazole and terbinafine, may be needed if the ringworm is more widespread, especially on the scalp. They are also sometimes taken for athlete's foot and nail infections. Your doctor can prescribe the drugs, which you will probably need to take for up to two months.

> **CAUTION**
>
> Antifungal drugs have a range of possible side-effects: ask your doctor to explain these to you.

Nutritional Therapy

PRIMARY TREATMENT **AN ANTI-CANDIDA DIET** may be a solution. Individuals with persistent ringworm or athlete's foot may also have an underlying problem with an overgrowth of *Candida albicans* in the intestine. There is insufficient research to confirm this, but clinical experience suggests that by controlling the overgrowth with an anti-*Candida* diet, it is usually possible to achieve long-term and even permanent relief from fungal infections, such as ringworm. (*For more details on* Candida *and anti-*Candida *diets, see p.40.*)

Western Herbal Medicine

MARIGOLD THERAPY is a proprietary treatment for foot problems. Prepared from marigold (*Calendula officinalis*) and French marigold (*Tagetes patula*), it is often effective for athlete's foot. Try to use the combination pack that includes a tincture, ointment and footwear spray.

BOOST IMMUNITY Help your immune system fight the various fungi that cause ringworm by regularly drinking a tea made from nettle (*Urtica dioica*), echinacea (*Echinacea spp.*), peppermint (*Mentha piperita*), burdock (*Arctium lappa*) and dandelion (*Taraxacum officinale*).

EXTERNAL TREATMENTS A herbal practitioner may recommend a number of herbs for external use. If you have athlete's foot, try soaking your feet in an infusion of golden seal (*Hydrastis canadensis*). Afterwards, dry your feet and then dust them with powdered golden seal.

The fungus *Microsporum gypseum* is found in the soil and causes ringworm on the scalp and the body. The yellow bullet-shaped structures produce the spores that spread the infection.

A cream prepared from marigold (*Calendula officinalis*) may relieve the itching. Another remedy that you can apply each day to athlete's foot is a mixture prepared from marigold ointment and the essential oil of either tea tree (*Melaleuca alternifolia*), clove (*Syzygium aromaticum*) or thyme (*Thymus vulgaris*).

For ringworm, try making a poultice from the green rind of the fruit of black walnut (*Juglans nigra*).

> **CAUTION**
>
> See p.69 before taking a herbal remedy and, if you are already taking prescribed medication, consult a medical herbalist first. Do not use thyme oil if you are pregnant.

PREVENTION PLAN

The following may help to prevent ringworm and athlete's foot:

- Keep your skin and feet dry.
- Don't walk barefoot in changing rooms.

Eyes & Ears

When our sight and hearing are reduced we can become disorientated, unnerved and isolated. Eating nourishing food, preventing excess strain and refraining from smoking can keep the senses intact. If an ailment does develop, there is a range of treatments available, from visual and hearing aids to medication, surgery and supplements.

CATARACTS

A cataract is a cloudy area in the normally clear lens of the eye. It stops light rays from passing through the lens, leading to a reduced clarity of vision and, in some cases, to blindness. One eye is often more severely affected, but cataracts may develop in both eyes. Since cataracts tend to develop over a long period, loss of vision is gradual and may not be noticed at first. Surgery is usually required, although you can help to slow cataract development with nutritional, homeopathic and environmental measures.

WHAT ARE THE SYMPTOMS?

- Blurred vision
- Colours appear faded
- Temporary improvement in near vision in long-sighted people
- Haloes and stars around bright light, which may be worse at night

WHY MIGHT I HAVE THIS?

PREDISPOSING FACTORS

- Low blood levels of antioxidants
- A diet lacking in antioxidants
- Increasing age
- Smoking
- Genetic factors
- Excessive sunlight, especially UV-B radiation

TRIGGER

- Free-radical damage

TREATMENT PLAN

PRIMARY TREATMENT

- Surgery

BACK-UP TREATMENTS

- Various nutritional supplements
- Environmental health measures

WORTH CONSIDERING

- Homeopathy

For an explanation of how treatments are rated, see p.111.

WHY DOES IT OCCUR?

Cataracts result from structural changes to protein fibres in the lens of the eye. The commonest type is an age-related cataract, the exact cause of which is not known. However, various factors, including sunlight exposure, general health and genes, are likely to play a role.

Other recognised causes of cataracts include eye injury, some medications (such as long-term corticosteroids), diabetes mellitus (*see p.314*) and inflammatory diseases of the eye. People with Down's syndrome are also at increased risk. In some people, the tendency to cataracts is hereditary and in rare cases, cataracts may be present from birth.

SELF-HELP

The following may help you while you wait for surgery or to manage without it:
- Have your eyes tested regularly to ensure your spectacles are correctly prescribed.
- Read in good light.
- Use a low-powered visual aid (from an optician or eye clinic), such as a magnifying glass (an attached light source is optional) or a mini-telescope to attach to glasses for looking across a room. A closed-circuit TV may help you to read – a camera aimed at a page produces a magnified image on a TV screen.

IMPORTANT

If the symptoms of a cataract develop quickly, or you have a painful eye, you should see a doctor urgently.

In a cataract, the lens of the eye becomes cloudy and opaque behind the pupil. The normally transparent lens loses its ability to transmit and focus rays of light, causing blurred or distorted vision.

TREATMENTS IN DETAIL

Conventional Medicine

PRIMARY TREATMENT **SURGERY** is the only treatment that can cure cataracts. However, your doctor will only recommend surgery if the problems with your vision interfere with everyday activities, such as driving and reading.

The operation is usually short, lasting around 15–30 minutes, and performed under a local anaesthetic. The surgeon makes a tiny cut – about 3mm (⅛in) long – in the eye and inserts a probe to remove the lens while leaving behind the lens capsule (the layer that encloses the lens). The surgeon places a plastic lens implant inside the lens capsule, which holds the new lens in the correct position.

After surgery, you may experience some blurring of vision and mild discomfort, both of which should last only a few days. Most people still need glasses after surgery, either for reading, distance vision or both.

The operation is relatively risk-free. However, infection is a possible complication of the surgery, affecting around 1 in 1,000 people. It may lead to permanent loss of vision in the affected eye. Very rarely, bleeding inside the eye during surgery causes permanent loss of vision. For 1 in 300 people, the operation is more complicated than expected – further surgery is needed to complete the treatment.

After routine surgery, some people develop scar tissue in the lens capsule. This causes the same symptoms as the original cataract, but is easily treated with a painless five-minute laser procedure at an eye clinic.

Nutritional Therapy

ANTIOXIDANTS The development of a cataract is believed to be related to damage caused by destructive molecules called free radicals. Antioxidants, such as beta-carotene (found in carrots, mangoes and apricots) and vitamins C and E, neutralise

the free radicals. People with few antioxidants in their blood or diet may be at high risk for cataracts.

Some research claims that certain antioxidants, such as vitamins A, C and E, may protect against the UV damage to the lens of the eye. Other evidence suggests that taking 3,000mg of N-acetylcysteine boosts levels of glutathione, which in turn neutralises the free radicals formed by UV light in the human lens. You could consider these supplements if you are exposed to sunlight on a regular basis.

CAROTENOID-RICH DIET Research shows that eating foods rich in nutrients known as carotenoids (especially lutein and zeaxanthin) is associated with a reduced cataract risk. In large epidemiological studies, lutein and zeaxanthin levels have been correlated with the risk of cataract and, in a small clinical trial, supplementation with lutein (15mg 3 times weekly for two years) appeared to improve the vision of people with cataracts.

Good sources of lutein include spinach, kale, collard greens, romaine lettuce, leeks, peas, egg yolks, kiwi fruit, squashes, black grapes, Brussels sprouts and green peppers. Zeaxanthin is found in mangoes, oranges, red peppers, nectarines, papayas, squashes, sweetcorn, honeydew melons and egg yolks. Eating plenty of these foods may help to prevent or slow down cataract formation.

NUTRITIONAL SUPPLEMENTS may slow the progression of age-related cataracts, but only if you take them for many years. A 2002 study found that, by taking a daily regime of 18mg of beta-carotene, 750mg of vitamin C and 600mg of vitamin E for three years, an age-related cataract will progress more slowly.

MULTIVITAMIN/MINERAL SUPPLEMENT A 2000 study revealed that people who took a multivitamin/mineral supplement that contained vitamin C and/or vitamin E for ten years enjoyed a 60 per cent reduction in

> ## Nearly two-thirds of all cases in developed countries are in people over the age of 65

the risk of cataract. Another study found that taking vitamin C supplements for ten years or more reduced the risk of cataract development by 70 per cent. On balance, the evidence suggests that if you take a daily dose of 500mg of vitamin C and 400IU of vitamin E, with a multivitamin/mineral supplement, you are likely to reduce the risk of cataract formation in the long term.

> **CAUTION**
>
> Consult your doctor before taking vitamin C with antibiotics or warfarin, or vitamin E with warfarin or aspirin (*see p.46*).

Homeopathy

The evidence that homeopathy can help to treat cataracts is not strong, but *Cineraria* eye drops are traditionally recommended. A number of other medicines may be given orally, including *Calcarea carbonica*, *Calcarea iodatum*, *Causticum* and *Silicea*.

CALCAREA FLUORICA pills may also be appropriate, particularly for people who generally have lax connective tissues. They may presently be (or have been when younger) hyperextensible (double-jointed), with sway-back knees (knees that go beyond straight) and a tendency to hernias. They may also be arthritic, with bony lumps on their fingers.

Environmental Health

UV-B RADIATION Exposure to UV-B (even in small amounts), primarily from the sun but also from welding or ironwork, causes a reaction in the lens that, over many years, contributes to the formation of certain types of cataracts. The risk may be increased because of holes in, or thinning of, the ozone layer. However, there is still some uncertainty about how serious the problem might be. Plastic or glass lenses in sunglasses block as much as 80–90 per cent of offending rays, and wearing a hat decreases exposure by 30–50 per cent.

INFRA-RED RADIATION may also cause cataracts. Exposure to damaging levels, such as the extreme heat in steel-making and glass-blowing, has been reduced through shorter work days, and the use of furnace shields and protective eyewear.

IONISING RADIATION, such as X–rays and nuclear fallout, causes cataracts that can take up to 20 years to develop. The risk from X–ray therapy for cancer can be reduced by using proper eye shields. Radiologists, radiation technicians and dentists should also use adequate protection.

SMOKING is directly toxic to the lens and decreases the availability of antioxidants, such as vitamins C and E, to the eye. Avoid smoky places and don't smoke.

> **PREVENTION PLAN**
>
> **The following may reduce your risk of developing a cataract:**
>
> - Eat fruit and green-leafed vegetables.
> - Minimise the exposure of your eyes to sunlight, especially UV-B radiation.
> - If you are a smoker, then stop.

MACULAR DEGENERATION

When the macula of the retina degenerates, central and detailed vision are progressively lost. People with macular degeneration have increasing difficulty reading and recognising faces. Both eyes are often affected. Of the two types, the dry form is the most common, but the wet form is more likely to severely affect vision. Both types affect women more than men, are more common in people over 70 and may run in families. The dry form can be treated with low-powered visual aids and a number of treatments are available for the wet form.

WHAT ARE THE SYMPTOMS?

In both the wet and dry forms of macular degeneration, the main symptoms are:

- A progressive deterioration in central vision
- Increasing difficulty reading, watching television and recognising faces
- Distortions of vision; for example, straight lines may appear wavy when looking at a crossword puzzle

In the dry form:

- Symptoms develop slowly

In the wet form:

- Symptoms develop more rapidly and the distortion of vision is more severe

WHY MIGHT I HAVE THIS?

PREDISPOSING FACTORS

- Increasing age
- Smoking
- High blood levels of cholesterol
- Excessive exposure to sunlight
- Low levels of zinc or vitamin E in the body
- Genetic factors
- Reduced carotenoid intake and subsequent reduction of macular pigment density

TRIGGER

- Free-radical damage

WHY DOES IT OCCUR?

The macula is the central and most sensitive area of the retina. An oval spot that is yellowish in colour and about 3mm ($^1/_8$in) to the side of the optic nerve, it is where the visual sense is at its best. Light-sensitive cells in the macula depend upon underlying supporting cells for their survival. Damage to these cells is the first stage in both wet and dry forms.

DRY MACULAR DEGENERATION The light-sensitive cells die in patches, leading to patchy loss of central vision. This dry form develops slowly over a period of between 5 and 10 years and accounts for about 85 per cent of the people with the disease.

WET MACULAR DEGENERATION In the wet form, blood vessels break through the damaged supporting cells and grow underneath the macula, where they may bleed or leak fluid. This eventually results in scarring in the cells of the macula. The wet form develops much more quickly – over a period of weeks or months.

UNDERLYING CAUSES What causes macular degeneration has yet to be established. However, increasing age, high levels of cholesterol in the blood and smoking all increase the risk, as may excessive exposure of the retina to sunlight.

One of the underlying causes of macular degeneration appears to be a reduction in the density of the macular pigment, which is related to dietary intake of carotenoids (specifically lutein and zeaxanthin).

LEGAL ISSUES Macular degeneration never causes total blindness, because an affected person's peripheral vision is preserved. However, if you have macular degeneration, you may be able to register as legally blind and therefore be eligible for financial and social support.

TREATMENT PLAN

PRIMARY TREATMENTS

- Low-powered visual aids (*see Self-Help*)
- AREDS formula supplements
- Laser therapy
- Macular relocation surgery
- Radiotherapy

BACK-UP TREATMENTS

- Various nutritional supplements
- Western herbal medicine

For an explanation of how treatments are rated, see p.111.

IMPORTANT

If you experience a sudden decrease in your vision, or a sudden onset or worsening of a distortion of your vision, you should seek a consultation with an eye specialist urgently, as these symptoms may indicate the wet form of macular degeneration.

HOW THE EYE WORKS

The cornea and lens of the eye focus light rays from an object and create an upside-down image on the retina. This image stimulates a multitude of light-sensitive cells (rods and cones), which generate a pattern of electrical impulses that are relayed by the optic nerve to the visual cortex at the back of the brain. Here, the pattern is decoded and the object is seen as being upright.

Anatomy of the eye

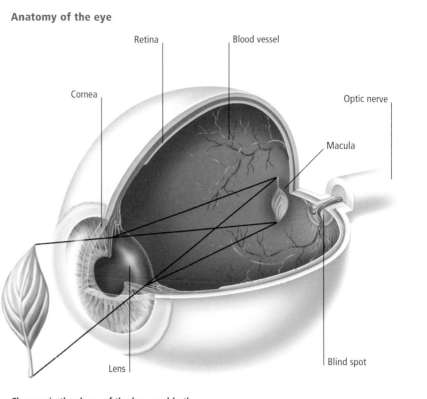

Changes in the shape of the lens enable the eye to focus the light rays on the macula, the most sensitive part of the retina.

Rod and cone cells

On the retina (coloured pink) are rod cells (blue), which detect light intensity, and cone cells (green-blue), which respond to colour.

SELF-HELP

PRIMARY TREATMENT If your sight is affected, the following advice may help:

- Read in good light.
- Use "low-powered visual aids" for reading or watching television, for example. These are available from an optician or a visual aid clinic, and include magnifying glasses and mini-telescopes (*see p.182*).

TREATMENTS IN DETAIL

Conventional Medicine

Your doctor can make a diagnosis of both forms of macular degeneration by testing your vision and looking at your retina with an ophthalmoscope.

Fluorescein angiography may be recommended to check for abnormal blood vessels in the retina and therefore to detect the wet form. The test involves dilating the pupils with drops and injecting a dye into an arm vein. Photos are taken with a special camera as the dye passes through the blood vessels of the eye.

PRIMARY TREATMENT **LASER THERAPY** may be recommended if you have wet macular degeneration. There are two kinds of laser therapy – conventional laser therapy and photodynamic therapy.

Conventional laser therapy employs a high-energy beam to destroy new blood vessels. However, the laser also damages retinal tissue in the targeted area, so the treatment is only used when the new vessels are a distance away from the centre of the macula. One result of the laser therapy will be a small blind spot that is close to your centre of vision.

Photodynamic laser therapy does not destroy retinal tissue but it can destroy new blood vessels at the very centre of the macula, preventing them from doing further damage. This treatment is successful only in a select group of patients. It takes about 30 minutes and can be carried out in an outpatient clinic.

If an eye specialist considers that you are suitable, you will be injected with a special light-sensitive dye 10 minutes before treatment begins. The dye will stick to the abnormal blood vessels in your eye, thereby helping the laser to single them out. You must avoid exposure to bright light for two days after treatment while your body eliminates the dye.

In both types of laser therapy, the blood vessels may grow back and treatment may need to be repeated. It is also important to realise that laser treatment aims to limit further visual loss and does not usually improve vision.

PRIMARY TREATMENT **MACULAR RELOCATION SURGERY** for the wet form of macular degeneration is the subject of ongoing research. It is the only treatment that can significantly improve your vision. Using keyhole surgery to get inside the eye,

People with macular degeneration experience a blurred central vision, as this image represents, yet they can see details around the centre because their peripheral vision remains unaffected.

the retina is detached, rotated and stuck back down so that the macula is relocated in an area of healthy supporting cells. In addition, the muscles that move the eye are adjusted to allow for the change in the position of the retina.

Sub-macular surgery is similar and involves removing the new blood vessels from underneath the retina with fine forceps and then replacing the retina in the same position.

PRIMARY TREATMENT **RADIOTHERAPY** Some people with the wet form of macular degeneration can benefit from a focused beam of radiotherapy.

Nutritional Therapy

PRIMARY TREATMENT **AREDS FORMULA** The Age-Related Eye Disease Study (AREDS), which reported in 2001, looked at a combined nutritional treatment for preventing macular degeneration.

Over 3,500 participants aged between 55 and 80, each with some degree of retinal changes, ranging from mild to severe, were followed by researchers over a six-year period. They received daily intakes of one of the following:

- antioxidants, including 500mg of vitamin C, 400IU of vitamin E and 15mg (25,000IU) of beta-carotene;
- 80mg of zinc and 2mg of copper;
- antioxidants plus zinc (no copper);
- no supplements at all.

Use of antioxidants reduced the risk of developing age-related macular degeneration by 17 per cent, while zinc lowered the risk by 21 per cent. An even more profound decline in risk was found when antioxidants and zinc were taken together, reducing the risk by 25 per cent.

In addition, the combination of antioxidants and zinc led to a 27 per cent decrease in the risk of worsening eyesight. Those with more severe retinal problems showed the largest drop in the risk of developing age-related macular degeneration.

This randomised, placebo-controlled clinical trial shows that the nutrient supplementation in the AREDS formula does have the potential to prevent and retard macular degeneration. Whether you will benefit from the AREDS supplement depends on the severity of your macular degeneration, which will need to be assessed by an eye specialist.

ANTIOXIDANTS, such as beta-carotene, can neutralise destructive molecules called free radicals that may be responsible for most cases of macular degeneration.

According to a study published in 1988, eating foods that are rich in beta-carotene, such as red and orange peppers, apricots, cantaloupe melon, kale and spinach, helps to reduce the overall risk of developing macular degeneration. Sometimes, taking 15,000–25,000IU of beta-carotene supplements each day is also recommended to prevent the ailment.

LUTEIN AND ZEAXANTHIN A variety of research studies show that the antioxidant carotenoids lutein and zeaxanthin may provide protection against macular degeneration. A 2001 study, for example, found that individuals with the highest level of lutein and zeaxanthin in their retinas had an 82 per cent lower risk of macular degeneration compared to those with the lowest levels of these nutrients.

Taking lutein supplementation in high doses of 10mg a day for a year has been shown to reverse symptoms of age-related macular degeneration.

As well as having potent antioxidant properties, lutein and zeaxanthin preferentially absorb blue light and therefore protect cells from this most damaging part of the visible spectrum (and hence they appear to be red, yellow and orange). Zeaxanthin is specifically concentrated in the yellow spot at the back of the retina where fine detailed vision is discriminated.

Lutein and zeaxanthin are important fat-soluble antioxidants that are absorbed along with fats in the diet. Therefore, supplements containing them should be taken with a fat-containing meal.

Good sources of lutein include spinach, kale, collard greens, romaine lettuce, leeks, peas, egg yolks, kiwi fruit, yellow squashes, Brussels sprouts and green peppers. Foods that are rich in zeaxanthin include mangoes, oranges, sweetcorn, red peppers, nectarines, papayas, squashes and honeydew melons.

You can also supplement your diet with lutein and zeaxanthin – the recommended dose is 6mg of each per day.

SPINACH Eating spinach seems to be particularly beneficial for people who have macular degeneration. A 1999 study, conducted in men aged between 61 and 79 with early indications of macular degeneration, found that eating 4–7 servings of spinach a week caused some improvement in visual function tests.

OMEGA-3 FATTY ACIDS Eating fish might prevent the development of macular degeneration, probably due to the presence of omega-3 fatty acids. A 2001 study found that eating four portions of fish per week was associated with a 35 per cent lower risk of macular degeneration compared to eating three or fewer portions each week. Try eating a portion of oily fish, especially salmon, trout, mackerel, herring or sardines, at least four times a week to help prevent the condition.

VITAMIN E AND ZINC also appear to have a protective role in macular degeneration. Studies show that low levels of both zinc and vitamin E are possible risk factors for the condition. Vitamin E is found in vegetable oils, nuts, seeds, egg yolk and green leafy vegetables, while zinc is found most readily in fish, seafood, meat, eggs and tofu. You may also be advised to take 400IU of vitamin E along with 15–30mg of zinc each day. Taking zinc supplements over a long period can deplete the body of copper, so take 1mg of copper for each 15mg of supplemental zinc.

RED WINE A recent study in the US also found evidence that consuming moderate amounts of wine – red wine contains appreciable levels of anthocyanins – was linked with a reduced incidence of macular degeneration.

> **CAUTION**
>
> Consult your doctor before taking AREDS formula or zinc with antibiotics, or omega-3 fatty acids, fish oils, vitamin E or vitamin C supplements with warfarin. (*see p.46*).

Western Herbal Medicine

Herbal medicine can help to maintain eye health and sight if it is taken over a long period. There are studies that indicate that anthocyanin antioxidants have a marked ability to slow or prevent the development of macular degeneration. Several herbal medicines – notably bilberry (*Vaccinium myrtillus*) – contain high levels of anthocyanins and have been demonstrated to strengthen and stabilise the circulation of blood within the eye, contributing to reduced free-radical damage to the retina and macula.

BILBERRY Studies indicate that workers can improve their night vision by eating bilberries. Uncorroborated reports from some pilots who flew in World War II reveal that their vision was improved after eating bilberry jam.

The high level of anthocyanosides in bilberry increases the rate of regeneration of light-sensitive pigments in the retina and improves night vision. Anthocyanosides strengthen the walls of capillaries, making them less liable to leak blood and so cause damage to surrounding tissue. This is particularly important within the eye, where leakage occurs close to the macula and other sensitive tissue in the retina.

Bilberry extracts have been found to reverse retinal damage in diabetics, which is a problem that commonly develops in longstanding diabetes.

OTHER HERBS WITH ANTHOCYANOSIDES Though the evidence suggests that bilberry is specifically helpful for the eyes, other similar herbs with significant anthocyanoside content may have the potential to help reduce or prevent macular degeneration. Three examples are the fruit of blackcurrant (*Ribes nigrum*), the seed extract of grape (*Vitis vinifera*) and the bark extract of pine (*Pinus spp.*).

GINKGO (*Ginkgo biloba*) is well known for its ability to treat glaucoma (raised pressure within the orbit of the eye). However, extracts of the herb also exert a positive effect on retinal tissue, according to clinical trials that demonstrate ginkgo improves clarity and range of vision in people with macular degeneration.

A standardised extract of ginkgo is known as GBE (ginkgo biloba extract), for which there is no recommended daily allowance. However, doses of 120mg of GBE a day (40mg taken 3 times a day) to 180mg of GBE a day (60mg taken 3 times a day) are recommended.

COMBINING BILBERRY AND GINKGO Both bilberry and ginkgo are routinely prescribed by practitioners. If there is concern about risk of retinal damage, taking a combination of them over a long period would be a good starting point in self-treatment. Try taking a combination of 120mg of a 50:1 ginkgo standardised extract with 3–6g a day of bilberry fruit.

OTHER HERBAL REMEDIES may also be useful in the treatment of macular degeneration. For example, hawthorn (*Crataegus spp.*), another herb with major anthocyanoside content, supports the health of

both arteries and capillaries. Cornflower (*Centaurea cyanus*), which is the traditional French herb for eye problems, also has appreciable levels of anthocyanosides in its sky-blue petals.

Eyebright (*Euphrasia officinalis*) is a much-valued remedy for eye problems ranging from cataracts to conjunctivitis. Research is beginning to uphold its traditional usage.

> **CAUTION**
>
> See page 69 before taking a herbal remedy and, if you are already taking a prescribed medication, consult a medical herbalist first.

Environmental Health

SMOKING According to research, people who smoke cigarettes are four times more likely than non-smokers to go blind in old age. Smoking is thought to be linked to a reduced amount of pigment in the macula, which is essential for clear vision.

Of the 13 million cigarette smokers in the UK in 2004, many will develop age-related macular degeneration (AMD) and, as a consequence, will probably lose some of their sight. People over 60 years old are particularly at risk from severe and irreversible loss of central vision.

Researchers at the University of Manchester estimate that about 54,000 people with AMD (over a tenth of the total) have developed it as a direct result of smoking. They conclude that giving up smoking reduces the risk of developing AMD in later life and may also improve the long-term effects of laser therapy.

> **PREVENTION PLAN**
>
> **The following may reduce your risk of developing macular degeneration:**
>
> - Eat plenty of oily fish and green-leafed vegetables such as spinach.
> - Limit your exposure to UV light and wear sunglasses in intense sunlight.
> - If you smoke, then stop.
> - Control high cholesterol.
> - Take antioxidant and carotene supplements.

TINNITUS

People with tinnitus hear sounds that originate in the ear itself. These noises may sound like roaring, ringing, buzzing, whistling or hissing. They are usually continuous, although their intensity may vary. Episodes of tinnitus may be brief in some people, but in others it is a permanent condition. Tinnitus may be helped by various measures, including drugs, the herb ginkgo, devices to mask the noises, dietary changes, acupuncture, chiropractic and other manipulation therapies. There are also psychological techniques to help you to cope better.

WHAT ARE THE SYMPTOMS?

- Noises originating within the ear that sound like roaring, ringing, buzzing, whistling or hissing

WHY MIGHT I HAVE THIS?

PREDISPOSING FACTORS

- Exposure to loud noises
- Temporomandibular joint disorder (*see p.280*)
- Ménière's disease
- Osteoarthritis in the neck
- Exposure to environmental hazards
- Treatment with certain drugs (e.g. aspirin and some antibiotics)

TREATMENT PLAN

PRIMARY TREATMENTS

- Masking devices or hearing aids
- Cognitive behavioural therapy

BACK-UP TREATMENTS

- Antidepressants (if depression is a factor)
- Ginkgo biloba
- Chiropractic and/or cranial manipulation
- Hypnotherapy

WORTH CONSIDERING

- Dietary changes
- Zinc and vitamin B12 (if deficiency is a factor)
- Homeopathy
- Environmental changes
- Acupuncture
- Relaxation training

For an explanation of how treatments are rated, see p.111.

WHY DOES IT OCCUR?

It is not known what causes the brain to perceive noises when none exist. Tinnitus sometimes occurs for no apparent reason, but is commonly associated with certain ear disorders, such as age-induced hearing loss (presbycusis); noise-induced hearing loss; or Ménière's disease (a disorder of the inner ear that causes episodes of dizziness, nausea and hearing loss, as well as tinnitus). A study of over 1,000 people with chronic tinnitus concluded that temporomandibular joint disorder (*see p.280*) is probably a causal factor in cases where no other cause can be determined.

The condition may also be associated with anaemia or hyperthyroidism (*see Thyroid Problems, p.319*) and nutritionists believe that it can sometimes be a symptom of blood-sugar fluctuation. Head injuries and treatment with certain drugs can also cause tinnitus.

Tinnitus may affect both ears or one ear only. Tinnitus in one ear may be caused by a tumour affecting the nerve that carries information from the ear to the brain.

People with tinnitus may find that the noises distract them and that they have difficulty concentrating. Some people with tinnitus have difficulty falling asleep at night (*see Sleep disorders, p.448*). If tinnitus causes problems with day-to-day living, it may lead to depression (*see p.436*) and anxiety (*see p.414*).

IMPORTANT

See your doctor if you develop tinnitus, especially if it affects one ear only.

TREATMENTS IN DETAIL

Conventional Medicine

Your doctor may arrange hearing tests and possibly investigations to look for an underlying cause, which will be treated where possible.

PRIMARY TREATMENT **MASKING DEVICES** Sometimes external noises, such as music, may help to distract you from the noises in your ears. In addition, masking devices are available that you can wear in or behind the ears. These emit sounds that may help distract from the tinnitus. Hearing aids may be beneficial if you also have hearing loss.

ANTIDEPRESSANTS Tricyclic antidepressants may help to relieve tinnitus when symptoms of depression are present.

CAUTION

Antidepressants can cause a range of possible side-effects. Ask your doctor to explain these to you.

Nutritional Therapy

DIETARY CHANGES Food sensitivity may occasionally be an underlying problem in tinnitus. People with Ménière's disease may find that their tinnitus improves when they receive treatment for a specific allergy. (*For more information on identifying food sensitivities, see p.456.*)

Tinnitus may also be related to general dietary factors. If you have tinnitus, it may help if you limit your intake of salt, red meat, dairy products and tea and coffee, and consume plenty of fresh fruits and vegetables, nuts, seeds, extra-virgin olive oil and water. One study showed significantly improved symptoms of Ménière's disease in people who had followed this regime for a year. Since tinnitus can be a symptom of blood-sugar fluctuation, controlling blood-sugar levels may help. *(For details of how to do this, see p.42.)*

NUTRITIONAL SUPPLEMENTS Some people who have tinnitus have an underlying zinc deficiency. Taking zinc (at a dose of about 50mg per day) seems to be effective in some cases, but not if blood zinc level is normal to begin with.

Vitamin B12 deficiency may also play a role in tinnitus. In one study, 47 per cent of tinnitus patients were found to be deficient in vitamin B12. This vitamin may be effective in the treatment of tinnitus because it can enhance the conduction of nerve impulses relating to hearing. If you have tinnitus, try taking 1mg of vitamin B12 each day.

> **CAUTION**
>
> Consult your doctor before taking zinc and vitamin B12 with existing medications. *(See also p.46.)*

Homeopathy

Although there is no convincing research to guide us, a number of homeopathic medicines may improve tinnitus.

CHININUM SULPHURICUM AND CHENO-PODIUM *Chininum sulphuricum* (quinine sulphate) is suitable when the tinnitus is part of Ménière's disease, with dizziness, ringing in the ears and deafness. The rarely used homeopathic medicine *Chenopodium* may be useful for people who experience the unusual symptoms of deafness, particularly to the human voice, when it is combined with sensitivity to loud sounds that hurt the ear.

GRAPHITES AND CAUSTICUM "Constitutional" features *(see p.73)* are important in prescribing *Graphites* and *Causticum*. People who respond to *Graphites* have ringing in the ears combined with deafness, which

---

TINNITUS MASKER DEVICE

A tinnitus masker is a small electronic device that fits in the ear, where it delivers a continuous "white" noise to block out the unwanted ringing and whistling sounds. To decide whether a masker may be useful, some specialists conduct a "tap test", in which the person with tinnitus stands close to a running tap. If the sound of the water is enough to block out the tinnitus, a masker may be appropriate. These devices are particularly useful during quiet periods in the day when the tinnitus noises tend to be at their most noticeable.

A tinnitus masker device fits neatly in the ear. Modern devices are unobtrusive.

---

improves when there is a lot of background noise. They may also have skin trouble affecting the outer ear. People who respond to *Causticum* have tinnitus with a peculiar sensation of echoing, particularly of their own voice, in the ear.

Western Herbal Medicine

There have been several clinical trials of ginkgo biloba for tinnitus and they have been reviewed. The better studies suggested that it helped. If you have tinnitus, try taking ginkgo biloba for two months at a dosage of 120–200mg per day.

Environmental Health

Environmental treatment for tinnitus consists first of identifying and avoiding any external causes of the condition.

HEAVY METALS If tinnitus may be the result of nerve damage, you should examine your environment as there is evidence that exposure to heavy metals can lead to nerve damage. In order to prevent worsening of damage to the nerves, you should scrupulously investigate your surroundings for lead or other heavy metals, such as mercury. Send a sample of your tap water to the public health authority to have them check the water quality, and investigate the possibility of toxic exposure at your workplace. Many foods contain mercury and other heavy metals, especially fish (particularly oily ocean fish, such as tuna, shark and swordfish) and products made from animal bones (such as some gelatins).

Although there are no definitive data to support chelation therapy (a treatment that lowers the levels of metals in the body), a visit to an environmental or functional medicine physician to determine the levels of iron and other heavy metals in your body and to discuss chelation therapy or other forms of reduction might be in order. Even if your present tinnitus is irreversible, you may be able to prevent further damage to nerves.

LOUD NOISES Injury to the cochlea in the inner ear is another frequent cause of tinnitus. One of the most obvious causes of cochlear damage is loud noise. If you know you will be exposed to loud noises, you should wear ear protectors (look for those approved by a regulatory body). Even children exposed to sounds from toy guns and fireworks can suffer auditory damage and resulting tinnitus.

OTHER CAUSES There are many other causes of tinnitus. Carbon monoxide poisoning is one, and a simple blood test to check for short- or long-term exposure to this deadly gas can determine whether it is responsible for your tinnitus. Many drugs are associated with tinnitus, especially some antibiotics and chemotherapeutic agents for cancer, quinine for leg cramps or malaria, and, most famously, salicylate drugs (such as aspirin). A careful review of your prescription and non-prescription medicines can help pinpoint potential tinnitus-causing factors – for example, several combination non-prescription and prescription pharmaceuticals contain acetyl salicylic acid, or aspirin. If you or your doctor are unsure whether you have had a significant exposure to one of these compounds, testing their levels in the blood, and other tests, may help.

HELPFUL STRATEGIES If tinnitus is disturbing your everyday life or interfering with sleep, consider using a masking device to "drown out" the sound in your head. These devices are worn in the ear and override the stimuli from the dysfunctional auditory nerve.

There are also some therapies for tinnitus that make use of sound or electrical stimulation in a similar way. Some people find that simply distracting themselves from the unwanted sound of tinnitus by

> ## Although tinnitus may be a distressing condition, the cause is almost always benign

using a ticking clock or static from the radio can provide relief. Cochlear implants to provide electrical stimulation are also an option, but there have been reports that these may actually make tinnitus worse in some people.

OXYGEN THERAPY If you have had tinnitus for less than three months, treatment with hyperbaric oxygen (oxygen at higher than normal pressure) can help to relieve it. In a study, over 80 per cent of people who started hyperbaric oxygen therapy between two and six weeks after the onset of tinnitus experienced improvement in the degree of tinnitus they experienced, while 35 per cent of those who started therapy between six weeks and three months gained relief to some degree.

Bodywork Therapies

CHIROPRACTIC AND CRANIAL MANIPULATION Temporomandibular joint (TMJ) problems (*see p.280*), which may cause tinnitus, can commonly be successfully treated by cranial osteopaths, cranio-sacral therapists, sacro-occipital practitioners and dentists, depending on the cause of the jaw dysfunction. An example of chiropractic treatment of tinnitus has been described,

involving a 41-year-old woman with ear pain, tinnitus, vertigo, some hearing loss and headaches. She had a history of ear infections, which had been treated with prescription antibiotics. Her complaints were attributed to TMJ syndrome and she had already been treated unsuccessfully by both a medical doctor and dentist. Treatment consisted of typical chiropractic adjustment manipulation to the upper neck. The woman's symptoms improved and she eventually recovered fully after nine treatments.

Chiropractic manipulation of the neck and cranium is also claimed to improve tinnitus in cases other than those relating to temporomandibular joint problems, especially in cases where the condition is associated with an imbalance between the sympathetic and parasympathetic nerve supply to the region.

Acupuncture

There have been some positive case reports of acupuncture being an effective approach for tinnitus, but the few clinical trials evaluating acupuncture for tinnitus have been largely negative. A traditional Chinese diagnosis is necessary if acupuncture is to be used to treat tinnitus, and it is always worthwhile trying four to six treatments to see if acupuncture can provide some relief. If acupuncture treatment is effective, then prolonged maintenance treatment may be required.

Mind–Body Therapies

PSYCHOTHERAPY AND RELAXATION EXERCISES Psychotherapy may be helpful for chronic tinnitus. Relaxation exercises may also be recommended (*for information, see p.99*). A 1999 article presented an overview of tinnitus, its psychological effects, and application of psychological therapies for its treatment. This study concluded that psychological treatment for tinnitus, particulary cognitive behavioural therapy, is

effective, but that aspects such as depression and sleep problems may need to be targeted in future studies.

In 2002 a research team investigated whether improving people's ability to manage stress would influence immunity in people with chronic tinnitus. The participants in the programme perceived that they had significantly less stress, anxious depression, anger and tinnitus disturbance. They also showed a reduction in stress on their immune systems. Overall, the study concluded that psychological training helped people manage stress better, which in turn reduced their tinnitus.

PRIMARY TREATMENT **COGNITIVE BEHAVIOURAL THERAPY** Several studies have confirmed an association between psychological factors, such as anxiety and depression, and severe tinnitus. Cognitive behavioural therapy can help tinnitus by enabling you to cope better with stress and by alleviating depression.

HYPNOTHERAPY Several good studies suggest that hypnotherapy may be a better treatment for tinnitus than either maskers or counselling.

OTHER THERAPIES Controlled studies have compared the effectiveness of cognitive behavioural training for tinnitus with other therapies, such as yoga. While yoga also helped tinnitus, cognitive behavioural therapy was shown to be of the greatest benefit and was the therapy that patients preferred. If you have tinnitus, you could consider having a course of cognitive behavioural therapy. You could also explore the possibility of incorporating yoga or another means of relaxing into your daily routine.

PREVENTION PLAN

To prevent tinnitus occurring:

- Avoid loud, persistent noises.

- Wear ear protectors during noisy activities.

- Avoid exposure to hazards, such as heavy metals and carbon monoxide.

- Review any long-term prescription drugs with your doctor.

EARACHE

Pain in the ear usually results from disease of the ear, most commonly infection in the middle or outer ear. Mild earache may be a symptom of a common cold. Sometimes, conditions affecting nearby structures may cause earache. Examples of this include temporomandibular joint disorder (*see p.280*) and shingles (*see p.165*) affecting the face. Depending on the cause, treatment for earache might involve drugs, dietary changes, herbal medicine and homeopathy. Cranial manipulation may also be helpful in some cases.

WHAT ARE THE SYMPTOMS?

Symptoms of middle ear infection include:
- Pain in the ear, which may be severe
- Fever
- Some hearing impairment
- A discharge from the ear if the eardrum ruptures

Symptoms of outer ear infection include:
- Itching and/or pain
- Discharge from the ear

There may be other symptoms associated with disorders affecting nearby tissues.

WHY MIGHT I HAVE THIS?

PREDISPOSING FACTORS

For inner ear infection:
- Upper respiratory tract infection, such as the common cold
- Food sensitivities

For outer ear infection:
- Swimming
- Eczema

TREATMENT PLAN

PRIMARY TREATMENTS
- Drugs for pain relief and to treat infection if necessary
- Dietary changes

BACK-UP TREATMENTS
- Western herbal medicine
- Homeopathy
- Cranial manipulation

For an explanation of how treatments are rated, see p.111.

WHY DOES IT OCCUR?

Earache is often due to germs that have spread up through the nasal passages and Eustachian tubes (which connect the middle ear to the back of the nose) to produce inflammation, swelling and pain within the middle ear. Middle ear infection (otitis media) is the most common cause of earache in children. It may be caused by a viral or bacterial infection. Recurrent middle ear infections may make a child more likely to develop glue ear (*see p.388*). Hearing may be impaired as a result of glue ear. Occasionally, earache results from a tumour in the ear or in a nearby area, such as the throat.

Inflammation of the outer part of the ear (otitis externa) may be caused by a bacterial, viral or fungal infection. Outer ear infections are often associated with swimming (and for that reason are known as "swimmer's ear"), because persistent moisture in the ear canal can increase the risk of an infection developing. Eczema may also be a factor in outer ear infection.

IMMEDIATE RELIEF

To reduce the pain of earache:
- Hold something warm against the ear, such as a hot-water bottle wrapped in a soft towel.
- Painkillers, such as paracetamol or ibuprofen, can also help. Never give aspirin to children under age 12.

IMPORTANT

If earache is severe or persistent, see your doctor without delay.

TREATMENTS IN DETAIL

Conventional Medicine

The doctor will examine your ears using a viewing instrument called an otoscope, and she will probably also look at your throat. If there is discharge from the ear, the doctor may take a sample of it with a swab and send it to the laboratory so the infection can be identified. In some cases, further examination and tests may be needed to look for diseases in nearby areas.

PRIMARY TREATMENT **DRUGS** Painkillers, either obtained over the counter or by prescription, may be taken to relieve the earache. The pain from a middle ear infection usually subsides in about a week. If hearing has been affected, mild hearing loss may persist for up to two weeks. Oral antibiotics may be prescribed for middle ear infection, in addition to painkillers.

To treat an outer ear infection, the doctor may carefully clean the outer ear and prescribe corticosteroid ear drops to relieve inflammation. If an infection is present, ear drops with an antibiotic or an antifungal drug may be prescribed. All of these ear drops may cause some local irritation. Oral antibiotics may be prescribed for more severe bacterial infections of the outer ear.

Other causes of ear infection will be treated whenever possible. For example, antiviral drugs may be given for shingles affecting the face.

CAUTION

Drugs for ear infection can cause a range of possible side-effects: ask your doctor to explain these to you.

ANATOMY OF THE EAR

The ears are organs of both hearing and balance. There are three distinct parts to the structure: the outer, middle and inner ear. The part of the ear that is visible is called the pinna; the outer part of the ear canal can also be viewed without an instrument. The ear canal, which is lined with hairs and secretes protective wax, channels sound. It leads to the eardrum, which vibrates in response to sound-waves. The middle ear lies beyond the eardrum and is filled with air. It contains three tiny bones – the malleus, incus and stapes – that transmit vibrations from the eardrum to the membrane of the oval window. This membrane separates the middle ear from the inner ear.

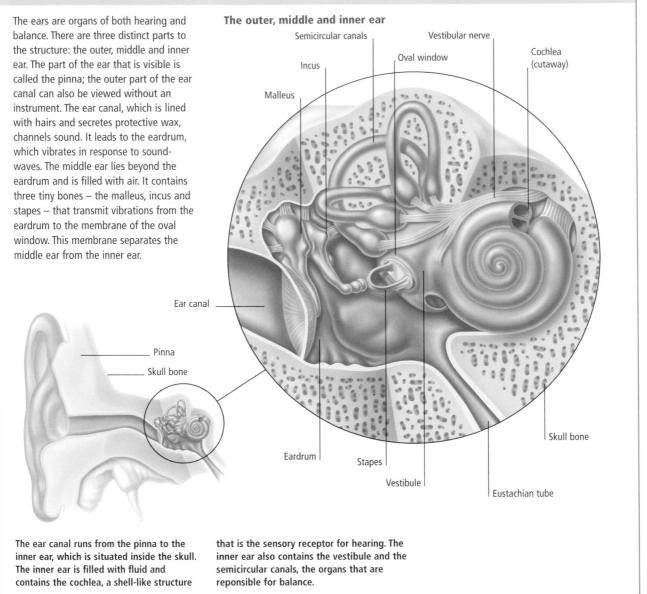

The outer, middle and inner ear

Semicircular canals · Vestibular nerve · Incus · Oval window · Cochlea (cutaway) · Malleus · Ear canal · Pinna · Skull bone · Eardrum · Stapes · Vestibule · Skull bone · Eustachian tube

The ear canal runs from the pinna to the inner ear, which is situated inside the skull. The inner ear is filled with fluid and contains the cochlea, a shell-like structure that is the sensory receptor for hearing. The inner ear also contains the vestibule and the semicircular canals, the organs that are reponsible for balance.

Nutritional Therapy

PRIMARY TREATMENT **DIETARY CHANGES** According to research, food sensitivity appears to be a common factor in children who have recurrent glue ear (*see p.388*) and ear infections. This also seems to be the case in nutritional practice.

In one study, the most common foods found to be associated with glue ear were milk, eggs, beans, citrus fruits and toma-toes. The elimination of the suspect food led to a significant reduction of glue ear symptoms in the majority of patients.

Moreover, the reintroduction of suspect foods back into the diet tended to provoke a recurrence of glue ear. (*For more information about food sensitivities, see p.39.*)

Some practitioners recommend restriction of dairy products and sugary foods because they believe that these impair immune function. If your child has recurrent ear infections, you could try restricting the amount of sugary foods he or she eats to see if this helps.

Certain nutrients may help maintain healthy immune function, which may help to keep ear infections at bay. Probiotic sup-

plements can also help counteract the effects on digestion that antibiotics prescribed for ear infections may cause. If your child has been given antibiotics for ear infection the number of beneficial gut bacteria may have become depleted. You may wish to try giving some "live" yoghurt, or a probiotic drink, each day. For more information about these and other nutritional approaches that may help, see Glue ear, p.388. Breast-feeding babies beyond the age of four months may also offer some protection against ear infection in babies and children.

Homeopathy

Clinical trials and outcome studies suggest that homeopathy is an effective treatment for acute otitis media.

A double-blind placebo-controlled study on the effectiveness of homeopathic treatment for ear infections looked at children between the ages of 18 months and 6 years who had infections of the middle ear. The children were divided into two groups, with 36 of the children receiving real homeopathic treatment and 39 receiving a placebo (sham treatment).

The study used eight different homeopathic remedies, which were prescribed for the children on an individual basis (*see p.73*). The most frequently used remedies were *Pulsatilla*, *Chamomilla*, *Sulfur* and *Calcarea carbonica*. Children receiving homeopathic treatment reported less pain and fever after 24 hours than those receiving the placebo.

For treatment at home, the remedies listed below may bring relief. However, if these do not work or seem inappropriate, you should consult a qualified homeopath for specific treatment. If no improvement is seen in 24 hours, consult your GP as soon as possible.

KALIUM SULPHURICUM The most commonly used medicine for middle ear infection is *Kalium sulphuricum*. This medicine is appropriate when there is deafness with clicking in the ears on swallowing during the infection. The affected child usually has a tendency to catarrh, with thick discharge, for instance down the back of the nose.

PULSATILLA *Pulsatilla* is appropriate when there are similar symptoms, but other characteristics: the affected child tends to be weepy, whingey and clingy, but quickly cheers up from a cuddle with Mum. These children tend to be timid and indecisive.

CALCAREA CARBONICA Perhaps the next most likely medicine for middle ear infection is *Calcarea carbonica*. Children who respond well to this get recurrent colds and tend to be large and chubby. They can be stubborn and tend to have many fears (such as being afraid of the dark). They may wake with frightening dreams and sweat freely, especially on the head.

Western Herbal Medicine

In serious acute cases of middle ear infection, where the onset is likely to be sudden and pain severe, conventional treatment with antibiotics is called for, rather than herbal medicine. Herbal treatment of earache and ear infection is appropriate where symptoms are relatively mild, or if earache is a recurrent problem that has not fully responded to antibiotic therapy.

The herbal approach seeks to determine the factors that have enabled the condition to develop. For example, a herbalist will look for signs of chronic nasal infection or allergy, or of chronic catarrh and congestion. All of these weaken the immune resistance of the mucus-secreting tissue within the upper respiratory passageways. A herbalist may also look for signs of an acute upper respiratory tract infection, either viral or bacterial.

HERBS TO FIGHT INFECTION For self-help measures where infection is present, echinacea (*Echinacea spp.*) and elderberry (*Sambucus nigra*) taken orally are appropriate and can prove effective. For acute infection and in cases of chronic recurrence, visit a practitioner who will prescribe a combination of herbs. The mix is likely to include natural antibiotics to counter infection, such as the antiviral garlic (*Allium sativum*) or the antibacterial golden seal (*Hydrastis canadensis*), and immune tonics (e.g. thyme, *Thymus spp.*) to strengthen non-specific immune activity (increase white blood cell activity).

It is usually also essential to include anti-inflammatory remedies such as liquorice (*Glycyrrhiza glabra*) to reduce swelling and ease pain, as well as plantain (*Plantago major*) or other astringents that work to tone mucous membranes and thus reduce the secretion of mucus.

HERBS FOR PAIN RELIEF Other herbs may be used specifically for pain relief. Lavender (*Lavandula angustifolia*) or German chamomile (*Matricaria recutita*) essential oil can be massaged gently into the area overlying the Eustachian tube, which is behind and in front of the ear, or 1–2 drops (preferably warmed) can be put on cotton wool and plugged into the ear.

> **CAUTION**
>
> See p.69 before taking a herbal remedy and, if already taking prescribed medication, consult a medical herbalist first.

Bodywork Therapies

CRANIAL MANIPULATION Recurrent earache and glue ear in children are often treated by cranial osteopaths, chiropractors and others who work on the cranio-sacral connection. Practitioners use very light pressure to evaluate the ease of motion and rhythm within the craniosacral system and to alter it if it is unbalanced. It is believed that this action can release stresses and tension throughout the body and assist the body's own healing ability.

Children have more ear infections due to their relatively horizontal Eustachian tubes

Although there is little research so far to back up the effectiveness of cranial manipulation for middle ear problems, it may be worth trying if either you or your child has a chronic condition affecting the middle ear. A major US research project has recently been funded for the purpose of examining the effectiveness of the cranial approach to ear problems.

> **PREVENTION PLAN**
>
> **The following may help prevent earache:**
>
> - Breast-feed babies beyond four months.
> - If problem foods may be contributing, try eliminating the most common ones (*see p.39*).
> - If you swim regularly, make sure you thoroughly dry your ears.

Respiratory
System

When breathing we literally take in the outside world. Environmental medicine protects the lungs from harmful chemicals, and herbal and nutritional therapies support the immune defences. Drugs change how the lungs work at a cellular level, but breathing is essentially physical. Bodywork therapies and exercises can optimise the process to help relieve asthma and other ailments.

CATARRH AND SINUSITIS

The sinuses are air-filled cavities in the head situated behind the nose and eyes and in the cheeks and forehead. They are lined with a mucus-secreting membrane and are connected to the nasal cavity by narrow channels. If the membrane in the sinuses and nose secretes too much mucus in response to infection or allergy, the condition may be called catarrh. If the membrane in the sinuses becomes inflamed, the condition is known as sinusitis. Drugs, lifestyle changes, homeopathy and manipulation therapy can all help to resolve these conditions.

WHAT ARE THE SYMPTOMS?

Symptoms of catarrh include:

- Persistently runny nose
- Cough and irritation caused by mucus running down the back of the throat

Symptoms of sinusitis include:

- Pain and tenderness in the face that may be worse when bending forwards
- Nasal discharge
- Nasal congestion or blockage
- Headache and possibly toothache, if the sinuses behind the cheeks are affected

WHY MIGHT I HAVE THIS?

PREDISPOSING FACTORS

- Infection
- Allergy
- Polyps in the nose
- Deviated septum
- Food sensitivity
- Yeast infection
- High levels of histamine in the body
- Trigger points in jaw muscles
- Upper chest breathing

IMPORTANT

If symptoms of sinusitis worsen or do not improve within three days, see your doctor. If redness and swelling develop in the tissues around the eye, consult your doctor urgently.

WHY DOES IT OCCUR?

Catarrh is frequently caused by an allergy, as occurs in allergic rhinitis (*see p.459*). In this condition, excessive mucus is produced by the nose lining. In this case the catarrh usually stops once exposure to the allergen stops. Catarrh may also be due to a viral infection, such as a cold. The most common cause of sinusitis is a viral infection, such as a cold or flu. If the channels connecting the sinuses to the nose become blocked, mucus may collect in the sinuses, where it may become infected with bacteria, which makes the condition worse. Blockage of the sinus channels is more likely in people with an abnormality of the nose, such as a deviated nasal septum or nasal polyps. Rarely, the channels are blocked by a tumour.

Nutritionists' clinical experience suggests that food sensitivity is a common factor in catarrh and sinusitis. Some foods, particularly dairy products but also certain other foods, seem to induce mucus formation in the sinuses, causing catarrh and congestion. Osteopaths believe that sensitive areas known as trigger points in the face and jaw can also increase mucus secretions in the nose and sinuses, causing or worsening catarrh and sinusitis.

IMMEDIATE RELIEF

The following measures may help to relieve the discomfort:

- Add a few drops of pine or eucalyptus essential oil to a bowl of steaming hot water. Lean over the bowl with a towel over your head and inhale for 5–10 minutes. If using this method for children, do not leave them unsupervised.
- Take a hot bath or shower, or run hot water and inhale the steam.
- Use a humidifier in your house, or put bowls of water on radiators.
- Take over-the-counter painkillers and nasal decongestants.

TREATMENT PLAN

PRIMARY TREATMENTS

- Drugs such as decongestants (for catarrh)
- Drugs such as analgesics and possibly antibiotics (for sinusitis)
- Identification and elimination of problem foods (for both)

BACK-UP TREATMENTS

- Acupuncture
- Breathing retraining
- Surgery (if sinusitis is recurrent)

WORTH CONSIDERING

- Vitamin C and bromelain
- Homeopathy
- Western herbal medicine
- Environmental health measures
- Deactivation of trigger points and cranial manipulation
- Nasal specific technique

For an explanation of how treatments are rated, see p.111.

Conventional Medicine

Various treatments are available for catarrh and sinusitis, some of which can be obtained over the counter.

PRIMARY TREATMENT **DRUGS** Nasal decongestants may help people with catarrh in the short term. However, their effect can gradually wear off after a week or so and symptoms may worsen when they are stopped. Antihistamines may produce some improvement in runny nose and sneezing in colds. Pain relievers may be taken to relieve the discomfort of sinusitis.

Antibiotics may be prescribed for sinusitis, but opinions vary over whether this is appropriate. Studies have shown that taking them may be helpful in some cases, but the potential benefits need to be weighed against possible side-effects and developing resistance to antibiotics. Sinusitis often clears up without treatment.

SURGERY Surgical treatment may be recommended if sinusitis is recurrent or does not clear and becomes chronic. The doctor may first recommend further investigations, such as X-rays or ultrasound.

> **CAUTION**
>
> Drugs for catarrh and sinusitis can cause a range of possible side-effects: ask your doctor or pharmacist to explain these to you.

Nutritional Therapy

PRIMARY TREATMENT **FOOD SENSITIVITIES** Dairy products (especially milk and cheese) may have mucus-forming properties in certain individuals. Other common problem foods include white flour and bananas. Since food sensitivity varies, this problem is best assessed individually (*see p.39 for details*).

ELIMINATING YEAST FROM THE BODY Nutritional therapists believe that many people who have chronic (long-term) sinus inflammation may have a yeast infection in their sinuses. Taking steps to eradicate yeast from the body (*for details see p.40*) can often help.

ANATOMY OF THE SINUSES

The air-filled cavities in the skull known as the sinuses are located around the nose and eyes and in the cheeks and forehead. The sinuses are lined with glands that secrete mucus, which passes continuously through narrow channels leading from the sinuses to the back of the nose. This mucus traps small particles and moistens inhaled air. A further set of sinuses, called the sphenoid sinuses, is located deep within the skull behind the ethmoid sinuses.

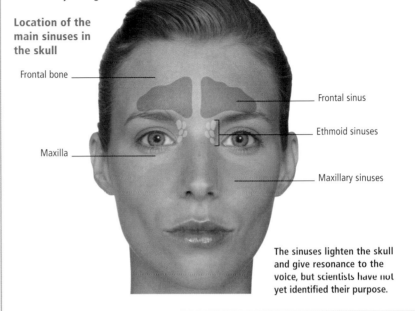

Location of the main sinuses in the skull

Frontal bone

Maxilla

Frontal sinus

Ethmoid sinuses

Maxillary sinuses

The sinuses lighten the skull and give resonance to the voice, but scientists have not yet identified their purpose.

VITAMIN C Histamine is associated with increased nasal and sinus congestion. There is some evidence to suggest that taking vitamin C (3,000mg per day) can reduce histamine levels in people whose levels of this chemical are naturally high or whose blood levels of vitamin C are low. Vitamin C taken at a dose of 2,000mg per day has been shown to help protect people who have allergic rhinitis (a significant predisposing factor for sinisitis) and are exposed to histamine. Research has also shown that people who have chronic sinusitis tend to have diminished antioxidant defences and taking extra vitamin C will remedy this.

BROMELAIN The enzyme bromelain, derived from pineapple, can be helpful in relieving the symptoms of sinusitis. Bromelain has the ability to break down protein in the body and may help to loosen and clear catarrhal congestion.

As a kind of natural nasal decongestant, 500mg of bromelain should be taken three times a day between meals to help prevent catarrh.

> **CAUTION**
>
> Consult your doctor before taking bromelain and vitamin C with antibiotics, or vitamin C with the blood-thinning drug warfarin. (*For more information, see p.46.*)

Homeopathy

Homeopaths believe that individualised homeopathic treatment can go further in treating catarrh and sinusitis than isopathy (treatment with homeopathic dilutions of allergens). As always with homeopathy, individualised treatment is important, and many different homeopathic medicines may be appropriate, depending on the type of catarrh and the person who has it (*see p.73 and also Allergic Rhinitis, p.459*).

ALLIUM CEPA AND EUPHRASIA OFFICINALIS For acute rhinitis, whether due to an allergy or a cold, the medicine *Allium cepa* (onion) provides a good illustration of the principles of homeopathy. The symptoms it is used to treat are exactly those you get from cutting onions: sore, streaming eyes and nose, often with sneezing. *Euphrasia* (made from the herb eyebright) may also be used, among others. In practice, these medicines are often used together in a homeopathic complex.

HEPARCALCAREUM SULPHURIS People for whom this medicine is appropriate usually have a sudden onset of sharp pain above the eyes, usually without a nasal discharge. This pain may be accompanied by a sore throat, with a sensation as if something sharp were stuck there, or a croupy cough and a chilly feeling.

KALIUM BICHROMICUM Perhaps the most frequently used medicine to treat chronic or recurring sinusitis is *Kalium bichromicum*. People who respond to this medicine have a headache either above the eyes or in the cheeks and a thick nasal discharge. Chronic sinusitis such as this often responds well to homeopathy.

PULSATILLA may also be used to treat chronic sinusitis. In people who respond to this remedy the discharge flows freely, and they feel better for being in the fresh air.

The sinuses are not present at birth, but develop gradually throughout childhood

The nose becomes blocked and uncomfortable in a stuffy, overheated room. The type of person who responds to *Pulsatilla* is usually mild-tempered, indecisive or dithery and easily moved to tears.

SILICEA is also given for sinusitis. People who respond to this remedy seem to get every cold that is going around and feel the cold excessively. They often have cold, clammy hands and feet, weak, ridged nails and fine or thinning hair.

LYCOPODIUM is another remedy for sinusitis. Typically, in people who respond to *Lycopodium* the sinuses on the right side are affected more, or the problem starts on the right and moves to the left. Again, "whole person" characteristics are important. People who respond to *Lycopodium*

are often rather reserved, intellectual types. They may get into a state of anxiety before doing anything important, because they set themselves high standards and may be quite depressed. They often have digestive problems, particularly wind and bloating.

> **CAUTION**
>
> Many homeopathic medicines are neutralised by strong smells, such as those of camphor, menthol, eucalyptus etc. If you are using homeopathic medicine, do not use products containing these substances.

Western Herbal Medicine

Acute sinus problems can respond well to herbal treatment. Herbalists consider catarrh and chronic sinus congestion to be commonly associated with poor digestive function, diet and metabolism. (In most traditional medicine systems, catarrh and congestion are thought to result from inadequate processing of food.) This gives rise to a build-up of waste products, which are eliminated via the mucous membranes. Dairy produce and sugar are among the foods linked to chronic catarrhal states and reducing or cutting them out of the diet is a good starting point. Preventing dehydration by drinking plenty of water and humidifying centrally heated air are also essential measures to help prevent catarrh and sinusitis from developing.

HERBS TO RELIEVE SYMPTOMS Plantain (*Plantago lanceolata*) and elderflower (*Sambucus nigra*) are suitable herbs for self-treatment. Both both act to reduce catarrhal secretion and inflammation within upper respiratory passageways. Elderflower also has antiviral activity, and both can be used where allergy may be a cause. Teas made with chamomile (*Matricaria recutita*) or limeflowers (*Tilia cordata*) are also helpful, easing sore and irritated nasal passageways. Limeflowers

are thought to be specifically helpful for sinus headaches. Warm chamomile tea (or warm salt water) may also be carefully inhaled up the nose as a nasal wash (*see Nasal Cleanse right*).

HERBS FOR DETOXIFICATION Practitioners are likely to prescribe herbs to promote detoxification and elimination, such as barberry (*Berberis vulgaris*) and golden rod (*Solidago virgaurea*) and will seek to correct any underlying causes of toxicity, such as constipation. In acute rather than chronic states, herbs with established antimicrobial activity, such as echinacea (*Echinacea spp.*) and golden seal (*Hydrastis canadensis*) will be suggested, often to be taken in combination with cayenne pepper (*Capsiucm annuum*) and liquorice (*Glycyrrhiza glabra*).

> **CAUTION**
>
> See p.69 before taking a herbal remedy and, if you are already taking prescribed medication, consult a medical herbalist first.

Environmental Health

ALLERGIES There are some conditions, such as allergic rhinitis (*see p.459*), which are frequently associated with sinusitis. A study done in New England linked a worsening of asthma and sinusitis with high pollen and mould counts caused by the wind El Nino in 1998, and environmental factors do seem to be a factor in both allergies and sinusitis. Inflammation of the nasal and sinus tissue typically precedes the actual infection of the sinuses.

AVOID DUST MITES AND MOULD If you are allergic to indoor allergens, such as dust mites or indoor moulds, remove upholstered furniture and carpeting and wash bed linens at high temperatures. You should also take steps to eliminate damp from your house.

AIR POLLUTION Numerous German studies demonstrate an association between air pollution and the prevalence of chronic sinusitis. Ozone levels can fluctuate in the air, and ozone can also irritate the mucous membranes and may therefore be important in the development of sinusitis.

If you have sinusitis regularly, limit your time outdoors on days when the pollution levels are high.

SMOKING Smoking is a strong risk factor for the development and prolongation of chronic sinusitis and catarrh. Many studies have supported this association, and the effects of tobacco smoke on the lining of the upper respiratory tract, which includes the nasal passages and the sinuses, is immense. If you have sinusitis or other respiratory disease and you smoke, quitting should be a top priority.

WORKPLACE CHEMICALS Vapours from amonia have been linked to the development of chronic sinus disease, and people exposed to chlorine at work (or maybe even in swimming pools) may be at risk of developing nasal congestion. In general, if you are prone to sinusitis, avoid swimming pools treated with chlorine, which irritates nose and sinus linings.

POLLUTANTS IN THE NOSE Nasal irrigation, preferably with a Neti pot or similar device, washes away many pollutants that are trapped in the nasal lining (*see below*).

AIR TRAVEL Travelling by air may worsen symptoms of sinusitis. With increasing altitude, the air pressure in a plane may be reduced, causing pressure to build up in your head and blocking your sinuses or the Eustachian tubes in your ears. Chewing gum or drinking water during take-off and landing may help the pressure in your sinuses and lessen pain. Some doctors recommend using decongestant nose drops or inhalers before your flight. Be sure to stay well hydrated by drinking plenty of non-caffeinated beverages while on board. Avoid drinking alcohol because it causes nasal and sinus membranes to swell. A saline nasal spray also helps to maintain moist nasal passages during a long flight.

Acupuncture

Acupuncture is widely used for the treatment of sinusitis and allergic rhinitis and is apparently effective. Treating specific points on the lung and large intestine channel, which runs over the affected area, can be useful, but a traditional Chinese diagnosis is required first. Four studies looking at acupuncture in allergic rhinitis suggest that it may be of value, but all the studies are of poor quality. A number of Chinese studies, again largely uncontrolled and of poor quality, also claim great benefit for acupuncture in rhinitis. There is one relatively poor study of acupuncture on sinus pain, which indicates significant benefit. As always with acupuncture, persistent treatment is required, particularly with a very chronic sinus infection.

Bodywork Therapies

NASAL SPECIFIC TECHNIQUE Many chiropractors, naturopaths and cranial osteopaths treat chronic sinusitis and sinus headaches with a combination of spinal manipulation, massage and a technique called "nasal specific" (NS). This involves inflating very small balloons within the nasal passages, creating a change of pressure and, theoretically, a realignment of nasal bones, which can relieve congestion. In a case study, a 41-year-old woman's sinus headaches resolved immediately following treatment involving NS. At the end of two months of care, her sinus headaches were reduced significantly in intensity and frequency.

TRIGGER-POINT DEACTIVATION Trigger points (particularly sensitive areas, *see p.55*) in the face and jaw may increase mucus production in the nose and sinuses. These can be deactivated by acupuncture, as well as by manual pressure from physiotherapists and other manual practitioners with a knowledge of neuromuscular techniques.

CRANIAL MANIPULATION This practice involves applying extremely gentle pressure to the bones of the head and face, sometimes working inside the mouth. There are a number of safe cranial techniques to help drain the sinuses.

Breathing Retraining

If breathing is shallow, the blood can become too alkaline. This makes histamine levels rise and allergic responses, which can contribute to catarrh and sinusitis, may result. Breathing retraining involves doing yoga-type diaphragmatic breathing exercises, which have been shown to be very effective in improving the mechanics and efficiency of breathing. (*For a breathing sequence, see p.62.*)

NASAL CLEANSE

Put a pinch of salt in 200ml (about 7oz) of warm water in a Neti pot. Stand over a sink, put your head back and pour the water into one nostril, allowing it to flow freely out through the other nostril. Repeat two to three times daily, increasing to four times daily during bouts of sinusitis. There is some evidence that a hypertonic (more concentrated) salt solution may be more effective, but the risk of damage to the mucosal tissue is increased, so do not increase the amount of salt.

COLDS AND FLU

The common infections known as colds and flu are caused by viruses. There are at least 200 different viruses that cause the common cold, while true flu (or influenza) is caused by just two principal types of influenza virus. Colds tend to have more minor symptoms than flu, which usually causes a high fever. Treatment is usually directed at relieving symptoms and might include painkillers for muscle aches and decongestants for a blocked nose. Vitamin supplements, homeopathic and herbal medicines and steam inhalations can also help.

WHAT ARE THE SYMPTOMS?

Symptoms of the common cold include:

- Sneezing
- Runny nose, with discharge that is initially clear but becomes thick and green later on
- Mild fever and headache
- Sore throat, and sometimes a cough

Symptoms of flu include:

- High fever, with sweating and shivering
- Aching muscles, especially in the back
- Severe exhaustion
- Frequent sneezing, runny nose, sore throat and cough

WHY MIGHT I HAVE THIS?

PREDISPOSING FACTORS

- Exposure to others who have colds or flu
- Overwork and being "run down"
- Low immune function

IMPORTANT

If cold or flu symptoms persist for more than a week, or if symptoms of a secondary infection (such as earache or coughing up green or yellow sputum) develop, see your doctor. Babies, young children, the elderly and those with reduced immunity who develop flu symptoms should see a doctor immediately.

WHY DOES IT OCCUR?

Cold and flu viruses affect the upper respiratory tract and cause symptoms such as sneezing, runny nose, sore throat and cough. Secondary bacterial infections, often affecting areas such as the ears, throat or sinuses, may develop as complications of either colds or flu.

The viruses responsible for colds and flu are all highly infectious and are spread in tiny airborne droplets from the coughs and sneezes of infected people. They can also be spread by direct contact, often from hand to hand, and may live for hours on inanimate objects such as door handles, towels or telephones.

Some people mistake a heavy cold for flu. The difference between them is that flu tends to cause a high fever along with muscle aches and pains, symptoms that are not usually present in a cold.

Most people can expect to have between two and four colds a year. Children are more susceptible to colds than adults because they have not yet developed immunity to the viruses that cause colds.

There is no cure for colds or flu. Both tend to run their course in one to two weeks if no secondary infection develops.

TREATMENT PLAN

PRIMARY TREATMENTS

- Rest and fluids
- Painkillers, NSAIDs and decongestants
- Vitamin C and zinc
- *Oscillococcinum* and other homeopathic medicines
- Echinacea

BACK-UP TREATMENTS

- Western herbal medicine
- Regular exercise
- Environmental health measures

WORTH CONSIDERING

- Chinese herbal medicine
- Bodywork therapies
- Acupuncture
- Mind–body therapies

For an explanation of how treatments are rated, see p.111.

SELF-HELP

PRIMARY TREATMENT The following measures will help bring some relief:

- Get plenty of rest.
- Drink lots of fluids, especially water.
- Take over-the-counter painkillers and decongestants for symptom relief.

TREATMENTS IN DETAIL

Conventional Medicine

It will probably not be necessary to see your doctor if you develop a cold or flu, unless a secondary bacterial infection develops. Colds and flu are caused by viruses, which cannot be treated with antibiotics. Elderly people and people with chronic conditions, such as chronic lung conditions and diabetes mellitus, may be offered immunization against flu. This needs to be repeated each year.

PRIMARY TREATMENT **OVER-THE-COUNTER DRUGS** Colds and flu may be relieved by medication from the pharmacist such as analgesics and non-steroidal anti-inflammatories (NSAIDs) including paracetemol and ibuprofen. Also available are decongestants and cough remedies to soothe a tickly throat. With both colds and flu, it is important to drink plenty of fluids.

PRESCRIPTION DRUGS Antibiotics may be prescribed if a secondary bacterial infection develops. However, this does not usually happen. If you only have a cold, antibiotics do not help. They can cause side-effects, such as diarrhoea, and there is concern that over-prescription of antibiotics is leading to increasing bacterial resistance to them.

Antiviral drugs, such as neuraminidase inhibitors, may be prescribed in some cases. In the UK, these drugs are recommended for people with suspected flu who are over the age of 65 and those considered at risk because they have certain chronic illnesses, such as chronic lung disease or diabetes mellitus, or because they are immunocompromised (their ability to fight infection is impaired).

> **CAUTION**
>
> Over-the-counter and prescription drugs for colds and flu can cause side-effects: ask your doctor or pharmacist to explain these to you.

Nutritional Therapy

PRIMARY TREATMENT **VITAMIN C SUPPLEMENTS** can help to treat the common cold, reducing the severity and duration of symptoms in individuals who become infected with the viruses that cause it. One systematic review of 30 placebo-controlled trials found fair evidence for high doses of vitamin C as a treatment that shortened the duration of colds, but no evidence to support the use of vitamin C to prevent colds. Taking large doses of vitamin C can sometimes cause diarrhoea, but this side-effect resolves once the dose is reduced. You could try taking 500mg vitamin C per day to treat a cold.

You can eat foods rich in vitamin C as well as taking supplements. Watercress is an excellent source of vitamin C. Drink

This electron scanning micrograph shows one of the flu viruses multiplying on a mucous membrane.

watercress soup, eat fresh watercress or juice it and take the juice. You can also juice oranges and grapefruit and drink them each morning for extra vitamin C.

PRIMARY TREATMENT **ZINC** Taking zinc lozenges may shorten a common cold, but the research results are unclear. Two systematic reviews came to slightly different conclusions. One found that zinc lozenges reduced symptoms after seven days, but there were no differences after three or five days. The second review (covering most of the same trials) showed no improvement in any cold symptoms after one week. A subsequent study of people using an over-the-counter zinc nasal gel within 24 hours of a cold beginning showed they had a shorter period of symptoms than did those using a placebo. Start taking zinc gluconate lozenges within 24 hours of the onset of cold symptoms. Suck one lozenge every two hours throughout the day until the symptoms disappear.

Although zinc gluconate is the most commonly used form of zinc for treating the common cold, there is good recent scientific evidence that zinc acetate may be an even better form of zinc for this purpose. Forms of zinc other than gluconate and acetate should be avoided because they may not release sufficient quantities of zinc

to exert a significant effect. Also, the lozenge should not contain citric acid, tartaric acid, mannitol or sorbitol, since these can inactivate the zinc.

> **CAUTION**
>
> Consult your doctor before taking vitamin C with antibiotics or warfarin, or zinc with antibiotics. (*For more information, see p. 46.*)

Homeopathy

No clinical trials of homeopathy for colds have been done but the following homeopathic treatments may be helpful. Take two 6C pills four times per day.

ACONITE AND BELLADONNA are the most commonly used single homeopathic medicines for the early stages of colds and flu. Both should be started within a few hours of the onset of symptoms. People who respond to *Aconite* feel chilly, although they may have a high fever, and are anxious. The skin is hot, red and dry. They may be very thirsty for cold drinks and feel tingling on the tip of the tongue or lips.

People who respond to *Belladonna* often have a fever; the face is flushed and sweaty, and they may be confused; children may even hallucinate. The pupils are dilated and bright light and loud noises hurt; sudden movement is painful. (Be aware that these symptoms can also be a sign of meningitis, *see p.391*).

GELSEMIUM may be useful after the initial stage of a cold or bout of flu when the patient feels tired, weak and tremulous and has profuse sweat but usually no thirst. *Coldenza*, made by Nelsons, contains *Gelsemium* and is a speciality for colds and flu. It is widely available in the UK.

MERCURIUS SOLUBILIS AND EUPATORIUM PERFOLIATUM *Mercurius solubilis* is one of the most useful homeopathic medicines for colds that have gone on for three or four days. Symptoms often include a sore throat with swollen glands or thick, green nasal discharge. People who respond to this medicine are always too hot or too cold. They may have a lot of perspiration and excessive saliva in the mouth. The tongue feels sore and swollen, imprints of the teeth may visible around the edge of the tongue, and there may be bad breath.

Eupatorium perfoliatum is a useful medicine for flu where there is a lot of muscular aching experienced, as well as backache and pain in the eyes.

PRIMARY TREATMENT **OSCILLOCOCCINUM**, a homeopathic speciality made by Boiron, has been shown to reduce the duration of flu and similar conditions. This medicine is available in the US, France and some other European countries, but not the UK.

> **CAUTION**
>
> Many homeopathic medicines are neutralised by very strong smells, such as those of camphor, menthol, eucalyptus etc. If you are taking homeopathic medicines, do not use remedies for colds containing these.

Western Herbal Medicine

Colds respond well to herbal self-help. Flu is more serious, but taking herbs as soon as you start to feel ill may shorten attacks.

This Schlieren photograph (which uses a specialised technique to show air turbulence) reveals what happens during a sneeze. Irritation of the nasal lining triggers a jet of droplets to erupt from the mouth and nose. An unprotected sneeze can travel 3 metres (9 feet).

GINGER Infuse three slices of fresh ginger (*Zingiber officinalis*) in a cup of boiling water for 10 minutes and drink. Drink a cup every three or four hours. Ginger has a warming, stimulating effect that brings on a therapeutic sweat. A recent study has shown it has a significant action against four different strains of bacteria that may cause secondary infection following colds or flu. Cinnamon, cloves and black pepper also have antibacterial properties.

PRIMARY TREATMENT **ECHINACEA** A review of 16 trials (eight prevention trials and eight trials of treatment of upper respiratory tract infections) suggested that overall, echinacea (*Echinacea spp.*) does work as a treatment but probably not as a preventive medicine. Take 10–15g per day at the first sign of a cold. Stop taking it when the cold has resolved; echinacea should not be used as a continuous preventive medicine except when someone has constant colds. In this case, echinacea can be used for between one and three months at a dosage of 1–3g per day.

ANDROGRAPHIS A promising new cold cure from India is the plant *Andrographis paniculata*, which is used in Ayervedic and Chinese medicine. In one double-blind study, 208 people with upper-respiratory tract infections were given either andrographis or a placebo (an inactive substance). By the second day, the andrographis group had improvement in cold symptoms (runny nose and sore throat) compared to those given just a placebo. By the fourth day, there was a significant improvement in other symptoms such as cough, headaches, earache and fatigue too.

STEAM INHALATION Put a few drops of Olbas oil, eucalyptus oil (*Eucalyptus globulus*) or some chamomile (*Matricaria recutita*) in a bowl, pour in boiling water and inhale the steam, covering your head with a towel.

OTHER TRADITIONAL MEASURES Tea made by infusing elderflower (*Sambucus nigra*) and peppermint (*Mentha piperita*) and adding 3–4 slices of ginger is effective for colds. Add yarrow (*Achillea millefolium*) if you have flu. Drink a teacupful every four hours. Alternatively, fresh hyssop (*Hyssopus officinalis*) tea is good for colds and flu. Add a teaspoonful of honey, especially manuka honey, to hot drinks. It has antibacterial properties and helps soothe sore throats.

Garlic (*Allium sativum*), mustard (*Brassica alba*) and horseradish (*Cochlearia armoracia*) have important properties that help combat colds and flu. As well as using them in cooking, you can try the old-fashioned remedy of taking a mustard footbath. Make these in a plastic bowl big enough to fit both your feet by pouring in three litres of hot water and mixing in three tablespoons of English mustard powder. Put your feet in the bowl for 10 minutes and cover your head with a towel while you do so to increase the heat in your head and sinuses. Do this morning and evening for the duration of your cold or flu symptoms.

Finally, tiger balm and olbas oil may help to ease congestion. Apply tiger balm to your chest and back, taking care not to get any in your eyes and washing your hands well afterwards. Alternatively, apply olbas oil to your temples and the back of your neck. Keep it away from your eyes.

> **CAUTION**
>
> See p.69 before taking a herbal remedy and, if you are taking prescribed medication, consult a medical herbalist first.

Chinese Herbal Medicine

Traditional Chinese Medicine (TCM) practitioners believe adverse climatic factors can breach the body's defence system (called *Wei Qi*), causing colds and flu. In particular, wind is said to be "the initiator of 100 diseases". Wind combines with other disease-causing factors, such as cold, heat and damp. Treatments aim to improve lung function, increasing the protection afforded by *Wei Qi*. Many treatments are said to "open the exterior" and produce a therapeutic sweat, which drives out the adverse climatic factors of wind, cold, heat or damp.

One simple general remedy is soya bean soup (*Cong Chi Tang*). This comprises stalks of green onion combined with prepared soya bean to which have been added perilla leaf (*Zi Su Ye* or *Perilla frutescens*), Quiang Huo (*Notopterygium incisum*), siler (*Fang Feng* or *Ledebouriella seseloides*) and schizonepeta (*Jing Jie* or *Schizonepeta tenuifolia*). In more severe wind-cold patterns TCM doctors use stronger prescriptions, such as Schizonepeta-Ledebouriella Defeat Poison Powder (*Jing Fang Bai Du San*).

WIND-COLD-DAMP INVASION If the pattern is wind-cold damp invasion, you will have a heavy feeling in the head and feel tired, possibly with nausea, loss of appetite, bloating and loose stools. In such cases a TCM doctor might prescribe Notopterygium Conquering Dampness Decoction (*Qiang Huo Sheng Shi Tang*).

WIND-HEAT INVASION Wind heat-cold/flu invasion is marked by feelings of cold and heat in which heat predominates. The person may have a blocked nose, a cough and a sore throat. The classical remedy is the famous Honeysuckle and Forsythia Powder (*Yin Qiao San*) available in pill form.

INVASION OF DRYNESS Another common pattern is invasion of dryness (said to be a feature of autumn colds and flus). The usual prescription is a variation of the Mulberry Almond Decoction (*Sang Xin Tang*).

INTERNAL DEFICIENCIES such as *Qi*, Blood, *Yin* or *Yang* deficiency are treated with specific formulas. Two remedies from the woad family that have antiviral properties, *Ban Lan Gen* and *Da Qing Ye*, are often added to cold formulas.

> **CAUTION**
>
> See p.69 before taking a herbal remedy and, if you are taking prescribed medication, consult a medical herbalist first.

Environmental Health

AVOIDING CROWDS AND CONFINED SPACES The most obvious way to avoid getting colds or flu is to avoid crowds and confined areas during the peak cold season, which is early autumn, and the peak flu season, which is in the winter. You are at greatest risk of getting infected in highly populated areas, such as in crowded living conditions and in schools or on public transport. People are most contagious from a day or so before they develop symptoms, making it difficult to identify contagious individuals.

Antibiotics have no effect against viruses, which are the cause of colds and flu

KEEPING YOUR HANDS AWAY FROM YOUR FACE Bear in mind that flu and colds can also be spread by inanimate objects such as towels, toys and door handles that carry disease-causing germs. Germs commonly live on these objects for minutes or hours or sometimes even longer. If you touch a contaminated surface, germs can easily pass from your hand to your nose or mouth and lead to infection. Keep your fingers away from your nose, mouth and eyes to avoid infecting yourself with virus particles that you may have picked up.

HANDWASHING Wash your hands regularly and thoroughly. One recent study done with hospital personnel showed the effectiveness of a newer "soap" for disinfection. The investigators promoted an alcohol-based handrub, which was distributed widely in patient care areas.

The result was a remarkable increase in hand disinfecting activity, and a corresponding huge drop in infection rates. The convenience of using this handrub was largely responsible for the results. The effectiveness of these alcohol-based instant soaps against cold and flu viruses has been demonstrated.

HUMIDITY When the mucous membranes become dry, it is easier for them to become infected with cold or flu viruses. An easy way to humidify your home is to put saucers of water on or near radiators throughout the house. A study emphasises the importance of maintaining an adequate humidity level at home to prevent the mucous membranes in the nose from drying out. Drinking plenty of water, or sipping drinks such as honey and lemon throughout the day also helps to keep the nasal membranes moist.

BREATHING THROUGH THE NOSE The same study also showed the benefits of breathing through the nose. When a virus enters the nose, it gives the immune system time to mount a defence before the virus reaches the lungs. When flu virus is given to laboratory mice whose gag and cough reflexes are repressed, half the dose of virus goes directly into the lungs and kills most of the mice within a week. However, when the virus is given to mice whose gag and cough reflexes are normal, these reflexes prevent the virus from reaching the lungs. One possible factor in the severity of flu is the initial site of infection (hence the development of the new nasal flu vaccine). Use your natural defences in the flu season and try to breathe through your nose.

Colds are more frequent in children, due to their lower resistance to infection

OTHER MEASURES When you have a cold or bout of flu, you can help to prevent the spread of infection by putting a second hand towel in the bathroom for healthy people to use. Remember to cover your nose and mouth with a tissue when you cough or sneeze, then throw the tissue away and wash your hands. Be sure to use tissues rather than a handkerchief.

If you need to travel by air during the cold and flu season, drink plenty of bottled water to combat dehydration. Wash your hands frequently while on board – you can use alcohol hand wipes. A nasal saline spray (preferably free of preservatives) can help to keep your nasal passages moist and prevent dryness and cracking.

Acupuncture

Acupuncture is frequently used in China to treat acute (sudden and short-lived) conditions that usually resolve on their own, such as colds and flu. People in China might be treated using acupuncture two or three times a day for colds and flu, often on the lung and large intestine meridian.

There are no clinical trials in this area, but the general experience of patients is very positive and suggests that acupuncture is an effective treatment. Practitioners believe that acupuncture can quickly stimulate an the immune system to respond, which is appropriate in acute viral infections such as colds and flu and would be likely to speed recovery.

Bodywork Therapies

LYMPHATIC DRAINAGE Osteopathic methods known collectively as lymphatic pump techniques aim to increase the immune system's response to infection.

These techniques work by increasing levels in the bloodstream of natural killer cells and B and T lymphocytes (important components of the immune system) for up to 24 hours after the techniques have been applied. The increased levels of these cells appear to offer very real advantages to the individual fighting colds, flu or infection of any sort.

MASSAGE, CHIROPRACTIC AND OSTEOPATHY Immune enhancement, in which levels of natural killer cells and B and T lymphocyte are significantly increased, has also been observed in people after they have received general, non-specific, massage. Similary, immune enhancement has been observed following specific chiropractic spinal manipulation.

The ways in which these methods improve immune function are not fully understood. However, it is thought that the osteopathic method stimulates production, or release from storage sites, of helpful immune substances. Massage is thought to reduce the presence of "stress hormones", thus improving the efficiency of the immune system.

Chiropractic treatment is thought to achieve its effect through the nervous system, in a similar way to osteopathic treatment. In order to benefit from these aspects of bodywork, consult a suitably qualified and licensed osteopath, chiropractor or massage therapist.

Exercise

Lifestyle factors, including exercise, can strengthen immune responses and it is suggested that if you have colds regularly, you could try taking some aerobic exercise. A study of 50 women showed that a group taking regular exercise (walking briskly for 45 minutes five days each week) had half as many colds as a group taking no exercise. People who exercise regularly had more natural killer cells, which are one of the body's first lines of defence against against viruses. However, most research suggests that while moderate exercise boosts immunity, too much is likely to leaves you prone to infection.

Mind–Body Therapies

Mental disharmony is known to undermine immunity. Big life events, such as moving house or bereavement, also undermine immunity, as do high levels of anxiety. The accumulation of daily stresses may also adversely affect the immune system, which is why adequate rest and self-care can help to boost immunity.

SELF-HYPNOSIS Stress reduces the immune responsiveness of the mucous membranes. Many studies have shown this. Self-hypnosis might help people who are prone to colds when they are under stress. A study of medical students at exam time found self-hypnosis incorporating imagery of the immune system can reduce the effects of stress on immune functions. Results showed that the students in the imagery group had heightened immune function, improvements in mood and fewer winter viral infections.

PREVENTION PLAN

The following may help to protect you against colds and flu:

- Eat a healthy diet rich in fresh fruit and vegetables.
- Wash your hands regularly and avoid crowds during cold and flu season.

ASTHMA

Asthma causes attacks of wheezing and shortness of breath. When someone with asthma inhales irritant particles, the immune system overreacts, producing histamine, making the airways narrow and swell. Unless your asthma is very mild, drugs are crucial for dilating the airways and reducing the inflammation. In integrated medicine, these are backed up with therapies to stretch the chest muscles and encourage easier breathing. Diet can play a part in susceptibility to asthma, so dietary change may be a key part of your plan.

WHAT ARE THE SYMPTOMS?

- Persistent dry cough, which may be the main symptom
- Wheezing
- Feeling of tightening in the chest
- Shortness of breath
- Difficulty exhaling

Symptoms may be accompanied by:

- Sweating
- Feelings of panic
- Inability to complete a sentence due to shortness of breath

If an attack is very severe, symptoms may include:

- Wheezing that is inaudible because so little air is entering the airways
- Inability to speak properly
- Blue lips, tongue and fingers due to lack of oxygen
- Exhaustion, confusion and coma

WHY MIGHT I HAVE THIS?

PREDISPOSING FACTORS

- Smoking
- Genetic tendency
- Food intolerance
- Diet low in fatty acids

TRIGGERS (FOR EXISTING ASTHMA)

- Irritants, such as pollen or polluted air
- Contact with birds or furry animals
- Stress
- Beta-blockers and other drugs
- Cold air and exercise
- Respiratory infection

IMPORTANT

If you have symptoms, see your doctor for a diagnosis. Severe asthma attacks can be life-threatening without immediate medical treatment. If you have an attack, see Immediate Relief (*overleaf*) and if necessary call a doctor or an ambulance. Never reduce or stop taking conventional medication for asthma without consulting your doctor.

WHY DOES IT OCCUR?

In an asthma attack, the immune system reacts to an inhaled substance and produces immunoglobulin E (IgE) antibodies. These substances stimulate the release of histamine in the lining of the airways, which consequently becomes inflamed and swollen. The excess mucus that is produced can block the smaller airways. The attacks of wheezing and shortness of breath that result can last for hours or days and be very exhausting and, in some cases, life-threatening. The airways of many people with asthma can become persistently inflamed over time. There is a wide range of factors that either trigger attacks or make you more susceptible to them (*see left*). In some people, asthma is triggered by exposure to an allergen, such as pollen, house-dust mites, animal dander or, less commonly, certain foods or food additives. This type of asthma tends to develop in childhood and can run in families. It may appear along with hay fever and eczema.

In some cases, the first asthma attack is triggered by a respiratory infection. Some people develop a form of the condition known as occupational asthma as a result of exposure to workplace substances such as glues, resins, latex and spray paints.

Air pollution does not seem to play a part in causing asthma to develop initially, but it may make existing asthma worse or act as a trigger for an asthma attack. Stress can also bring on asthma attacks. In some people, exercise triggers attacks (this is known as exercise-induced asthma).

ASTHMA RATES WORLDWIDE The numbers of people with asthma have soared in recent decades in Australia, New Zealand, the UK and the US. Australia has one of the world's highest asthma rates, with 14–16 per cent of children and 10–12 per cent of adults affected. In Melbourne, over 25 per cent of children have asthma.

Except in the big cities, asthma rates in Asian countries are half those of developed countries. Asthma rates are increasing the fastest among the poor and the young: in the US, for example, the disease is particularly prevalent among the inner-city ethnic minority youth. It would seem, therefore, that poverty, stress, pollution, race and urbanisation are all key factors in the increase of the disease.

TREATMENT PLAN

PRIMARY TREATMENTS

- Reliever and preventer drugs
- Avoiding environmental triggers
- Breathing retraining
- Stress-management programme

BACK-UP TREATMENTS

- Food exclusion diet
- Western and Chinese herbal medicine

WORTH CONSIDERING

- Low-salt diet and other dietary changes
- Homeopathy
- Acupuncture
- Bodywork therapies and exercise

For an explanation of how treatments are rated, see p.111.

- During an attack take your usual dose of reliever, preferably using a spacer device.
- Keep calm and relax (don't lie down).
- Try to breathe slowly for 5–10 minutes. If symptoms disappear, you can resume normal activities.
- If severe symptoms persist after several doses, call an ambulance immediately. Take your reliever every few minutes until help arrives.

TREATMENTS IN DETAIL

Conventional Medicine

Your doctor will discuss your symptoms and consider possible triggers. He may assess your breathing by asking you to blow into a peak flow meter, a device that records the maximum flow of air you can produce when you breathe out. This can be reduced if you have asthma, and there may be a marked difference in morning and evening readings if your asthma is not adequately controlled. Your doctor may also arrange for you to have lung function tests to test your breathing, and possibly some allergy tests.

You will be asked to keep a record of your peak-flow readings. In this way you can monitor your condition and adjust your treatment or see the doctor as appropriate. He will assess your progress and alter your treatment if your symptoms are not being adequately controlled.

Asthma drugs are mainly taken with an inhaler, sometimes used in combination with a "spacer" – a plastic device placed between the mouth and the inhaler that makes it easier to inhale the drug. Spacers are particularly useful for young children and elderly people. A nebuliser delivers drugs as a fine mist inhaled through a face-mask or mouthpiece. They are effective in acute attacks unrelieved by inhalers.

PRIMARY TREATMENT **RELIEVER AND PREVENTER DRUGS** Your doctor is likely to prescribe a reliever drug, such as salbutamol, to take when you have symptoms. These are short-acting bronchodilators, which means they relax the muscles of the airways, allowing air to pass in and out more easily. Reliever drugs usually start to work within 5–10 minutes of being

INHALING ASTHMA DRUGS

Inhaling is an efficient way of taking drugs for asthma because the chemicals reach the airways quickly and very little of the medication enters the bloodstream, so there are few side-effects. In an asthma attack, the walls of the airways of the lungs constrict and excess mucus collects, so less air can pass through, which consequently makes breathing difficult. A few minutes after taking a reliever drug, the airway walls dilate and breathing becomes easier.

Effects of asthma drugs on the airways

Asthma drug inhaled

Bronchi

Lung

BEFORE INHALATION

Contracted muscle

Narrowed air passage

Mucus-producing cells

The muscular walls of the airway have constricted, meaning less air can enter.

AFTER INHALATION

Relaxed muscle

Widened air passage

Mucus-producing cells

Once inhaled, asthma drugs travel swiftly to the network of airways in the lungs.

Following a dose of a bronchodilator drug, the airway wall has relaxed.

inhaled, but their effects last for only a few hours. The doctor may tell you to take a reliever drug before you exercise.

You may have to take preventer drugs regularly. These are mainly inhaled corticosteroids, such as beclometasone. You take them every day to reduce inflammation in the airway linings and make them less likely to narrow in response to triggers.

LONGER-ACTING BRONCHODILATORS, such as salmeterol, may be prescribed. They also relax the muscles of the airways, but unlike shorter-acting bronchodilators their effects last for up to 12 hours.

LEUKOTRIENE ANTAGONISTS may also be prescribed if asthma symptoms persist. These drugs work by dampening down the allergic response and preventing narrowing of the airways.

ORAL CORTICOSTEROID DRUGS Courses of these drugs may also be prescribed for very severe asthma.

CAUTION

Asthma drugs can have a range of possible side-effects: ask your doctor to explain these. People with asthma should avoid taking beta-blockers, aspirin and non-steroidal anti-inflammatory drugs (NSAIDs).

Nutritional Medicine

A FOOD EXCLUSION DIET is recommended (see p.39) since food sensitivities can often be an underlying factor, especially in childhood asthma. In one study, 91 per cent of children with respiratory allergy found their symptoms improved on a six-week diet that excluded common problem foods including grains and dairy products.

FISH OILS may help, since asthma may be related to imbalance in fatty acids in the diet. Excessive amounts of omega-6 fatty acids (found in vegetable oils) and a relative lack of omega-3 fats (found in oily fish and some nuts and seeds) may promote inflammation of the airways and aggravate asthma. Try cutting back on margarine and vegetable oils and eating at least two portions of oily fish a week (such as salmon or mackerel). Children should take 300mg of fish oil a day. A number of studies suggest that this is worth trying.

A LOW-SALT DIET might help to reduce asthma symptoms. Salt seems to increase the response of the airways to histamine, causing increased airway constriction. You should avoid adding salt to dishes and limit the amount of processed foods you eat. One study found giving an additional 6.1g of salt per day to a group of patients with asthma made their symptoms worse and increased their use of inhaled corticosteroid drugs. The authors concluded that a low-salt diet (5–6g of salt per day) appears to have a favourable effect on symptoms and reduces the need for anti-asthma drugs. In another study of people with exercise-induced asthma, a low-salt diet improved and a high-salt diet worsened post-exercise lung function.

AN ANTIOXIDANT-RICH DIET may be beneficial because high levels of flavonoids and antioxidants are linked to a lower risk of asthma and reduced severity of symptoms. To boost your intake of antioxidants, eat plenty of fruit and vegetables.

In children, eating fresh fruit has been related to fewer asthma symptoms and improved lung function. This protective effect was evident even in children who only ate fruit once or twice a week. You can try taking 500mg–1g of vitamin C a day and 100mcg of selenium (adult doses), both of which are potent antioxidants. Children who weigh 40kg should take half this dose; smaller children, less. Research from the 1990s suggested that vitamin C supplements improved asthma. More recent studies have shown no effect.

MAGNESIUM can be helpful for people with asthma. Magnesium is found in nuts, seeds and wholegrain foods. A study of children found low intakes of magnesium and potassium were associated with poorer lung function. In one study, asthma patients given 400mg of magnesium a day showed improved asthma symptom scores, but a more recent study showed no effect.

BREAST-FEEDING YOUR BABY may help to reduce the risk of childhood asthma. One study found an increased risk of asthma if exclusive breast-feeding was stopped before the baby was four months old. Also, taking probiotics during pregnancy and then giving them to your baby may help to prevent asthma. The gut microflora of infants who develop asthma appears to be different from that of those who do not develop it, according to studies. In one study, the probiotic *Lactobacillus GG* was given to pregnant women who at had least one first-degree relative (or partner) with an allergic condition such as atopic eczema, allergic rhinitis, or asthma. After birth, the probiotic was also given to their child for six months. Probiotic supplements were found to significantly reduce the risk of early allergic disease in children at high risk of developing it.

> **CAUTION**
>
> Consult your doctor before taking fish oil supplements with the blood-thinning drug warfarin. (For more information, *see p.46*.)

Homeopathy

There are three ways homeopathy can treat asthma: isopathy, acute treatment and constitutional treatment (*see p.73*).

Isopathy involves taking homeopathic dilutions of allergens (such as house-dust mites or pollen). You should not take isopathic remedies when you have symptoms, since they work best during the "plateau" phase. The evidence for isopathy's effectiveness is controversial; some is positive, some not. However, isopathy is only a small part of homeopathy and deeper effects can be achieved by whole-person, individualised treatment.

Homeopathy can also be used for acute attacks of asthma, when it is generally prescribed on the basis of a small number of typical "keynote" symptoms. There is a fairly small amount of scientific research into individualised homepathy for asthma. It is generally positive though not conclusive. Outcome surveys of the results of homeopathic treatment, however, are consistently positive.

ISOPATHY is helpful if you are sensitive to a known single substance (if you do not have allergic asthma or have multiple sensitivities, it is unlikely to help). For house dust sensitivity, take *House dust mite* 30C, two pills weekly. Do not take it during a flare-up as it works best during the quiescent phase. If asthma is triggered by pollen, start isopathy several months before the pollen season starts and stop a couple of weeks before the start of the season.

ARSENICUM ALBUM is a medicine that is commonly used to treat asthma. *Arsen. alb.* is appropriate when the person affected feels chilly and very frightened during an asthma attack. People who respond to it frequently have eczema, psoriasis or dry skin.

KALIUM CARBONICUM, IPECACHUANA AND ANTIMONIUM TARTARICUM *Kalium carbonicum* is another frequently used medicine, particularly for asthma that persists after a chest infection. Typically asthma that responds to *Kali. carb.* is worse at 3–4 a.m. *Ipecachuana* is mostly given to children with asthma, particularly if they cough up a lot of mucus and feel sick. *Antimonium tart.* may be appropriate if the child is coughing but little mucus is brought up. The recommended dose is two pills of the 6C dilution every half hour when the child is having an attack. For long-term asthma, give two 6C pills three times a day.

Western Herbal Medicine

Herbal medicine can help people with asthma signficantly, but the guidance of an experienced medical herbalist is vital. A

Surprising but true: asthma rates in Cornwall and central London are the same

Western medical herbalist will assess your symptoms and prescribe a mixture of herbs to support easier breathing and reduce underlying allergy. The use of conventional medicines, such as inhalers, must be adjusted only in collaboration with your doctor.

LOBELIA AND EPHEDRA are the most commonly prescribed herbs for asthma. Lobelia (*Lobelia inflata*) is an antispasmodic and expectorant, which rids the body of mucus. Ephedra (*Ephedra sinica*) is a bronchodilator, which eases spasm of the airways. Your herbalist may prescribe a mix that also includes other expectorants such as thyme (*Thymus serpyllum*), elecampane (*Inula helenium*) and hyssop (*Hyssopus officinalis*). The herbal treatment of asthma must be carefully handled, as some of the herbs used can be toxic.

OTHER HERBS Anti-allergic herbs, such as nettle (*Urtica spp.*) and ginkgo (*Ginkgo biloba*) leaf, are usually also prescribed, and so too are herbs such as marshmallow (*Althea officinalis*), which soothes irritated mucous membranes lining the respiratory tract. Coltsfoot (*Tussilago farfara*) and wild cherry bark (*Prunus serotina*) may be recommended to ease coughing. Calming herbs such as chamomile (*Matricaria recutita*) and cramp bark (*Viburnum opulus*) are useful for relieving anxiety and goldenseal (*Hydrastis canadensis*) is often given for its anticatarrhal and anti-inflammatory properties and echinacea (*Echinacea spp.*) to support the immune system.

> **CAUTION**
>
> See p.69 before taking a herbal remedy. Do not self-treat with herbs for asthma; many are strong-acting with a range of side-effects and can be dangerous if misused. Do not combine herbal and conventional asthma treatments without expert advice.

Chinese Herbal Medicine

In Traditional Chinese Medicine (TCM), asthma is equivalent to *Xiao Chuan* (wheezing and shortness of breath). TCM perceives asthma as primarily caused by phlegm that blocks the airways. TCM doctors distinguish between "cold" asthma

(characterised by wheezing, shortness of breath and a cough producing frothy white or clear sputum) and "hot" asthma (characterised by hoarse breathing, a hacking cough and yellow sticky sputum which may be difficult to cough up).

"COLD" ASTHMA *Xiao Qing Long Tang* (Lesser Blue Dragon Decoction) is the classic treatment for "cold" asthma. It warms the lungs, dispels cold and wind, relieves cold phlegm and eases breathlessness.

"HOT" ASTHMA In "hot" asthma, the patient's tongue is red with a sticky, yellow coat and the pulse is rapid. Typically *Ding Chuan Tang* (Stop Asthma Decoction) is prescribed, which clears lung heat, relieves phlegm and "descends lung *Qi*".

> **CAUTION**
>
> Do not self-treat with Chinese herbs.

Environmental Health

PRIMARY TREATMENT Environmental substances can trigger asthma attcks. The small airways of the lungs are susceptible to allergens, toxins and irritants, and these should be avoided as far as possible. Nonetheless, it seems that early exposure to "normal" amounts of dirt, dust and hair probably reduces the likelihood of developing asthma.

PETS If you have tested positive for allergy to pets (usually cats), the best option would be to avoid having them. If this is not possible, the bedroom at least should become a "pet-free" zone. Regular pet bathing seems important. A vacuum cleaner with a high-efficiency particle air (HEPA) filter may be useful.

DUST MITES These microscopic organisms live in bedding, upholstered furniture and carpeting and leave behind highly allergenic droppings. A recent study suggests that using a mite-impermeable mattress cover as a single intervention is not effective. However, as part of a systematic approach that includes weekly washing of bed linens in hot water, removal of as much carpeting from the house as is practical, elimination of stuffed toys on beds,

and maintenance of home humidity levels below 40 or 50 per cent, this measure may be very valuable. It is likely that reducing exposure to mites in the home will help people with allergies. Installing a highly filtered closed vacuum system or using a vacuum cleaner with a HEPA filter are better alternatives than simple vacuuming.

MOULD AND COCKROACHES Numerous species of mould live around leaky pipes and in bathrooms that are not adequately ventilated. Removing obvious mould on surfaces and increasing ventilation in rooms where mould is found are useful steps. Also, the cockroach has been shown to be a significant asthma trigger. Appropriate removal, preferably without harmful pesticides, is an important step.

POLLEN Outdoor allergens are less controllable than indoor allergens and present more of a problem. Tree pollens, for example, can be blown for hundreds of miles, making life miserable for allergic individuals who do not even live near trees. Keep windows closed on days when the pollen count is high and use an air conditioner with an electrostatic micron-range furnace filter if possible. People with asthma should also avoid grass as much as possible and should not mow lawns or be present when grass is being mowed. In the autumn, susceptible people should not rake leaves, since allergenic moulds live in decomposing leaves and these have been implicated as a leading cause in cases of life-threatening asthma.

COLD AIR In cold weather, wearing a mask or scarf that allows the air to be humidified and warmed is useful, since cold, dry winter air can cause airway constriction in nearly all types of asthma. Alternatively, breathing through the nose provides a little humidification and warming.

ODOURS Many people with asthma find that strong odours can trigger wheezing or chest tightness. These include odours from strong cleaning solutions, perfumes and exhaust fumes. Where possible, avoid exposure to strong-smelling substances, especially if you are in a confined area with inadequate ventilation. If exposure cannot be avoided, make sure that you wear a respirator mask.

Acupuncture

There have not been many reliable trials into the efficacy of acupuncture for asthma, but clinical practice supports its use: it is widely given and appears to benefit a significant proportion of its recipients. A review of acupuncture in asthma concludes that the trials are on balance positive, but in fact very limited.

An acupuncturist will first make the traditional Chinese diagnosis (see p.82). The "pathogen cold" is frequently part of the diagnosis. He or she will then insert acupuncture needles into various meridian points and will probably also use cupping and moxibustion in order to provide heat on the relevant acupuncture points. Some acupuncturists in China use embedded or permanent needles to treat asthma, but this is not common in developed countries. You will probably need a weekly treatment for 10–12 weeks to evaluate whether acupuncture is going to help you.

Bodywork Therapies

SOFT-TISSUE MANIPULATION (deep massage-type manipulation) can relax the breathing muscles and mobilise the spine and ribs, making breathing easier. A recent study showed these methods can improve movement of the chest, increase air flow and ease chronic asthma symptoms. Osteopaths, chiropractors or physiotherapists can provide soft-tissue manipulation.

If the nervous system is in "alarm" phase, as it may be when you are anxious, breathing becomes rapid and shallow and asthma symptoms increase. The vagal nerve, which runs from the neck, has branches that influence breathing function. Stimulation of the vagal nerve has been shown to help normalise the excessive degree of activity of the nerves that accompanies asthma. A practitioner can manipulate the thoracic spine (the first four or five vertebrae below the neck) and the first joint of the neck to influence the activity of the vagal nerve, relax the diaphragm and help ease asthma symptoms. In one study, three months of chiropractic manipulation involving 20 treatments reduced the symptoms of persistent childhood asthma, with benefits still present a year after treatment finished. However, the two best research studies showed disappointingly small benefit of chiropractic for asthma.

MASSAGE given regularly may help reduce symptoms and stress. In a recent study, children with asthma were given either 20 minutes of massage or relaxation instruction from their parents. Anxiety and lung function in the children aged six to eight who were massaged improved more in the short-term than those in the relaxation group. Children aged nine to 11 improved whether they had massage or relaxation.

Exercise

Research shows that exercise helps people with asthma by improving fitness and breathing rate and increasing the amount of air movement through the lungs, which in turn improves oxygen supplies.

Breathing Retraining

PRIMARY TREATMENT **PURSED-LIP EXERCISES** These improve the mechanics and efficiency of breathing. Breathe in slowly through your nose and then, pursing your lips as if blowing up a balloon, exhale slowly (taking 4–6 seconds) through your mouth. Practise for several minutes each day. In a study, patients who were taught basic yoga breathing, similar to the pursed-lip breathing described above, used less medication and had improved breathing function, an improvement still apparent four years after the study finished.

PRIMARY TREATMENT **THE BUTEYKO METHOD** is a similar method of breathing training (with specific variations, including controlled breath-holding). An Australian study of this Russian method showed that it reduced use of corticosteroid drugs and improved breathing.

Yoga

Yoga is recommended for asthma. It has been shown to be helpful, especially when used in combination with breathing exercises and meditation.

Mind–Body Therapies

Although the exact mechanisms are not fully understood, stress may increase the demand for oxygen throughout the body, especially in the brain. If lung capacity is reduced due to asthma, this increased demand for oxygen cannot be met, which in turn intensifies the stress.

Research also shows a link between emotional distress and poor compliance with taking prescription medications. Taking asthma medication incorrectly is a common problem and can increase the severity of asthma symptoms. Studies have also shown that when stress increases, asthma symptoms may become exaggerated. At the same time, people may be less able to judge their symptoms accurately and more likely to underestimate their severity.

PRIMARY TREATMENT **STRESS-MANAGEMENT PROGRAMME** A recent trial showed that a four-week self-administered programme was very effective for people with asthma.

AUTOGENIC TRAINING AND MEDITATION Autogenic training, a programme in which you learn six mental exercises with a view to being able to relax at will, can be useful in managing asthma. Alternatively, you could try meditation (see p.98). A study of transcendental meditation (TM) suggested that people taught to meditate had less severe asthma symptoms.

> Swimming is good exercise for asthma. The moist pool environment may be a helpful factor

---

PREVENTION PLAN

The following may help:

- Avoid known allergens.
- Do not smoke; relax regularly.

Digestive & Urinary Systems

The digestive and urinary systems convert food into fuel and nutrients, then excrete anything unwanted. Our nutrition, immune defences, state of mind, and habitual posture can all affect these core systems. The holistic approach of integrated medicine works to counter stresses and to support the digestive system's natural healing processes.

PEPTIC ULCER AND GASTRITIS

A peptic ulcer is an eroded area in the lining of the stomach or the duodenum, which is the first part of the small intestine. Gastritis is inflammation of the stomach lining, which may begin suddenly and be short-lived (acute) or may develop gradually and persist (chronic). Though once considered a stress-related disorder, doctors now realise most people with ulcers or chronic gastritis have the bacterium *Helicobacter pylori* in their stomachs. Eradicating *H. pylori* is key to treating ulcers and chronic gastritis. Natural medicines may also help.

WHAT ARE THE SYMPTOMS?

Symptoms of peptic ulcer include:
- Pain or discomfort in the middle of the upper abdomen, which is sometimes relieved by eating
- Loss of appetite and weight loss
- Nausea and occasionally vomiting

Symptoms of gastritis include:
- Discomfort or pain in the middle of the upper abdomen, often felt after a meal

WHY MIGHT I HAVE THIS?

PREDISPOSING FACTORS
- Infection with *H. pylori*
- Smoking
- Drinking alcohol excessively
- Taking nonsteroidal anti-inflammatory drugs (NSAIDS)
- Foods that increase stomach acid secretion

IMPORTANT

If you develop symptoms of peptic ulcer or chronic gastritis, see your doctor. Gastritis that is accompanied by gastroesophageal reflux (GOR), in which stomach contents are regularly regurgitated back up into the oesophagus, should be treated by a doctor. GOR can contribute to oesophageal cancer if it is left untreated.

WHY DOES IT OCCUR?

The bacterium *Helicobacter pylori* has been found to be associated with chronic inflammation and ulceration of the stomach and duodenal lining. The discovery of *H. pylori* in the early 1980s revolutionised the treatment of peptic ulcers. The *H. pylori* bacterium may be found in the stomach lining of about half the population, but it is not known why it causes digestive problems in some people and not others. It is thought that the bacteria may be transmitted orally.

TREATMENT PLAN

PRIMARY TREATMENTS
- Drugs
- Lifestyle and dietary changes
- Surgery

BACK-UP TREATMENTS
- Nutritional therapy
- Acupuncture
- Western herbal medicine

WORTH CONSIDERING
- Homeopathy
- Bodywork therapies
- Exercise and yoga

For an explanation of how treatments are rated, see p.111.

How *H. pylori* contributes to peptic ulcers and gastritis is not known, but it may be that the body's immune response to the bacteria causes inflammation of the stomach lining.

Other factors that may play a role in the development of peptic ulcer and chronic gastritis include drinking large amounts of alcohol, smoking, and taking aspirin or non-steroidal anti-inflammatory drugs, such as diclofenac. Acute gastritis may follow an alcoholic binge or a severe illness. Stress is not a cause of ulcers, but it can reduce or increase acid production in the stomach and so may have an effect on ulcers and gastritis.

Chronic gastritis and stomach ulcers tend to be more common in people over the age of 50, while duodenal ulcers tend to be more common in men between the ages of 20 and 45. Possible complications of peptic ulcers include bleeding, which can turn the stools black and tarry. The person might also vomit blood. Perforation, in which the ulcer penetrates the full thickness of the stomach or duodenum and allows the contents to leak into the abdomen, is a surgical emergency.

Long-term infection with *H. pylori* may be associated with an increased risk of stomach cancer.

SELF-HELP

PRIMARY TREATMENT If you have mild, infrequent gastritis, try these measures:
- Eat small, regular meals.
- Avoid spicy foods, caffeine and alcohol.
- Sit down when you eat and eat slowly.

- Do not lie down right after eating; allow your body time to digest before going to bed after an evening meal.
- Use antacids judiciously.

TREATMENTS IN DETAIL

Conventional Medicine

Your doctor may suspect that you have a peptic ulcer or chronic gastritis from a description of your symptoms, but tests are needed to confirm the diagnosis. These might include endoscopy, in which a flexible viewing instrument is passed down the throat to examine the stomach and duodenum and contrast X-rays of these areas. Endoscopy also allows the doctor to exclude the presence of stomach cancer, which may produce similar symptoms to those of a peptic ulcer. Other tests may be done to look for the presence of *H. pylori.* For acute gastritis, the doctor may recommend stopping alcohol and NSAIDs. Short-term treatment may be needed, for example with antacids and H2-receptor antagonists, such as ranitidine.

| PRIMARY TREATMENT | **TESTS FOR H. PYLORI** There are two main tests that look for the presence of *H. pylori.*

In the breath test, the patient drinks a substance that is broken down if bacteria are present in the stomach and then breathed out. A breath analyser can then be used to detect whether or not the bacteria are present.

Alternatively, a sample of the stomach lining (a biopsy) is taken during endoscopy. This can then be examined for the presence of *H. pylori.* A blood test that looks for antibodies to the bacteria is also available. However, a positive result in this test can indicate either a current or a previous infection.

Eradication of *H. pylori* (if present) and lifestyle changes, such as giving up smoking, reducing alcohol intake and avoiding foods that exacerbate the symptoms, are likely to be recommended.

| PRIMARY TREATMENT | **DRUG THERAPY** Studies have shown that eradicating *H. pylori* is beneficial both in healing a peptic ulcer and in preventing its return. People with chronic gastritis may also benefit from *H. pylori* eradication.

COMMON SITES OF PEPTIC ULCERS

The upper part of the digestive tract includes the oesophagus, the stomach and the duodenum. (The duodenum is the first part of the small intestine and is located just below the stomach.) Peptic ulcers affect the stomach and duodenum and are among the most common digestive disorders. Most peptic ulcers occur in the area known as the duodenal bulb. In the stomach itself, the most common site for ulcers is the lesser curvature.

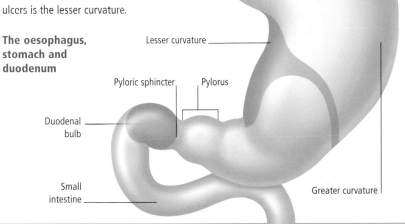

The oesophagus, stomach and duodenum

Your doctor will prescribe combination therapy, which may comprise a proton pump inhibitor (PPI), such as omeprazole, which reduces stomach acid, together with two different antibiotics. These are all taken for one to two weeks. You may have to continue to take the PPI for several weeks afterwards.

Sometimes, the drug bismuth or an H2-receptor antagonist may be prescribed instead of a PPI as part of combination therapy. Bismuth not only plays a role in healing the ulcer but also in treating *H. pylori.* Like PPIs, H2-receptor antagonists reduce the amount of acid produced.

Overall, these regimes for eradicating *H. pylori* are successful in around 90 per cent of patients, although the infection may recur. More than one antibiotic is given as part of the treatment because some strains of the bacteria are resistant to certain antibiotics. If you smoke, you will be advised to stop, because smoking slows the healing process.

| PRIMARY TREATMENT | **SURGERY** With all the treatments available, surgery is now reserved for treating ulcer complications, such as perforation.

CAUTION

Drugs for peptic ulcer and gastritis can cause a range of possible side-effects: ask your doctor to explain these to you.

Nutritional Therapy

DIETARY CHANGES Certain foods may interfere with the healing of an ulcer. Sugar, alcohol, coffee, decaffeinated coffee and tea have all been reported to increase stomach acidity, which may worsen or prolong an ulcer. There is also evidence to suggest that salt consumption is a risk factor for gastric ulcers. Research also suggests that eating salty food increases the risk of developing *H. pylori* infection and so increases the risk of gastritis and peptic ulcers. Avoiding these foods may help people who have a peptic ulcer.

VITAMIN A This vitamin is needed in the healing of mucosal tissue, including the linings of the stomach and intestines. One study found that vitamin A helped healing in people with stomach ulcers. A very high dose of vitamin A (50,000 IU, three times daily) was used in this trial, although clinical experience suggests that vitamin A at a much lower and safer dose of 10,000 IU per day for women and 25,000 IU for men might be helpful for people with peptic ulcers. If you have a peptic ulcer, you could try taking vitamin A supplements at these lower doses.

ZINC This mineral is another nutrient that may help people with peptic ulcers. Like vitamin A, zinc enhances tissue healing. Animal studies suggest that zinc can protect rats from stomach ulceration. In one study, when people with gastric ulcers took zinc (at a dose of 88mg, three times daily), their ulcers healed three times faster than those taking a placebo. Clinical experience suggests that supplementing with 30mg of zinc per day (balanced with 2mg of copper per day) may help people with peptic ulcers. If you have a peptic ulcer, try taking zinc and copper at these dosages for three months to see if it helps.

> **CAUTION**
>
> Consult your doctor before taking vitamin A and zinc supplements with prescribed medications. Pregnant women and women trying to conceive should not take vitamin A supplements. (*See also p.46.*)

Homeopathy

The three most commonly used homeopathic medicines for gastritis and peptic ulcer are *Kalium bichromicum, Nitric acid* and *Phosphorus.*

KALIUM BICHROMICUM People who respond to *Kalium bichromicum* have burning stomach pain, with a sensation of heaviness, nausea and vomiting; the vomit often contains stringy mucus. They may crave beer, although it makes their symptoms worse. These patients often also suffer from sinusitis or chronic catarrh.

NITRIC ACID The pains of people who respond to *Nitric acid* are typically described as sharp or piercing. They may crave rich or spicy food, although this makes the symptoms worse. Other symptoms include cracking at the edges of the mouth and also anal fissures, causing

severe pain after passing stool. These people may also have warts and hard unforgiving personalities.

PHOSPHORUS is often appropriate, especially if the ulcers bleed easily. People who respond to this medicine vomit easily. They are thirsty, especially for iced drinks, yet vomit even water a few minutes after drinking it. The pain is of burning character, and the symptoms are usually better in the morning and after a short nap. Those who respond to this medicine often have irrational fears and phobias, particularly of being alone in the dark and of storms. They may be may be oversensitive, "picking up vibes" too readily.

Western Herbal Medicine

Although self-treatment with herbal remedies can be helpful in treating ulcers and gastritis, professional treatment is recommended. Practitioners will combine key herbs to promote repair of mucous membranes, stimulate mucus secretion, counter inflammation and infection and relieve associated symptoms such as acidity, indigestion and pain. In the process, digestive health as a whole – including that of the stomach and duodenum – will normally be improved. Treatment will vary depending on the site of ulceration and severity of symptoms, although suppression of acid production within the stomach is not usually a central aim. The herbal approach typically focuses on strengthening the stomach lining.

DEMULCENT AND ASTRINGENT HERBS Liquorice (*Glycyrrhiza glabra*), marshmallow root (*Althea officinalis*) and slippery elm (*Ulmus fulva*) are demulcent herbs, which have the ability to soothe and coat the stomach lining. They reduce inflammation and stimulate the rate of healing in the stomach lining.

As well as being a demulcent, liquorice is also a powerful anti-inflammatory. Clinical

research indicates that liquorice extracts are as effective as conventional treatments for treating peptic ulceration, with fewer relapses occurring on discontinuation of the treatment.

Side-effects of liquorice can be avoided by taking special de-glycyrrhizinated extracts, now available.

> Only about half of people with duodenal ulcers have the typical symptoms of pain and soreness

Astringent remedies, such as agrimony (*Agrimonia eupatoria*) and cranesbill (*Geranium maculatum*), may be used to tone mucous membranes, increasing resistance to inflammation and infection.

ANTIBACTERIAL AND OTHER HERBS Where infection, as with *H. pylori*, is suspected or confirmed, antibacterial and immune-stimulant herbs may also be selected, such as echinacea (*Echinacea spp.*) and garlic (*Allium sativum*). Anti-inflammatory and carminative remedies, such as chamomile (*Matricaria recutita*) and marigold (*Calendula officinalis*), can also be important elements in balanced treatment. However, there is as yet little research to confirm the effectiveness of such herbs against *H. pylori*.

St John's wort (*Hypericum perforatum*) macerated oil, which is a safe and effective anti-inflammatory and wound healer, is a common treatment for stomach ulceration and inflammation in Germany.

> **CAUTION**
>
> See p.69 before taking a herbal remedy and, if you are already taking prescribed medication, consult a medical herbalist first.

Acupuncture

Acupuncture is used frequently in China for peptic ulcers, and a number of non-randomised studies have been done, all indicating a "good response". In one, over 90 per cent of people treated felt significant improvement with acupuncture alone. Experiments have also suggested acupuncture may prevent duodenal ulcers in rats.

Spiral-shaped *H. pylori* bacteria burrow into the mucous lining of the stomach in order to survive the strongly acidic environment. They also produce urease, an enzyme that neutralises gastric acids.

It is unlikely that acupuncture can help to eradicate *H. pylori* where this is the cause of ulcers. However, it may help quite substantially with the symptoms of peptic ulcers and gastritis. A traditional Chinese diagnosis is required to prescribe and treat appropriate acupuncture points.

If you are going to use acupuncture for these conditions, you will need to persist with treatment for at least six to eight sessions on a weekly basis. If the condition is very acute, treatment may be given every day, or every other day. When symptoms settle, long-term constitutional acupuncture may be required to prevent their recurrence, perhaps on a monthly basis.

Bodywork Therapies

MASSAGE THERAPY There is some surprising research evidence from China that massage is valuable in treating peptic ulcers. The question for researchers is: does it relieve stress, thus influencing acid production in the stomach, or does it work on the autonomic nervous system in some way to reduce acid production directly? We do not know, and we must treat this research cautiously until we do. More recently, massage and exercise (*see right*) have been reported by Russian researchers to be at least as effective in treating peptic ulcer patients as medication.

In earlier research, the Russian team had compared conventional treatment with deep reflex muscular massage, combined with exercise, for the treatment of peptic ulcer patients. The results, they suggested, "may result in prolongation of the remission and in a decreased number of recurrences of ulcer and associated gastrointestinal diseases."

OSTEOPATHY AND CHIROPRACTIC For about a century, osteopaths and chiropractors have manipulated the region of the spine from which the nerves to the stomach and duodenum emerge to treat uncomplicated peptic ulcers, as an adjunct to normal medical treatment.

Researchers in one study concluded: "If there is no evidence of an extraordinary or complicating event, the routine use of medication, along with osteopathic manipulative treatment for symptomatic relief, is generally sufficient."

TRIGGER POINT DEACTIVATION Trigger points (sensitive areas, *see p.55*) in the abdominal muscles can cause referred pain in the digestive organs. Abdominal pain may originate in either the muscles or the internal organs themselves. It is very easy for trigger-point activity to produce symptoms, especially pain, that can be confused with actual organ disease.

Since the joints of the spine and pelvis can be the cause of the muscular stresses that lead to trigger points developing in the first place, a comprehensive evaluation of pelvic and spinal mechanics, as well as of the muscles of the region, would clarify whether or not bodywork would be worth trying in a case of peptic ulcer.

Treatment to restore normality to dysfunctional joints and muscles, including deactivation of trigger points, might include osteopathic, chiropractic, physiotherapy or massage/neuromuscular therapy.

Exercise

A number of research studies have shown that taking regular exercise can help to heal peptic ulcers and, in the case of men, may even act as a preventive measure. Russian research, for example, suggests that cycling is helpful in the healing process: "Introduction of bicycle exercise in the treatment of ulcer promoted acceleration of ulcer defects healing."

Yoga

Doing yoga on a regular basis, particularly relaxing poses such as the corpse pose (*see p.226*), may be of benefit if you have a peptic ulcer. Although stress is no longer thought to be the primary cause of peptic ulcers, persistent stress may make the pain of peptic ulcers worse and may be a factor in bringing on attacks. Learning to relax through regular yoga practice each day may make it easier to cope. You should be sure to wear loose clothing that does not restrict your waist and to avoid doing any exercises for an hour after a meal.

PREVENTION PLAN

The following may help you avoid peptic ulcers:

- Avoid using aspirin and NSAIDs.
- Do not smoke.
- Moderate your alcohol intake.
- Eat small, regular meals and avoid overeating and caffeine.

CROHN'S DISEASE

WHAT ARE THE SYMPTOMS?

- Weight loss
- Loss of appetite
- Diarrhoea
- Abdominal pain
- Fever

WHY MIGHT I HAVE THIS?

PREDISPOSING FACTORS

- Genetic tendency
- Cigarette smoking

TRIGGERS FOR CROHN'S DISEASE RELAPSES

- Bowel infections
- Stress
- Food sensitivities

IMPORTANT

If you experience unexplained weight loss and/or abdominal pain, see your doctor without delay.

The condition known as Crohn's disease is one of the inflammatory bowel diseases, in which the lining of the bowel becomes inflamed (*see also Ulcerative colitis, p.227*). Crohn's disease can affect any part of the digestive tract from the mouth to the anus. However, it most commonly affects the last part of the small bowel (the ileum). There is no cure for Crohn's disease, but a variety of approaches, including drugs, dietary changes and relaxation training, may help to control symptoms and reduce the frequency of recurrences.

WHY DOES IT OCCUR?

It is not known why Crohn's disease develops, but many theories have been proposed and there may be several causes. The disease sometimes runs in families and a number of genes have been identified that increase the risk of developing the disease. Past exposure to certain infections may also play a role. Most people who develop the disease do so before the age of 30, with the majority being between 15 and 30 when symptoms first appear.

TREATMENT PLAN

PRIMARY TREATMENTS

- Drugs for relapse and remission including corticosteroids, aminosalicylates and azathioprine
- Liquid feeds

BACK-UP TREATMENTS

- Surgery (in severe cases)
- Eliminating sugar and problem foods
- Probiotics
- Vitamin supplements

WORTH CONSIDERING

- Fish oils
- Homeopathy
- Bodywork and movement therapies
- Acupuncture

For an explanation of how treatments are rated, see p.111.

Crohn's disease is a life-long condition, which is characterised by periods of remission (being well) and relapse (being ill). It is not known what factors trigger relapses. However, in some circumstances an acute bowel infection may be a trigger. Stress may also have a detrimental effect, as may certain foods. Smokers are more likely to develop Crohn's disease and their disease may also be more difficult to control.

People with Crohn's disease may also be likely to have other disorders, including joint disease, uveitis (inflammation of the eye) and erythema nodosum (a skin condition in which tender swellings appear, usually on the shins).

Those with Crohn's disease may have complications including the development of anal abscesses and fistulae (abnormal connecting channels between the bowel and surrounding areas). Intestinal narrowing or obstruction may also occur. Over a long period of time, people with Crohn's disease may also have a slightly increased risk of developing colorectal cancer.

TREATMENTS IN DETAIL

Conventional Medicine

If symptoms suggest Crohn's disease, the doctor will arrange several investigations in order to make the diagnosis. These include endoscopy, in which flexible viewing instruments are passed into the upper part of the bowel through the mouth and into the lower bowel through the anus. Doctors view the bowel lining to look for the characteristic changes of the disease. Biopsies (small samples of tissue) will be taken from the lining of the intestines for examination under a microscope.

In this colour-enhanced contrast X-ray showing an intestinal tract affected by Crohn's disease, affected areas appear ragged and narrowed (top and right). In the centre is healthy tissue.

A barium X-ray will also be performed, in which a radio-opaque fluid, which is either swallowed or passed down the digestive tract via a tube, outlines the lining of the bowel on a series of X-rays. This allows imaging of areas that cannot be viewed by standard endoscopy.

Treatment for Crohn's disease can be divided into treatment of relapse and maintenance of remission. More recent drugs may have a role to play in both these aspects of treatment. All treatments aim to reduce bowel inflammation and so reduce symptoms. Occasionally, simple antidiarrhoeal drugs such as loperamide may be prescribed to help control diarrhoea. They work by slowing the passage of faeces through the bowel.

PRIMARY TREATMENT | **DRUGS AND LIQUID DIETS FOR RELAPSE** Corticosteroids and special liquid feeds are mainly used to treat relapses and will gradually be stopped over time. Corticosteroids reduce inflammation in the bowel. Liquid feeds contain precisely measured amounts of dietary components such as fats, carbohydrates and proteins. In some cases, long-term steroids or frequent courses of steroids may be needed. In children, there is a risk of these drugs affecting growth, which is therefore carefully monitored. Corticosteroids should not be stopped suddenly.

PRIMARY TREATMENT | **DRUGS FOR REMISSION** Remission is maintained by longer-term use of certain drugs. These drugs may be combined with corticosteroids and liquid feeds in some cases, depending on the severity of the disease, the part of bowel involved and the presence of other associated problems, such as abscesses or fistulae, which are abnormal connecting channels that may develop, often between different sections of the bowel or between the bowel and the anus. These additional drugs range from those with mild anti-inflammatory properties, such as aminosalicylates, to immunosuppressant drugs, such as azathioprine.

New drugs are being developed that target specific chemicals in the body known to play a part in inflammation. However, the understanding of when to use these medicines is only in its early stages. Antibiotics also have a role to play, especially for disease around the anus.

SURGERY Every effort is made to avoid surgery, but it may be necessary. If symptoms persist despite the use of every suitable medication, a portion of diseased bowel may have to be be removed. Surgery is also used to remove areas of the bowel that are narrowed if they are causing problems. A repair operation may also be carried in some situations where fistulae or abscesses have formed.

In some cases of Crohn's disease, an operation known as an ileostomy (in which the ileum, which is the last part of the small bowel, is connected to an artificial opening in the abdomen) may be necessary. Less commonly, a surgeon may have to carry out a colostomy (in which a similar procedure is followed with the colon – the large bowel).

> **CAUTION**
>
> Drugs for Crohn's disease can cause a range of possible side-effects: ask your doctor to explain these to you.

The American gastroenterologist Burrill B. Crohn first identified the disease in 1932

Nutritional Therapy

ELIMINATING SUGAR People who have Crohn's disease may find it useful to eliminate refined carbohydrates from their diet, particularly the sugar sucrose. Experiments suggest that a low-carbohydrate diet can be effective in controlling the condition. In one study done in the 1970s, people with Crohn's disease who followed a low-sugar, high-fibre diet led had a 79 per cent reduction in relapses requiring hospitalisation compared to people with the disease who did not change their diet. In another study, people with Crohn's disease were fed either a high- or a low-sugar diet. Those with more active Crohn's disease fared better on a low-sugar diet compared to those eating larger amounts of sugar. Several people on the high-sugar diet had to stop eating sugar entirely because their condition worsened while on this regime.

AVOIDING PROBLEM FOODS Identification and treatment of food sensitivities is often used in clinical practice to treat Crohn's disease. There is some scientific evidence to suggest that food intolerance can be a factor. In one study, 77 patients were put on a diet excluding foods to which they were thought to be sensitive. Fifty-one of them (66 per cent) remained well on the diet alone for periods of up to 51 months and had an annual relapse rate of less than 10 per cent. The most frequent symptom-provoking foods in this study were wheat, dairy products, brassicas (cabbage, broccoli, cauliflower, Brussels sprouts and so forth), sweetcorn, yeast, tomatoes, citrus fruits, and eggs. (*For more information on food sensitivity, see p.456.*)

VITAMIN SUPPLEMENTS People who have Crohn's disease may have multiple nutritional deficiencies because they tend not to be able to absorb nutrients very effectively. Nutrients that are of particular importance are zinc, vitamin B12 and folic acid, both because they can help in the repair of the cells that line the intestinal tract and because people with Crohn's disease have been shown to be deficient in them. If you have Crohn's disease, try taking 30–45mg of zinc (balanced with 2–3 mg of copper), 800mcg of vitamin B12 and 800 mcg of folic acid each day.

FISH OILS Crohn's disease is an inflammatory condition. Excessive amounts of omega-6 fatty acids (found in vegetable oils and most processed and fast foods) and a relative lack of omega-3 fatty acids (found in oily fish, walnuts and linseeds) seems to promote inflammation. Maintaining a balance between omega-6 and omega-3 fatty acids in the diet by avoiding excessive amounts of margarine, processed foods and vegetable oils and including oily fish (such as salmon, sardines, trout and mackerel), walnuts and flaxseeds in the diet may be helpful in controlling the symptoms of Crohn's disease. One two-year study found that a diet that was high in oily fish (85–200g/3.5–7oz per day) substantially reduced the relapse rate in people with the condition. In addition, fish oil supplements, which contain the omega-3 fatty acids EPA and DHA, might help to control Crohn's disease due to their anti-inflammatory effect. If you have Crohn's disease, try taking 1g of concentrated fish oil one to three times a day.

PROBIOTICS Probiotic organisms (healthy bacteria) are believed to be important for maintaining a healthy lining in the gut. Probiotic supplements may help people with Crohn's disease. Studies of probiotics in children with Crohn's disease have been positive. One study showed that probiotic treatment may allow the dosage of steroids given to patients to be reduced.

> **CAUTION**
>
> Consult your doctor before taking fish oil, zinc or folic acid supplements with existing medications. (*See also p.46*.)

Homeopathy

The treatment of Crohn's disease using homeopathy is likely to require skilled, individualised treatment from a qualified practitioner. Many different medicines may be appropriate in the treatment of this disease, including *Nitric acid*, *Sulphur* and *Phosphorus*.

NITRIC ACID In people who respond to *Nitric acid*, there are likely to be painful splits in the skin (fissures) around the anus, which may cause pain for some time after passing a stool. There is also often a tendency to small, painful mouth ulcers (known as aphthae). The pains of the fissures and aphthae are splinter-like. People who respond to *Nitric acid* are said to be rather bad-tempered, to bear grudges and to be anxious about their health.

SULPHUR In people who respond to the homeopathic remedy *Sulphur*, diarrhoea feels hot and is often worst in the morning, forcing the patient out of bed; the odour of the diarrhoea may be very offensive. These people also often have skin trouble, particularly itchy skin. In terms of personality, they are untidy and they may be outgoing, "larger than life" characters. They frequently feel the heat excessively.

PHOSPHORUS is useful when diarrhoea is frequently bloody. Indeed, in people who respond to *Phosphorus* there is a general tendency to easy bleeding, including nosebleeds and easy bruising of the skin.

In people who respond to *Phosphorus* there are sometimes accompanying liver problems, such as hepatitis. The patient often feels run-down and tired, but is briefly better from rest and so usually feels better first thing in the morning. Mentally these people tend to be characteristically sensitive and sympathetic both to the human as well as to the physical environment. They may have fears of such things as storms or being alone in the dark.

> ## Crohn's disease has become more common throughout the world in the past few decades

Bodywork and Movement Therapies

General relaxation and massage as well as anti-anxiety breathing exercises are useful in easing the stress associated with inflammatory bowel disease.

Exercise

Osteoporosis (*see p.308*) is a common complication of inflammatory bowel disease because the absorption of nutrients by the intestine is reduced. People with Crohn's disease are at particular risk of developing osteoporosis.

If you have Crohn's disease, research indicates that taking regular weight-bearing exercise is beneficial. In a study on the effects of exercise on bone loss in people with the condition, participants following a low-impact exercise programme for 12 months showed significant increase in bone density. This was sufficient to reduce their risk of osteoporotic fracture.

Acupuncture

In order to treat Crohn's disease, a traditional Chinese diagnosis needs to be made, and patients will often require quite lengthy treatment courses. While there are a number of case studies indicating that acupuncture may be of benefit, there are no good-quality clinical trials available in this field. Acupuncture may help in the treatment of Crohn's disease, in conjunction with other approaches, and may be particularly valuable in symptom control.

Acupuncture has been reported as being effective in managing very acute symptoms, and treatment may be required daily or every other day. Generally, however, people seek acupuncture for chronic and more persistent complaints, and for Crohn's disease it would be appropriate to have treatment weekly for eight to ten weeks, in order to assess whether there is some benefit. Further maintenance treatments may be required to avoid relapse.

> **PREVENTION PLAN**
>
> • Do not smoke.

INDIGESTION AND NON-ULCER DYSPEPSIA

The term indigestion is usually used to describe pain or discomfort in the upper abdomen that tends to occur after a meal, particularly one that includes fatty, rich or spicy foods. Indigestion may also be known as non-ulcer dyspepsia (NUD) if no underlying cause can be found. Simple lifestyle and dietary changes can do a great deal to help indigestion. Other approaches, including drugs, homeopathy, breathing retraining, bodywork and relaxation and hypnosis can all help to bring relief and prevent future episodes of indigestion.

WHAT ARE THE SYMPTOMS?

- Pain or discomfort in the upper part of the abdomen
- Excessive wind
- Bloating in the abdomen

WHY MIGHT I HAVE THIS?

PREDISPOSING FACTORS

- Hypochlorhydria (low levels of acid in the stomach and/or low levels of digestive enzymes in the small intestine)
- Lactose intolerance
- Smoking
- Being overweight

TRIGGERS

- Irritation of the digestive tract
- Stress
- Excessive air swallowing (aerophagia)
- Alcohol
- Caffeine

IMPORTANT

See your doctor if you develop persistent indigestion, particularly if it begins around or after age 40 or is accompanied by loss of appetite, weight loss, vomiting or gastro-esophageal reflux (GOR), in which food is regurgitated into the oesophagus. Untreated GOR can contribute to oesophageal cancer.

WHY DOES IT OCCUR?

Indigestion occurs when the digestive tract becomes irritated. Food, especially rich, fried or spicy food, alcohol, coffee and certain drugs, such as aspirin and non-steroidal anti-inflammatory drugs (e.g. ibuprofen), can all irritate the digestive tract and cause indigestion. Smoking and being overweight increase a person's risk of developing indigestion. Stress can also cause the condition.

Indigestion may be accompanied by gastroesophageal reflux (GOR; also called acid reflux or heartburn), in which partially digested food is regurgitated from the stomach back up into the oesophagus. If GOR is persistent, digestive acids from the stomach can erode the oesophageal lining, which is not protected by a layer of mucus as is the stomach. Left untreated, this erosion may cause pain and can also lead to bleeding from the oesophagus.

The body can digest only so much food at once, so eating large meals increases the risk of indigestion. Eating smallish meals regularly may help to prevent indigestion.

Osteopaths and chiropractors believe that mechanical stress resulting from spinal restrictions or from trigger points in the back or abdomen can affect digestive function and may cause indigestion.

TREATMENT PLAN

PRIMARY TREATMENTS

- Lifestyle changes
- Drugs such as antacids
- Chewing properly; breathing retraining

BACK-UP TREATMENTS

- Food combining
- Nutritional supplements and probiotics
- Homeopathy
- Bodywork therapies

WORTH CONSIDERING

- Psychological therapies

For an explanation of how treatments are rated, see p.111.

IMMEDIATE RELIEF

- Press the "belch button" to induce belching. This is located in the lower back just below the lowest rib *(see p.221)*.
- Take the homeopathic medicines *Nux vomica* or *Carbo vegetalis*.
- Take over-the-counter antacids.
- Drink a cup of peppermint, fennel or ginger tea; suck a peppermint sweet.

TREATMENTS IN DETAIL

Conventional Medicine

PRIMARY TREATMENT **LIFESTYLE CHANGES** Indigestion may be relieved by reducing intake of fatty and spicy foods, limiting or eliminating coffee and alcohol, reducing stress, stopping smoking and eating smaller, more frequent meals. Avoid

INDIGESTION AND GASTROESOPHAGEAL REFLUX (GOR)

Indigestion is often accompanied by gastroesophageal reflux (also known as acid reflux or heartburn), in which partially digested stomach contents are regurgitated up into the oesophagus. GOR occurs when the lower oesophageal sphincter does not work properly and allows acidic stomach contents back up into the oesophagus. Too much food in the stomach or increased pressure in the stomach can cause the sphincter to relax. Long-standing GOR can result in pain and bleeding.

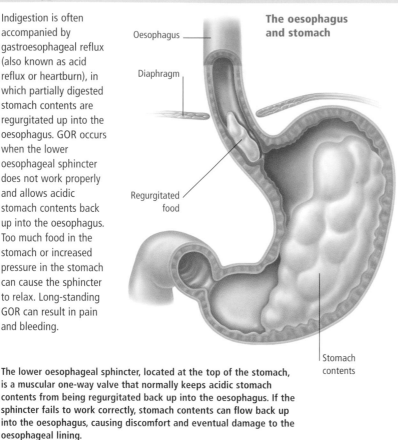

The oesophagus and stomach

Oesophagus

Diaphragm

Regurgitated food

Stomach contents

The lower oesophageal sphincter, located at the top of the stomach, is a muscular one-way valve that normally keeps acidic stomach contents from being regurgitated back up into the oesophagus. If the sphincter fails to work correctly, stomach contents can flow back up into the oesophagus, causing discomfort and eventual damage to the oesophageal lining.

taking aspirin or non-steroidal anti-inflammatory drugs (NSAIDs), such as ibuprofen. You could also try sleeping with your upper body propped up on pillows. These lifestyle changes may be combined with antacid drugs when necessary.

For persistent symptoms, the doctor may recommend investigations to exclude an underlying cause. These might include endoscopy, in which a flexible viewing instrument is inserted through the mouth to examine the oesophagus and stomach. The doctor may also arrange for contrast X-rays of these areas. He or she may then prescribe one of the various treatments described below.

PRIMARY TREATMENT **DRUGS** Various drugs are available that reduce stomach acid secretion. These include proton pump inhibitors (PPIs), such as omeprazole, and H2-receptor antagonists, such as rantidine. Prokinetic agents, such as domperidone, reduce the time food spends in the stom-ach and may also be prescribed. Studies suggest that these drugs may be helpful for some patients with indigestion.

ELIMINATING HELICOBACTER PYLORI *H. pylori* is a bacterium that is often found in the stomach and is associated with certain disorders of the stomach and duodenum (the first part of the small intestine, just below the stomach), including chronic gas-tritis (inflammation of the stomach lining) and peptic ulcer (*see p.212*).

The role of *H. pylori* in ordinary indiges-tion is less clear and the impact on symptoms of treating the infection (with a course of antibiotics, usually in combina-tion with a proton pump inhibitor drug) is probably small.

> **CAUTION**
>
> Drugs for indigestion can cause a range of possible side-effects: ask your doctor or pharmacist to explain these to you.

Nutritional Therapy

PRIMARY TREATMENT **CHEWING PROPERLY** The simple measure of making sure you chew food thoroughly before swallowing it can improve symptoms of indigestion. Ideally, each mouthful should be chewed to the consistency of a cream before it is swallowed.

FOOD COMBINING involves eating pro-tein-based foods (such as meat, fish and eggs) at different times from carbohydrate-based foods (such as bread, potatoes, rice and pasta). The theory is that the body digests proteins and carbohydrates in rela-tively distinct ways, so in theory, keeping them apart can make lighter work for the digestive tract. Food combining seems to be most useful in the evening, when the body's digestive capacity naturally tends to be lower. (*For more information, see p.39.*)

LOW ACID LEVELS Sometimes, indigestion may be the result of hypochlorhydria (low levels of acid in the stomach and/or low levels of digestive enzymes in the small intestine). A nutritionist may be able to suggest nutritional supplements to help remedy this.

PROBIOTIC SUPPLEMENTS (which contain healthy gut bacteria) can promote healthy digestion and may be worth trying. In one study, 30 patients with indigestion were given *Lactobacillus acidophilus* (one capsule containing two billion live bacteria), in the morning after breakfast. Symptoms of indigestion such as pain, pressure, bloating, flatulence and appetite improved within two weeks.

Homeopathy

A range of homeopathic medicines may be used for indigestion. If the following fail to bring relief, consult a practitioner.

NUX VOMICA is the most frequently used homeopathic medicine for indigestion. It has been shown to be effective in clinical trials by Messinger (1976) and by Ritter (1966) in Germany. *Nux vomica* is useful for indigestion triggered by too much food, especially when it is rich or fatty, or by alcohol. People who respond to *Nux vomica* often have nausea (sometimes with vomiting) and a bitter taste in the mouth. They are irritable and annoyed by inefficiency; their sleep may be poor, they often wake early and feel terrible in the morning.

CARBO VEGETABILIS is another possible treatement for indigestion. In people who respond to it, digestion seems to be slow and the stomach is bloated, with a lot of burping.

LYCOPODIUM may be used when the symptoms include a lot of wind, a craving for sweets, feeling full quickly and, often, anxiety or depression.

> **CAUTION**
>
> Coffee can nullify the effect of *Nux vomica*; do not drink it if you are using this homeopathic medication.

Western Herbal Medicine

Digestive teas made from herbs such as peppermint (*Mentha piperita*), fennel (*Foeniculum vulgare*), chamomile (*Matricaria recutitia*) and ginger (*Zingiber officinale*) may soothe the stomach.

Bodywork Therapies

The spinal nerves that govern digestive function can speed up or slow down the organs of digestion. The sympathetic and parasympathetic nerves control the body's unconscious actions, such as heartbeat. The sympathetic nerves, which emerge from the upper spine, slow digestive function, while the parasympathetic nerves, which emerge from the top and bottom of the spine, speed it up.

CHIROPRACTIC AND OSTEOPATHY A chiropractic survey of almost 1500 people showed that fully 70 per cent of those with mechanical restrictions of the upper back reported symptoms of indigestion. Of these, 22 per cent were relieved by spinal manipulation.

DEACTIVATION OF TRIGGER POINTS Trigger points, or sensitive areas, in the abdominal muscles can produce symptoms of indigestion that affect the upper abdomen. Heartburn and a feeling of full-

Pressing the "belch button" can ease indigestion by releasing trapped wind. Find the lowest rib on your back and feel for a tender point just below it. Press firmly for 5 seconds.

ness are common effects of trigger points that lie close to the centre of the chest, on or just below the breastbone. Trigger points can be deactivated by acupuncture, as well as by manual pressure and stretching techniques as used by osteopaths, massage therapists (particularly those with neuromuscular therapy training) and some physiotherapists and chiropractors. A specific trigger point located in the lower back on either side and just below the lowest rib is known as the "belch button", since this is the common effect of pressing it (*see illustration, above*).

Breathing Retraining

PRIMARY TREATMENT | **LEARNING TO BREATHE CORRECTLY** Bloating and heartburn may be caused by swallowing too much air (aerophagia). This is a common side-effect of eating too quickly or rapid upper-chest breathing. It can usually be improved or corrected by breathing rehabilitation techniques which involve slow, diaphragmatic (yoga type) breathing. It also usually requires correction of restrictions that may have developed in overused and stressed muscles and joints. See p.62 for a breathing sequence and, if indigestion troubles you regularly, visit an osteopath, who can relieve restrictions in overstretched joints.

Psychological Therapies

PSYCHOTHERAPY In 1990 a study was done to determine whether brief psychodynamic-interpersonal (PI) psychotherapy was more effective than a psychological control treatment for patients with chronic, intractable non-ulcer dyspepsia, and whether patients with abnormal gastric function responded differently from those with normal gastric function. At the end of treatment, there were significant advantages for the people who had received PI psychotherapy compared with the people in the control group. One year after treatment, the advantages remained.

A review of all available research into psychological treatments for indigestion concluded psychodynamic psychotherapy and cognitive behavioural therapy may be useful treatments for non-ulcer dyspepsia.

MOOD-IMPROVING TECHNIQUES If you have indigestion regularly, you may want to try psychological techniques such as guided imagery (*see p.100*) to improve your mood. A 2001 Cochrane review found that people who regularly had indigestion were more likely to be anxious, depressed and pessimistic than the rest of the population. The review determined that psychological treatments, including psychotherapy, psychodrama, cognitive behavioural therapy, relaxation therapy, guided imagery or hypnosis, improved patients' digestion. However, more studies to assess the role of psychological intervention in treating indigestion are needed in order to give a clearer picture.

> ## PREVENTION PLAN
>
> **If you are prone to indigestion, try the following measures:**
>
> - Eat small meals regularly.
> - Sit at a table to eat rather than lounging on a sofa.
> - Eat slowly and chew food thoroughly to the consistency of cream.
> - Keep to a normal weight.
> - Avoid alcohol, coffee, carbonated water and spicy foods.

IBS involves abdominal pain that is relieved by defecation. Related symptoms may include:

- A change in the frequency of stool
- A change in the appearance of the stool

There may also be:

- Fewer than three bowel movements a week or more than three a day
- Hard or lumpy stools
- Loose (watery) stools
- Straining during a bowel movement
- Urgency (having to rush to have a bowel movement)
- A feeling that the bowel has not emptied completely
- Passage of mucus during defecation
- A feeling of fullness and bloating

WHY MIGHT I HAVE THIS?

PREDISPOSING FACTORS

- Anxiety
- Depression
- Food sensitivities
- Imbalance of organisms in the digestive tract
- Lactose and fructose intolerance
- Sorbitol (an artificial sweetener)
- Trigger-point activity from muscles of the abdomen or back
- Smoking

IRRITABLE BOWEL SYNDROME

Irritable bowel syndrome (IBS) describes a combination of intermittent abdominal pain, constipation and/or diarrhoea. The condition usually develops in people between the ages of 20 and 30 and is twice as common in women as in men. The symptoms typically persist for many years. Although it can be very distressing, IBS does not lead to serious complications. There is no single treatment for IBS, but a combination of therapies such as drugs, dietary changes, relaxation and herbal preparations may bring relief.

WHY DOES IT OCCUR?

The cause of irritable bowel syndrome, which accounts for more referrals to gastroenterologists than any other digestive disorder, is unknown. It is classed as a "functional disorder", which means that the intestines appear normal but do not function normally. One theory is that it may result from abnormal contractions of the intestinal walls. Another factor may be food sensitivity. In particular, an increased sensitivity to certain foods such as fruit or the artificial sweetener sorbitol may contribute to the condition. IBS sometimes occurs after a gastrointestinal infection and the condition seems to run in families. Stress, anxiety or depression may be associated with IBS and can make it worse.

In making a diagnosis of IBS, the doctor may ask whether the pain is relieved by defecation, whether you experience a change in the frequency of passing stools, and whether there is a change in the appearance of the stools. Many doctors will diagnose IBS if two out of three of these features are present.

IBS is not typically associated with pain or diarrhoea that interferes with sleep, blood in the stool (either visible or on laboratory examination), weight loss, fever or any physical abnormality. If any of these symptoms is present, you should see your doctor without delay. IBS rarely begins after the age of 40. Any change in bowel habits that happens in middle age should be investigated at once by a doctor.

TREATMENT PLAN

PRIMARY TREATMENTS

- Antidiarrhoeal drugs and bulking agents
- Food elimination diet

BACK-UP TREATMENTS

- Antimuscarinics and antispasmodics
- Probiotics and anti-yeast diet
- Western and Chinese herbal medicine
- Acupuncture
- Mind–body therapies

WORTH CONSIDERING

- Individualised homeopathy
- Breathing retraining
- Bodywork and movement therapies

For an explanation of how treatments are rated, see p.111.

IMPORTANT

- Consult your doctor if your IBS symptoms are severe, persistent or recurrent, or if you have rectal bleeding, blood in the stool, pain that interferes with sleep, or have unexpectedly lost weight.
- Consult the doctor if you are over 40 when symptoms first appear, as some gastrointestinal disorders have similar symptoms.

- Keep a food diary to help you identify foods that bring on attacks so you can avoid them.
- Make sure you get some exercise on a regular basis.
- If stress is a factor in your IBS, practise relaxation or meditation daily.
- Take a daily probiotic supplement.
- Try peppermint oil capsules.
- If constipation is a problem, take a gentle bulk-forming laxative regularly, but avoid bran and bran-based laxatives, which can make IBS worse.
- Do not smoke, because smoking irritates the gastrointestinal tract.

TREATMENTS IN DETAIL

Conventional Medicine

Clinical guidelines for diagnosis of IBS say the person should have had a total of 12 weeks of unexplained abdominal pain in last 12 months (the 12 weeks do not have to be consecutive). The pain will have two out of three of the following characteristics: it is relieved by defecation; it is related to a change in frequency of stools; it is related to a change in the stools' appearance.

The doctor will review your symptoms and may refer you for investigations, such as bowel X-rays or endoscopy, to exclude underlying disorders. Often, no medication is needed and the symptoms can be controlled with some lifestyle and dietary changes and relaxation techniques. However, if treatment is needed, there are various options.

PRIMARY TREATMENT **ANTIDIARRHOEAL DRUGS AND BULKING AGENTS** Antidiarrhoeal drugs, such as loperamide, may be helpful for people with diarrhoea. There is some evidence to support the use of bulking agents, such as ispagula husk, in the treatment of constipation associated with IBS. These drugs act by increasing the bulk of the stool, so stimulating normal contractions in the wall of the gut.

ANTIMUSCARINICS AND ANTISPASMODICS Studies have shown that some antimuscarinics, such as hyoscine butylbromide, and antispasmodics, such as mebeverine, can help relieve the pain of IBS. These drugs are thought to reduce abnormal contractions in the gut by relaxing the muscles in the wall.

Nutritional Therapy

PRIMARY TREATMENT **ELIMINATION DIET** Studies have shown that many people with IBS have food sensitivities. Wind and other IBS symptoms diminish when these sensitivities are discovered and the offending foods are eliminated from the diet. Clinical experience suggests that wheat is one of the most common food sensitivities in people with IBS, and this is supported by some scientific evidence.

Some people with IBS-like symptoms may not in fact be able to digest the sugars lactose (found in milk) and fructose (found in high concentrations in fruit juice and dried fruit). The artificial sweetener sorbitol (found in diabetic and sugar-free products) can make diarrhoea worse. Research shows that in a large majority of IBS patients with lactose malabsorption, a lactose-restricted diet can improve symptoms markedly both in the short term and the long term. Fructose- and sorbitol-reduced diets in people with fructose malabsorption reduce gastrointestinal symptoms such as bloating, cramps, diarrhoea and other IBS symptoms. People with IBS should consider the possibility that milk, fruit juice, dried fruit and products containing sorbitol might make their IBS symptoms worse. *(For more information about food sensitvities, see p.456.)*

PROBIOTICS AND ANTI-YEAST DIET An imbalance in the organisms in the gut (gut dysbiosis) is common in people with IBS. One study found reduced numbers of "friendly" bacteria such as lactobacilli and bifidobacteria and higher numbers of harmful bacteria in those with symptoms of IBS. Overgrowth of yeast organisms, such as *Candida albicans*, also seems very common in people with IBS. Reducing yeast in the gut is often effective in improving IBS symptoms *(for details see p.40).*

Probiotics appear to help people who have IBS. Some studies have shown improvements in symptoms of pain and flatulence when people with IBS took supplements.

FIBRE may help in IBS, but it depends on the type of fibre. Most studies find that people with IBS will generally not benefit by adding wheat bran to their diets. In fact, some people feel even worse after taking wheat bran supplements. However, fibre from other sources, such as psyllium (20–30g per day of psyllium seed husk fibre), may alleviate symptoms.

Homeopathy

The evidence for the effectiveness of homeopathy in treating IBS is quite strong – two controlled studies in Germany published in the 1970s showed positive results. However, these looked only at a single homeopathic medicine and, as with homeopathic treatment for many conditions, several medicines may be appropriate. To start with, two pills of all of the medicines discussed below should be taken twice daily in the 6C strength.

ARGENTUM NITRICUM may be indicated when anxiety is associated with IBS. The affected person has a lot of bloating and a craving for sweet food.

PHOSPHORIC ACID may be indicated, particularly if a person's symptoms have been triggered by emotional stresses, such as relationship difficulties or bereavement, and are associated with weak memory. Diarrhoea is usually a prominent symptom.

NUX VOMICA may be given if there is a frequent urge to pass faeces, often without result, as well as irritability and poor sleep.

Western Herbal Medicine

Even though insufficient research has been carried out, many people with IBS turn to herbal remedies to ease their symptoms.

There are many traditional herbal remedies that can help a great deal in IBS. Since patients tend to react to remedies at a very low dose, it is always a good idea to start any remedy at low doses, gradually increasing the strength as necessary.

CARMINATIVE HERBS Most important in easing spasms of the gut associated with IBS are so-called carminative (flatulence-relieving) herbs. Teas of mixtures of the following carminative remedies may relieve pain, bloating and flatulence: chamomile (*Matricaria recutita*), caraway (*Carum cari*), fennel (*Foeniculum vulgare*), aniseed (*Pimpinella anisum*), cardamom (*Elletaria cardamomum*), peppermint (*Mentha piperita*), spearmint (*Mentha spicata*), garden mint (*Mentha arvensis*), dill (*Anethum graveolens*), lemon balm (*Melissa officinalis*), rosemary (*Rosemarinus officinalis*) and lovage (*Levisticum officinalis*).

These remedies combine well with bitter aromatics such as angelica root (*Angelica archangelica*), tangerine peel (*Citrus reticulata*) and bitter orange (*Citrus aurantium*). The bitter, aromatic combination is particularly calming to the disordered gut.

The carminative herb chamomile also combines well with other relaxing herbs, such as valerian, to relieve IBS aggravated by anxiety. Peppermint oil is the main ingredient in several over-the-counter products for symptoms of IBS. A meta-analysis of five randomised controlled trials of special peppermint oil capsules for IBS suggests that this preparation can be effective in relieving symptoms.

HERBS TO AID BILE OUTPUT A painful, bloated feeling after eating fatty foods may be due to poor bile output. In stimulating bile production and flow, these remedies enable the body to digest fats. Some herbs have an especially bitter action, which aids digestion. Wormwood (*Artemisia absinthium*), gentian (*Gentiana lutea*) and hops (*Humulus lupulus*) are extremely bitter and are given in small doses. Hops are sedative and relaxing to the bowel in low doses. Other bitter herbs effective for treating IBS include milk thistle (*Silibum marianum*), dandelion root (*Taraxacum officinale*) and globe artichoke (*Cynara scolymus*) leaves.

ARTICHOKE LEAF EXTRACT shows promise in treating IBS as well as dyspepsia (indigestion). It is an ingredient in many over-the-counter remedies for IBS and apparently relieves IBS symptoms in some patients. There have been no randomised controlled trials yet, but researchers at the University of Reading suggest "there is a growing body of evidence which indicates

Irritable bowel syndrome is thought to affect 10–20 per cent of the general population

therapeutic properties for artichoke leaf extract". In their small study, IBS patients had significant reductions in the severity of their symptoms after taking the extract. Both the patients and their doctors felt that it was effective, and 96 per cent of the patients rated the extract as better than or as good as other therapies they had tried.

CONSTIPATION REMEDIES Aloe vera (*Aloe vera*) juice has a gentle, soothing effect on the bowel and is particularly appropriate for people with IBS who have chronic constipation. Take a tablespoon of the commercially extracted juice twice daily.

Other remedies for the constipation of IBS include psyllium seeds. Psyllium is a soluble fibre, similar to oat bran, and has a gentle, bulk-forming effect on the stool. Psyllium has been researched for more than 20 years in the treatment of IBS and many people with constipation find it effective. One reliable trial showed that both psyllium and wheat bran were effective in normalising stool consistency and frequency in IBS, but that psyllium was better for improving frequency and reducing abdominal distension. However, results of research trials have been inconsistent, and better research is needed.

Dark psyllium seeds often work best stirred into a little warm water as a bulk laxative. Pale psyllium seeds, also known as isphagula seeds, and linseeds are other alternatives (linseed must be crushed to obtain its full effect). A tablespoon a day taken with porridge or natural yoghurt is likely to ease constipation without any side-effects. For these bulk laxatives to work effectively, drink a glass or two of water with them.

The use of anthraquinone-containing stimulant laxatives, such as rhubarb root (*Rheum officinale*), senna (*Senna alexandrina*) and cascara (*Rhamnus purshiana*), is generally to be avoided in the treatment of constipation associated with IBS. These remedies are likely to make it worse in the long term.

SOOTHING HERBS There are several herbs that soothe the bowel. Slippery elm (*Ulmus fulva*) powder contains an abundance of mucilage (a sticky substance). When mixed with powdered ginger (*Zingiber officinale*), cinnamon (*Cinnamomum cassia*) and caraway, it helps to reduce abdominal bloating. Slippery elm powder combines well with cooked porridge oats. Other herbs that soothe an irritated bowel are marshmallow root (*Althea officinalis*) and fenugreek (*Trigonella foenum-graecum*). They work best if combined with pungent warming spices, such as ginger and/or cinnamon, when they can be used to treat both diarrhoea and constipation in people with IBS by helping to restore normal bowel function.

HERBAL COMBINATION PRODUCTS Over-the-counter herbal products for IBS are popular in many countries. A recent randomised controlled trial compared two herbal combination products, both containing a mixture of several plant extracts, including bitter candytuft (*Iberis amara*), chamomile and other extracts, with a bitter candytuft extract and a placebo (inactive substance). The patients taking the combination medicines had significantly fewer IBS symptoms than those taking either the bitter candytuft extract or the placebo.

OTHER REMEDIES A useful remedy for loose stools is arrowroot (*Pueraria labata*), which can be taken up to three times a day, flavoured with a little ground cinnamon or nutmeg. Stir two teaspoons of arrowroot into a paste with water or chamomile tea, or combine it with live yoghurt. Commercially formulated charcoal tablets can also be effective for reducing the swing from loose bowel movements to constipation. It also helps to reduce flatulence too.

> **CAUTION**
>
> • See p.69 before taking a herbal remedy and, if you are already taking prescribed medication, consult a medical herbalist first.
> • Aloe vera juice should not be confused with aloes, which is a violent cathartic.
> • Do not take hops if you have depression.

Chinese Herbal Medicine

There is no disease equivalent to IBS in Traditional Chinese Medicine (TCM). Strategies for treating IBS are to be found in the discussions of treatment of three diseases well known in China: diarrhoea, constipation and abdominal pain. The traditional treatment of these diseases allows modern TCM practitioners to discern a number of effective lines of treatment for IBS. TCM doctors will give appropriate dietary advice and, in common with Western doctors, will recommend that eating patterns must be regular. Meals should not be missed or eaten on the run.

RESEARCH There is important research that supports the use of Chinese medicine for IBS. A randomised controlled trial followed 116 patients with the condition. One-third were given capsules of a herbal formulation that was prescribed individually for them, another third were given a standard Chinese herbal mixture, and the final group were given a placebo (inactive substance). Treatment continued for 16 weeks and those who received the Chinese herbal medicines showed significant improvement. The people receiving individualised herbs did not benefit more than those taking the standard Chinese herbal preparations. However, on follow-up 14 weeks after completing treatment, only the group that received individualised treatment had maintained their improvement.

TREATMENTS Chinese practitioners diagnose and then prescribe herbs for a variety of conditions. The first is liver *Qi* (energy) stagnation. The most usual cause of this is emotional disturbance. Long-term resentment, anxiety, worry or depression blocks the flow of liver *Qi* that in turn disrupts the smooth flow of stomach, spleen and large intestine *Qi* (digestive *Qi*), causing bloating, pain, flatulence and diarrhoea and/or constipation. In women, there may be accompanying PMS marked by mood swings as well as worsening IBS.

A second common pattern of symptoms is that of deficiency of Spleen and Stomach with stagnation of *Qi*. In this case the patient is tired, especially after eating, and experiences bloating and dull pain after meals. A third pattern is deficiency of spleen with accumulation of "damp". People with this syndrome have loose stools and are fatigued. A fourth common pattern is "damp heat" in the large intestine. People with this syndrome may have bloating and abdominal pain and may complain of rather explosive, bad-smelling bowel movements that may burn on passing. Lastly, if there is Spleen and Stomach *Yin* deficiency, the patient may complain of feeling hungry but not being able to eat much, abdominal bloating, dry lips, a dry mouth and irregular bowel movements with difficulty in passing stools.

> **CAUTION**
>
> Do not self-medicate with Chinese herbs for IBS. Consult a herbalist.

Bodywork and Movement Therapies

The spinal nerves that govern digestive function can either speed up or slow down the organs of digestion. The sympathetic nerves that emerge from the spine roughly between the shoulder blades, down to the low back, slow down digestive functions, while the parasympathetic nerves, which emerge from the very top and very bottom of the spine, restore digestive function to normal, or speed it up. Another branch of the nervous system exists in the abdomen itself, and this contains almost as many nerve cells as are found in the spine itself. Mechanical stress resulting from spinal restrictions, or from trigger points in the muscles of the back or abdomen, can influence these "slowing down" or "speeding up" processes. Since IBS may involve a speeding up of the activities of the bowel (diarrhoea) and sometimes a slowing down (constipation), either branch of the nervous system might be involved.

CHIROPRACTIC AND OSTEOPATHY There have been no reliable clinical trials of chiropractic and osteopathic treatments for IBS. Clinical experience however suggests they can be useful. A case report illustrates the possible benefit of spinal treatment. The patient was a 25-year-old woman with a history of five years of diarrhoea, abdominal pain and cramping. On examination her spine was found to have a number of areas of marked restriction, in the neck, middle and lower back. She reported sustained improvement after chiropractic

Although irritable bowel syndrome may recur throughout life, it does not usually get worse

treatment that mobilised the restrictions in the spine. If you have IBS, a chiropractor or osteopath should be able to tell you whether spinal restrictions are contributing to your condition, and should also be able to treat them if they are.

DEACTIVATION OF TRIGGER POINTS Trigger points are sensitive areas in muscles that usually cause pain or discomfort, not only where they are situated but also in areas some distance away. Those in the spinal or the abdominal muscles can cause symptoms in the intestinal tract itself. Research conducted nearly 50 years ago and confirmed by recent evidence shows that trigger points in the lower abdomen can cause or encourage diarrhoea, one of the common symptoms of IBS. Trigger points can be deactivated by acupuncture as well as by manual pressure and stretching techniques as used by osteopaths, massage therapists (particularly those with neuromuscular therapy training) and some physiotherapists and chiropractors.

RELAXATION FOR IBS

Visualisation and relaxation have both been shown to help relieve IBS symptoms. Each day, lie on the floor with a slim paperback under your head and a rolled towel under your knees. Close your eyes and relax fully for 20 minutes, visualising a soothing image such as a beach on a sunny day. Breathe deeply, exhaling slowly.

Breathing Retraining

IBS and fibromyalgia (*see p.298*) co-exist in many patients. Studies have shown that patients with IBS may also have significantly more tender points in muscles than normal. Some experts suspect that the link between IBS and fibromyalgia might be a breathing-rate disorder, such as hyperventilation. A common side-effect of rapid upper-chest breathing is elimination of too much carbon dioxide from the body. This can cause your bloodstream to become too alkaline (a condition known as respiratory alkalosis), making the smooth muscle layer around the digestive tract contract. Sluggish or interrupted digestion may result, which can lead to constipation.

Breathing-pattern disorders, such as a tendency to breathe using only the upper chest, can usually be improved or corrected with breathing rehabilitation, which involves learning slow, diaphragmatic (yoga-type) breathing methods (*for a sequence, see p.62*). Osteopathic correction of restrictions that may have developed in overused and stressed muscles and joints can also help.

Acupuncture

There are very few studies of acupuncture as a treatment for irritable bowel syndrome. One is a series of case reports that does suggest benefit, and the other is a randomised controlled trial that showed benefits for acupuncture in the short term. This study looked at the effects of acupuncture in seven IBS patients. The study found significant improvement in general well-being and in the patients' experience of bloating following acupuncture. However, this study did not include a placebo group, making it difficult to determine the degree to which acupuncture treatment really helped.

Acupuncture is certainly a reasonable treatment option for IBS, with some evidence to sustain claims of benefit. However, the benefits of real and "sham" acupuncture treatment appear to be the same, so it is difficult to tell whether true acupuncture is really useful.

Mind–Body Therapies

Depression is prevalent in IBS patients, as is diminished quality of life. IBS can affect sleep, sexual functioning, business and personal obligations and social life. The condition may be complicated by other conditions, such as fibromyalgia, chronic fatigue syndrome (*see p.474*) and thyroid problems (*see p.319*).

Since there are no definitive diagnostic tests, IBS is a diagnosis of exclusion. Drug treatment is geared toward symptom management, not cure. If you have IBS, you might want to consider mind–body therapies, such as relaxation or hypnosis (*see p.99*), since research supporting their use is very positive indeed.

PSYCHOTHERAPY AND ANTIDEPRESSANTS are very effective in patients with severe IBS. A study randomly allocated 257 patients with severe IBS to receive either eight sessions of individual psychotherapy, 20mg daily of the antidepressant paroxetine, or routine care. Patients having either psychotherapy or paroxetine did not feel better psychologically, but reported feeling better physically than those getting routine medical care. During the follow-up year, the patients who had psychotherapy maintained the improvement in that they were less likely to need other medication or to see doctors. The improvement was not maintained in the paroxetine group.

RELAXATION, BIOFEEDBACK AND HYPNOSIS Relaxation and biofeedback have shown success in improving symptoms of IBS and preventing the condition from recurring. One approach using relaxation therapy and medication was effective in two-thirds of patients who had not found relief using medication alone. Another approach using progressive muscle relaxation, thermal biofeedback, cognitive therapy and education had a 50 per cent success rate, and four years later those patients still showed improvement. Hypnosis has been shown to improve IBS symptoms, even in severe cases and in cases where psychotherapy had failed.

OTHER THERAPIES Mind–body therapies are effective in alleviating depression and improving quality of life. A self-help programme that includes meditation and visualisation can improve abdominal pain and reduce or eliminate symptoms, so less medication may be needed. (*For details of these therapies, see pp.98–100.*)

> Around 50 per cent of people with IBS had their first attack during a major life event

PREVENTION PLAN

The following may help prevent IBS:

- Reduce stress.
- Take regular exercise.
- Avoid known problem foods.

ULCERATIVE COLITIS

Ulcerative colitis is an inflammatory bowel disease (*see also Crohn's disease, p.216*), in which the colon (the large bowel) and/or the rectum (to which the large bowel leads) becomes inflamed and ulcerated. The disease may affect the rectum alone or may extend from the rectum up into the colon. Treatment involves a range of drugs and sometimes surgery. Dietary changes and supplements, homeopathic medicines and acupuncture may also play a useful role in controlling the symptoms and progress of ulcerative colitis.

WHAT ARE THE SYMPTOMS?

In a mild attack, symptoms may include:

- Diarrhoea, sometimes with mucus and blood in the faeces
- Abdominal pain
- Fatigue
- Loss of appetite
- Weight loss

In a more severe attack, the diarrhoea is more frequent and may be accompanied by:

- Pain and swelling in the abdomen
- Fever

WHY MIGHT I HAVE THIS?

PREDISPOSING FACTOR

- Genetic tendency

TRIGGER (IN EXISTING DISEASE)

- Gastrointestinal infection

WHY DOES IT OCCUR?

The exact cause of ulcerative colitis is not known. Since about one in ten people with ulcerative colitis has a relative with the condition or another inflammatory bowel disease, such as Crohn's disease, it is possible that genetic factors are involved. Overactive immune responses have also been proposed as a causative factor.

Ulcerative colitis usually starts between the ages of 15 and 35 and is a life-long condition that is characterised by periods of relapse (being ill) followed by periods of remission (being well). The symptoms vary from being mild to severe and generally become apparent over several days.

People who have ulcerative colitis often have other associated disorders, including liver disease, joint disease, uveitis (inflammation of the eye) and erythema nodosum

IMPORTANT

If you experience unexplained weight loss and/or abdominal pain, see your doctor without delay.

(a skin condition in which tender swellings appear, usually on the shins).

Unlike Crohn's disease, ulcerative colitis affects only the large intestine and/or the rectum and never affects the small intestine. People with ulcerative colitis whose disease is confined to the rectum alone tend to experience the fewest complications and have the best prognosis.

People who have ulcerative colitis are also at increased risk of developing colorectal cancer. The risk becomes significant about 10 years after the onset of the illness and is greatest when the whole colon is involved and there is also associated liver disease.

TREATMENT PLAN

PRIMARY TREATMENTS

- Drugs, such as aminosalicylates
- Fish oils

BACK-UP TREATMENTS

- Nutritional therapy
- Surgery

WORTH CONSIDERING

- Acupuncture
- Individualised homeopathy

For an explanation of how treatments are rated, see p.111.

TREATMENTS IN DETAIL

Conventional Medicine

The doctor will arrange investigations. Ulcerative colitis is diagnosed using colonoscopy, in which a flexible viewing instrument is passed up the bowel to examine its lining. Tissue samples (biopsies) are also taken for examination.

If ulcerative colitis is diagnosed, the aim is to control the disease with medical treatment. Several drugs are used to treat ulcerative colitis. The choice of drug depends on how much of the large bowel is involved, how severe the disease is and whether the aim is to treat a relapse or to maintain a remission.

PRIMARY TREATMENT **DRUGS FOR LIMITED DISEASE** If disease is limited to the last 25–30cm of the colon or less, it can be treated by liquid or foam enemas or suppositories which are given directly into the rectum. These may contain mild anti-inflammatory agents, such as amino-salicylates or corticosteroids.

PRIMARY TREATMENT **DRUGS FOR EXTENSIVE DISEASE** If the disease affects a large portion of the colon, oral drugs are required. Aminosalicylates can be used if the disease is mild. However, their main role is in the long-term maintenance of remission and possibly to protect against the development of cancer.

Generally, for more extensive disease or for symptoms that fail to respond to aminosalicylates, a course of cortico-steroids will be recommended. These drugs reduce inflammation. The starting dose will be continued for a few weeks and then the dose will be gradually reduced; corti-costeroids should not be stopped suddenly. For some people with ulcerative colitis, long-term steroids or frequent courses of steroids may be necessary, too. In children, there is a risk that steroids may affect growth and, for that reason, their use is carefully monitored.

DRUGS TO MAINTAIN REMISSION Aza-thioprine is an immunosuppressant drug, which helps maintain remission and which may be prescribed for persistent disease as it is thought that ulcerative colitis may be due in part to autoimmune factors. Azathioprine is also known as a steroid-sparing agent and may allow reduction of the steroid dose in people who require high doses or prolonged use of steroids.

PROBIOTICS Some early research has suggested that probiotics ("friendly" micro-organisms that are present naturally in the large bowel) may help maintain remission in ulcerative colitis (see Nutritional Therapy, opposite).

SURGERY Surgery may be considered for severe disease that persists despite medical treatment or when high doses of steroids are needed on a regular basis to control the symptoms. There are various options. For example, the colon may be removed but the rectum left in place. The ileum (lower

This double contrast X-ray shows a large intestine affected by mild ulcerative colitis. An abnormal mucosal pattern appears as mottling in the ascending colon, which can be seen on the left side of the X-ray. The white areas show barium, the contrast medium.

end of the small bowel) is then connected to an opening on the abdominal wall to form an ileostomy and the stools are collected in bags placed over the opening. It may be possible to reconnect the small bowel and the rectum at a later date or to remove the rectum and connect the small bowel to the anus. In some cases, the ileostomy is permanent. If part of the colon is left in place, the disease may recur in the remaining section.

Toxic megacolon is a serious condition that occurs in very severe cases of ulcerative colitis. In toxic megacolon, the motion of the intestinal wall stops and the colon rapidly becomes distended. Immediate admission to hospital is necessary and the patient is monitored very closely. If the condition does not improve after a few

days of treatment with intravenous steroids and antibiotics, surgery to remove most or all of the colon (known as colectomy) will be required. An ileostomy will be necessary if the entire colon is removed.

COLONOSCOPY Regular surveillance with colonoscopy is recommended for individuals with ulcerative colitis from about 10 years after the onset of the illness. This is done to check for the development of colorectal cancer.

Regular colonoscopy is especially important if the disease affects the entire colon and is accompanied by liver disease. Even if most of the colon has been surgically removed, surveillance is still needed because cancer may develop in the small amount of colon left in place.

Nutritional Therapy

ELIMINATING PROBLEM FOODS People affected by ulcerative colitis may benefit from identifying and eliminating problem foods from their diet (*For more information, see p.39.*)

PRIMARY TREATMENT **FISH OIL SUPPLEMENTS** Ulcerative colitis is an inflammatory condition. Excessive amounts of omega-6 fatty acids (found in vegetable oils) and a relative lack of omega-3 fatty acids (found in oily fish, walnuts and linseeds) seems to promote inflammation.

Maintaining a balance between omega-6 and omega 3-fatty acids in the body may be helpful. This can be achieved by avoiding excessive amounts of margarine and vegetable oils and including oily fish (such as salmon and mackerel), walnuts and flaxseeds in the diet. Studies suggest that taking fish oil (which has anti-inflammatory properties) might be useful in treating ulcerative colitis. In one study, ulcerative colitis patients taking fish oils were able to reduce their dosage of steroid medication by 50 per cent. However, the relapse rate after one year was the same as in another group taking olive oil capsules.

It was found that fish oil supplementation also resulted in weight gain and reduced intestinal inflammation in those taking it. If you have ulcerative colitis, you could try taking fish oil providing 3g EPA and 2g DHA per day.

PROBIOTICS Supplements of beneficial gut bacteria, such as *lactobacillus* and *bifidobacteria*, may be useful in treating ulcerative colitis. One study found that a probiotic supplement was effective in preventing flare-ups of chronic pouchitis (a major long-term complication in ulcerative colitis) in ulcerative colitis patients.

In another study, a group of 15 patients were treated with a mix of beneficial bacteria for one year. Eighty per cent of these patients were still in remission from the condition at the end of the year-long study.

FOLIC ACID Ulcerative colitis is linked to an increased risk of colon cancer, especially when the disease is long-standing. Studies show that people with ulcerative colitis who have been taking folic acid supplements or who have high blood levels of folic acid have a reduced risk of colon cancer compared to people with the condition who do not. People with ulcerative colitis who are taking the drug sulphasalazine, which inhibits the absorption of folic acid, appear to be at particular risk of developing folic acid deficiency. Folic acid supplementation may therefore be important for people with ulcerative colitis, especially for those taking sulphsalazine. If you are taking this drug, try taking 1mg of folic acid per day.

Homeopathy

Records of patients treated at the Tunbridge Wells Homeopathic Hospital suggest that most patients treated with individualised homeopathy (*see p.73*) for ulcerative colitis were helped considerably.

Among the most important homeopathic treatments for this condition are *Mercurius corrosivus*, *Arsenicum album* and *Phosphorus*.

MERCURIUS CORROSIVUS This homeopathic medicine is indicated when the condition is acute and the "keynote" symptom is tremendous tenesmus, which is a constant but ineffective urge to pass a stool, often at its worst just after having passed a stool. Only a little faeces may actually be passed, but they often contain a lot of blood. People affected may also have bladder tenesmus accompanied by a very sore mouth or throat.

ARSENICUM ALBUM can be very helpful in the acute situation when the patient feels very ill, cold and anxious, and may even fear he or she is about to die. Although the patient may indeed be quite ill, they generally feel worse than they are. The stool is typically thin, watery and foul-smelling and there is burning pain in the rectum. It can also be useful in a less acute situation for tense, anxious, chilly patients who may also have skin trouble or at least very dry, flaky skin.

> Doctors suspect ulcerative colitis may be an autoimmune disease, but there is no proof as yet

PHOSPHORUS In patients who respond to *Phosphorus* there is a lot of bleeding; the stools may be copious but often there is not much pain. The patient is tired and weak, although a bit better for rest, and hence feels better in the morning. The patient is often thirsty, especially for cold, refreshing drinks. In terms of personality, *Phosphorus* types are very sensitive, both to the physical and human environment. They are emotionally "up and down", but can be sympathetic and vivacious.

Acupuncture

There are a number of Chinese trials that have looked at the use of acupuncture for inflammation of the colon, but often the diagnosis is unclear and the quality of the trial is poor. There are no good controlled trials analysing the use of acupuncture in proven ulcerative colitis, although acupuncture is widely used for this condition. A traditional Chinese approach is needed for both diagnosis and treatment. It is essential to visit a qualified practitioner and to tell them of any prescribed drugs taken.

Circumstantial evidence and case reports suggest that acupuncture may be of real value in treating acute colitis, but treatment may need to be quite prolonged. Initially, treatment should be given on a weekly basis, or more frequently if the condition is very acute. If there is no obvious improvement after six to eight sessions, it is questionable whether continuing acupuncture treatment will be of value.

GALLSTONES

Hard masses that form from substances in the gallbladder are known as gallstones. They are made from the digestive juice bile, which is stored in the gallbladder and contains cholesterol, pigments and salts. Most gallstones consist of a mixture of cholesterol and pigments. Gallstones are more common in women and in people of Scandinavian and Native American origin. Surgery may be a necessary measure if gallstones are troublesome or cause the gallbladder to become infected. Other options include lithotripsy, dietary changes and acupuncture.

WHAT ARE THE SYMPTOMS?

- Upper abdominal pain, which may range from mild to severe
- Nausea and vomiting

WHY MIGHT I HAVE THIS?

PREDISPOSING FACTORS

- Being overweight
- Pregnancy
- Diabetes mellitus
- Diet high in fat
- Genetic factors
- Certain blood disorders

TRIGGERS

- Changes in spinal joints
- Trigger points in abdominal muscles

IMPORTANT

If you develop any of the symptoms of gallstones, see your doctor without delay.

WHY DOES IT OCCUR?

In many cases there is no obvious reason for gallstone formation. However, stones made up mainly of cholesterol are more likely in people who are very overweight, and a diet high in animal fat may increase the risk of developing this type of gallstone. A tendency to develop gallstones may run in families, suggesting that a genetic component may be involved. Stones made up mainly of pigment may form if there is excessive destruction of red blood cells, as occurs in some heredi-

tary blood disorders. Symptoms arise if a gallstone blocks the ducts that carry bile from the gallbladder to the gut. Symptoms tend to occur after a fatty meal, which causes the gallbladder to contract. In some cases gallstones cause no symptoms.

TREATMENTS IN DETAIL

Conventional Medicine

If your doctor suspects that you have gallstones, he or she will arrange tests that are likely to include an ultrasound scan of the upper abdomen. Gallstones that are not causing symptoms (those that are picked up incidentally during other tests) do not require treatment.

If you have gallstones, your doctor will probably advise you to eat a diet low in animal fat. If you are overweight, he or she may advise you to lose weight.

PRIMARY TREATMENT | **SURGERY** If gallstones are causing symptoms, cholecystectomy (removal of the gallbladder) may be recommended. This may be performed by traditional or more often by laparoscopic ("keyhole") surgery. Occasionally, stones develop in the remaining bile duct.

PRIMARY TREATMENT | **SHOCKWAVE LITHOTRIPSY** Other treatments are used less often and tend to be reserved for people for whom surgery would be hazardous. They include shockwave lithotripsy, in which ultrasound waves are used to shatter stones so that the fragments can pass through the bile ducts and into the gut.

OTHER TREATMENTS Occasionally, drugs such as ursodeoxycholic acid are given that

TREATMENT PLAN

PRIMARY TREATMENTS

- Weight-loss diet (if overweight)
- Surgery to remove gallbladder
- Shockwave lithotripsy

BACK-UP TREATMENTS

- Endoscopic retrograde cholangiopancreatography (ERCP)
- Dietary changes
- Western herbalism
- Acupuncture

WORTH CONSIDERING

- Vitamin C and phosphatidyl choline
- Homeopathy
- Bodywork therapies

For an explanation of how treatments are rated, see p.111.

aim to dissolve cholesterol stones, but this is a slow process that takes several months or even years and is only rarely used.

Gallstones in the bile duct may be treated using a procedure known as endoscopic retrograde cholangiopancreatography (ERCP), in which a flexible viewing tube with surgical attachments is passed down the oesophagus to view and treat the stones.

> **CAUTION**
>
> Surgery and other procedures for gallstones carry some risks. Ask your doctor to explain them to you.

Nutritional Therapy

PRIMARY TREATMENT **WEIGHT LOSS** Obesity is often a factor in gallstone formation, and obese women have been found to have seven times the risk of developing gallstones compared to women of normal weight. Losing weight may help to reduce the risk of gallstone problems. However, extreme, rapid weight loss has been shown actually to increase the risk of gallstone formation, so if you need to lose weight, do so slowly and sensibly.

Other risk factors for gallstone formation during weight loss include very low-calorie diets with no fat and a high level of certain blood fats called triglycerides. People who want to lose weight should follow a sensible eating plan and avoid extreme, "crash" diets. Slow, steady weight loss will probably help reduce the risk of gallstones in the long term. (*See p.444 for more information on obesity and weight loss.*)

DIETARY CHANGES In general, your diet should be rich in fibre, since this may reduce the risk of developing gallstones. A diet high in refined carbohydrates (such as sugar, white bread and white rice) appears to increase risk of gallstones. Refined carbohydrates may increase the production of cholesterol in the liver, which in turn may increase the risk of gallstone formation by raising the level of cholesterol in the gallbladder. For the best protection, your diet should be based on whole foods such as wholemeal bread, brown rice, beans, fruits and vegetables.

FORMATION AND LOCATION OF GALLSTONES

Gallstones usually result from an imbalance in the chemical composition of bile, a substance produced by the liver that is stored in the gallbladder. Gallstones form in the gallbladder but may travel from there into the cystic duct. They may also pass into the common bile duct and from there into the duodenum. If stones become lodged in a duct, they cause severe upper abdominal pain and nausea.

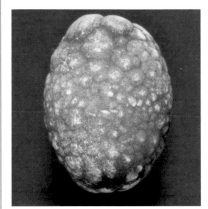

Cholesterol precipitates out of the bile to form crystals, which coalesce together to create a gallstone.

The gallbladder and bile ducts

Cystic duct

Gallbladder

Gallstone in cystic duct

Gallstones

Gallstone in common bile duct

Gallstones form in the gallbladder but may then travel to the bile ducts, where they sometimes become impacted.

Many people with gallstones, particularly those who are overweight, are advised to avoid fat in the diet. However, dietary fat stimulates the gallbladder to empty, which may help the flow of bile and reduce the risk of gallstone development.

In one study, obese individuals on a weight-loss programme had no gallstone formation. The authors of the study attributed this to the fact that their diet contained significant amounts of fat (26g of fat per day). In another study, two groups of obese people were put on very low-calorie diets (a known risk factor for gallstone formation). One group was only given only 3g of fat per day, while the other was allowed 12.2g of fat per day.

Weight loss was achieved in both groups, but while gallstones developed in more than 50 per cent of people following the lower-fat diet, no one on the higher-fat regime developed gallstones.

The type of fat eaten also seems to be important in the development or prevention of gallstones. There is some evidence that a diet high in vegetable fat is a risk factor for gallstone formation, while fat that comes from fish (omega-3 fatty acids) seems to be protective.

Include oily fish (such as salmon, mackerel and sardines) as part of your weight-loss regime to help prevent the development of gallstones.

VITAMIN C could theoretically help to prevent gallstones. It helps to convert cholesterol into substances called bile acids that are involved in the digestion of fat in the body. Studies on animals show that vitamin C supplementation can reduce the formation of gallstones.

A study on humans demonstrated that vitamin C (2,000mg per day for four weeks) altered bile acid formation in a way that would be expected to reduce cholesterol gallstone formation. Vitamin C supplement use has also been associated with a decreased prevalence of gallstones. If you are prone to developing gallstones, try taking 2,000mg vitamin C a day.

PHOSPHATIDYL CHOLINE (a purified extract of lecithin) is one of the components of bile that may help to protect against gallstone formation. If there is too little phosphatidyl choline or too much cholesterol in the bile, the risk of gallstones increases. Some studies have shown that 300–2,000mg of phosphatidyl choline per day may be helpful in preventing and treating gallstones.

If you have gallstones or are concerned about developing them, try taking a daily supplement of phosphatidyl choline within this dosage range.

> **CAUTION**
>
> Consult your doctor before taking vitamin C with antibiotics or the blood-thinning drug warfarin; it may enhance the effects of these drugs. (*See also p.46.*)

Homeopathy

Several homeopathic medicines are said to help with the tendency to form stones in the gallbladder. *Berberis vulgaris* and *Chelidonium majus* are prescribed based on symptoms, while *Calcarea carbonica*, *Lycopodium* and *Natrum sulphuricum* are prescribed on a "constitutional" basis (*see p.73*). *Colocynthis* may also be given in certain cases.

BERBERIS Where *Berberis* is indicated, there is often nausea and drowsiness after eating, along with a tendency to kidney stones and gout.

CHELIDONIUM In people for whom *Chelidonium* is indicated, there may be intermittent slight jaundice and pain radiating to the tip of the right shoulder blade, which may be accompanied by headache, which is usually right-sided.

CALCAREA CARBONICA The person who responds to *Calcarea carbonica* is typically stocky and solidly built, with a tendency to be overweight. People who respond to this remedy are phlegmatic types, solid, stubborn, and hard-working, but this calm exterior may conceal anxieties and fears about things such as serious illness. These people may also have bad dreams. They tend to be chilly and yet sweat a lot, especially on the head and neck. They often crave eggs, especially soft-boiled.

This colour-enhanced X-ray shows a gallbladder containing gallstones, which appear as red masses in the centre of the picture. Gallstones cause problems when they become stuck in the bile ducts, where they create pain and may block the flow of bile to the duodenum.

LYCOPODIUM The type of person who responds to *Lycopodium* is typically rather quiet and reserved, disliking large social gatherings. They are often thoughtful, conscientious people who worry in advance of important occasions and may be quite depressed. They take their responsibilities very seriously. They often crave sweets and may feel hungry when they start eating, but quickly feel full. These people often suffer from bloating and wind. They tend to be at their worst in the afternoon, typically between 4 and 8pm.

NATRUM SULPHURICUM People who resond to this remedy feel worse when they are exposed to damp in any form (examples include such things as wet weather, damp housing and so forth). Apart from gallstones, these people may also have a cough that produces sputum, along with stiff joints and a stiff back, all of which are made worse by damp. They may also have warts.

COLOCYNTHIS Finally, *Colocynthis* may be indicated in gallstone colic, when a stone gets stuck in the bile duct. It is a severe, colicky pain that comes in waves and is relieved by doubling up.

Western Herbal Medicine

Several herbs can improve bile flow, but when gallbladder health is generally poor and gallstones are either large or have been in place for a long time, conventional treatments (including surgery) may well be the the primary remedy.

Herbal treatment is most effective when it is started when scans show relatively few, small stones. At this time, the primary problem may be gallbladder congestion and remedies can be selected to help flush our debris from the gallbladder and bile ducts. Self-help treatment can be safely undertaken in the early stages of gallstone formation, but professional treatment is best, not least due to the sheer number of herbs available for treatment.

HERBS TO CLEAR THE GALLBLADDER There have been no clinical trials of herbal medicines for gallstones. However, many herbal remedies, known as choleretics, directly stimulate bile production by the liver. This means that increased and more dilute bile flows through the bile ducts into the small intestine.

Over time, the increased bile flow encourages cleansing of the gallbladder, reducing the size of stones so that they can be passed without discomfort. Choleretic herbs form the basis of treatment when multiple small gallstones are present.

Clinical research since the 1930s confirms that globe artichoke (*Cynara scolymus*) has a marked ability to increase

it is also an antioxidant and choleretic herb. Peppermint (*Mentha piperita*), which has long been used to relieve nausea and dyspepsia, appears to relax the bile ducts and gallbladder and thus increase the scope for clearance of gallstones. Finally, turmeric (*Curcuma longa*) is a valuable remedy for gallbladder inflammation and is a powerful anti-inflammatory and choleretic remedy.

OTHER MEASURES Other approaches may also be appropriate, especially those improving diet and digestive function.

> **CAUTION**
>
> See p.69 before taking a herbal remedy and, if you are already taking prescribed medication, consult a medical herbalist first.

Acupuncture

TRADTIONAL CHINESE TREATMENT While acupuncture treatment for gallstones is common in China, it is far less common in the West. The Chinese usually give daily treatment to help expel the gallstones under close medical supervision. There have been several large, non-randomised clinical studies that have clearly demonstrated the discharge of gallstones after treatment with acupuncture.

It is thought that acupuncture works by dilating the common bile duct and causing the gallbladder to contract simultaneously.

Treatment needs to be intensive over a relatively short period of time, with two or three hours of treatment given on a daily basis for three or four days.

Bodywork Therapies

Osteopaths believe that improvement in gallbladder function, including reduction of associated discomfort and pain (both before and after surgery) can be achieved by appropriate osteopathic manipulation of the spine.

GALLBLADDER DYSFUNCTION AND THE SPINE The theory is that there is a connection between the way the gallbladder functions and the condition of the middle of the thoracic spine (the part of the spine that runs through the chest), from which the gallbladder derives its nerve supply. Osteopaths and chiropractors think that dysfunction of the gallbladder is linked to changes in the spinal joints, due to a feedback from the distressed organ to the tissues in and around the nerve root emerging from the spine.

DEACTIVATION OF TRIGGER POINTS Pain relating to active trigger points (sensitive areas) in the abdominal muscles can mimic symptoms that are almost identical to the pain experienced in the gallbladder region when gallstones are present.

Relief from this pain is often possible when these trigger points in the abdominal muscles are deactivated. Research has shown that trigger-point activity can have far-reaching effects that spread beyond the muscle housing the trigger point itself.

Symptoms that may be caused by trigger points, such as pain in the gallbladder region, can often be relieved by acupuncture (*see above*) as well as by manual pressure and stretching techniques as used by osteopaths, massage therapists (particularly those who have training in neuromuscular therapy) and some physiotherapists and chiropractors.

> # Some gallstones are as small as a grain of sand, but they can grow to the size of a plum

bile production, lower cholesterol levels (which is important in cholesterol-based gallstones) and relieve dyspepsia (indigestion-like pain) and other symptoms.

Greater celandine (*Cheldonium majus*) is beginning to be used in the same way, although it has traditionally been viewed as a treatment for spasmodic pain arising from the gallbladder.

Milk thistle (*Silibum marianum*) may also be used to treat gallstones. It is best known for its ability to protect the liver but

Ultrasound scans show that acupuncture treatment results in 7 to 10 per cent of people having complete clearance of stones and a further 15 per cent having a significantly reduced number of stones.

A dramatic increase in gallstones eliminated in the stool is also found after acupuncture treatment. Stones pass through the common bile duct and into the duodenum, from where they pass through the remainder of the digestive system and are eliminated.

> **PREVENTION PLAN**
>
> **To reduce your risk of gallstones:**
> • Keep to a normal weight.

HEPATITIS

Inflammation of the liver, whatever the cause, is known as hepatitis. The liver has a variety of vital functions including processing nutrients, regulating blood-sugar levels, breaking down toxic chemicals, making proteins needed for blood clotting and producing the digestive juice bile. Hepatitis may be acute (short term), lasting less than six months, or chronic (long term), lasting for more than six months. Hepatitis requires medical attention, but there are also things you can do to help yourself, such as changing your diet and taking supplements.

WHAT ARE THE SYMPTOMS?

Initial symptoms of acute hepatitis may include:

- Fatigue and a feeling of ill health
- Poor appetite
- Nausea and vomiting
- Fever
- Pain or discomfort in the upper right side of the abdomen

Several days later, the following symptoms may appear:

- Yellowing of the whites of the eyes and the skin (jaundice)
- Pale faeces and dark urine

Symptoms of chronic hepatitis may include:

- Loss of appetite and weight loss
- Fatigue
- Yellowing of the whites of the eyes and the skin (jaundice)
- Widespread itchiness
- Abdominal discomfort and possibly swelling

WHY MIGHT I HAVE THIS?

PREDISPOSING FACTORS

- Poor hygiene (hepatitis A)
- Consuming contaminated water or food in high-risk areas (hepatitis A)
- Contact with blood (hepatitis B, C)
- Needle sharing (hepatitis B, C)
- Unprotected sexual intercourse (hepatitis B, C)
- Excessive alcohol consumption
- Exposure to chemicals that are toxic to the liver (e.g. toluene)
- Exposure to drugs or herbs that are toxic to the liver (e.g. phenytoin)

WHY DOES IT OCCUR?

Many conditions can cause hepatitis, but the most widespread of these is infection with a hepatitis virus. There are several viruses, of which the most common are hepatitis A, hepatitis B and hepatitis C. Other, lesser-known types of hepatitis virus include hepatitis D and hepatitis E. Additional hepatitis viruses are likely to be discovered. Non-infectious causes include excessive alcohol consumption, medication side-effects and paracetamol overdose.

Hepatitis A virus is transmitted via contaminated food or water and can be found in the urine and faeces of infected people. Infection with the hepatitis A virus is always acute and does not become chronic.

The hepatitis B virus is spread by contact with infected bodily fluids, such as blood. Modes of transmission include sharing of needles by drug abusers and sexual intercourse. Infection with the hepatitis B virus can cause acute or chronic hepatitis.

The hepatitis C virus is transmitted mainly by needle sharing, blood transfusions (although all blood is now tested for hepatitis C in the UK) and less commonly by sexual intercourse. It can cause either acute or chronic hepatitis and is the most common cause of chronic hepatitis.

ACUTE HEPATITIS may cause no symptoms, or symptoms may be so mild that they go unnoticed. If hepatitis is caused by a virus, the time from infection to appearance of symptoms varies from 2–3 weeks for hepatitis A to 1–5 months for hepatitis B. Acute hepatitis may become severe and in some cases may progress to liver failure, a life-threatening condition in which the liver is unable to carry out its functions. Severe acute hepatitis is relatively common after a paracetamol overdose, but rarely occurs with hepatitis A and B infections.

CHRONIC HEPATITIS Roughly one-third of chronic hepatitis cases develop following infections with type B or C viruses. In the

TREATMENT PLAN

PRIMARY TREATMENTS

- Drugs, including antivirals and corticosteroids

BACK-UP TREATMENTS

- Liver-supporting diet
- Liver transplant (for liver failure)
- Vitamin C
- Milk thistle, glycyrrhizin and other liver-protective herbs

WORTH CONSIDERING

- Homeopathy
- Acupuncture

For an explanation of how treatments are rated, see p.111.

IMPORTANT

If you develop symptoms that suggest hepatitis, see your doctor without delay. If left untreated, some types of hepatitis can lead to irreversible liver damage.

THE LIVER AND ITS FUNCTIONS

The liver converts digested food molecules and toxins from the bloodstream into chemicals that the body can use, store or excrete. The liver consists of thousands of lobules, which are tiny units about 1 mm (¹⁄₂₅in) wide that process blood. Each lobule is surrounded by branches of the portal vein, hepatic artery and bile duct. Processed blood is returned to the bloodstream through the inferior vena cava. The liver also produces the digestive juice bile, which is then stored in the gallbladder.

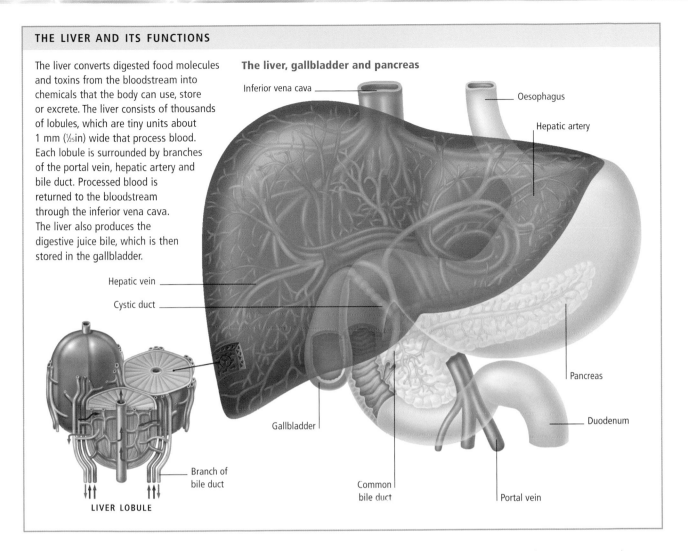

The liver, gallbladder and pancreas

Inferior vena cava

Oesophagus

Hepatic artery

Hepatic vein

Cystic duct

Pancreas

Duodenum

Gallbladder

Branch of bile duct

LIVER LOBULE

Common bile duct

Portal vein

---

other two-thirds of cases of chronic hepatitis, the condition develops with no apparent previous illness. Some people may be unaware of having a previous episode of acute viral hepatitis until the symptoms of chronic hepatitis appear or until routine blood tests assessing liver function are found to be abnormal. Other causes of chronic hepatitis include autoimmune diseases (in which the body's immune system produces antibodies against its own tissues).

Chronic hepatitis can progress to cirrhosis (irreversible liver damage that may cause liver failure). Both of these conditions are associated with an increased risk of developing liver cancer.

Some people with hepatitis caused by hepatitis B, D and possibly C continue to carry the virus in their blood. They can pass on the virus, although they do not develop symptoms themselves.

TREATMENTS IN DETAIL

Conventional Medicine

The precise treatment of acute hepatitis depends on the underlying cause. In many cases of acute hepatitis, no specific treatment is necessary.

Hepatitis A requires no specific treatment. It usually lasts 3–6 weeks and in most cases the prognosis is good. Similarly, acute hepatitis B requires no treatment; most people make a complete recovery.

PRIMARY TREATMENT **ANTIVIRAL DRUGS** People who develop chronic hepatitis may be treated with antiviral agents, such as interferon, which is given by injection, usually for about four months. (Interferons are proteins produced by the body in response to viral infections; synthetic versions are used to treat certain diseases.)

Interferon produces a response in up to half of those treated, but relapses may occur. The antiviral drug lamivudine is also used. It is taken orally for about a year and is generally well tolerated. If hepatitis C is diagnosed in the acute phase, interferon is sometimes given. Treatment with a combination of antiviral drugs (often including interferon), usually for about six months, may be appropriate and is effective for some cases of chronic hepatitis C.

OTHER MEASURES In other types of chronic hepatitis the underlying conditions are treated. For example, hepatitis that results from autoimmune disease is treated with long-term corticosteroids and sometimes azathioprine, which reduces the activity of the immune system.

If liver failure occurs in either acute or chronic hepatitis, a liver transplant may be needed.

Nutritional Therapy

LIVER-SUPPORTING DIET People with hepatitis should avoid anything that puts stress on the liver, such as high-dose vitamin A, paracetamol, alcohol and fatty foods. Drinking plenty of water (about two litres per day) helps to reduce the toxic load on the body. *(For more information on a diet to support the liver, see p.42.)*

VITAMIN C Vitamin C may be helpful to people with hepatitis. In addition to its immune-stimulating and antiviral properties, this nutrient is also known to promote tissue healing, and may therefore help to reduce the risk of damage to the liver in the longer term.

Vitamin C may also be useful for combating the free radical damage that seems to be a factor in people with hepatitis. Clinical experience suggests that 2,000mg of vitamin C taken three times a day while symptoms persist may be helpful. In the longer term, individuals with hepatitis

CATECHIN This bioflavonoid compound, which is found in green tea, has an antioxidant action and may help to neutralise the free radicals generated by substances toxic to the liver. One study found that catechin supplementation was effective in treating hepatitis in some individuals. Try taking 500–750mg catechin, three times a day if you have hepatitis.

Homeopathy

PHOSPHORUS is the usual homeopathic medicine for acute hepatitis, particularly for hepatitis A and acute alcoholic hepatitis. People for whom *Phosphorus* is indicated are tired and weak, although a bit better for rest and hence feel more energetic in the morning. Those who respond to this medication often have pain under the right ribs and loss of appetite, although are often thirsty, especially for cold, refreshing drinks. They like ice cream.

LYCOPODIUM AND NATRUM SULPHURICUM can both be indicated for hepatitis. People who respond to *Lycopodium* often have a lot of bloating and indigestion along with right-sided migrainous headaches. Patients are typically rather reserved and their symptoms are worse between 4 and 8pm.

People who respond to *Natrum sulphuricum* often have pale, bulky stools with diarrhoea, especially in the morning. They are always worse when the weather is wet and may be very depressed.

Western Herbal Medicine

In conjunction with conventional treatment, herbal medications are of great interest as treatments for acute and chronic hepatitis. Self-treatment with herbal medicines for hepatitis is not appropriate, however, and affected individuals should always seek treatment from a qualified herbal practitioner.

In determining treatment for hepatitis of all types, the herbal practitioner will assess and prioritise specific areas requiring treatment. These include support and protection of liver function, stimulating the elimination of toxins other than via the liver (e.g. by the kidneys or through sweating), managing fever, stimulating immune function and countering viral infection.

HERBS TO FIGHT INFECTION If treating an acute condition, the herbal practitioner will usually put greater emphasis on countering infection than if treating chronic hepatitis. The first priorities will be to stimulate immune resistance and support normal liver function.

Echinacea (*Echinacea spp.*), garlic (*Allium sativum*), phyllanthus (*Phyllanthus amarus*) and St John's wort (*Hypericum perforatum*) will figure prominently in prescriptions. All four have broad anti-infective properties, while St John's wort and its active constituents hypericin and pseudohypericin may have specific actions against the hepatitis A, B and C viruses.

Schisandra (*Schisandra chinensis*) is a plant used in traditional Chinese and Japanese medicine, usually in herbal mixtures. One small study of a Japanese herbal mixture (called TJ-108) containing schisandra found that it may be an antiviral that is effective in hepatitis C.

> Liver specialists report a worrying increase of acute alcoholic hepatitis in people in their 20s

might benefit from taking 1,000mg of vitamin C, twice a day. If you have hepatitis, try taking vitamin C at these dosages.

VITAMIN E Vitamin E is another antioxidant vitamin that may help people with hepatitis, who often have low levels of this nutrient. A study demonstrated the ability of vitamin E (1,200 IU per day of the d-alpha-tocopherol form for eight weeks) to prevent one aspect of liver damage (fibrogenesis cascade) in hepatitis C patients. Another study found that vitamin E supplementation might be effective in the treatment of chronic hepatitis B. People with hepatitis may benefit from taking 800–1,200 IU vitamin E per day.

ARSENICUM ALBUM is another possible medicine for acute hepatitis. In this case, the "picture" is similar to that of *Phosphorus*, but the people who respond to *Arsenicum album* are also very anxious and chilly and there may be oedema (accumulation of fluid) and ascites (accumulation of fluid in the abdomen). *Ars. alb.* may also be appropriate for chronic hepatitis.

LACHESIS may be indicated if the patient's face is flushed (often a dark reddish-blue hue). People who respond to it may also have bleeding gums and haemorrhoids. They tend to be talkative and may be aggressive or paranoid. *Lachesis* may also be indicated for chronic hepatitis.

While in hepatitis A full recovery can be expected, in hepatitis B and C herbal treatment aims principally at preventing the development of chronic hepatitis.

LIVER-PROTECTIVE HERBS For sub-acute or chronic hepatitis, the practitioner will mainly use liver-protective herbs, which have specific antioxidant action on liver tissue, protecting against damage and cirrhosis (scarring of the liver) and normalising liver function.

Key liver-protective herbs include milk thistle (*Silybum marianum*), dandelion root (*Taraxacum officinale*), bupleurum (*Bupleurum falcatum*) and globe artichoke (*Cynara scolymus*). Milk thistle and its flavanolignans (known collectively as silymarin) may protect the liver from toxicity and have some anti-hepatitis B virus activity. However, many other herbs and medicinal foods, including wormwood (*Artemisia absinthium*) and beetroot (*Beta vulagaris*), also have antioxidant and liver-protective activity.

LIQUORICE A review of several randomised trials suggested that glycyrrhizin (an extract of the liquorice plant, *Glycyrrhiza glabra*) may reduce complications in chronic hepatitis C in patients who do not respond adequately to the conventional drug interferon.

Several trials showed that the liver did its job better after treatment with glycyrrhizin. In addition, two studies in 1997 and 2002 showed that long-term treatment with glycyrrhizin might prevent liver cancer in patients with chronic hepatitis C.

> **CAUTION**
>
> Hepatitis is not suitable for self-treament with herbs. Always consult a medical herbalist. See also p.69 before taking a herbal remedy.

Environmental Health

The liver is the body's chemical factory. It is responsible for breaking down and metabolising drugs and for processing environmental and other toxins. These activities can bring it into contact with a variety of hepatotoxins (compounds that are toxic to the liver).

Many hepatotoxins have specific effects on just one area of the liver or on one type of cell in the liver. Others cause a certain type of damage to the liver, such as fatty changes or fibrosis, which are not technically classified as hepatitis but nevertheless put the organ under stress.

People with existing hepatitis should avoid hepatotoxins and anything else that could further injure, or cause stress to, the cells of the liver. In practice, this means eating organically grown foods, avoiding smoky atmospheres, drinking filtered water and not taking drugs or supplements that may be metabolised through the liver, such as alcohol and many common over-the-counter medicines that contain the drug paracetamol.

HEPATOTOXIC MEDICINES Many drugs are hepatotoxic. The most common medications to cause acute or chronic cases of hepatitis are methyldopa, isoniazid, nitrofurantoin, phenytoin and oxyphenisatin.

If you are taking any of these medications, your doctor will routinely test your blood to check your liver enzymes. You should discuss with your doctor the possibility of changing medications if these test show any evidence of liver damage.

HEPATOTOXIC CHEMICALS AND METALS Certain chemicals and metals can also damage the liver. If your job involves working with hepatotoxic chemicals (such as toluene, chloroform, solvent mixtures or trichloroethylene) or heavy metals (such as lead, mercury and manganese), it is very important to follow safety guidance. This might involve protective gloves or suits, glasses, or respirators, which should be used at all times.

If you are exposed to these chemicals or metals heavily or on a regular basis, you should have a blood test to check your liver function for possible damage. An environmental health practitioner can help you take stock of the chemicals you are exposed to and offer avoidance advice. Taking a daily supplement of the herb milk thistle (*see Western Herbal Medicine, above*) can help to protect the liver from damage caused by exposure to toxins.

OTHER HEPATOTOXINS There are certain natural compounds from plants that may be hepatotoxic and should be avoided.

Examples include alflatoxin, which comes from a fungus that infects peanuts and tree nuts, and certain bacteria. To protect yourself from naturally occurring hepatotoxins, be sure that you discard any nuts that appear old, shrivelled or mouldy. Since alcohol is also considered a hepatotoxin, limit the amount of alcohol you drink and avoid it altogether if you have hepatitis.

Acupuncture

Acupuncture is of no proven value in acute infective hepatitis, although it has been used to improve symptoms in a number of patients with hepatitis B and C. It may provide symptom relief, but there is little hard evidence to sustain these claims.

If acupuncture is to be used to help constitutionally with chronic hepatitis, weekly treatments should be provided for at least eight to ten weeks. If after this period there appears to be clinical benefit, then regular constitutional acupuncture may be required on a monthly, or three-monthly basis to help maintain the improvement.

Remember that you should always inform your practitioner if you have an infective form of hepatitis. Particular care should be taken with respect to exposure to blood products and needle disposal when using acupuncture on patients who have hepatitis, so that the infection is not transmitted to others.

> **PREVENTION PLAN**
>
> **The following measures will help to protect you from hepatitis:**
>
> - Observe the rules of hygiene carefully. Always wash your hands after using the toilet and before eating. Make sure your children do this too.
> - Drink alcohol only in moderation.
> - Practise safe sex.
> - If you use intravenous drugs, never share needles.
> - Follow immunisation advice if you are travelling to a developing country where hepatitis A may be prevalent.
> - If you are a healthcare worker, get immunised against hepatitis B.
> - Minimise your use of drugs and herbs that are toxic to the liver.

CYSTITIS

In cystitis, the lining of the bladder becomes inflamed, causing frequent, painful urination. About half of all women have at least one attack of cystitis in their lives, and some women have recurrent attacks. In men, cystitis is rare and is often associated with a disorder of the urinary tract. In some cases of cystitis, short courses of antibiotics may be given. Painkillers may help with any discomfort. There are also herbal, homeopathic, dietary and other strategies to help prevent cystitis from recurring.

WHAT ARE THE SYMPTOMS?

- Burning pain when urinating
- Frequent and urgent need to urinate, with only a little urine passed each time
- A feeling that the bladder has not been emptied completely

If a bacterial infection is causing cystitis, symptoms may also include:

- Pain in the lower abdominal region and sometimes in the low back
- Fever and chills
- Smelly or cloudy urine
- Blood in the urine

WHY MIGHT I HAVE THIS?

PREDISPOSING FACTORS

- Wiping incorrectly after a bowel movement
- Menopause
- Yeast overgrowth
- Diabetes mellitus

TRIGGERS

- Sexual intercourse
- Diaphragm use
- Trigger points in muscles in the pelvic area

IMPORTANT

If you suspect that your child may have cystitis, see a doctor immediately. In children, cystitis needs prompt treatment because it may otherwise progress to a kidney infection and eventually to kidney damage.

WHY DOES IT OCCUR?

Cystitis is often caused by a bacterial infection, most commonly by infection with *Escherichia coli*, which normally lives in the intestines. Women are more likely to be affected than men, probably because they have a shorter urethra (the tube that leads from the bladder to outside the body) which makes it easier for the bacteria to pass up into the bladder. Bacteria from the vaginal or anal areas may enter the bladder during sex or when wiping after a bowel movement. The risk of bacterial cystitis is increased if the bladder is not emptied fully and urine remains in the bladder, where bacteria can multiply.

People with mellitus diabetes may be particularly susceptible to cystitis (among other reasons their urine may contain glucose which the bacteria can feed on). Postmenopausal women may also be at increased risk, due to changes in the urinary tract that occur with age and as a result of lower levels of female sex hormones in the body.

Recurrent bouts of cystitis are often associated with yeast overgrowth in the body. Beneficial bacterial organisms are thought to exert a controlling effect on organisms around the female genitalia that may cause bladder infections, such as *E. coli*. In yeast overgrowth, lower levels of healthy organisms around the urethra make it more likely that unwanted organisms can infect the bladder.

Pelvic pain and frequent urination that do not respond to antibiotics may be due to interstitial cystitis, an uncommon condition in which the lining of the bladder becomes chronically inflamed.

TREATMENT PLAN

PRIMARY TREATMENTS

- Antibiotics (for bacterial cystitis)
- Pure cranberry juice (unsweetened or extract)
- Increased water intake

BACK-UP TREATMENTS

- Bearberry and other Western herbs
- Probiotics
- Dilating the urethra for intersitial cystitis

WORTH CONSIDERING

- Anti-candida diet
- Individualised homeopathy
- Chinese herbal medicine
- Trigger point deactivation

For an explanation of how treatments are rated, see p.111.

SELF-HELP

There are a number of measures that you can take to relieve the discomfort of cystitis.
- Drink plenty of fluids (around two litres per day and more in hot weather). This helps to flush the bacteria out of the bladder. Drinking cranberry juice may be particularly helpful (*see p.240*).
- Pass urine shortly after intercourse and before going to bed.
- Take painkillers and hold something

warm, such as a heating pad or hot water bottle, against your abdomen.

- Avoid caffeinated beverages, which may further irritate the bladder.

TREATMENTS IN DETAIL

Conventional Medicine

PRIMARY TREATMENT **ANTIBIOTICS** The doctor may send a urine sample to be tested for evidence of infection. While waiting for the results he or she may prescribe an antibiotic, which studies show resolve the majority of cases of bacterial cystitis. Another antibiotic may be prescribed once the results are back.

Studies have shown that a long course of low-dose antibiotics, usually for 6–12 months, significantly reduces the rates of recurrent cystitis. Alternatively, if cystitis seems to be related to sexual intercourse, some women may be prescribed antibiotics to take postcoitally. Studies have shown that these can prevent cystitis.

OTHER TREATMENTS Further tests, such as ultrasound scanning, may be recommended to look for an underlying disorder of the urinary tract in women who have recurrent bacterial cystitis or for men who have a single episode. If your doctor suspects that you have interstitial cystitis, he or she may recommend that you see a specialist. Dilating the urethra during cystoscopy (viewing the inside of the bladder through an instrument inserted into the urethra) may be one treatment option. Postmenopausal women may find oestrogen creams applied around the urethra helps to relieve their symptoms.

Nutritional Therapy

PRIMARY TREATMENT **DRINKING WATER** throughout the day can help to flush out organisms in and around the bladder and the urethra before they can cause infection. Aim to drink at least two litres of water each day.

ELIMINATING YEAST FROM THE BODY Clinical experience suggests that taking steps to control yeast organisms, such as *Candida albicans*, in the body can help to prevent recurrent urinary tract infections (*for information, see p.40*).

THE URINARY TRACT

The kidneys filter waste products from the blood and pass them into the bladder, with excess water, as urine. The urinary tract consists of the two kidneys, the ureters (which connect the kidneys and bladder), the bladder and the urethra (which leads from the bladder to outside the body). The lower urinary tract differs in men and women. In men, the urethra is longer and passes through the prostate gland. In women, the shorter urethra passes directly to the opening in front of the vagina.

Sexual differences

The male bladder sits above the prostate gland and the male urethra passes through it. The male urethra is about 20cm (8in) long and carries either urine or semen out through the penis.

The female bladder sits below the uterus and the female urethra carries urine directly to an opening located in front of the vagina. In women, the urethra is about 4cm (1½ in) long.

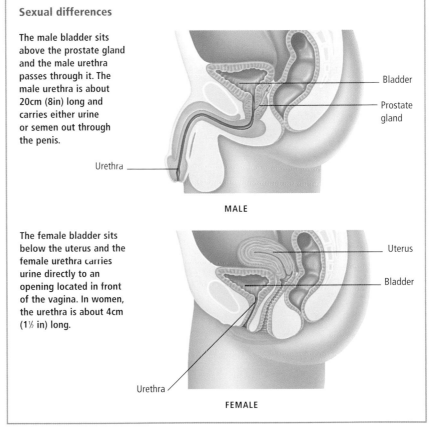

MALE

FEMALE

PROBIOTICS are supplements containing "healthy bacteria" which seem to be particularly useful in controlling unwanted organisms. Probiotic organisms are believed to compete with and crowd out the unhealthy organisms around the vagina, hence helping to prevent infection. Probiotic micro-organisms, such as *lactobacilli*, also make the bladder environment more acidic, and this helps to prevent the growth of unwanted organisms. In one study, weekly probiotic pessaries containing *lactobacillus* reduced the recurrence rate of cystitis infections in women.

Herbal Medicine

TRADITIONAL HERBS for cystitis and urinary tract infections (UTI) include agrimony (*Agrimonia eupatoria*), barleywater (made from barley, *Hordeum distychum*), bearberry (*Arctostaphylos uva ursi*), bilberry (*Vaccinium myrtillus*) fruit and leaves, buchu (*Agathosma betulina*), couchgrass (*Agropyron repens*), cranberry (*Vaccinium macrocarpon*), garlic (*Allium sativum*), goldenrod (*Solidago virgaurea*), golden seal (*Hydrastis canadensis*), heather flowers (ling, *Calluna vulgaris*), horsetail (*Equisetum arvense*), hydrangea (*Hydrangea arborescens*), juniper (*Juniperus communis*), ladies mantle (*Alchemilla xanthochlora*), marshmallow root (*Althea officinalis*), matico leaves (*Piper angustifolia*), nettle (*Urtica dioica*), parsley (*Petroselinum crispum*), parsley piert (*Alchmilla arvensis*), pellitory of the wall (*Parietaria judaica*), pipsissewa (*Chimaphila umbellata*), plan-

The bacterium *E. coli.* is one of the main causes of cystitis. It normally inhabits the intestines without causing problems, but may infect the bladder by travelling up the urinary tract.

tain (*Plantago lanceolata*), shepherd's purse (*Capsella bursa-pastoris*), wild carrot (*Daucus carota*) and yarrow (*Achillea millefolium*). To date, few of these herbal remedies have been investigated for the treatment of UTI, but given the emergence of strains of bacteria resistant to antibiotic treatment, research should be carried out into this largely untapped and potentially invaluable resource.

PRIMARY TREATMENT **CRANBERRY JUICE** is perhaps the best-researched remedy for the treatment of UTI. It is a nutraceutical (functional food), bought as much for its reputation for allaying urinary tract infections as for its taste. It was once assumed that cranberry was effective because it acidified the urine, thereby inhibiting bacterial growth. However, it has been discovered recently that its action is probably due to its condensed tannins, (proanthocyanidins), which appear to prevent the adherence of harmful bacteria to urinary epithelial cells. If bacteria cannot stick to the walls of the urinary tract, they are washed out of the system.

Conclusions are mixed. A Cochrane systematic review of research on the use of cranberry juice for urinary infections has highlighted significant flaws in the accumulated data. The reviewers commented that the small number and poor quality of the trials gave no reliable evidence for the use of cranberry juice or other cranberry products in the treatment of UTI. Nevertheless, data from laboratory studies and clinical trials (including one published after the Cochrane review) seem to support the use of cranberry. More research, however, is needed to test its efficacy.

People who are subject to recurrent UTI who are prescribed long-term antibiotic therapy, are ideal candidates to try cranberry treatment. Two to three glasses of juice a day should be sufficient. Those with diabetes should use sugar-free prepara-

tions. A recent Canadian trial revealed that cranberry tablets provided the most cost-effective prevention for UTI.

OTHER REMEDIES Bearberry is a close relative of cranberry with a similar longstanding reputation for curing UTI. It has exhibited an antibacterial action on a wide range of infecting organisms including *Staphylococcus aureus*, *Bacillus subtilis*, *Escherichia coli*, *Mycobacterium smegmatis*, *Shigella sonnei* and *Shigella flexneri*.

In a study, a herbal mix that included bearberry, hops (*Humulus lupulus*) and peppermint (*Mentha piperita*) was used to treat patients with enuresis and painful and difficult urination. About 70 per cent of the 915 patients who participated reported improvement after six weeks of treatment with this regime..

Buchu (*Agathosma betulina*) is a traditional remedy of the indigenous people of South Africa and was taken for UTI by the early Dutch settlers there. In a laboratory study an alcoholic extract of buchu was found to be effective against infecting organisms causing UTI.

Nettle leaf has been approved in Germany for inflammatory disease of the lower urinary tract and prevention of kidney gravel, and is useful for chronic cystitis. Couchgrass (*Elymus repens*) is also recommended in Germany for UTI.

Golden seal has a reputation as a urinary antiseptic. This herb contains a substance known as berberine, which has a broad-spectrum action against many bacteria, including *E. coli*.

CAUTION

● See p.69 before taking a herbal remedy. If you are already taking a prescribed medication, consult a herbalist first.

● Do not take bearberry for more than 10 days. Do not take it if you are pregnant, breast-feeding or trying to conceive.

● If symptoms do not ease within two days of taking herbal remedies, see your doctor.

Almost half of all women will have an attack of cystitis at some point in their lives

Chinese Herbal Medicine

In Traditional Chinese Medicine (TCM), *Lin* disease (*Lin Zheng*) includes a variety of disorders characterised by pain associated with urination, some of which correspond to cystitis and UTI.

There are several varieties of *Lin* disease, but heat is characteristic of most of them. TCM doctors distinguish between "full" (*Shi*) and "empty" (*Xu*) conditions. There are three varieties of heat *Lin*: damp heat, heart fire and liver fire.

Some people repeatedly have persistent symptoms of cystitis despite several courses of antibiotics. In such cases it may be that there are no harmful bacteria causing the condition; in western medicine this is known as interstitial cystitis. This phenomenon may be due to other *Lin* patterns, one of which is liver *Qi* stagnation (*Qi Lin*). Once again, this has an emotional basis. The classic prescription for this condition is Aquilaria Powder (*Chang Xiang San*). Another pattern that may occur in chronic cystitis which may not respond to antibiotic treatment is fatigue *Lin*. After making a diagnosis, the TCM doctor would treat the underlying cause, which may be kidney *Yin*, *Qi* or *Yang* deficiency or spleen deficiency.

> **CAUTION**
>
> Consult a Chinese herbal practitioner before taking a remedy for cystitis. (*See also p.69.*)

Homeopathy

Homeopathy can be particularly helpful in interstitial cystitis, in which no infective organism can be found but urination is frequent and painful nonetheless.

STAPHYSAGRIA (made from a type of wild delphinium) is the most frequently used treatment. A clinical trial conducted by Ustianowski in the UK showed it to be effective. It helps when symptoms include a constant desire to pass urine. Symptoms are frequently triggered by trauma (including sexual intercourse), and there may be a background of anger or indignation that is sometimes related to previous sexual assault or abuse. The anger may be apparent or suppressed.

OTHER REMEDIES *Equisetum* is often helpful in chronic or recurrent cystitis in children, which may be associated with bed wetting. Pain at the end of urination is typical of the type of cystitis that responds to this medicine.

Cantharis is the classical homeopathic medicine for acute cystitis with severe pain on passing urine and tenesmus, which is the sensation of needing to urinate again as soon as you have finished.

Bodywork Therapies

TRIGGER POINTS are sensitive spots in the muscles which can refer pain to other parts of the body (*see p.55*). As far back as the early 1950s there were reports that symptoms similar to those of cystitis could be the result of trigger-point activity in the muscles of the abdomen.

The leading researchers into trigger points report: "Urinary frequency, urinary urgency and 'kidney' pain may be referred from trigger points in the skin of the lower abdominal muscles. Injection of an old appendectomy scar… has relieved frequency and urgency, and increased the bladder capacity from 240ml to 420ml.

More recent research confirms these findings and has shown how the effects of trigger-point activity can spread. In some cases trigger-point activity may have effects that reach well beyond obvious muscle and joint pain.

TRIGGER-POINT DEACTIVATION Symptoms resulting from trigger points, such as those of cystitis, may be relieved manually, as well as by injection. A recent study involved 42 people with "chronic cystitis" whose main symptoms were painful urgency and frequency. Following manual treatment of trigger points in the pelvic muscles, 35 of these people (83 per cent) reported moderate to marked improvement, with some being completely relieved, after up to 14 years of experiencing these symptoms.

Trigger points can be deactivated using acupuncture as well as by using various manual pressure and stretching techniques. These are used by osteopaths, massage therapists (particularly those with neuromuscular therapy training) and some physiotherapists and chiropractors. Check whether your practitioner uses these techniques before commencing on a course of treatment.

CHIROPRACTIC AND OSTEOPATHY If you experience recurring attacks of cystitis, it may be that you have a back problem that is either causing or contributing to it. The nerve supply to the bladder derives from the low back, and some studies have suggested that irritation of these low back nerves can also affect bladder function. A chiropractor, osteopath or a physiotherapist trained to use manipulative techniques could evaluate your condition and advise or treat you accordingly, depending on what is found.

> ### The South African herb buchu was first exported to the UK as a remedy for cystitis in 1790

> **PREVENTION PLAN**
>
> **If you are prone to cystitis, try the following:**
>
> - Drink plenty of fluids, especially in hot weather. Drinking cranberry juice may help in particular.
> - Avoid sugar and tea and coffee.
> - Always wipe from front to back after a bowel movement.
> - Avoid wearing tight jeans or trousers.
> - Urinate after intercourse and before going to bed.
> - Empty your bladder frequently and completely.
> - Do not use perfumed toiletries or bubble baths.
> - Do not use douches.
> - Avoid becoming constipated.

Circulatory System

Circulating blood carries food and oxygen to all parts of the body. Problems can develop if the heart loses its power or rhythm, or if the flow through the vessels is disrupted. Surgery and powerful drugs are available for certain circulatory illnesses and a healthy lifestyle and complementary therapies help to restore health and well-being.

WHAT ARE THE SYMPTOMS?

High blood pressure does not usually cause symptoms, but if your blood pressure is very high you may have:

- Headaches
- Nosebleeds
- Dizziness
- Blurred vision

WHY MIGHT I HAVE THIS?

PREDISPOSING FACTORS

- Smoking
- A diet high in salt
- Lack of exercise
- Excess weight
- Being over 60
- Drinking too much alcohol
- Excess caffeine
- Nutrient deficiency

TRIGGERS

- Stress

TREATMENT PLAN

PRIMARY TREATMENTS

- Lifestyle changes (*see Self-Help*)
- Oral drugs

BACK-UP TREATMENTS

- Nutritional therapy
- Aerobic exercise
- Hawthorn

WORTH CONSIDERING

- Homeopathy
- Western herbal medicine
- Environmental health
- Acupuncture
- Bodywork therapies
- Yoga-type breathing
- Mind–body therapies

For an explanation of how treatments are rated, see p.111.

HIGH BLOOD PRESSURE

Persistently high blood pressure, also known as hypertension, affects as many as 1 in 5 adults in the UK. It puts strain on the heart and arteries, and can damage delicate tissues, such as the eyes and kidneys. The higher the pressure, the greater the risk that serious complications, such as a heart attack or stroke, will develop. Integrated treatments offer very real ways of lowering blood pressure. They include lifestyle changes, drugs, supplements, regular exercise, osteopathy, chiropractic, massage, herbs, homeopathy, yoga and other stress-reduction techniques.

WHY DOES IT OCCUR?

Blood pressure varies naturally with activity, rising during exercise or times of stress and falling when we rest. It also varies among individuals and increases with increasing weight.

In most people with high blood pressure, there is no obvious cause for the condition. However, lifestyle and genetic factors may both contribute. High blood pressure increases with age and is more common in men than women. It tends to run in families, and people of Asian and Afro-Caribbean descent are more at risk of developing high blood pressure than Caucasians. Risk factors for the condition include stress, a high alcohol intake, a diet high in salt and excess weight.

Older people are more prone to high blood pressure because the arteries become less flexible with age. The condition may be aggravated by too much stress. In a few cases, kidney disease or a hormonal disorder may be the cause. Some drugs, including combined oral contraceptives and corticosteroids, may also cause high blood pressure.

BLOOD PRESSURE IN PREGNANCY High blood pressure may occur in pregnancy, for reasons that are largely unknown. The high blood pressure may form part of pre-eclampsia, which is a condition that may occasionally cause convulsions if the blood pressure becomes very high, and must be monitored closely by a doctor. However, not all pregnant women with high blood pressure have pre-eclampsia. Blood pressure usually returns to normal after the birth, but the condition may recur in subsequent pregnancies.

IMPORTANT

If you are experiencing symptoms that suggest your blood pressure may be high, consult your doctor as soon as possible to have it checked.

SELF-HELP

PRIMARY TREATMENT Try the following to reduce the risk of high blood pressure and coronary artery disease (*see p.252*):

- Achieve a healthy weight.
- Eat a diet low in salt and saturated fat, and rich in vegetables, fruit and oily fish.
- Drink alcohol in moderation (less than 21 units per week for men and 14 units per week for women).
- Take regular exercise (mainly dynamic exercise, such as brisk walking).
- If you smoke, stop.

TREATMENTS IN DETAIL

Conventional Medicine

When your blood pressure is raised, your doctor will make an assessment to exclude an underlying cause, to look for risk factors and to assess whether vulnerable organs – in particular the heart, eyes and kidneys – have been damaged.

Your blood pressure, unless it becomes very high, will be monitored on a number of occasions. Your doctor will also advise you on self-help measures to lower your blood pressure before drug treatment is considered. These include maintaining a healthy weight, moderate alcohol intake and taking regular exercise.

| PRIMARY TREATMENT | **ORAL DRUGS** If the self-help measures (*see left*) fail to lower |

ORAL DRUGS If the self-help measures (*see left*) fail to lower your blood pressure sufficiently, or if your blood pressure is very high, your doctor may prescribe drugs. When you start the drugs, and which drugs you take, depends on various factors, including the level of your blood pressure, your age and the presence of other diseases. Various drugs can control blood pressure and so reduce the risk of organ and tissue damage.

Thiazide diuretics, such as bendroflu-azide, are often the first drugs to be prescribed. They have been found to reduce the risk of stroke associated with hypertension. They cause the kidneys to excrete more water and salts than usual, so reducing the volume of circulating blood.

Antihypertensives may be prescribed in preference, or in addition, to diuretics. Antihypertensives work in various ways – most dilate (widen) the blood vessels throughout the body or reduce the force with which the heart pumps blood. Your doctor will weigh the side-effects of anti-hypertensives against the potential benefits, such as reducing the risk of a stroke or coronary artery disease.

Groups of antihypertensives include:
- Beta-blockers, such as atenolol, which have been shown to reduce the risk of complications in people with hyperten-sion. These block the effect of adrenaline and noradrenaline, two chemicals pro-duced by the body that increase heart rate and raise blood pressure.
- Angiotensin-converting enzyme (ACE) inhibitors, such as captopril, which dilate the body's blood vessels so that the blood pressure falls.
- Calcium-channel blockers, such as nifedipine, which block the entry of cal-cium ions into the muscle in arterial walls. The muscles relax, thereby allow-ing the walls to dilate and causing the blood pressure to fall.
- Others include alpha-blockers, such as doxazosin, and angiotensin II receptor blockers, such as losartan.

Aspirin (75mg) may be prescribed for some people with high blood pressure. It is not suitable for everyone as there may be a risk of bleeding from the digestive tract. However, it is often recommended for those who are shown to be at particular risk of coronary artery disease (*see p.252*) and stroke (*see p.148*).

HOW THE HEART PUMPS BLOOD

In every heart beat there are two main phases as the blood is pumped out of the ventricles (systole) and then as blood fills the atria (diastole). One-way valves between the chambers of the heart open and close in sequence, controlling the direction of blood flow. The timing of the systolic contractions and diastolic relaxation are synchronised by the heart's pacemaker (known as the sino-atrial node), which sends out electrical impulses to the muscles in the atria and ventricles.

The cycle of the beating heart

In systole, the left ventricle pumps oxygenated blood into the aorta and the right ventricle pumps deoxygenated blood into the pulmonary arteries.

Aorta

Pulmonary artery

Mitral valve

Oxygenated blood entering the aorta

Left ventricle

Pulmonary valve

Deoxygenated blood entering the pulmonary arteries

Right ventricle

SYSTOLE

In diastole, the heart relaxes, allowing the right atrium to fill with blood from the body and the left atrium to fill with blood from the lungs.

Aorta

Left atrium

Oxygenated blood from the lungs

Mitral valve

Right atrium

Tricuspid valve

Deoxygenated blood returns from the body

DIASTOLE

Lipid-lowering drugs, such as statins, may also be prescribed where appropriate, to reduce the risks of atherosclerosis.

> **CAUTION**
>
> Drugs to combat high blood pressure have a range of side-effects: ask your doctor to explain these to you.

Nutritional Therapy

LOWER SALT LEVELS Some people have salt-sensitive hypertension, which responds well to reducing dietary salt. One meta-analysis that pooled the results of several trials showed that reducing salt in the diet to around 5g per day had a significant effect on blood pressure in individuals

MEASUREMENT OF BLOOD PRESSURE

Blood pressure is expressed as two values given as millimetres of mercury (mmHg). The upper figure, known as the systolic pressure, refers to the pressure of the blood when the heart contracts. The lower figure, known as the diastolic pressure, refers to the pressure of the blood when the heart muscle relaxes between contractions. The blood pressure of a young adult should not be more than about 120/80 mmHg. Definitions vary but, in general, high blood pressure is defined as being higher than 140/90 mmHg.

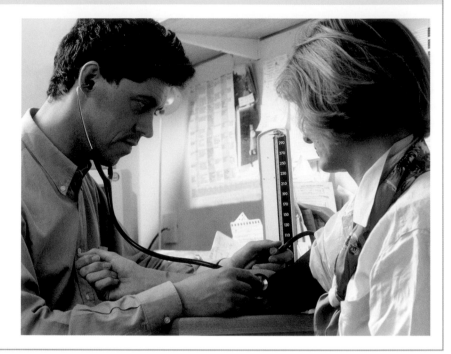

An inflatable cuff is wrapped around the upper arm. The doctor listens to the blood flow through a stethoscope. When he can hear the heart beat he records the systolic pressure, when the sound disappears he notes the diastolic pressure.

both with and without high blood pressure. If possible, reduce your salt intake by not adding salt during cooking or at the table. Avoid processed and packaged foods as these tend to have a high salt content.

RAISE POTASSIUM LEVELS While the sodium in salt tends to raise blood pressure, potassium tends to lower it. One study shows that eating a diet that is rich in potassium (one with plenty of fresh fruits and vegetables), in conjunction with a low-sodium diet, can help to reduce blood pressure.

REDUCE CAFFEINE A review of many trials indicates that coffee consumption (average five cups a day) increases blood pressure and could therefore contribute to hypertension. In trials with younger participants, the effect of coffee drinking on blood pressure was greater than normal. People with hypertension are recommended to reduce or eliminate coffee from their diet.

SUPPLEMENTS Calcium has been reported to help reduce blood pressure, although not by much. However, individuals seemingly sensitive to salt may get significant benefit. Try taking 1,000mg of calcium supplements per day for a 12-week period.

Magnesium supplements may also help to reduce blood pressure. The recommended dose is 300–500mg of magnesium supplements per day. Another nutritional agent that may help is Coenzyme Q10. The recommended dose is 50mg of Coenzyme Q10 supplements, taken twice a day.

One systematic review has found that fish-oil supplementation in doses of 3g daily modestly lowers blood pressure.

> **CAUTION**
>
> Consult your doctor before taking fish oil, calcium, magnesium and CoQ10, because they can interfere with other medications (see p.46).

Homeopathy

If you have high blood pressure, consult a practitioner for a suitable remedy.

BARYTA CARBONICA, according to one study, helps to reduce high blood pressure in certain people. The medicine is effective in patients with arteriosclerosis (hardening of the arteries) and helps people who are mentally slow and timid, and whose feet sweat offensively.

SULPHUR People who respond to *Sulphur* are sensitive to heat. They also dislike it. They tend to have congestive phenomena, such as congested haemorrhoids, red lips, congestive headaches and burning feet. (*See also Constitutions and constitutional prescribing, p.73.*)

AURUM MURIATICUM People who respond to *Aur. mur.* often have palpitations or extrasystoles. They may be deeply depressed, lacking in self-confidence and bad tempered – they can get very angry over small things. They feel worse in winter and may suffer from sinusitis.

LACHESIS is often appropriate for women with high blood pressure that starts in the perimenopausal period, although it can also be used for men. People who respond to *Lachesis* are generally excitable and loquacious. (*See also Constitutions and constitutional prescribing, p.73.*)

GLONOINUM is a symptomatic medicine that is usually given in fairly low dilution (6C), two or three times daily. The kind of symptoms that suggest *Glonoinum* may be appropriate include throbbing or pulsating in the head or neck, and attacks of glowing heat in the face.

Western Herbal Medicine

DIAGNOSIS Herbal practitioners use a wide range of medicinal plants to normalise blood pressure, whether it is high or low. As in most cases no identifiable cause can be found for raised blood pressure, the selection of specific remedies depends upon assessment of immediate needs, such as relaxation and weight loss, and of underlying factors, such as constipation.

The herbal practitioner assesses your pulse and blood pressure over several visits, as well as checking your cholesterol, LDL, HDL and triglyceride levels (*see p.34*). These are linked to other signs that reflect your overall state of health. Important factors here include signs of oxidative damage and atherosclerosis; the tone of the capillaries; venous congestion; constipation; and nerve and muscle tone. When kidney or endocrine factors lie behind raised blood pressure, these require treatment in their own right.

HAWTHORN Regarded as a "food for the heart", hawthorn (*Crataegus spp.*) is an antioxidant that also tones the heart (cardiotonic) and dilates the blood vessels (vasodilator). As a result, it is a key treatment for hypertension associated with atherosclerosis. It is also a recommended treatment whenever there is a long-term increased load on the heart (*see Coronary artery disease, p.252*).

OTHER REMEDIES Garlic (*Allium sativum*) has been intensively investigated for its ability to lower raised cholesterol and triglycerides (often present alongside high blood pressure) and several studies support its use as an antihypertensive.

Dandelion (*Taraxacum officinale*) leaf has traditionally been used as a diuretic, which helps to reduce blood pressure. Clinical studies since the 1950s have confirmed this activity. Rich in potassium, dandelion leaf is thought to minimise the risk of potassium loss that is commonly associated with diuretics.

Cramp bark (*Viburnum opulus*) is an antispasmodic herb that herbalists use to relax the muscles in the walls of arteries. Limeflowers (*Tilia europea*) are diaphoretic (they promote sweating) and relaxant, with the potential to lower elevated systolic blood pressure.

> **CAUTION**
>
> See page 69 before taking a herbal remedy and, if you are already taking a prescribed medication, consult a medical herbalist first. Extracts of hawthorn may interact with other medicines.

Environmental Health

The causes of high blood pressure are difficult to ascertain, as conventional medicine acknowledges when using the generic term "essential hypertension" to describe the seemingly complex and undescribed causes of this common problem. However, there are some compelling environmental associations with high blood pressure that warrant a close look.

LEAD As with so many other diseases, there is ample evidence that some hypertension is linked to long-term lead exposure. Do the following to minimise your exposure:
- Limit your exposure to lead-containing paints in older homes.
- Before using, run water for at least a minute through household pipes that may contain lead-containing solder.
- Only drink cold, not hot, tap water (or filter your water with an approved portable filter or reverse osmosis system).
- Avoid leaded crystal or improperly glazed ceramic dishes for eating or drinking.
- Check that remedies, including calcium supplements, are free from lead.
- Take precautions if you use lead solder either in a hobby or professionally.

Exposure to significant amounts of lead can be detected by testing the blood or, in cases of long-term exposure, by measuring the amount of lead that as been incorporated into bone. Chelation (binding a metal and filtering it from the bloodstream by chemical means) is one way of dealing with lead in the body, but there is no guarantee that this will work, even in acute high-dose lead poisoning.

Supplementing your diet with calcium (*see Osteoporosis for RDA table, p.309*) may work, since it takes preference over lead when the metals are absorbed and incorporated in the body.

CADMIUM Several studies suggest that cadmium may be involved in causing some high blood pressure. To limit your level of cadmium, avoid zinc-processing plants and eat organ meats and shellfish only in moderation. If you are a smoker, stop.

If you are exposed to cadmium, take lead-free calcium supplements in recommended amounts (*see Osteoporosis for RDA table, p.309*). Do not exceed the recommended daily allowance for calcium because too much calcium can cause cardiac and other problems.

POLYCHLORINATED BIPHENYLS (PCBS) A strong incentive for everyone to convert to a vegetarian diet is the correlation between PCB levels and high blood pressure. PCBs are most often found in animal fat and in certain fish.

AIR POLLUTION Some evidence suggests that exposure to air pollution directly relates to elevated blood pressure. People with heart disease are more susceptible to worsening cardiac problems and even death from dangerous levels of air pollution. There are several reports of unexpectedly large numbers of people succumbing to heart disease during periods of intense air pollution.

COLD WEATHER Exposure to cold temperatures may be linked with one of the dreaded complications of high blood pressure – ischaemic stroke (*see p.148*). Blood pressure varies more than normal in colder temperatures, which may account for the increase in cardiac and stroke afflictions during the winter. If you are likely to be affected, then you should "take it easy" and avoid strenuous exercise during especially cold weather.

Each kilogram of weight you lose can lower your blood pressure by 2.5/1.5 mmHg

Acupuncture

Established high blood pressure may produce a range of different symptoms, some of which can clearly be relieved by acupuncture. These may include excessive fatigue and headaches. However, there is no evidence that the use of acupuncture alone, even in the long term, will produce a sustained and safe normal blood pressure.

Acupuncture may help if it is combined, in a prolonged treatment, with appropriate dietary and conventional medicine. Occasionally, acupuncture treatment may relieve the adverse reactions from antihypertensive drugs.

Acupuncture really needs to be used on a weekly basis, and probably for eight to ten weeks, to obtain a consistent initial

as effective in lowering blood pressure in people with mild hypertension as the use of medication.

As well as the breathing benefits, the movements and postures of traditional yoga can produce a significant lowering of blood pressure, often sufficient to allow a reduction in medication.

Aerobic Exercise

In one study, mildly hypertensive white women who exercised aerobically for 30 minutes could reduce their blood pressure for up to seven hours. A later study showed this response to be different in black women, whose blood pressure rose or stayed the same – in fact, aerobic exercise may adversely affect their blood pressure.

blood pressure, but who reported high baseline levels of hopelessness, were three times as likely to develop high blood pressure over four years of follow-up.

In many respects, anger–hostility, depression–hopelessness and anxiety can be viewed as the emotional and behavioural consequences of stress. In other words, they are what happens when people perceive that they do not have the internal or external resources to meet the demands or challenges of life.

Experiencing occasional feelings of anger, worry and sadness is normal. However, when these mood states become more frequent or even chronic, it is a clue that normal life stresses and challenges are no longer being managed effectively. This chronic activation of the stress response can not only wear away at the quality of mental and emotional health and well-being, but can also have a significant effect on physical health and well-being, especially cardiovascular health.

> # High blood pressure affects approximately three-quarters of people over the age of 75

response. If acupuncture treatment is proving effective, then it will often need to be repeated on a monthly basis for a very prolonged period, in order to help control blood pressure.

Bodywork Therapies

There is evidence to suggest that osteopathic manipulation, focused on those spinal areas where the nerve supply to the kidneys emerges, may help to reduce high blood pressure. This manipulation encourages the kidneys' role in fluid elimination. Cranial manipulation (chiropractic sacrooccipital technique) can reduce high blood pressure to normal in some cases.

Any therapy that reduces stress will probably lower high blood pressure, if only temporarily. For example, massage has been shown to effectively reduce diastolic blood pressure (the lower of the two figures when blood pressure is measured).

Yoga-type Breathing

A simple yoga-type breathing method may help to lower your blood pressure after a stressful episode. Slowing the rate of breathing (see Anxiety, p.414) appears to be

Weight loss is helpful in reducing high blood pressure. Exercise is better than dieting – research reveals that aerobic exercise is more effective at helping reach a healthy weight than a low-calorie diet alone.

Finally, there is another benefit of exercise for people with high blood pressure. Between 20 per cent and 45 per cent of people experience "white coat hypertension" – their blood pressure rises when tested by a nurse or physician. Research has shown that this tendency reduces markedly if they take regular exercise.

Mind–Body Therapies

STRESS Each day the relationship between stress, emotions, such as anger and hostility, and cardiovascular health are becoming increasingly clear. The link between anger–hostility and heart disease is well documented (see Coronary artery disease, p.252). In addition, people who are very hostile are also more likely to engage in unhealthy lifestyle behaviour, such as smoking and eating a high-fat diet.

Studies have also shown a link between increased feelings of hopelessness and cardiovascular disease. One Finnish study showed that men who did not have high

JOB STRAIN is a type of stress characterised by situations of high demand (excessive amounts of work) but low control (little input about the workload). One study focused on 40 men who had mild to moderate high blood pressure while they were at work. When these men were faced with tasks they felt were dictated by external demands they had little control over, their blood pressures increased. When they were faced with tasks that they felt they could meet with their own self-pacing (internal control), their blood pressures remained normal to borderline high.

SENSE OF CONTROL Practising mind–body skills, such as relaxation and yoga, can help to restore a sense of control and calm. They provide a safe and effective means of maintaining normal blood pressure levels, even in demanding work situations.

PREVENTION PLAN

To prevent high blood pressure:

- Eat a diet low in salt and saturated fat, high in fruit, vegetables and oily fish.
- Exercise regularly.
- Give up smoking if you are a smoker.

ANGINA

Angina is a chest pain that is often brought on by physical activity and is relieved by rest. The pain is due to an inadequate supply of oxygen to the heart muscle that usually results from coronary artery disease (*see p.252*). The flow of oxygen-rich blood to the heart may be adequate when the body is at rest, but becomes inadequate during exertion. The integrated approach to treatment combines lifestyle measures and drugs, such as aspirin, beta-blockers and nitrates, with nutritional supplements and stress-relieving therapies, such as relaxation.

WHAT ARE THE SYMPTOMS?

- A heavy or tight pain in the middle of the chest that may spread to the neck and down one or both arms, usually the left
- The pain may be accompanied by breathlessness
- If severe, angina may also occur when resting

WHY MIGHT I HAVE THIS?

PREDISPOSING FACTORS

- Smoking
- A diet high in fats
- Lack of exercise
- Excess weight
- High blood pressure
- Diabetes mellitus

TRIGGERS

- Physical exertion
- Cold, windy weather
- Extreme emotions, such as excitement
- Blood-sugar imbalance

IMPORTANT

If you develop the symptoms of angina, see your doctor without delay. If you have established angina, and attacks become more frequent than usual or occur at rest, or if you have a severe attack or pain that is not relieved by your fast-acting nitrate spray or tablets, seek medical help immediately.

WHY DOES IT OCCUR?

When deposits of fatty acids build up on the internal walls of the coronary arteries – a process called atherosclerosis – they form plaques that consequently restrict the flow of blood to the heart. Angina is likely to occur when the coronary arteries are too narrow to allow the heart muscle to receive the oxygen it needs during exercise.

Angina is less common in women than in men until the age of 60. This is thought to be due to the protective effect of the female hormone oestrogen. After the menopause, the protective effect wears off.

Smoking, a diet high in fats, lack of exercise and excess weight are all risk factors for coronary artery disease and angina, as are high blood pressure (*see p.244*) and diabetes mellitus (*see p.314*). Angina is often brought on by physical exertion, but may be triggered or worsened by exposure to cold temperatures, windy weather and extreme emotions, such as excitement.

IMMEDIATE RELIEF

Angina is usually relieved by rest and using a fast-acting nitrate spray or tablet. If the pain persists despite these measures, seek medical attention urgently.

TREATMENTS IN DETAIL

Conventional Medicine

TESTS If your doctor suspects angina, you will need to undergo various investigations. Blood tests will look for various conditions, such as high cholesterol levels and diabetes mellitus.

An electrocardiogram, or ECG, is a recording of the electrical rhythm of the heart that is routinely taken when heart problems are suspected. It is likely to be normal between episodes of angina. However, an ECG taken while you exercise on a treadmill may indicate the presence of coronary artery disease and its severity.

TREATMENT PLAN

PRIMARY TREATMENTS

- Lifestyle changes
- Oral drugs for symptom relief and prevention

BACK-UP TREATMENTS

- Angioplasty
- Coronary artery bypass grafting
- Blood-sugar stabilising diet
- Magnesium and coenzyme Q10 supplements

- Breathing retraining
- Mind–body therapies

WORTH CONSIDERING

- L-arginine and L-carnitine
- Exercise
- Bodywork therapies
- Acupuncture

For an explanation of how treatments are rated, see p.111.

Echocardiography (ultrasound scanning of the heart) may be used to assess the functioning of the heart muscle. Sometimes, coronary angiography may be needed. This involves injecting a dye into a blood vessel in the arm or groin. The dye's progress through the coronary arteries is monitored on a screen and recorded on X-rays. Coronary angiography may be used to confirm the diagnosis and will show where and to what extent the arteries have become narrow.

PRIMARY TREATMENT | **LIFESTYLE CHANGES** You will need to take stock of your lifestyle and make real changes: if you are a smoker, then stop; if you lead a sedentary life, take regular exercise (under medical advice); and, if you need to, lose weight. Your doctor may prescribe drugs to help lower your lipid levels as well as suggest a low-fat diet (*see Cardioprotective Diets, p.254 and The Ornish approach, p.256*).

PRIMARY TREATMENT | **ORAL DRUGS** Taking 75mg of aspirin every day can reduce the risk of a myocardial infarction (heart attack). Fast-acting nitrate drugs, in the form of a spray or tablet, are used to relieve the pain when it occurs.

You may be prescribed one of a variety of drugs to prevent angina from occurring. There are three main drug groups.

Beta-blockers, such as atenolol, reduce the heart's rate and the force with which it contracts. This puts less stress on the heart muscle, reducing its demand for oxygen.

Long-acting nitrates, such as isosorbide mononitrate, relax the walls of the coronary arteries (so improving the blood supply to the heart muscle) and widen the blood vessels around the body, making it easier for the heart to pump blood.

Calcium-channel blockers, such as amlodopine and diltiazem, also relax the walls of the coronary arteries and reduce the force of contraction of the heart. Some also make the heart beat more slowly.

ANGIOPLASTY aims to relieve angina by widening the affected arteries (*see p.253*). A catheter with a deflated balloon at its end is inserted through an artery in the groin and then passed through the circulation to the affected coronary artery. It is inflated several times to widen the narrowed artery. The doctor is guided by images on a

An angiogram is a contrast X-ray that is used to detect abnormalities, such as narrowing, in the coronary arteries. Dye is injected into the blood vessels to make them clearly visible on an X-ray.

screen. There is a relatively small risk of myocardial infarction or of a split in the artery, which necessitates bypass grafting. Sometimes, a tube called a stent is placed in the artery to keep it open and to reduce the risk of it becoming narrowed again.

CORONARY ARTERY BYPASS GRAFTING A blood vessel taken from the leg or chest is used to bypass the narrowed part of the artery. This graft, which may last 8–10 years, may be offered if symptoms are still present despite drug therapy and if angioplasty is inappropriate. There may be a small risk of a stroke.

> **CAUTION**
>
> Drugs for angina can cause side-effects: ask your doctor to explain them to you.

Nutritional Therapy

A BLOOD-SUGAR BALANCING DIET may help to control angina. When blood-sugar levels fall, adrenaline stimulates the liver to release sugar but may trigger angina because it increases the oxygen demands of the heart muscle and can induce spasm in the coronary arteries. (*See also p.42.*)

MAGNESIUM SUPPLEMENTS are often useful in treating angina. Important for energy production in the body, magnesium also enhances the function of the heart muscle and reduces the risk of spasm and constriction in the coronary arteries. There is some evidence that magnesium deficiency may be a factor in angina. A randomised, double-blind trial performed in the US, Israel and Austria found that taking 365mg of magnesium citrate a day for six months lessened exercise-induced angina and increased exercise duration. The recommended dose is 500–1,000mg of magnesium per day.

COENZYME Q10 (COQ10) is another nutrient that is essential for energy production in the body. One study showed that taking 150mg of CoQ10 per day significantly lengthened the amount of time it took for angina to come on during exercise.

L-ARGININE, an amino acid, may be useful for people with angina. It appears to operate by helping blood vessels dilate, which might enable more blood to reach the heart muscle. L-arginine supplements have been shown to help people with angina to exercise without pain. The recommended dose is 2g of L-arginine per day.

L-CARNITINE supplements can help transport fat into parts of the body's cells called mitochondria, where energy is produced. Studies show that taking 1g of L-carnitine twice a day can improve heart function and reduce angina symptoms.

> **CAUTION**
>
> Consult your doctor before taking magnesium or Coenzyme Q10 with either warfarin or ciproflaxin (*see p.46*).

Breathing Retraining

There is evidence that spinal or soft-tissue problems can produce symptoms identical to those of "real" (i.e. cardiac) angina. Called pseudoangina, chest pains that mimic angina can occur in people with or without coronary artery disease, when excessive upper-chest breathing causes spasm in otherwise normal blood vessels of the heart. Pseudoangina may be diagnosed when the usual indicators, following blood tests and ECGs, are absent.

One study suggests that up to 90 per cent of non-cardiac chest pain is brought on by hyperventilation (HVS) and other breathing pattern disorders (BPD) (*see p.57*). It is therefore important that chest pain associated with HVS/BPD is investigated, so that heart disease can be excluded as a diagnosis and breathing retraining started (*see p.62*).

People with a history of chest pain whose symptoms can be provoked by an exercise test (the chest pain comes on within six minutes) but who have normal cardiac arteries may be diagnosed with Prinz-Metal angina. More common in women than men, this condition is also helped by breathing retraining (*see p.62*).

Exercise

People with angina should follow a graduated and prescribed exercise programme that is based on research evidence of benefit in cardiovascular rehabilitation.

Bodywork Therapy

TREATING PSEUDOANGINA Spinal restrictions and disc degeneration can cause symptoms identical to angina, without any cardiac involvement at all. A series of 164 such cases of pseudoangina were reported in the medical literature, with all patients experiencing angina symptoms, as well as neck pain, headaches and arm pain. About a quarter needed spinal surgery, but most were successfully treated with non-surgical methods, such as intermittent traction, hard collars, stretching of neck muscles and anti-inflammatory medication.

In a 1976 report, the lower neck region was involved in seven pseudoangina cases. Relief was achieved in five cases, either by surgically removing the damaged discs or by using soft collars.

The thoracic spine can also be a major source of pseudoangina. In a coronary unit at a Swedish hospital, pseudoangina resulting from thoracic spinal dysfunction (known as T4 Syndrome) was the third most common diagnosis after coronary thrombosis and true angina. Treating the spinal causes by manipulation has been shown to relieve "angina-like" symptoms, often in as little as one treatment, with no return of symptoms up to ten years later.

DEACTIVATE TRIGGER POINTS Many cases of pseudoangina result from trigger points (*see p.55*) in the pectoral muscles, as well as in various shoulder and neck muscles. In one report, angina-like pain, palpitations and shortness of breath were cleared up following treatment of the trigger points by lidocaine injections, as well as massage, hydrotherapy (hot packs, ice packs and whirlpool) and muscle stretching.

Trigger points can also be deactivated by acupuncturists, osteopaths, massage therapists (those with neuromuscular therapy training in particular) and some physiotherapists and chiropractors.

Acupuncture

Several small studies suggest acupuncture can help angina symptoms over a two-year period of continuous treatment and follow-up. Surgery was avoided in 61 per cent of cases and heart attacks possibly halved. However, there is no proof that acupuncture is an effective alternative to surgery. While acupuncture does not alter the underlying coronary artery disease (*see p.252*) that triggers angina, it may modify its predicted outcome. The treatment is usually given weekly for two months.

Mind–Body Therapies

STRESS MANAGEMENT combined with exercise yields tangible, positive benefits for the reduction of angina. According to research, those with angina should take up mind–body techniques, such as meditation, deep breathing or guided imagery (*see p.99*). Results from a 1997 study suggest that mind–body techniques that induce relaxation can reduce the frightening and dangerous chest pain of angina.

Approximately 1.8 million people in the UK experience the symptoms of angina

Many people with angina in the UK report a poor quality of life, including higher levels of anxiety and depression. In 1999 and 2000, newly diagnosed patients from York followed the "Angina Plan", a cognitive behavioural disease management programme. They suffered less anxiety and depression, and, most significantly, had fewer angina episodes, a reduced need of glyceryl trinitrate and none of the physical limitations they reported at the beginning of the study. Participants also changed their diet and increased their daily walking.

> **PREVENTION PLAN**
>
> **The following should reduce your risk of developing angina:**
>
> - Eat a diet that is high in vegetables, fruit and oily fish, but low in salt and saturated fat.
>
> - Take regular exercise, such as brisk walking or cycling, for 30 minutes on five or more days of the week.
>
> - If you smoke, give it up.

WHAT ARE THE SYMPTOMS?

- In the early stages of CAD there may be no symptoms
- Later, angina (*see p.249*) may develop

If a heart attack occurs, the individual may experience:

- Persistent, severe pain in the chest that may spread up into the neck and down the arm – the pain may come on while at rest
- Sweating
- Shortness of breath
- Nausea and vomiting

WHY MIGHT I HAVE THIS?

PREDISPOSING FACTORS

- Smoking
- Genetic factors
- A diet high in certain fats
- Lack of exercise
- Excess weight
- High blood pressure
- Diabetes mellitus
- High intake of trans-fatty acids
- Oxidised cholesterol
- Raised triglyceride levels
- Raised homocysteine levels
- Anger, hostility, anxiety, depression

TRIGGERS (IN EXISTING DISEASE)

- Physical exertion, cold, windy weather, extreme emotions, excitement
- Blood-sugar imbalance

CORONARY ARTERY DISEASE

In coronary artery disease (CAD), sometimes called coronary heart disease, one or more of the coronary arteries becomes narrowed and blood flow to the heart is restricted. Exertion or stress, which increase the oxygen demands of the heart muscle, may bring on symptoms, such as chest pain (*see Angina, p.249*), and even a heart attack. Primary treatments include lifestyle changes, aspirin and lipid-lowering drugs. In some cases, angioplasty or bypass surgery may be recommended. Various nutritional therapies will help, as will managing stress.

WHY DOES IT OCCUR?

The coronary arteries branch from the aorta and supply the heart muscles with oxygenated blood. Coronary artery disease (CAD) is usually due to atherosclerosis, in which fatty deposits build up on the internal lining of the coronary arteries. These deposits narrow the arteries and restrict the flow of blood through them, reducing the supply of oxygen to the muscles. If one of the arteries becomes blocked, a heart attack (myocardial infarction) occurs and the heart muscle is damaged.

CAD due to atherosclerosis is more likely if you have a high level of cholesterol in your blood and if you eat a diet that is high in fats. Smoking, a lack of exercise, excess weight, high blood pressure (*see p.244*) and diabetes mellitus (*see p.314*) are all risk factors.

CAD is more common with increasing age and may sometimes run in families. The risk of developing CAD is generally lower in women than in men – until women reach the age of 60, when the risk for both sexes becomes approximately the same. The lower risk of CAD for a woman is thought to be due to the protective effect of the female hormone oestrogen during the fertile part of her life. This protection against CAD wears off gradually after the menopause (*see p.339*).

CAD may be an underlying factor in arrhythmias (*see Palpitations, p.258*) and heart failure, in which the heart becomes too weak to pump blood around the body effectively. Chronic heart failure may occur in the elderly, causing excess fluid in the lungs and tissues, as well as shortness of breath and swollen ankles.

TREATMENT PLAN

PRIMARY TREATMENTS

- Lifestyle changes (*see Self-help*)
- Thrombolytic, anti-angina and other drugs, surgery
- Cardiac rehabilitation programme

BACK-UP TREATMENTS

- Nutritional therapy
- Cardio-protective diets
- Western herbal medicine
- Moderate aerobic exercise
- Breathing retraining
- Mind–body therapies
- Ornish approach

WORTH CONSIDERING

- Acupuncture

For an explanation of how treatments are rated, see p.111.

IMPORTANT

If you experience any of the symptoms of CAD, consult your doctor immediately. (*See also Angina, p.249.*)

PRIMARY TREATMENT If you have CAD, or wish to reduce the risk of CAD, take the following measures:

- Stop smoking.
- Eat a diet low in saturated fats.
- Maintain your cholesterol levels at a desirable level.
- Lose weight if necessary.
- Exercise regularly according to your doctor's advice.
- Take a blood-pressure lowering drug if your blood pressure is high.
- Consider taking a low dose of aspirin (75mg) every day to reduce the risk of a heart attack. (Check with your doctor as taking aspirin is not appropriate for everyone – for example, for some people with asthma.)

TREATMENTS IN DETAIL

Conventional Medicine

TESTS If you are experiencing chest pain, your doctor may suspect CAD and will probably organise tests. These may include an electrocardiogram (ECG) to record the electrical rhythm of the heart and an exercise test to discover how your heart performs under stress. If the tests indicate your heart is not receiving enough blood, you may need a coronary angiography. A dye injected intravenously highlights the coronary arteries under X-ray and reveals where they are blocked or narrowed. If tests confirm CAD and that you are having angina episodes, various treatments may be prescribed (*see Angina, p.249*).

If your doctor suspects that you had a myocardial infarction, your heart rhythm will be recorded on an ECG at regular intervals. The ECG recordings will enable the doctor to look for changes characteristic of a heart attack and to monitor progress. A series of blood tests will measure the levels of certain enzymes that are produced by damaged heart muscle.

PRIMARY TREATMENT **THROMBOLYTIC DRUGS**, such as streptokinase, may be given if a heart attack is confirmed. These aim to break down the clot (thrombus) that is blocking the coronary artery in order to minimise the damage to the heart muscle. Taking aspirin can also help the process.

ANGIOPLASTY

In an angioplasty, which is a less invasive alternative to open-heart surgery, a tiny balloon is inflated to open up a coronary artery that has become clogged with fatty deposits. The patient, who is usually awake throughout, has a mild sedative and a local anaesthetic. Then a catheter (a hollow tube) carrying the balloon is inserted into a blood vessel in the groin and guided, with the help of X-rays, through the arteries to the blockage. The surgical procedure follows four stages.

The four stages of an angioplasty

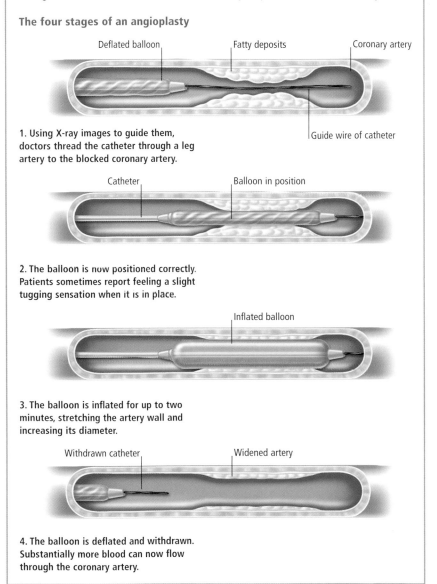

Deflated balloon — Fatty deposits — Coronary artery — Guide wire of catheter

1. Using X-ray images to guide them, doctors thread the catheter through a leg artery to the blocked coronary artery.

Catheter — Balloon in position

2. The balloon is now positioned correctly. Patients sometimes report feeling a slight tugging sensation when it is in place.

Inflated balloon

3. The balloon is inflated for up to two minutes, stretching the artery wall and increasing its diameter.

Withdrawn catheter — Widened artery

4. The balloon is deflated and withdrawn. Substantially more blood can now flow through the coronary artery.

PRIMARY TREATMENT **SURGERY**, such as an angioplasty or a coronary bypass (*see Angina, p.249*), may be needed to widen or bypass narrowed coronary arteries.

CORONARY CARE After a heart attack, you may need to be monitored on the coronary care unit for about two days, where you may be given oxygen and a pain-relieving drug, such as diamorphine. In the short term, you may need intravenous drugs, such as beta-blockers, which aim to slow the heart rate and may help relieve the pain.

PRIMARY TREATMENT **LONG-TERM TREATMENT** for CAD may include aspirin and beta-blockers, which can help to reduce the risk of a myocardial infarction. Drugs called angiotensin-converting enzyme (ACE) inhibitors may also improve the prognosis in some cases. They dilate (widen) blood vessels around the body, making it easier for the heart to pump blood round the body.

Lowering cholesterol with drugs and diet (*see Cardioprotective diets, below*) can also reduce the risk of further myocardial infarctions and strokes.

Following a myocardial infarction, you can gradually increase your activity levels. Take appropriate exercise and follow a cardiac rehabilitation programme, which will focus on various aspects of life after a heart attack, such as diet and stopping smoking. Emotional support is also very important.

> **CAUTION**
>
> Heart drugs can cause side-effects: ask your doctor to explain these to you.

Nutritional Therapy

PRIMARY TREATMENT What you eat partly determines whether or not your coronary arteries will gradually accumulate cholesterol and other fats on their internal walls. (*See also Angina, p.249.*)

HEALTHY AND UNHEALTHY FATS The type of fat we eat has an important bearing on the development of CAD (*see p.34*). While much emphasis has been placed on the need to avoid saturated fat in the diet – for example, in red meat, dairy products and eggs – some evidence suggests that the role it plays in heart disease may not be so important after all.

There is mounting evidence to suggest that fats known as "partially hydrogenated" and trans-fatty acids (*see p.34*) are a more important risk factor for CAD. These hard fats, which are found in many fast foods, baked goods, processed foods and margarine are associated with an increased risk of heart disease. You should avoid these fats if possible.

The omega-3 fatty acids in oily fish, such as salmon, trout, mackerel, sardine and herring, have several effects in the body that would be expected to reduce the risk of CAD. For example, they can raise the levels of "healthy" high-density lipoprotein (HDL) cholesterol, reduce blood pressure

and thin the blood. According to experts, eating one or two portions of fish each week, or supplementing your diet with 1g of concentrated fish oils per day, is likely to reduce the risk of heart disease.

TRIGLYCERIDES Raised levels of blood fats known as triglycerides appear to be another risk factor for CAD. Raised triglycerides often occurs in conjunction with accumulation of body fat around the middle of the body and a condition called insulin resistance (which may lead to diabetes in time). Together, these risk factors are a metabolic syndrome (known sometimes as Syndrome X), which is present in about 25 per cent of the UK's middle-aged population. Its importance as a risk for CAD development is well established. Fish-oil supplements can help here, too.

HOMOCYSTEINE LEVELS Raised levels of a substance called homocysteine appear to be a major risk factor for CAD and heart disease. Homocysteine is a breakdown

Vitamin E may also help to prevent heart disease through its ability to thin the blood. Two studies (one on men and one on women) found that taking vitamin E supplements (100 IU or more per day) for two or more years was associated with a 20–40 per cent reduction in the risk of CAD. However, other studies do not back up these findings.

VITAMIN C Evidence is starting to emerge that vitamin C may protect against CAD, especially if taken with vitamin E. But the protection probably applies only to people with poor dietary intake of the vitamins.

A 16-year follow-up study of over 80,000 nurses in the US suggested that increased vitamin C intake reduced the risk of CAD. After factoring out other risks for CAD, such as age, smoking and exercise, the women who took vitamin C still had a significantly lower risk of CAD. As a result, taking 1g vitamin C each day in conjunction with vitamin E supplements may help to reduce the risk of CAD.

88 per cent of men and 83 per cent of women in the UK consume too much saturated fat

product of the amino acid methionine, and is normally converted in the body to a harmless substance called cystanthionine. However, this conversion is dependent on the presence of vitamins B6, B12 and folic acid. A deficiency of one or more of these nutrients might cause homocysteine levels to rise. Higher intakes of folic acid and vitamin B6 in the diet are associated with a decreased risk of CAD.

Anyone with a raised homocysteine level (as determined by a blood test) should take 10mg of vitamin B6, 50mcg of vitamin B12 and 400mcg of folic acid per day.

VITAMIN E When trying to prevent CAD, medical attention focuses on the need to control the level of cholesterol in the blood. However, it is when cholesterol becomes damaged through a process known as oxidation that it has the propensity to settle on the inside of the body's arteries. Vitamin E is an antioxidant nutrient that can protect cholesterol from oxidation.

MULTIVITAMIN/MINERAL SUPPLEMENT taken daily may be a good way to protect against CAD. Studies have found that a daily intake of a multivitamin is associated with a lower risk of CAD. Many nutrients within the mineral supplement, such as vitamin E, vitamin C, copper and selenium, may be beneficial in reducing the risk of CAD.

BIOFLAVONOIDS are phenolic compounds that are present in a wide range of foods and medicinal plants. Many studies indicate that flavonoids are anti-inflammatory, antiviral and able to dilate blood vessels. Most importantly, they are antioxidants, able to neutralise free radicals and reduce their formation.

Bioflavonoids are found in nuts, cereals, olive oil, vegetables, fruits, berries, tea, red wine, dark chocolate and many herbs (*see Western herbal medicine, below*). Many of these foods are part of the so-called Mediterranean diet.

Polyphenols extracted from the purple grape skins in red wine have been shown to inhibit the formation of endothelin-1, a chemical that makes blood vessels constrict. It seems that the polyphenols reduce the stickiness of blood and protect the lining of the blood vessels of the heart by producing nitric oxide. In this way, both wine and dark grape juice can reduce atherosclerosis and heart disease.

CHINESE RED-YEAST RICE is a supplement that contains lovastatin, a naturally occurring statin. Other compounds that lower cholesterol include cholestin, which has been shown to lower raised levels of cholesterol and triglycerides in blood serum.

> CAUTION
>
> Consult your doctor before taking omega-3 fatty acids or fish oils with warfarin, or zinc with antibiotics, or vitamin E with warfarin or aspirin, or vitamin C with antibiotics or warfarin (*see also p.46*).

Cardioprotective Diets

In parts of France and other Mediterranean countries, death from heart disease is significantly lower than in other developed countries, despite a high consumption of fat and saturated fats. The reason advanced for this cardio-protective effect is the diet accompanied by regular consumption of red wine. A long-term study of 89,299 male physicians in the US found that drinking

> An estimated 2.7 million people in the UK are living with coronary heart disease

moderate amounts of red wine (one or two glasses a day) reduced overall mortality. However, there was no benefit from drinking more!

The people of Okinawa, a collection of islands between Japan and Taiwan, commonly live active, independent lives well into their 90s and 100s. Their rates of obesity, heart disease, osteoporosis, memory loss, menopause and breast, colon and prostate cancer rank far below those in

other industrialised countries. Researchers point to their mainly vegetable diet, which includes plenty of onions and soya, giving high levels of antioxidant bioflavonoids and carotenoids. In addition, a slower decline in sex hormones, which appears to be linked to diet and lifestyle, is believed to contribute to the impressive cardiovascular health of the Okinawans.

WHAT DIET? In 2002, a review looked at 147 studies of dietary factors and their relationship to CAD. The factors included fat, cholesterol, omega-3 and omega-6 (polyunsaturated) fatty acids, carbohydrates, glycaemic index, fibre, folate and dietary patterns.

The review concluded that there are apparently three effective strategies for preventing CAD. First, replace saturated fats with unsaturated fats in the diet. Second, increase the amount of omega-3 fatty acids derived from fish, fish oil supplements or plant sources in the diet. Third, eat a diet that is high in fruits, vegetables, nuts and whole grains, but one that is also low in refined grain products.

As yet, it is unclear just how much or in what proportion each of these is important. Nor is there certainty about the precise role played by essential plant substances, such as antioxidant vitamins, minerals, flavonoids and lycopenes. However, the authors suggest that a diet containing these components, combined with regular exercise, no tobacco and remaining at your ideal body weight, could prevent most cases of CAD.

GARLIC AND ONIONS contain organosulphur compounds that reduce the stickiness of human blood platelets and appear to confer cardiovascular benefits on those who eat them regularly. In addition, they reduce levels of unhealthy fats in the blood and can help to lower blood pressure.

The protective effect of garlic (*Allium sativum*) is attributed to its ability to reduce arterial plaque and atherosclerosis, and to protect the lining of the blood vessels in the

heart. Garlic also appears to inhibit cholesterol manufacture in the liver and to increase the excretion of cholesterol. It may also relax the heart muscle and maintain the elasticity of the aorta.

TEA (*Camellia sinensis*) has cardioprotective properties because it is rich in catechins and polyphenols which are antioxidants. A study carried out on black tea consumption found that tea-drinking appeared to improve the function of the coronary blood vessels in patients with CAD. In a Japanese study, people drinking over ten cups of green tea a day had a decreased risk of death from cardiovascular disease.

TOMATOES contain lycopene, an antioxidant carotenoid which has the ability to inhibit cholesterol synthesis and prevent heart disease. Tomatoes are also a good source of beta-carotene, flavonoids, potassium, folic acid, vitamins C and E – all of which may work together to maintain a healthy heart.

OTHER CARDIOPROTECTIVE FOODS Several studies suggest that eating plenty of fruit and vegetables is associated with a reduced risk of CAD.

Substantial epidemiological evidence indicates that diets rich in fibre and whole grains are associated with decreased risk of CAD. Studies show that eating whole-grain foods can also help to reduce the risk of CAD, by up to 30 per cent if you eat more than three servings per day.

Legumes also seem to have a beneficial effect on the heart. Soya has been shown to reduce "bad", low-density cholesterol (LDL), while increasing the ratio of "good", high-density cholesterol (HDL).

> CAUTION
>
> Consult your doctor before taking medicinal doses of garlic at the same time as anticoagulant drugs (*see p.69*).

Western Herbal Medicine

From across the world, epidemiological evidence makes the case that common chemical compounds found in traditional plant remedies help to maintain a healthy heart. If you have coronary artery disease, a herbalist may prescribe one or more of the following plant remedies.

HAWTHORN (*Crataegus monogyna* or *Crataegus laevigata*) flowers are rich in bioflavonoids while the spring leaves are particularly high in oligomeric proantho-cyanidins (OPCs). These OPCs are bioflavonoid antioxidants that are about 20 times as potent as vitamin C and 50 times as potent as vitamin E.

OPCs protect the heart by binding to the surface of blood vessel (endothelial) cells where they neutralise harmful free radicals. OPCs can also be found in grapeseed (*Vitis vinfera*) extract.

Hawthorn extract strengthens the power of the heart muscle, increases blood flow through the coronary arteries and appears to keep the rhythm of the heartbeat regular. This research demonstrated that those patients with heart disease who were taking hawthorn found their breathlessness and fatigue improved significantly compared to patients taking a placebo.

GINKGO (*Ginkgo biloba*) can improve circulation and is used to treat CAD. Standardised ginkgo biloba extract (GBE) helps to normalise the circulation of the blood and exerts a beneficial effect on the lining and tone of the blood vessels. GBE reduces the stickiness of blood platelets that can lead to coronary artery blockage and heart disease.

MOTHERWORT (*Leonurus cardiaca*) is another herb with a long folk use for treating cardiac debility, rapid heartbeat and anxiety affecting heart function.

OTHER HERBS AND SPICES Several kitchen herbs and spices also have a beneficial effect on the heart. They include rosemary (*Rosmarinus officinalis*), which contains phenolic diterpenes that reduce "bad" low-density lipoprotein (LDL) cholesterol in the blood. The antioxidants in cinnamon (*Cinnamon verum*) bark can lower blood fat levels. Turmeric (*Curcuma longa*) has antioxidant activity that can help to lower cholesterol levels and has demonstrated reduction of the symptoms of angina pectoris. Ginger (*Zingiber officinale*), a close relative of turmeric, prevents the aggregation of blood platelets in patients with coronary artery disease.

TERMINALIA ARJUNA The bark of this Ayurvedic remedy is a source of OPCs and bioflavonoids that strengthen the power of heart muscle as well as relieving angina and the frequency of angina attacks.

> CAUTION
>
> See p.69 before taking a herbal remedy and, if you are already taking prescribed medication, consult a medical herbalist first.

Aerobic Exercise

Performing aerobic exercise on a regular basis is commonly associated with protection against heart disease. However, exercise is usually beneficial for people with existing heart disease, too. Among the benefits of aerobic and general exercise are decreased risk of thrombosis, myocardial ischaemia (involving symptoms such as angina) and stroke. If you have CAD, you should should follow a graduated exercise programme that is based on research evidence in cardiovascular rehabilitation and prescribed by a physiotherapist.

One remarkable study that lasted 33 years revealed that aerobic exercise, when performed 3–4 times each week, slows down the ageing process of the heart. Another long-term (13-year) research study involving 10,000 men showed that regular exercise helps to prevent strokes as well as helping people recover from strokes. In the study, walking, stair climbing, dancing, cycling and gardening all reduced the risk of stroke. However, the lowest risk was associated with walking 20km or more a week. The research also strongly suggests that regular participation in moderate-intensity (non-aerobic) lifestyle activities, such as walking, stair-climbing, vigorous housework and gardening, for not less than 60 minutes per week, give almost the same heart health benefits as regular and more intense aerobic activity.

It is current exercise levels that protect the heart, rather than an earlier history of physical exercise. Researchers send a clear message when they say it may never be too late to start exercising.

Breathing Retraining

Hyperventilation and altered breathing patterns can aggravate existing cardiovascular disease by reducing oxygen delivery to the tissues, including the heart itself, and by causing contractions of the smooth muscles surrounding the blood vessels. Breathing retraining (*see p.62*) may therefore be a useful way of easing these stresses to the heart, as well as lowering general levels of anxiety. Physiotherapists and yoga instructors can help you learn better breathing habits.

Acupuncture

Acupuncture cannot treat the primary causes of CAD, but it can treat the pain and may act to dilate the coronary arteries, sometimes providing effective long-term treatment. A study using coronary arteriograms has shown that acupuncture can dilate coronary arteries. The authors suggested that this might be the basis of a useful treatment for angina and CAD.

Within the next two minutes, someone in the UK will experience a heart attack

Mind–Body Therapies

STRESS can have a "double whammy" effect in cardiovascular health. First, it can impact the body directly – for example, the chronic overproduction of stress hormones, such as adrenaline and cortisol, negatively affect the cardiovascular system.

Second, stress can indirectly contribute to poor cardiovascular health when people respond to it with unhealthy behaviour, such as poor diet, lack of exercise, smoking and excessive alcohol.

PHYSIOLOGICAL EFFECTS Stress affects the cardiovascular system in a number of ways. It speeds up the heart rate, raises blood pressure and increases the tendency for blood clots to form. Blood vessels throughout the body become narrow and the arteries that supply blood to the heart muscle constrict.

As blood flow becomes more turbulent it can injure the lining of the arteries and, over time, lead to blockage of the arteries as the body attempts to heal these injuries.

HOSTILITY AND ANGER Numerous studies have demonstrated a strong link between higher levels of hostility and anger and heart disease. In one of the most famous studies, physicians who scored high in a measure of hostility at the age of 25 were seven times more likely to have died from heart disease (as well as from other causes) 25 years later than physicians who had a calmer disposition.

People who express higher levels of hostility are also more likely to engage in unhealthy lifestyle behaviours, such as smoking, drinking alcohol and eating a diet that is high in fatty acids. In a 1983 study, Finnish men with the highest levels of expressed anger were found to be at twice the risk of having a stroke during eight years of follow-up.

Overall, the clinical and research literature suggests that symptoms of depression represent a significant risk factor for developing cardiovascular disease. For example, a study of 1,190 medical students found that the incidence of clinical depression was a risk factor for coronary artery disease later in life.

THE MANAGEMENT OF STRESS In many respects anxiety, hostility–anger, depression–hopelessness can be viewed as the emotional and behavioural consequences of stress, or what happens when people perceive that they do not have the internal or external resources to meet the demands or challenges of life.

Experiencing occasional feelings of anger, worry and sadness is normal. However, when these mood states become more frequent or even chronic, it is a clue that normal life stresses and challenges are no longer being managed effectively. Not everyone who is clinically "stressed" reacts this way: the tendency to do so may be genetically determined.

The chronic activation of the stress response can not only wear away at the quality of mental and emotional health

management, which included instruction in a variety of relaxation techniques (*see* p.99) and stress-coping strategies, were significantly less likely to have a recurrent coronary event, such as a heart attack, at the five-year follow-up.

If you have coronary artery disease, ask your doctor about a stress-management programme or take up meditation or guided imagery (*see p.98*).

THE ORNISH APPROACH The Lifestyle Heart Trial was initially published in 1990 and updated in 1998. It follows the approach devised by American doctor Dean Ornish in the 1980s and entails a low-fat diet, combined with a programme of stopping smoking, aerobic exercise, stress-management training and psychological support.

The Ornish approach is a good example of the benefits of integrating mind–body therapies with nutritional changes. Patients exercise for an hour three times a week, participate in group therapy sessions and learn to manage their stress with techniques adapted from yoga and meditation. They also follow a rigorous high-fibre diet that provides the following calorie breakdown: 10 percent comes from fat, 15–20 per cent from protein and 70–75 per cent from complex carbohydrates.

Research suggests that the Ornish approach can reverse and prevent coronary artery disease without the need for either drugs or surgery. These findings have been replicated at many different places throughout the US since 1983. The longer the regime is maintained, the more heart scans show that the atherosclerosis continues to reverse.

Vegetarians have a lower mortality rate from coronary heart disease than meat-eaters

Research published in 1996 examined a sample of 1,305 men who did not have coronary artery disease at the beginning of the study. Among these men, those reporting the highest levels of anger were three times as likely to experience either a non-fatal heart attack or fatal heart disease at follow-up seven years later.

ANXIETY AND DEPRESSION Studies have also demonstrated a link between both anxiety and depression (including hopelessness) and cardiovascular disease. For example, several large-scale, community-based studies have shown significant relationships between anxiety disorders and deaths from heart disease. Other studies have shown the relationship between both anxiety disorders and worry and coronary artery disease.

and well-being, it can also have a significantly negative effect on the quality of physical health and well-being, especially cardiovascular health.

Given the clear link between stress and cardiovascular health, it is not surprising that clinical research shows that stress-management techniques, such as relaxation (*see* p.99) can be effective in treating and preventing coronary artery disease.

One of the best examples of this comes from a study, published in 2002, by Professor James Blumenthal and his team of researchers at Duke University in north Carolina. They conducted a trial in which individuals with documented coronary artery disease followed an exercise programme, a stress-management programme or the usual medical treatment for five years. Those who were trained in stress-

PREVENTION PLAN

The following measures should reduce your risk of developing coronary artery disease:

- Eat a diet that is high in vegetables, fruit and oily fish, and low in salt and saturated fat.

- Take regular exercise, such as brisk walking or cycling, for 30 minutes on five or more days of the week.

- If you smoke, give it up.

PALPITATIONS

Palpitations are an awareness of the heartbeat, which may be felt either as normal in rate and rhythm or may be sensed as irregular and/or rapid. It is normal to sense the heartbeat when nervous, excited or as a result of exertion, but sometimes there is a trigger that needs eliminating or an underlying arrhythmia that needs medical attention, so diagnosis is essential. Treatment may include drugs to control the rhythm of the heart, as well as supplements, manipulation therapy, breathing retraining and mind–body therapies, such as relaxation.

WHAT ARE THE SYMPTOMS?

- Awareness of the heartbeat

Additional symptoms may be experienced, depending on the cause:

- Palpitations with panic attacks may be associated with nausea and increased sweating
- Palpitations associated with atrial fibrillation may be accompanied by light-headedness and shortness of breath
- Palpitations associated with other rapid arrhythmias may be accompanied by shortness of breath, fainting and chest pain

WHY MIGHT I HAVE THIS?

PREDISPOSING FACTORS

- Underlying arrhythmia
- Overactive thyroid gland
- Anaemia

TRIGGERS

- Caffeine
- Nicotine
- Alcohol
- Anxiety
- Panic attacks
- Calcium-channel blockers

IMPORTANT

Consult your doctor if you experience palpitations, especially if they are irregular or recurrent. Seek urgent medical attention if they are accompanied by other symptoms, such as chest pain.

WHY DOES IT OCCUR?

Rapid, regular palpitations may occur repeatedly in people who are prone to persistent anxiety and panic attacks (*see p.414*), as well as in people with certain medical disorders, such as an overactive thyroid gland (*see Hyperthyroidism, p.319*) and anaemia. Palpitations may also occur as a side-effect of certain medications, such as calcium-channel blockers, which are used to treat angina (*see p.249*) and high blood pressure (*see p.244*). Palpitations may also be triggered by stimulants, such as caffeine and nicotine.

ARRHYTHMIAS There are two types of arrhythmia that commonly cause palpita-

tions. When premature ectopic beats occur there is an early heartbeat, which means that the next normal heartbeat appears to be delayed and may be felt as a "thud" in the chest.

Ectopic beats are usually no cause for concern and are often associated with stress (*see p.408*) or the use of stimulants, such as nicotine, caffeine and alcohol. However, occasionally ectopic beats may cause discomfort or may be a symptom of an underlying heart disorder, such as coronary artery disease (*see p.252*).

The second arrhythmia is atrial fibrillation, in which the atria (the upper heart chambers) contract irregularly and very rapidly. Some of the electrical impulses that cause these contractions trigger rapid irregular contractions of the ventricles (the lower heart chambers). This arrhythmia is often present continuously and may be symptomless. However, it may cause palpitations when it occurs in episodes.

Less commonly, rapid and regular palpitations are a symptom of other arrhythmias.

TREATMENT PLAN

PRIMARY TREATMENT

- Drugs, such as beta-blockers

BACK-UP TREATMENTS

- Nutritional therapy
- Homeopathy

WORTH CONSIDERING

- Bodywork therapies
- Breathing retraining
- Acupuncture
- Relaxation and other mind–body therapies

For an explanation of how treatments are rated, see p.111.

TREATMENTS IN DETAIL

Conventional Medicine

DIAGNOSIS Your doctor may arrange tests to exclude causes that are not related to the heart, such as hyperthyroidism. If the doctor suspects an underlying arrhythmia, your heart rate may be recorded over a 24-hour period by a portable monitor attached to a strap that can be worn around your body.

Whether palpitations are due to panic attacks, anxiety, an excess of a stimulant, such as coffee, a disrupted heart rhythm (arrhythmia) or another medical disorder, such as anaemia, the underlying cause needs to be avoided or treated.

PRIMARY TREATMENT **DRUGS** Some types of arrhythmia require treatment with drugs. Ectopics are not usually treated

unless they are bothersome, in which case the doctor may prescribe beta-blockers. Recurrent episodes of atrial fibrillation may also be treated with beta-blockers or certain anti-arrhythmic drugs, such as flecainide or propafenone.

CAUTION

Beta-blockers and anti-arrhythmic drugs have a range of side-effects: ask your doctor to explain these to you.

HEART RHYTHMS

An electrocardiograph (ECG) is a machine that measures the electrical activity of the heart. It is safe and painless, and can show whether a heartbeat is normal or is affected by a disrupted rhythm (arrhythmia). Electrical activity in various parts of the heart is detected by electrodes attached to the skin on the chest, ankles and wrist, and is recorded on paper in the ECG machine. The sino-atrial node (the hearts pacemaker) initiates electrical currents that pass through the heart's chambers, triggering contractions in the muscles.

Normal and disrupted heart rhythms

NORMAL

A normal ECG shows a small peak as the current passes through the atria, a large peak as it passes through the ventricles (yellow); and a third when the ventricles relax.

SINUS TACHYCARDIA

In sinus tachycardia ("tachy" means fast), the rhythm of the electrical pulse from the sinoatrial node is over 100 beats per minute (30 more than normal).

ATRIAL FIBRILLATION

In atrial fibrillation, the pulse from the node is chaotic and the heart rate rapid and irregular. The atria contract weakly between 300 and 500 beats a minute.

Nutritional Therapy

CAFFEINE can increase the pulse rate and may even trigger abnormal heart rhythms. If you experience palpitations, reduce or eliminate caffeine (in coffee, tea, cola, mate, guarana, ephedra) from your diet.

OMEGA-3 FATTY ACIDS There is some evidence to suggest that eating fish and fish oils (omega-3 fatty acids) may help to maintain a normal heart rhythm. If you suffer from palpitations, eating oily fish (salmon, mackerel, sardines, herring and trout) or taking fish oil supplements may benefit you.

MAGNESIUM seems to be important for maintaining a normal heart rhythm, with several studies showing that intravenous magnesium may be useful in the treatment of various types of arrhythmia. One study of people who had abnormal heart rhythms (and heart failure) found that taking oral magnesium helped. Taking 300–600mg of magnesium supplements per day may be an effective dose for people with palpitations and/or arrhythmia.

COENZYME Q10 (COQ10) seems to possess the ability of stabilising the heartbeat of individuals with arrhythmias. In one study, 100mg per day of CoQ10 (in addition to standard treatment) was effective in reducing palpitations in the majority of patients with congestive heart failure.

CAUTION

Consult your doctor before taking either CoQ10 or omega-3 fatty acids/fish oils with warfarin (*see p.46*).

Homeopathy

SPIGELIA ANTIHELMIA is frequently used by homeopaths to treat palpitations, at times with other medicines chosen to suit the individual. It is most effective when the palpitations are accompanied with facial pain or migraine, usually left-sided and involving the eye. Sometimes, in those whom the medicine benefits, a hot drink seems to help control the palpitations.

LACHESIS The palpitations in people who respond to *Lachesis* are often accompanied by a sensation of constriction in the chest and/or hot flushes. In women, the problem often starts at the menopause and tends to be at its worst just after waking in the morning. In general, the patient is hot and hates tight clothes, especially collars. They may be depressed, moody or irritable and are sometimes very talkative.

NATRUM MURIATICUM People who may find *Natrum mur.* useful have palpitations that seem to be triggered by mental exertion, or sometimes by lying down. Typically, the heart seems to "skip a beat" every few beats. But the key to this medicine is the "mental profile": people who respond to it often have masked depression – they may be very depressed, but they hide it. This profile may have been triggered by a psychological trauma: a bereavement or relationship break-up, for instance, which they have never talked about. They put on a brave face, but privately feel desperately depressed.

NUX VOMICA Overindulgence in food or alcohol may trigger off the palpitations in people who respond to *Nux vom.* The problem is often worse early in the morning (between 5 and 6 a.m.). The person is often very bad tempered; indeed, the palpitations may be triggered by a fit of bad temper or a frustrating incident.

Bodywork Therapies

Much of the heart's regular rhythmic contraction is triggered by an internal nerve supply, which is rather like a local generator that is independent of the overall power supply. The external nerve supply to the heart that helps it adapt to the demands of life come from different areas of the spine. The sympathetic nerves that "speed up" the heart rate arise from the first five spinal segments below the neck (thoracic spine), while the parasympathetic nerves that slow down the heart rate come from the vagus nerve, which emerges from the spine in the

neck region. Imbalances in nerve supply, sometimes associated with spinal dysfunction can disturb the rhythm of the heart, and palpitations may be one result of this.

OSTEOPATHY AND CHIROPRACTIC Someone with a heart problem will almost always have identifiable and palpable changes in those areas of the spine that feed the nerves to the heart. Appropriate osteopathic or chiropractic manipulation of the spinal joints of the neck and upper back can influence and, at times, assist in returning irregular heart rhythms to normal.

DEACTIVATE TRIGGER POINTS Another reason for an uneven heart rhythm can be trigger-point activity (*see p.55*) between the 5th and 6th ribs, in the intercostal or pectoral muscle fibres a little to the right side of the breast bone. Pressure into, and stretching of, the local contractions surrounding the trigger point can deactivate it and ease the symptoms it may be causing.

Breathing Retraining

People who habitually breathe just from the upper chest automatically exhale excessive carbon dioxide and so increase the alkalinity of their blood. The biochemical changes that follow can disrupt the normal oxygen supply to the heart, at times causing it to beat abnormally.

An upper-chest breathing pattern also creates a great deal of additional work for particular muscles, including the intercostals and pectorals, that may house trigger points involved in heart arrhythmia (*see p.258*). Breathing retraining (yogic-type patterns) can help to restore normal nerve and oxygen supply to the heart, easing disturbances such as palpitations.

Acupuncture

Case reports and studies published in China suggest that acupuncture may be able to treat some causes of palpitations. Certainly,

acupuncture relieves anxiety; it appears to have a powerful effect on the parts of the nervous system, particularly the autonomic nerves, that may trigger palpitations.

Acupuncture can sometimes be used to relieve palpitations as they occur, but may also have an effect on more chronic and persistent symptoms. Try six to eight treatment sessions on a weekly basis to see if the palpitations improve. If they do, your acupuncturist can decide, depending on symptoms, on further treatment.

Mind–Body Therapies

Palpitations can be a symptom of organic ischaemic heart disease, such as coronary artery disease, or of anxiety, social phobia and the tendency to manifest anxiety in

> One type of palpitation – atrial fibrillation – affects 3–5% of people over the age of 70

physical symptoms. They are more prevalent in people who are both highly sensitive to bodily sensations and who experience a greater number of minor daily irritants. Research suggests that people who are more anxious or under more stress tend to report more intense palpitations than others.

RELAXATION AND BIOFEEDBACK are two mind–body techniques that, with regular practice under medical supervision and/or used regularly at home, can help an individual prevent the onset of heart palpitations. Although the research is still not definitive, it seems very likely that practising them regularly could help people with palpitations cope better and perhaps reduce the severity of palpitations when they occur.

PREVENTION PLAN

The following may help to prevent palpitations:

- Practise relaxation regularly.
- Avoid stimulants such as caffeine.

VARICOSE VEINS

Varicose veins are swollen veins just beneath the skin that occur mainly in the legs. They may cause discomfort and look unsightly, but they are not harmful to health. If left untreated, they often get worse. If self-help measures, such as losing weight and regular walks, do not prevent the veins from worsening, surgery may be needed. Eating foods rich in anthocyanidins, hydrotherapy, compression stockings, homeopathic medicines and herbal remedies may also help relieve the symptoms and halt the progression of the condition.

WHAT ARE THE SYMPTOMS?

- Easily visible, blue, swollen and distorted veins that bulge beneath the skin and are more prominent when standing
- Aching or pain in the affected leg, especially after prolonged standing
- In severe cases, the skin over a varicose vein may become thin, dry and itchy – eventually, an ulcer may form

WHY MIGHT I HAVE THIS?

PREDISPOSING FACTORS

- Excess weight/obesity
- Inherited tendency
- Pregnancy
- Prolonged standing
- Straining while constipated

TREATMENT PLAN

PRIMARY TREATMENTS

- Self-help measures (*see right*)
- Surgery (sclerotherapy or stripping)
- Compression stockings

BACK-UP TREATMENTS

- Horse chestnut and other Western herbal remedies
- Exercise
- Hydrotherapy

WORTH CONSIDERING

- Nutritional therapy
- Homeopathy

For an explanation of how treatments are rated, see p.111.

WHY DOES IT OCCUR?

Normally, blood in the legs collects in the superficial veins just below the skin and is transferred to deep-lying veins by small blood vessels called perforating veins. Valves in the veins prevent the blood from flowing backwards away from the heart. If valves in the perforating veins do not close properly, the blood flows back into the superficial veins, causing them to become swollen and distorted. These are the varicose veins. (*See illustration, p.262.*)

Weakness of the valves in the veins may be inherited, but often the reason why varicose veins develop is not known. The condition is more common in people who are overweight or obese. It is also more common in women, especially during pregnancy when the female hormone progesterone, which causes veins to dilate, is produced in greater quantities.

Standing in one position for a prolonged period of time may encourage the development of varicose veins, and some people believe that straining while constipated may also be a predisposing factor.

SELF-HELP

| PRIMARY TREATMENT | The following measures may prevent varicose veins from appearing or worsening and may help to relieve aching and discomfort:

- Lose weight if necessary.
- Avoid standing for long periods.
- Take regular daily walks.
- Keep your legs elevated above your hips while you are sitting.
- Avoid crossing your legs.
- Avoid clothes that constrict the circulation in your legs.

TREATMENTS IN DETAIL

Conventional Medicine

Your doctor will be able to diagnose varicose veins from the appearance of your legs. If they are not severe, the doctor will advise the self-help measures (*see Self-Help, left*) in the first instance.

| PRIMARY TREATMENT | **SURGERY** may be needed if the varicose veins are unsightly or causing you discomfort, or if an ulcer develops. In sclerotherapy, a chemical is injected into the affected veins, causing their walls to stick together and thus preventing blood from entering.

Alternatively, the perforating veins of the affected varicose vein may be tied off, so that blood cannot enter. In some cases, the whole of an affected vein is removed (known as stripping).

CAUTION

Surgical procedures for varicose veins may lead to complications: ask your doctor to explain these to you.

Nutritional Therapy

PREVENT CONSTIPATION Some evidence suggests that a cause of varicose veins is constipation. The theory is that straining to pass faeces during constipation raises the pressure in the abdomen, which is transmitted to the veins of the legs. If you are susceptible to varicose veins, you may benefit from a high-fibre diet, containing fruit, vegetables, beans, pulses, oats, seeds and nuts, to prevent constipation.

PROANTHOCYANIDINS (or procyanidins) may help to alleviate varicose veins, possibly by strengthening the walls of the veins. Studies have shown them to be useful in treating varicose veins. If you have varicose veins, incorporate proanthocyanidins in your diet. Good sources include red wine, dark chocolate, cranberry juice, apples, blueberries, grapes (especially the skins), peanuts and bilberries.

Homeopathy

If you have varicose veins, consult a practitioner who can recommend the most appropriate remedy for you.

POIKIVEN A clinical trial has shown that the homeopathic complex *Poikiven* is effective for varicose vein symptoms.

HAMAMELIS is among the most commonly used medicines for varicose veins. It may be taken by mouth or can be applied as a cream or lotion to the affected areas. In individuals who respond to *Hamamelis*, there is a feeling of heaviness and distension, made worse by the heat, as well as easy bruising.

VIPERA is a very useful medicine for inflamed varicose veins – a condition called thrombophlebitis in which a person feels a throbbing pain that can be relieved by elevating the legs.

CALCAREA FLUORICA People who respond to this deeper-acting constitutional medicine (*see p.73*) may have lax connective tissues. When younger, they may have been hyperextensible (double-jointed) or had swayback knees (knees that go beyond straight). Alternatively, they may have a tendency to develop hernias.

PULSATILLA is a constitutional medicine (*see p.73*) in which the pain of varicose veins is relieved by elevating the legs. People who respond to *Pulsatilla* may also have a tendency to develop chilblains.

LACHESIS A marked feature in people who respond to *Lachesis* is that they are intolerance of wearing anything tight around their legs. In women, the symptoms are worse before a period and may also be triggered by the menopause.

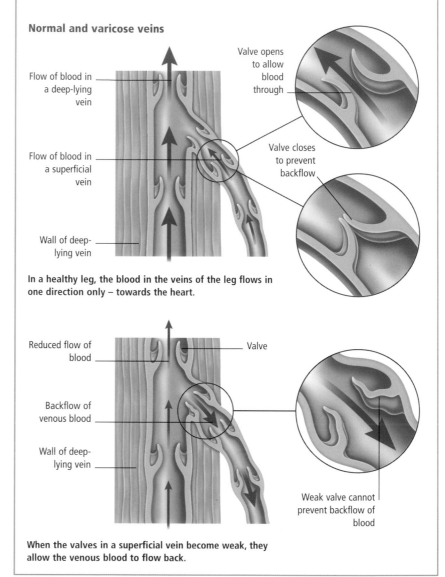

HOW VARICOSE VEINS DEVELOP

The veins that lie deep in the leg collect deoxygenated blood and return it to the heart. The contraction of the leg muscles helps this process. Within every vein, there are one-way valves that prevent the blood from flowing backwards. Blood at the surface of the legs is channelled into the deep veins by superficial veins. Sometimes the valves in the superficial veins fail, causing the vein to bulge.

Normal and varicose veins

Flow of blood in a deep-lying vein

Valve opens to allow blood through

Flow of blood in a superficial vein

Valve closes to prevent backflow

Wall of deep-lying vein

In a healthy leg, the blood in the veins of the leg flows in one direction only – towards the heart.

Reduced flow of blood

Valve

Backflow of venous blood

Wall of deep-lying vein

Weak valve cannot prevent backflow of blood

When the valves in a superficial vein become weak, they allow the venous blood to flow back.

Western Herbal Medicine

Herbal medicine can be used to strengthen vein walls, reduce fluid leakage resulting from varicose veins and improve venous circulation to and through the liver. When prescribing, practitioners take into account the health of the affected veins and the cardiovascular system as a whole. They assess your weight, speed of healing and tissue repair, and liver function. Treatment generally needs to be continued for a long time. For example, you may need to take butcher's broom (*Ruscus aculeatus*) and apply a remedy, such as witch hazel (*Hamamelis virginiana*) water, to the affected leg for a minimum of six months.

HORSE CHESTNUT (*Aesculus hippocastanum*) is the herb of choice for chronic venous insufficiency, a different and more serious condition than varicose veins and which is associated with swollen, discoloured legs. It contains a complex mix of saponins and other active constituents. Many clinical trials confirm its ability to strengthen and tone the walls of veins, reduce swelling (oedema) and fluid leakage from incompetent veins, and decrease the permeability of the capillaries. Horse chestnut extract also reduces the risk of deep vein thrombosis (DVT).

Clinical trials endorse the extract's use in the treatment of varicose veins during pregnancy, and in the treatment and relief of haemorrhoids, which have similar causes to varicose veins.

OTHER REMEDIES include butcher's broom, which is an anti-inflammatory with strong clinical evidence for use in chronic venous insufficiency and increased vascular permeability. Though poorly researched, yarrow (*Achillea millefolium*) is a traditional herb that can widen blood vessels, stimulate tissue healing and provide a tonic for veins. Bilberry (*Vaccinium myrtillus*) is a powerful antioxidant and capillary tonic.

EXTERNAL TREATMENTS include aloe vera (*Aloe vera*) juice to promote tissue repair, witch hazel for its astringent and anti-inflammatory properties when applied to the skin, and butcher's broom extract.

Varicose in Ancient Greek means grape-like, referring to the appearance of the veins

Gotu kola (*Centella asiatica*) is a well-researched Ayurvedic herb that improves the tone and function of varicose veins and recover the tone of connective tissue.

> **CAUTION**
>
> See page 69 before taking a herbal remedy and, if you are already taking a prescribed medication, consult a medical herbalist first.

Exercise

German research reveals that medically supervised exercise can relieve pain and reduce the tendency for the legs to swell. It can also heal leg ulcers, which are sometimes associated with varicose veins.

Hydrotherapy

Exercise with hydrotherapy appears to help varicose veins. A Swiss study showed that thermal hydrotherapy (balneokinesis) with sulphurous water and elastic compression of the legs reduces pain and leg swelling.

Italian hydrotherapy research examined the effect of spa treatment on 2,504 patients with primary or secondary varicose veins. For 15–20 days, the patients were treated under water with active and passive physical therapy using mineral waters. As many as half the patients returned to the spa a year later for the same treatment. The researchers concluded that "The occurrence of acute venous episodes, working days missed, number and duration of hospital admissions, consumption of drugs and physical therapies were all significantly reduced in the year after thermal therapy."

Compression Therapy

PRIMARY TREATMENT **COMPRESSION STOCKINGS** assist the circulation and help to reduce the symptoms of varicose veins by offering mechanical support.

According to a leading Swiss researcher, minor forms of varicose veins affect approximately 40 per cent of the population, while a further 10 per cent show major varicose veins and about 3 per cent suffer from the advanced stages of chronic venous insufficiency.

Elastic bandages may be more effective at creating a a degree of pressure in a particular area, whereas support stockings press uniformly. Compression therapy using elastic bandages can tackle the swelling during the acute phase, with compression stockings used to maintain the result. In more severe cases, joint mobilisation, walking exercises and draining the lymph from the affected areas may reduce the swelling.

EXERCISES TO PREVENT VARICOSE VEINS

Whenever you need to sit for long periods, it is important to exercise the leg muscles every 30 minutes or so. If you sit still for hours at a time, the veins in the legs become compressed, and it becomes harder to return blood to the heart. Blood begins to pool in the veins, putting pressure on the valves.

Slip off your shoes and raise your left foot slightly off the ground. Gently flex your foot up and down ten times. Then repeat with the other foot.

Rotate your left ankle ten times to the left, as if drawing a circle with your big toe, and then ten times to the right. Repeat with the other foot.

PREVENTION PLAN

The following may help to prevent varicose veins from developing:

- Reduce your weight if necessary.
- Avoid standing for long periods.
- Take regular exercise.

RAYNAUD'S DISEASE

In Raynaud's disease, spasm of the arteries supplying the fingers or toes restricts their blood supply, causing them to become pale. In addition, there may be feelings of numbness or tingling in the affected fingers or toes. Exposure to cold and handling frozen items can trigger an attack. Treatment involves keeping the hands and feet warm and taking the drug nifedipine and circulation-enhancing supplements, such as niacin or inositol hexaniacinate. Occasionally, surgery may be needed.

WHAT ARE THE SYMPTOMS?

- Numbness or tingling in the fingers or toes that may develop into a painful burning sensation
- Change of colour in the affected fingers or toes – they first become pale, then bluish and finally red as blood flow is restored to the tissues
- In severe cases, ulcers may form at the tips of the fingers or toes

WHY MIGHT I HAVE THIS?

PREDISPOSING FACTORS

- Autoimmune disorder
- Beta-blockers and other drugs

TRIGGERS

- Exposure to cold

TREATMENT PLAN

PRIMARY TREATMENTS

- Keeping hands warm and stopping smoking (see Self-Help)
- Nifedipine (in some cases)

BACK-UP TREATMENTS

- Low back surgery (occasionally)
- Niacin or inositol hexaniacinate
- Ginkgo extracts
- Acupuncture

WORTH CONSIDERING

- Magnesium supplements
- Homeopathy
- Exercise
- Mind–body therapies

For an explanation of how treatments are rated, see p.111.

WHY DOES IT OCCUR?

The name of the condition can be confusing. If there seems to be no apparent cause, it is called Raynaud's disease. However, when the cause is known, it is called Raynaud's phenomenon.

A variety of disorders may underlie this condition. These include autoimmune disorders (in which the body's immune system produces antibodies that attack its own tissues), such as rheumatoid arthritis (see p.293) and systemic sclerosis, a rare connective tissue disease that affects many organs and tissues of the body, including the blood vessels. Buerger's disease, a rare condition in which the small arteries of the legs become inflamed as a result of long-term smoking, can also cause Raynaud's phenomenon. Some drugs, such as beta-blockers, can produce the symptoms of Raynaud's phenomenon as a side-effect.

SELF-HELP

PRIMARY TREATMENT The following measures may help the symptoms:

- Wear plenty of layers and keep your hands and feet warm with special thermal gloves and socks.
- If you are a smoker, stop. This is because nicotine constricts the arteries.
- If you are taking beta-blockers, consult your doctor about stopping.

TREATMENTS IN DETAIL

Conventional Medicine

A diagnosis is made from a description of the symptoms and an examination. The doctor may arrange tests to see if there is an underlying cause.

When Raynaud's disease affects the hands, the blood supply to the tips of the fingers is restricted, causing them to turn white.

PRIMARY TREATMENT **NIFEDIPINE** Your doctor may prescribe nifedipine, a calcium-channel blocker that helps to relax blood vessel walls. The drug is also used to prevent angina attacks and to treat high blood pressure.

LOW BACK SURGERY may, in very severe cases of Raynaud's, be needed to cut the nerves that control constriction of the arteries supplying the feet.

CAUTION

Nifedipine may have side-effects: ask your doctor to explain these to you.

Nutritional Therapy

MAGNESIUM People with Raynaud's disease may have low levels of magnesium or suffer from abnormal magnesium metabolism. Magnesium deficiency can cause spasms in small blood vessels and hence worsen the symptoms. Taking 300–500mg of magnesium per day may reduce the frequency and severity of your condition.

VITAMIN B3/NIACIN Vitamin B3 is known to enhance circulation. Niacin, a form of this nutrient, can induce flushing in the skin in doses as low as 50–100mg per day.

An alternative is inositol hexaniacinate, which is a compound of inositol (loosely classified as a B vitamin) and niacin. It appears to help enhance the circulation without the side-effects that commonly occur with niacin. Taking 500mg of inositol hexaniacinate 2–4 times a day may help to control the symptoms of a poor circulation, although it may be two months before you see any improvement.

> **CAUTION**
>
> Consult your doctor before taking magnesium with ciproflaxin, warfarin or spironolactone (*see p.46*), and ask about the possible side-effects of niacin.

Homeopathy

Raynaud's disease can respond well to homeopathy. Among the more frequently indicated medicines are *Agaricus*, *Carbo vegetabilis*, *Secale* and *Silicea*.

AGARICUS is appropriate when the symptoms are very painful and like "splinters of ice". The individual may also have itchy chilblains or suffer from twitching or tics.

CARBO VEGETABILIS People who respond to *Carbo veg.* have a sluggish circulation: their fingers and toes turn a blotchy reddish-blue, often with burning pain. They may have varicose veins (*see p.261*) or piles, too. Their digestion is also sluggish, with bloating and wind, or they may be short of breath. They often look flushed and congested, and feel better if there is a breeze.

SECALE People who respond to *Secale* have spasm of the blood vessels: the fingers go white and feel very cold to the touch. There is a burning pain that strangely gets worse, at least in the short term, from warming up.

SILICEA People who respond to *Silicea* are said to have a "frog handshake" – their hands are cold and damp. Although cold, their hands and feet are sweaty; their nails are weak with length-wise ridges. People who respond to *Silicea* may have other "constitutional" features (*see p.73*).

Bodywork Therapies

Crowding, compression and irritation of the nerves and blood vessels in the narrow space between the collar bone, the shoulder blade and the first rib are collectively known as thoracic outlet syndrome, or TOS. Although TOS usually causes pain, it can sometimes produce symptoms virtually identical to Raynaud's – extremely cold hands that appear sweaty and blue. This condition may sometimes follow injury, but may also be the result of other causes, including excessive growth of the first rib.

Chiropractic manipulation aimed at relieving the crowded space between the upper ribs, the shoulder blade and the collar bone, can sometimes relieve TOS and so improve the circulation to the hands.

Western Herbal Medicine

GINKGO A randomised, controlled trial of a standardised ginkgo extract showed it to be more effective than a placebo in reducing the number of weekly attacks of Raynaud's.

> **CAUTION**
>
> See page 69 before taking a herbal remedy and, if you are already taking a prescribed medication, consult a medical herbalist first. Ginkgo may interact with other medicines.

Acupuncture

Four clinical trials of varying quality all conclude that acupuncture is of value in treating Raynaud's disease. It particularly helps in the short term but also possibly offers a preventive effect. The clinical improvement in "attacks" correlates well with an improved flow of blood flow through the hands.

When you know you are likely to experience Raynaud's symptoms – for instance, in the winter – a course of treatment over a period of six to eight weeks may help. If there is no obvious benefit, then acupuncture is unlikely to prove of value.

Mind–Body Therapies

Stressful life events can influence the sympathetic nervous system, which is responsible for spasms of the small blood vessels (vasospasms) that are associated with Raynaud's disease. As a result, the spasms, which can be quite painful, may be amenable to mind–body treatment.

Research has demonstrated that a number of mind–body therapies, such as clinical biofeedback, autogenic training and progressive relaxation, can help with treatment. However, there does not appear to be any distinct advantage of one technique over the other.

These mind–body techniques can be combined with conventional drugs, such as sympathetic blocking agents, that reduce the impact of stress on the nervous system.

TEMPERATURE BIOFEEDBACK or regular relaxation may help improve symptoms of Raynaud's disease. A 1979 study examined the possible benefits of relaxation and finger temperature (FT) biofeedback in people with Raynaud's disease.

After six weeks, both the combined treatment groups and the relaxation-only groups demonstrated consistent increases in the finger temperatures with a resulting decrease in Raynaud's symptoms and discomfort. However, there was no difference between the groups. At a two-year follow-up, many of the patients reported that the improvements were sustained: they had less severe and less frequent episodes of Raynaud's discomfort.

A 1987 research summary of the use of mind–body interventions with Raynaud's disease revealed that temperature biofeedback reduces reported symptom frequency and enables patients to voluntarily increase finger temperature and capillary blood flow for upwards of one year after treatment. Moreover, the improvement in the symptoms persists for up to three years.

> **PREVENTION PLAN**
>
> **The following may help to prevent Raynaud's disease:**
>
> - Avoid cold conditions.
> - If you are a smoker, then stop.

Musculoskeletal System

We rarely appreciate the amazing engineering of the muscoloskeletal system until something goes wrong. Integrated medicine aims to keep muscles, bones and joints working well throughout life. Acupuncture can be as effective as painkillers for certain conditions, and surgery can sometimes be avoided with appropriate bodywork and movement therapies.

BACK AND NECK PAIN

Back and neck pain may have a variety of causes and descriptions. The pain is usually centred around the vertebrae of the spine, from the neck to the sacroiliac joints of the pelvis. Causes include muscle and ligament injuries, problems derived from habitually poor posture and chronic joint disorders. Back pain more commonly affects the low back. Treatment focuses on resolving the underlying problem or, at the very least, bringing short-term relief or organising the long-term management of chronic pain.

WHAT ARE THE SYMPTOMS?

- Pain in the back or the neck, which may be mild or severe
- The pain may come on suddenly or develop over a period of days or weeks
- Persistent numbness in one limb or a persistent weakness of certain movements may reflect pressure on a nerve root

WHY MIGHT I HAVE THIS?

PREDISPOSING FACTORS

- Habitual poor posture
- Stress
- Certain occupations, such as working on computers
- Pregnancy
- Joint dysfunction or muscle spasm
- Prolapsed disc
- Muscle and ligament pain
- Degenerative disease

TRIGGERS

- Sports injury
- Whiplash
- Lifting a heavy object awkwardly

TREATMENT PLAN

PRIMARY TREATMENTS

- Rehabilitation programme
- Chiropractic, osteopathy and massage
- Acupuncture

BACK-UP TREATMENTS

- Postural therapies and exercise
- Homeopathy
- Mind–body therapies

WORTH CONSIDERING

- Nutritional therapy

For an explanation of how treatments are rated, see p.111.

WHY DOES IT OCCUR?

The spine is an intricate network of bones, nerves, muscles, ligaments, tendons and cartilage. Back and neck pain can result from acute physical injury, such as a pinched nerve, strained muscle, torn ligament or compressed cartilage. These can be caused by various means, such as whiplash – often from a car accident – (see right), lifting a heavy object, engaging in a strenuous, unaccustomed activity or exercising without warming up. Back pain and the injury causing it may become worse with continued activity, so it is best to consult a doctor about the level of activity that is appropriate for you.

Low back pain can accompany pregnancy, due to changes in posture and the softening of ligaments in the pelvis. Adopting a bad posture for a prolonged period of time (a common occurrence in people who work on computers) can cause either neck or back pain. Stress can also result in neck pain, often in combination with tension headaches.

Persistent pain in the back or neck may also be caused by joint disorders such as osteoarthritis (see p.289) and ankylosing spondylitis (see p.305). Vertebral fractures resulting from osteoporosis (see p.308) may also cause severe back pain. (See also Sciatica, p.272 and Prolapsed disc, p.274.)

SELF-HELP

The following may bring relief from an acute attack of back and neck pain:

- Apply an ice pack or bag of frozen peas, wrapped in a cloth, to the area of maximum pain for 5–10 minutes each hour.
- Hold a hot-water bottle wrapped in a cloth and over the painful area if the pain is in muscles or ligaments.
- Take painkillers, such as ibuprofen.
- Rub in tiger balm or a liniment containing wintergreen or camphor.
- Practise therapeutic exercises for low back pain, such as the pelvic tilt and the passive extension.

TREATMENTS IN DETAIL

Conventional Medicine

Your doctor will examine your spine and posture, testing your reflexes and looking for areas of tenderness and numbness. You may need to have tests, such as X-rays, to look for an underlying condition, which will be treated if possible.

PRIMARY TREATMENT **REHABILITATION** If your pain is due to an injury, you may require only painkillers, rest and, in some cases, physiotherapy to help you recover. However, fractures and other damage may need specific treatment.

If your pain is thought to be related to posture or stress, you may need a prescription for either painkillers or non-steroidal

IMPORTANT

If back pain is associated with difficulty controlling your bowel or bladder, you may have a disorder putting pressure on the spinal cord and should see a doctor at once. If you have an area of persistent numbness, consult a doctor immediately.

WHIPLASH

A car accident in which the collision comes unexpectedly from behind is the most familiar cause of whiplash. Anyone who is in the car will feel their head thrown violently backwards and forwards. Their neck vertebrae curve one way and then the other and the ligaments take the strain because the muscles were not primed for the impact. The ligaments are overstretched and may be torn. Vertebral discs, muscles and facet joints may all be damaged in the process.

Strain on the neck

Soft tissues at the back of the neck are stretched and may be damaged

Soft tissues at the front of the neck are damaged

Neck vertebrae curve backwards

Vertebrae close up

When the force of the collision comes from behind, the head is suddenly thrown back. The strain is felt most by the soft tissues at the front of the neck's vertebrae.

When the force of the collision comes from in front, the head is suddenly thrown forwards. The soft tissues at the back of the neck feel the strain most of all.

---

anti-inflammatory drugs (NSAIDs) for a short period. Physiotherapy may also be recommended to relieve muscle spasms and help to relieve the pain.

As part of your rehabilitation programme, you may also need expert advice on posture, appropriate relaxation techniques and, in some cases, counselling to help you cope with stress. Occupational therapists can help if the pain appears to be work-related.

CAUTION

NSAIDs may have side-effects: ask your doctor to explain these to you.

Nutritional Therapy

VITAMIN C Collagen is largely responsible for the strength and resilience of the discs of cartilage located between the vertebrae in the spine. One report found that a daily dose of 1,500–2,500mg of vitamin C, which plays an important part in the formation of collagen, can alleviate back pain and reduce the need for disc surgery. If you are experiencing back or neck pain, you may benefit from long-term supplementation with 1,000mg of vitamin C, taken twice a day.

GLUCOSAMINE SULPHATE is a constituent of intervertebral discs. Clinical experience suggests that taking 500mg of glucosamine sulphate two or three times a day may help to stimulate healing and repair within damaged discs. Glucosamine hydrochloride may also be used.

VITAMIN D Evidence suggests that vitamin D may help in the treatment of chronic back pain. One study in 2003 examined individuals who had experienced low back pain with no obvious cause for more than six months. After treatment with 5,000 or 10,000 IU of vitamin D each day for three months, every individual with a previously low level of vitamin D showed clear signs of improvement. Vitamin D supplements may have special significance for those who have little exposure to sunlight, since most of our vitamin D supplies come from the action of sunlight on the skin.

CAUTION

Consult your doctor before taking vitamin C with antibiotics or warfarin, or vitamin D with verapamil (*see p.46*).

Homeopathy

In a clinical trial published in 2002, individualised homeopathy was shown to be at least as effective as physiotherapy for low back pain. Evidence from clinical trials also suggests that different forms of homeopathic medicines may help in various conditions underlying back pain, including osteoarthritis and fibromyalgia. These include topically applied creams and gels, such as SRL gel (which contains *Symphytum*, *Rhus toxicodendron* and *Ledum*).

RHUS TOXICONDENDRON AND BRYONIA
Rhus tox. is one of the most commonly appropriate medicines for back pain, particularly if there is rapid stiffening up, with waking at night due to stiffness. By contrast, if the pain is relieved by keeping very still, and hence by a support (for example, a collar or corset) then *Bryonia* may help.

OTHER MEDICINES may be helpful, but they will need to be prescribed on constitutional grounds (*see p.73*). These include *Sepia*, often useful for inflammation that involves the sacroiliac joints, and *Natrum muriaticum*. Those for whom *Sepia* and *Nat. mur.* is indicated find that they get relief from a firm cushion in the small of the back. They may also be depressed but hide their feelings. *Nux vomica* may help with pains where muscle spasm is an important factor.

Bodywork and Movement Therapies

Short- and long-term treatment solutions need to be found for back and neck problems that involve either joint dysfunction or complex imbalances between different muscle groups. These may be brought on by: injuries, such as whiplash (*see above*); years of misuse of the body (for example, bad sitting postures, or awkward working and sporting postures); or by disuse (for example, a general lack of exercise).

PRIMARY TREATMENT **CHIROPRACTIC, OSTEOPATHY AND MASSAGE** In the short term, it is important to ease your symptoms and return to normal activity as soon as possible. Once your doctor has ruled out a serious disorder, a number of body-work approaches may help: chiropractic, osteopathy and massage, as well as deactivation of local trigger points (which can be responsible for much neck and back pain), yoga, stretching, ultrasound, hydrotherapy and exercise. A 2002 review of eight randomised controlled trials of massage for low back pain concluded that massage may be beneficial, especially in combination with exercise and education.

AVOID BED REST Evidence suggests that there is no point in taking to your bed to rest (unless it is totally necessary – for example, if you have an acute disc prolapse). A review of many studies concluded that bed rest has no positive effect for low back pain and may even be slightly harmful. The recommendation is that you should start to move around as soon as your pain will allow. Most people with backache recover in three to four weeks, with or without treatment.

POSTURAL THERAPIES AND EXERCISE If backache is a recurring problem, you need to learn how to keep your spine and pelvis supple (and the supporting muscles strong and stable). You also need to avoid movements and positions that put the joints at risk of strain, which means being particularly careful when lifting and bending.

Experts cannot agree whether, in both the short and the long term, manipulation of the body is more effective than exercise, and/or re-education, in helping to relieve back pain. In the short term, there is evidence that osteopathic and chiropractic manipulation can help your period of recovery from back pain to be more comfortable at least.

However, because acute back pain is a feature that commonly recurs in the long term, re-educating your posture by learning new ways of standing, walking, sitting and working has been shown to be very important in preventing further episodes of back and neck problems.

TREATMENT TO RESTORE FUNCTION once the back has become painful may usefully involve the stretching of tight muscles, the mobilisation of restricted joints and the learning of better habits of use, such as postural re-education using the Alexander technique (*see p.62*).

ACHIEVING CORE STABILITY There is very good evidence that the maintenance of strong abdominal muscles – the transversus abdominis, in particular – as well as spinal supporting muscles, such as the multifidi, is the key to a back that remains pain-free. Most back-care professionals now teach basic exercises to achieve this so-called "core stability". The Pilates exercise system is one good example of a programme that can help to prevent back pain recurring.

AVOID RISKY POSTURES Sometimes, simple changes can reduce the chance of the back pain recurring. For example, one of the most vulnerable times for the low back is early morning, soon after getting out of bed. Some movements, such as bending forwards (for example, putting on socks), can strain the back.

Avoiding such "high-risk" activities early in the morning, or after sitting for any length of time, can help to prevent both injury and re-injury. Research has shown that avoiding early morning bending helps recovery from acute low back pain.

TRIGGER POINTS

People who strain the muscles of the neck and shoulder region, through poor posture or overuse of the area, may develop trigger points (*see p.55*). These are sensitive areas of tension that cause radiating or referred pain, both locally and often at a distance from the trigger point, when pressed or stretched. Ways of relaxing these trigger points include massage, dry needling by an acupuncturist, passive stretching exercises or physiotherapy.

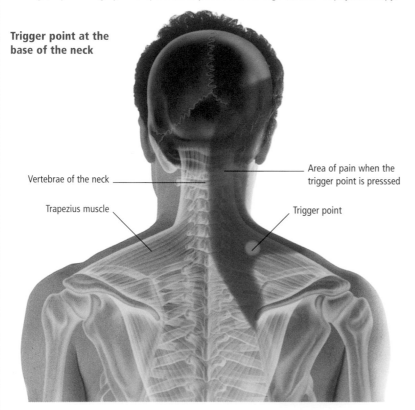

Trigger point at the base of the neck

Vertebrae of the neck

Trapezius muscle

Area of pain when the trigger point is presssed

Trigger point

When a person feels a pain in the muscles down one side of the neck or in the top of the trapezius muscle, a trigger point may develop at the point where the base of the neck meets the shoulder. When this sensitive knot of tension is touched or pressed, a wave of pain may spread through the same muscles that were hurting in the first place, from the base of the skull to the tip of the shoulderblade.

Acupuncture

PRIMARY TREATMENT There is strong evidence that acupuncture is an effective treatment for both back and neck pain. Studies with long-term follow-ups have suggested that it achieves 60–70 per cent of pain relief even a year after treatment.

A limited number (usually between four and eight) of acupuncture treatments can have a prolonged benficial effect on chronic back or neck pain. Moreover, the requirement for painkillers or anti-inflammatory drugs can be substantially reduced for prolonged periods.

However, scientists continue to debate how much of acupuncture's effect is due to activating the right acupoints and whether "sham" acupuncture – in other words, placing the acupuncture needles at random places on the body – would have exactly the same effect.

Treatment for back or neck pain is usually given on a weekly basis. Anybody contemplating acupuncture for this condition should assume that six to eight treatment sessions will produce some initial benefit. Further treatment should be based solely on the need for symptom relief and continued improvement.

Mind–Body Therapies

In both the UK and the US, back pain is a leading cause of absenteeism from work and one of the most common reasons why people visit their doctors.

The psychosocial symptoms that are a feature of chronic pain have been well documented and include anger, anxiety, depression, low perceived quality of life and poor coping skills.

HELPFUL APPROACHES Daily relaxation, meditation or guided imagery (*see pp.98– 100*) may help. Studies demonstrate the effectiveness of cognitive behavioural measures, including relaxation, meditation and guided imagery, in reducing pain perception, visits to the doctor and narcotic use, and increasing feelings of well-being in painful conditions.

A Swedish study of 253 people with neck and back pain found that cognitive behavioural intervention, including relaxation and imagery, reduced progression to chronic disability by 88 per cent.

PAIN-FREE WAYS TO SIT DOWN AND GET DRESSED

Bending from the waist first thing in the morning is a "high-risk activity" (*see left*) that can exacerbate back pain. Here are some tips on how to get dressed and get up from a chair without stressing the back. In addition, choose clothes that are easy to put on and take off, such as slip-on shoes and loose trousers.

Sitting down and leaning over to put on socks or trousers can strain the back. Instead, try getting dressed standing against a wall. Raise one knee to your chest to put on a sock or other garment. With practice this movement becomes easier.

If you have back pain, choose chairs with arms. To sit down or get up, position your feet close to the chair legs. Place your hands on the arms and lever yourself up or down. Try to keep your back as straight as you can.

PAIN RELIEF Research evidence shows that mind–body therapies (*see p.94*) as well as the use of home-based practices, such as meditation and guided imagery, can be effective treatments for relieving pain from back and neck conditions. For example, at the University of Massachusetts School of Medicine, meditation was found to be successful in a mixed group of chronic pain patients, including those with back pain. The actual location of the pain did not appear to make a difference.

In a study into the relief of tension headaches, a group practising relaxation and imagery were three times as likely to report major pain reduction – a very striking difference.

Relaxation and imagery has also significantly reduced pain in studies involving patients with cancer, arthritis, fibromyalgia, haemophilia, and migraine headaches. In all follow-up studies, improvements in pain, function and mental outlook were sustained for as long as 18 months.

Overall, it is clear from this research that mind–body interventions as well as the use of mind–body practices, such as meditation and guided imagery, by patients at home can be an effective complementary treatment for general chronic pain conditions, including back and neck pain.

PREVENTION PLAN

The following may help you to prevent back and neck pain:

- Practise warm-up and cool-down exercises before and after sport or physical activity.

- Develop good postural habits – for example when sitting for long periods of time or moving heavy objects.

- Practise back exercises to keep your body supple and flexible.

SCIATICA

Sciatica is pain that can occur anywhere along the course of the sciatic nerve, which runs from the buttock down the back of the leg (*see also Back and Neck Pain, p.268*). Most people have at least one episode of sciatica in their lives. Often, only one leg is affected. The pain usually disappears gradually over the course of a week or two, but it may recur. Treatment aims to treat the underlying cause where possible, to relieve the pain and to encourage the patient to remain active through exercise training programmes.

WHAT ARE THE SYMPTOMS?

Symptoms may be mild or severe, and include:

- Shooting pain down one or both legs, made worse by movement
- Tingling or numbness in the affected leg
- Muscle weakness in the affected leg
- Difficulty in walking if the sciatica is severe

WHY MIGHT I HAVE THIS?

PREDISPOSING FACTORS

- Changes in the spinal column due to a prolapsed disc or osteoarthritis
- Changes in posture during pregnancy
- Anatomical abnormality in the path of the sciatic nerve

TRIGGER

- Sudden heavy strain in the back

TREATMENT PLAN

PRIMARY TREATMENTS

- Treatment of underlying cause
- Pain-relieving and muscle-relaxant drugs
- Physiotherapy, osteopathy or chiropractic

BACK-UP TREATMENTS

- Homeopathy
- Dynamic back exercises
- Acupuncture

WORTH CONSIDERING

- Mind–body therapies

For an explanation of how treatments are rated, see p.111.

WHY DOES IT OCCUR?

The sciatic nerves are the largest nerves in the body and the main nerve in the legs. Their roots nerve emerge from the lower spinal cord, merge together in the buttock, and run down the back of the thigh. They branch above the knee and then extend to the lower leg and the foot.

Severe sciatica is usually caused by compression of, or damage to, the sciatic nerve, usually where the roots emerge from the spine. A prolapsed disc that presses on a spinal nerve root (*see p.274*) is the most common cause of the compression, particularly among 20–40-year-olds. This kind of sciatica is usually sharp and well delineated, and may be accompanied by tingling or numbness in the affected leg. Sitting in an awkward position for long periods is a possible cause. In some cases, the cause is unknown.

Very often, leg pain is less sharp. It may still be due to a prolapsed disc, but some complementary practitioners believe that it can also be produced by irritation or trigger points in the low back or buttocks muscles, or by strain or inflammation in the ligaments of the sacroiliac joint.

Changes in posture that put extra pressure on the sacroiliac joint may cause pregnant women to develop sciatica during the last few months of pregnancy. This usually disappears after childbirth.

IMPORTANT

The pain of sciatica normally starts to subside after a few days, but if it is severe or does not improve within two weeks consult your doctor.

SELF-HELP

The following measures may help to bring relief from the pain of sciatica:

- Apply an ice pack wrapped in a cloth to the low back or buttock for 5–10 minutes each hour.
- Hold a hot-water bottle wrapped in cloth over the painful area.
- Take painkillers, such as paracetamol.
- Practise low back exercises, such as pelvic tilt and passive extension.

TREATMENTS IN DETAIL

Conventional Medicine

Your doctor will carry out a full examination to assess your spinal column and legs. This may be followed by X-rays of the low back and other tests, such as magnetic resonance imaging (MRI), if a disc prolapse is suspected (*see p.274*).

PRIMARY TREATMENT **DRUGS** Your doctor will treat the underlying cause where possible. Painkillers and NSAIDs may both relieve the pain of sciatica. Keeping mobile (under medical advice) may help relieve the pain and increase the speed of recovery. You may need physiotherapy.

Muscle relaxants, such as diazepam, are sometimes prescribed for acute sciatica to relax muscles in the back if there is spasm, but only on a short-term basis due to the risk of dependence.

CAUTION

NSAIDs and muscle relaxants have various side-effects: ask your doctor to explain these to you.

SCIATIC NERVE

A sharp pain shoots down one leg when one of the roots of the sciatic nerve is pinched as it leaves the spinal cord between the second sacral vertebra and the fourth lumbar vertebra. The area of pain may stretch from hip to toe.

Back view showing sciatic nerve

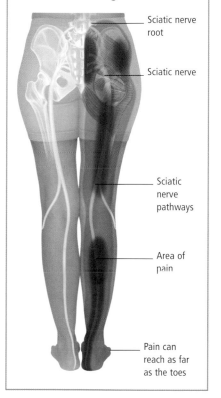

Sciatic nerve root

Sciatic nerve

Sciatic nerve pathways

Area of pain

Pain can reach as far as the toes

Nutritional Therapy

VITAMIN B12 A study found that 1mg of vitamin B12, injected daily into the muscle for two weeks, effectively alleviated the low back pain associated with lumbago or sciatic neuritis. In addition, the recipients did not need to take so much paracetamol.

Homeopathy

The following homeopathic medicines may help with sciatica. Each should be taken in the 6C dilution. Take two pills four times daily.

BRYONIA ALBA is useful for people whose sciatica improves when their back is supported (for example, with a corset) and when they keep still. It is also appropriate if movement (for example, a sneeze or a cough) makes the sciatica worse or when they are thirsty, with a dry mouth and a headache.

COLOCYNTHIS may be for people whose sciatica improves if they lie on the affected side and are in the warm. Symptoms are accompanied by bad temper and irritability.

NUX VOMICA If warmth makes the sciatica feel better, but stress or overwork makes it worse and the pain makes them irritable, *Nux vomica* may help. It is also indicated when the pain is worse in the morning.

RHUS TOXICODENDRON If gentle movement, limbering up or warmth relieves the pain, or if immobility and cold, wet weather make it worse, then *Rhus tox.* is indicated. It is also appropriate for people who sleep restlessly or who have a skin rash with fine blistering.

OTHER REMEDIES *Hypericum* suits those who have a shooting pain down the course of the sciatic nerve or whose symptoms started after a back injury. *Magnesia phosphorica*, on the other hand, is useful when sciatica is better for heat or pressure, worse for cold or is accompanied by cramps.

> **CAUTION**
>
> Do not drink coffee if you are taking *Colocynthis* and *Nux vomica.*

Exercise

DYNAMIC BACK EXERCISES All the available evidence suggests that prolonged bed rest can be harmful, so people with sciatica are recommended to remain active. But the question is, how active?

A 1991 study revealed that, irrespective of sex, age, duration and degree of severity of the back trouble, or of pre-existing sciatica or X-ray findings of damage, people with sciatica derived most benefit from a dynamic training programme of back exercises. The study did not include people with clinical signs of current lumbar nerve root compression (disc herniation).

In 1999, research revealed that people with low back pain and sciatica had a sig-nificant reduction in symptoms after a programme of Mensendieck exercises. Named after a Danish therapist, these functional exercises correct body postures and make people more body-conscious so they can prevent injuries and sore muscles. They may be available from physiotherapists and specialist teachers.

Bodywork Therapies

PRIMARY TREATMENT **PHYSIOTHERAPY AND CHIRO-PRACTIC MANIPULATION** are equally beneficial for individuals with low back pain. However, in a 1998 study, even people who followed the advice of an educational booklet on the best ways to look after the spine (such as posture) experienced benefits that were almost as good.

OSTEOPATHY Sometimes the sciatic nerve runs through the small piriformis muscle that connects the sacrum to the top of the leg rather than under it. The nerve may be compressed here by muscle spasm, causing sciatica (*see Neuropathy, p.127*). Effective osteopathic soft-tissue manipulation can release the muscle in many cases. When this fails, surgery may be required.

Acupuncture

Acupuncture is promising for low back pain, but it is not proven. The cause of sciatica makes a difference. If it is generated by mechanical back pain, then acupuncture should be effective, often with relatively few treatments. If it is caused by nerve compression as a result of a prolapsed disc, then acupuncture is likely to be less effective with more treatments required. A Western acupuncture technique is usually used: the tender areas are needled and sometimes electrical stimulation is given following the pain from the low back down to the foot. Treatment is given twice a week for very acute pain, or weekly for less acute pain. If there is no benefit after six to eight sessions, it is probably wise to stop.

> **PREVENTION PLAN**
>
> **To reduce the risk of sciatica:**
> - Follow a back exercise programme.

PROLAPSED DISC

A prolapsed disc occurs when the soft core of the cartilage between two vertebrae pushes outwards. The disc inflames the surrounding tissue, causing swelling. If its outer coat ruptures, it is called a herniated disc. In both conditions, the bulge produced presses on local nerves, causing pain, commonly in the leg (*see Sciatica, p.272*). Prolapsed (slipped) discs occur most commonly in the lower back, but discs in the neck and, rarely, in the upper back may also prolapse or herniate. Treatment aims to relieve the pain and restore the health of a damaged disc.

WHAT ARE THE SYMPTOMS?

Symptoms may appear gradually over a period of weeks or can appear suddenly. They may include:

- Pain in the affected area
- Muscle spasm and stiffness around the affected area that make movement difficult

If a spinal nerve is affected, the following symptoms may also be present:

- Severe pain, tingling, or numbness in a leg, or, if the neck is affected, an arm
- Weakness or restricted movement in the leg or arm

In a few cases, when a disc herniates it puts pressure on the cauda equina (a bundle of nerves that emanate from the lower parts of the spinal cord). This requires emergency treatment. Symptoms of this may include:

- Inability to pass urine
- Loss of bowel control
- Numbness around the anus
- Shooting pains down the legs

WHY MIGHT I HAVE THIS?

PREDISPOSING FACTORS

- Bad posture

TRIGGERS

- Lifting a heavy weight

IMPORTANT

If you develop impaired bladder or bowel function combined with other symptoms of a prolapsed or herniated disc you should get immediate medical attention.

WHY DOES IT OCCUR?

The vertebrae of the spine are separated and cushioned by shock-absorbing discs consisting of a strong, fibrous outer coat and a soft, gelatinous core. When a prolapse or herniation occurs, the shape of the disc is distorted. Pain results when the inflamed and swollen surrounding tissues and the disc itself press upon a spinal nerve as it emerges from the spinal cord or press on the spinal cord itself. The initial symptoms are often back pain and spasm. These gradually fade over several days but leg pain gets more severe.

From about the age of 25, the discs begin to dry out and become more vulnerable to prolapse or herniation due to the normal stresses of daily life and minor injury. A disc may sometimes be damaged by a sharp bending or twisting movement or by lifting a heavy object incorrectly. From about the age of 45, fibrous tissue forms around the discs, eventually stabilising them and making them less prone to damage.

SELF-HELP

PRIMARY TREATMENT If you have the symptoms of a prolapsed or herniated disc, try the following:

- Take analgesics, such as aspirin, paracetamol or ibuprofen, to ease the pain.
- Relax and lie flat on your back on a comfortable surface to reduce the pressure on your spine. If this is still uncomfortable, bend your knees at right angles and support your calves with pillows.
- In the short-term, soothe tight muscles with a hot-water bottle held against the most painful part of your back. Or wrap a pack of crushed ice cubes in a cloth and apply to the area for 15 minutes every couple of hours.
- Get up and move about carefully as soon as the pain allows.
- Avoid lifting anything heavy for three months as advised by your doctor. Avoid heavy lifting in the long term and don't drive for long periods.

TREATMENT PLAN

PRIMARY TREATMENTS

- Analgesics and relaxation (*see Self-Help*)
- Treatment for cervical disc prolapse
- Treatment for lumbar disc prolapse
- Anaesthetic injections
- Surgery (if severe or if symptoms are dangerous)

BACK-UP TREATMENTS

- Bodywork therapies

WORTH CONSIDERING

- Nutritional therapy
- Acupuncture

For an explanation of how treatments are rated, see p.111.

TREATMENTS IN DETAIL

Conventional Medicine

The doctor can usually make a diagnosis from a description of the symptoms and an examination of the back. In some cases, an X-ray may be needed to exclude other

Nerves supplying the limbs, and those providing bowel and bladder control, run through the spinal cord in the neck. A prolapsed cervical disc in the MRI scan (above) may cause pain and weakness in the neck and arm or lower down the body.

causes of pain. Tests, such as magnetic resonance imaging (MRI) may then be arranged to establish the site and severity of the prolapse. A prolapsed or herniated disc commonly returns to normal spontaneously.

PRIMARY TREATMENT **TREATMENT FOR CERVICAL DISC PROLAPSE** Symptoms caused by a cervical disc prolapse (in the neck) often settle with rest and painkillers. A collar for the neck may be needed for support. Sometimes, a period of traction in hospital may help to relieve pain and other symptoms.

Occasionally, for very severe persistent pain, surgery may be performed to remove the affected disc. Vertebrae in the neck may be fused to avoid making them unstable and to prevent some of the original symptoms persisting. However, this restricts the movements of the cervical spine.

PRIMARY TREATMENT **TREATMENT FOR LUMBAR DISC PROLAPSE** Symptoms of a lumbar disc prolapse (in the low back) tend to settle with rest, painkillers and, sometimes, muscle relaxants, such as diazepam (only for a short period due to the risk of dependence). Physiotherapy is often recommended to help relieve muscle spasm and so speed up recovery.

PRIMARY TREATMENT **ANAESTHETIC INJECTIONS** To relieve the pain of a prolapsed disc, a local anaesthetic may be injected into the epidural space (the space surrounding the membranes that envelop the spinal cord). Alternatively, a local anaesthetic, sometimes in combination with a corticosteroid drug, may be injected into the area of the affected disc to help relieve pain and swelling.

PRIMARY TREATMENT **SURGERY** should only be considered if the symptoms persist after several weeks or if they are worsening, or if the pain or weakness is very severe. If there is pressure on the cauda equina (a bundle of nerves at the base of the spine), surgery must be carried out urgently.

A disc may be removed either by traditional surgery or by microdiscectomy, a relatively new procedure in which the surgeon removes the disc through a small incision, while watching images of the procedure provided by a camera inserted through another small incision.

The results from these two types of surgical approach are thought to be similar in terms of the relief of symptoms, although the recovery period following traditional surgery is likely to be longer. Following removal of a disc, there may be some residual pain, and stiffness may develop due to new stresses placed on the back.

In some cases, rather than removing the disc to relieve the symptoms, the affected disc may be softened by an injection of a softening agent called chymopapain, a protein-digesting enzyme prepared from the papaya fruit. The procedure is known as chemonucleolysis.

> **CAUTION**
>
> Drugs and surgery for prolapsed disc may have side-effects: ask your doctor to explain these to you.

Nutritional Therapy

GLUCOSAMINE SULPHATE is a basic building block of disc tissue. Clinical experience suggests that taking 500mg of glucosamine sulphate supplements, 2 or 3 times a day, may help to stimulate healing and repair within damaged discs. (*See also Back and neck pain, p.268.*)

Bodywork Therapies

RESOLVING DISC-RELATED LOW BACK PAIN Studies show that various strategies can all assist in the early resolution of disc-related, low back pain. These include supervised "McKenzie-concept" exercises (involving repetitive extension, or arching, of the back when lying face down and strengthening the "core stability" of abdominal and low back muscles), traction, use of a cold pack on the affected area and mobilisation of the muscles and joints.

CHIROPRACTIC The success of chiropractic treatment of herniated lower back and neck discs is supported by a great deal of evidence (including scan images). In one study, CT scans showed that the resolution of symptoms following manipulation was accompanied by a reduction in disc prolapse in 75 per cent of larger herniations and 40 per cent of smaller ones.

PENS UNITS The pain of sciatica (*see p.272*) caused by disc prolapse has been shown to be effectively controlled with the use of PENS units. This involves passing a mild electrical current through needles inserted into the tissue so that the current passes through the painful area. PENS is more effective than the more widely used TENS, which involves passing the current over the pain area. PENS is available at pain control clinics and some acupuncturists use it. However, it is not recommended for self-use.

ALTERNATIVES TO SURGERY Intradiscal electrothermal therapy (IDET) is an alternative surgical intervention that heats the damaged tissues in order, it is thought, to speed up the process of reabsorption of disc fragments.

Results of a 2002 study revealed that, two years after IDET, a significant improvement in pain levels, physical functioning (sitting, standing and walking) was observed, and overall quality of life was much improved. More than 80 per cent of the patients reported they were satisfied with the procedure.

When disc prolapse occurs in the neck (often causing major pain in the arms) a 2002 Swedish study found that supervised, intermittent, on-the-door, neck traction resulted in complete symptom resolution

THERAPEUTIC BACKCARE EXERCISES

Regular strengthening exercises are a key part of a backcare programme to avoid further injury, but you should always first consult a physiotherapist or doctor. The following exercises help to strengthen the extensors (the muscles used to straighten the back and limbs) as well as the deep stabilising muscles of the abdomen so they can protect the spine. Do ten repetitions each day to begin with. For best results, you should combine them with exercises to stretch your hamstrings as tight leg muscles contribute to back problems.

Horizontal raise

Start on all fours, with your knees hip-width apart. Breathing out, pull in your abdomen tightly. Carefully stretch out a leg, keeping your pelvis stable. Hold for 5 seconds. Repeat 5 times on each side.

Cycling

Do not lower the leg beyond this angle

Lie on the floor, with your knees bent. Engage the deep stomach muscles to stabilise your pelvis. Slowly straighten one leg. Bend the knee and then straighten the other leg as if cycling.

---

within three weeks. On-the-door traction is widely available for self-use and involves a person, either seating or standing, using a harness or other form of material attached to a piece of equipment that hooks on to the top of a door.

RECOVERY AFTER SURGERY Surgery definitely has a place in treating prolapsed discs. In a 2001 study, 294 patients with disc degeneration were treated by surgery or by different types of physical therapy. Two years after treatment, 63 per cent of the surgical group reported they were "much better" or "better" after surgery and that their "back to work rate" was also significantly better. After surgery, exercise is an essential part of your rehabilitation

plan. A systematic review of research made the following recommendations:

- Starting 4–6 weeks after surgery, intensive exercise programmes get faster results than mild exercise programmes. In the long term, however, there is no difference between intensive and mild exercise programmes with regard to overall improvement.
- There is no strong evidence for the effectiveness of supervised training as compared to peforming home exercises.
- It is not known whether active rehabilitation programmes should start immediately after surgery or later.
- There is no evidence that patients need to have their activities restricted after first-time lumbar disc surgery.

Acupuncture

If a prolapsed disc impinges on a nerve root and causes neurological signs, acupuncture can help manage the pain, but it is not effective for the underlying condition.

PREVENTION PLAN

The following may help you to keep your spine healthy:

- Mackenzie exercises or a course of Pilates or other core-strengthening exercises.
- Advice on posture and lifting.

SPORTS INJURIES

Athletes and other people who exercise strenuously risk sports injuries, such as strains, sprains, bursitis (*see p.284*), ligament injuries, stress fractures and joint dislocations. Such injuries often occur in people who are new to a sport, begin exercise after a long period of inactivity or fail to warm up properly before exercising. Sports injuries may occur suddenly or may develop more gradually as a result of repeated stresses. Treatment aims to relieve pain and restore function; options include using painkillers, physiotherapy, manipulation and homeopathy.

WHAT ARE THE SYMPTOMS?

Depends on the injury

- Pain
- Swelling
- Stiffness

WHY MIGHT I HAVE THIS?

PREDISPOSING FACTORS

- Lack of fitness
- Failure to warm up/cool down properly

TRIGGERS

- Violent contact
- Overuse of a joint or muscle
- Accidental injury

TREATMENT PLAN

PRIMARY TREATMENTS

- Rest, Ice, Compression, Elevation (*see Immediate Relief*)
- Painkillers and NSAIDs
- Treatment for dislocated joints, fractures, ruptured Achilles tendons and other specific injuries
- Physiotherapy, osteopathy and chiropractic

BACK-UP TREATMENTS

- Nutritional therapy
- Acupuncture
- Homeopathy

For an explanation of how treatments are rated, see p.111.

WHY DO THEY OCCUR?

Any part of the musculoskeletal system can be injured while you are playing a sport. Bone injuries commonly occur in contact sports, such as rugby. Repeated jarring of small bones in the feet can lead to stress fractures in runners. Joint injuries can happen in any sport that puts joints under strain, and dislocation of a joint is also a risk in contact sports.

Injuries to ligaments and tendons, the fibrous bands of tissue that hold the musculoskeletal system together, are also common and often result from falling or jumping. Tendons may become inflamed in tendinitis. Inflammation of the tissues at the point where a muscle, via a tendon, attaches to a bone is called enthesitis.

Two common types of enthesitis are tennis elbow and golfer's elbow, which affect the outer and inner sides of the elbow respectively – they are named after the sports in which they classically occur, although they are not restricted to these. Plantar fasciitis, common in long-distance runners, affects the sole of the foot. Less commonly, tendons may rupture; the Achilles tendon at the back of the ankle is particularly susceptible to this.

Finally, muscle injuries, such as strains, can occur in any sport, especially if you fail to warm up properly before starting.

DIFFERENT SPORTS Each sport has its own hazards, no matter how much time is spent training. For example, golf produces the highest level of back problems in any professional sport. Many are spine-related because the spine absorbs a great deal of the strain caused by rotation of the hips, knees and shoulders.

Low back pain, as well as shoulder and neck pain, are commonly reported by runners. Gymnastics is the sport most connected with lumbar spinal injuries.

In swimming, certain strokes, such as the butterfly, produce enormous stress on the bones and muscles of the low back, especially in young swimmers. Thoracic pain and round back deformities are common in young women who do breast stroke because of the repeated round shoulder-type stroke motion.

More young players experience injuries in football than in any other sport. Too much repetitive activity damages certain bones, muscles or tendons over time. Gifted youngsters are asked to train and play competitively at ever-younger ages, which can lead to tragic consequences.

IMMEDIATE RELIEF

| PRIMARY TREATMENT | **RICE** is the best immediate treatment for most injuries:

- Rest – sit or lie down with the injured part comfortably supported.
- Ice – apply ice or a bag of frozen peas to the injured part for 10–15 minutes.
- Compression – bandage a thick layer of cotton wool around the injured part.
- Elevation – raise and support the injured part to reduce blood flow and prevent further swelling.

IMPORTANT

If you think you have injured yourself while involved in a sport or physical activity, don't carry on regardless – stop, get immediate relief and seek a medical opinion.

Conventional Medicine

Your doctor can often make a diagnosis from the symptoms and an examination, although X-rays may be needed to look for fractures. Sometimes, additional investigations, such as CT scanning, enable a doctor to look at the affected area in more detail.

PRIMARY TREATMENT **PAINKILLERS AND NSAIDS** The treatment varies depending on the injury. In all cases, analgesics are likely to be needed. Tendinitis, ligament damage and muscle strains are usually treated by rest and sometimes with NSAIDs.

PRIMARY TREATMENT **TREATMENT FOR FRACTURES** involves holding the fragments of bone in position, often with a cast, so that they heal strongly; surgery may first be needed to return displaced fragments to their original position.

PRIMARY TREATMENT **TREATMENT FOR DISLOCATED JOINTS** In a dislocation, the displaced joint may need to be manipulated into the correct position and then held immobile, so that the tissues around it can heal and once again keep the bones of the joint in position.

PRIMARY TREATMENT **TREATMENT FOR RUPTURED ACHILLES TENDON** If an Achilles tendon ruptures, the two ends of the tendon are held together with a plaster cast; this is sometimes preceded by surgery. You will need to avoid exercise for around four months.

PRIMARY TREATMENT **PHYSIOTHERAPY**, and sometimes ultrasound treatment (to cool or heat tissues), form a part of the treatment for many injuries. Following injuries, you will be given advice on when to resume a gradually increasing exercise programme. When exercising, always wear the correct clothing and use quality equipment. Warm up and cool down, and avoid overusing your muscles and joints.

BURSITIS A bursa is a fluid-filled sac that separates tendons and prevents them rubbing or from rubbing bone. They are found throughout the body and are easily inflamed and irritated by strong repetitive movements (*see also Bursitis, p.284*). For example, the psoas bursa over the hip joint is commonly injured in hurdlers and people who do martial arts and step classes. Injection with a long-lasting cortisone usually cures bursitis. Doctors who specialise in sports injuries can recommend training modifications to avoid recurrences.

> **CAUTION**
>
> NSAIDs have side-effects: ask your doctor to explain these to you.

Nutritional Therapy

BROMELAIN For joint or ligament sprains, take 500mg of bromelain (a pineapple extract), 3 times a day on an empty stomach. A study shows that fluid retention and inflammation may be reduced if you do this as soon as possible after a sprain.

CHONDROITIN AND GLUCOSAMINE are important components of cartilage and may help recovery from cartilage, ligament or tendon damage. In a 1984 study, athletes with damaged knee cartilage who received 1,500mg of glucosamine sulphate per day for 40 days, followed by 750mg of glucosamine sulphate per day for a further 100 days, either experienced a complete cure or were at least able to resume training.

In a 2003 study, people with regular knee pain that may have been caused by prior injury experienced some degree of pain relief and improved function after receiving 2,000mg of glucosamine each day for eight weeks. No studies have looked specifically at chondroitin sulphate in sports injury, though in practice, 1,200mg per day seems to be an effective dose for many.

> **CAUTION**
>
> Consult your doctor before taking bromelain with amoxicillin (*see p.46*).

Homeopathy

Many different medicines may be indicated due to the wide range of injuries, strains and overuse problems.

ARNICA MONTANA is frequently the most appropriate homeopathic medicine. It is used for muscle overstrain and bruising, and is particularly suitable if you feel achey all over and even your bed feels too hard.

OTHER REMEDIES The most common medicine for enthesitis is *Ruta graveolens*, but others including *Bryonia alba* and *Rhus toxicodendron* may be needed. People who respond to *Bryonia* typically feel a sharp pain from particular movements, so that they may suddenly drop a heavy object. The symptoms are relieved by firm support, such as an elasticated brace. Similar symptoms elsewhere – for instance, in the knees (a common injury in footballers) – may also respond to *Bryonia*, if they improve with support. *Rhus tox.* can help a range of different injuries when the characteristic marked improvement from limbering up is found.

TISSUE AFFINITIES Some homeopathic medicines have specific tissue affinities. For example, *Symphytum* is used for bone fractures, such as the stress fractures of the metatarsal bones of the feet common in professional footballers and long-distance runners. *Ledum* is used for black eyes.

A 10-minute warm-up before exercise may help to prevent most sports injuries

---

Bodywork and Movement Therapies

PRIMARY TREATMENT **PHYSIOTHERAPY, OSTEOPATHY AND CHIROPRACTIC** These manipulation treatments, as well as sports massage and neuromuscular therapy, aim to rapidly resolve sporting injuries and restore optimal function.

A practitioner will assess the injury and take the action that is needed – for example, freeing and loosening whatever is tight

STRETCHING TO PREVENT INJURIES

Recent opinion is that stretching does not prevent injuries or soreness. However, most athletes report that they feel better if they gently stretch before and after exercise and physical activity. The muscles in the legs and feet work hard during sports, so protect them with the following exercises. Stretch before your activity for a few minutes to warm the muscles and afterwards for at least 10 minutes to reduce soreness.

Ankle stretch

Your feet should touch from the toes to the heels. Breathe deeply and hold for 10 seconds.

Sitting tall, bend your knees and place the soles of your feet together. Grasp the ankles and allow your knees to fall towards the floor.

Achilles tendon

Achilles tendon stretch

Step your right foot back. Leaning forwards, bend the left knee. Rise on the ball of your foot to stretch the tendon. Hold for 10 seconds and repeat on the other side.

Hands on the knee

or restricted, and toning and improving both the strength and function of whatever tissue is weak. However, the most basic advice for dealing with a recent injury is known as RICE – rest, ice, compression and elevation (*see Immediate relief, p.277*).

An osteopathic perspective on sporting-related injuries and dysfunction starts from the principle that the human body has an in-built capacity to cope with, and successfully adapt to, most of the normal (and many abnormal) demands placed upon it (*see Adaptation, p.53*).

One major mistake made in treating sports injuries is neglecting to respect the natural healing process. Practitioners advise against returning to activity too soon after an injury – time is needed to allow tissue inflammation to calm and tissue repair to be consolidated.

The body's response to soft-tissue injury follows a predictable sequence: there is an inflammatory phase, a repair phase and a maturation (or remodelling) phase. Manual therapy should not start until tissue repair is well established – usually about four weeks after injury. The timing of the three phases is fairly predictable, but varies with the severity, extent and type of tissue injured, as well as according to the age, general health and nutrition of the injured person.

Within that framework, treatment needs to avoid retarding repair and recovery, while at the same time avoiding too much rest and inactivity which would lead to loss of strength and muscle bulk.

Acupuncture

Acupuncture in sports injuries is directed both at relieving pain and accelerating healing. It is widely used by sports physiotherapists and can be very effective in the treatment of injury to joints and the surrounding ligaments and tendons as well as muscle. It is vitally important that a clear diagnosis is made: acupuncture may take away the pain of a stress fracture but in the long term it may cause more damage.

Trigger points (*see p.55*) commonly occur in injured muscles. They cause pain that can be local or referred (experienced some distance away). Acupuncture (or local anaesthetic injection) can successfully treat trigger point pain. As with all acute conditions, the more acupuncture that can be given quickly the better. Initial daily treatment is ideal, followed by weekly, or twice weekly, treatment as the injury settles.

PREVENTION PLAN

The following should help you to prevent sports injuries:

- Warm up and cool down properly.
- Exercise regularly.

TEMPOROMANDIBULAR JOINT DISORDER

The temporomandibular joint connects the lower jawbone (mandible) to the temporal bone of the skull. In temporomandibular joint disorder (TMJ), the joint and its associated muscles and ligaments do not work together properly, causing pain. Treatment may involve orthodontic work, painkillers, chondroitin and glucosamine supplements, acupuncture, physical manipulation and mind–body therapy.

WHAT ARE THE SYMPTOMS?

- Tenderness in the jaw muscles
- Headaches
- Aching pain in the face and sometimes the ears – the pain may be caused by chewing or opening the mouth widely, as when yawning

There may also be other symptoms, including:

- Difficulty opening the mouth
- Locking of the jaw
- Clicking noises from the joint when the mouth is opened or closed

WHY MIGHT I HAVE THIS?

PREDISPOSING FACTORS

- Osteoarthritis
- Malocclusion

TRIGGER

- Stress

TREATMENT PLAN

PRIMARY TREATMENTS

- Orthodontic treatment
- Paracetamol or NSAIDs for pain and muscle spasms (*see Self-Help*)
- Chondroitin and glucosamine

BACK-UP TREATMENTS

- Physical therapy (mouth-opening exercises)
- Chiropractic and other bodywork therapies
- Acupuncture
- Mind–body therapies
- Surgery (rarely)

For an explanation of how treatments are rated, see p.111.

WHY DOES IT OCCUR?

The temporomandibular joint allows the jaw to move in all directions so that the teeth can bite and chew food efficiently. TMJ disorder is often due to spasm of the muscles responsible for chewing. The spasm is commonly a result of clenching the jaw or grinding the teeth. Stress may be a factor in both of these. If the teeth do not meet properly (malocclusion), there may be additional stress on the temporo-mandibular joint.

TMJ disorder may also be the result of an injury that displaces the joint. Rarely, the condition is due to arthritis. The condition is more common in women.

SELF-HELP

PRIMARY TREATMENT The following measures may help you to reduce muscle spasm and relieve pain:

- Massage the muscles of the jaw.
- Apply heat to the painful area with a warm towel or a covered hot-water bottle containing warm water.
- Ease the pain with analgesics such as paracetamol or NSAIDs.
- Eat soft foods until the pain settles. Avoid chewy foods, such as bagels, and do not chew gum.

TREATMENTS IN DETAIL

Conventional Medicine

Your doctor or dentist may arrange X-rays of your jaws and teeth. Other imaging tests, such as magnetic resonance imaging (MRI), may also be needed to accurately diagnose TMJ disorder.

PRIMARY TREATMENT **ORTHODONTIC TREATMENT** The underlying causes are treated where possible. For example, orthodontic treatment appliances may be recommended to improve the bite (how the teeth come together) and a device is available that can be fitted over the upper or lower teeth at night to prevent grinding and clenching.

SYMPTOM RELIEF Treatment aims to reduce muscle spasm and relieve pain (*see Self-Help*). Relaxation techniques may help to relieve associated stress.

SURGERY Occasionally, in severe cases when symptoms persist and there is an underlying problem in the joint, surgery is recommended to restructure the joint.

CAUTION

NSAIDs may cause side-effects: ask your doctor to explain these to you.

Nutritional Therapy

PRIMARY TREATMENT **CHONDROITIN AND GLUCOS-AMINE** supplements may help people with TMJ. Glucosamine is believed to help regenerate cartilage, while chondroitin is said to enable cartilage to remain hydrated and hence keep its resilience. Clinical experience and scientific studies suggest that a combination of both can help people with TMJ who might have osteoarthritis of this joint. In one study, people with osteoarthritis of the temporomandibular joint took 1,500mg of glucosamine hydrochloride and 1,200mg of chondroitin sulphate daily for 12 weeks. The supple-

THE TEMPOROMANDIBULAR JOINT

The temporomandibular joint is located where the temporal bone meets the mandible (jaw) bone. Between the two bones lies a disc of cartilage called the meniscus that allows the joint to open and close like a hinge, but also to move backwards, forwards and from side to side. The two temporomandibular joints bear a great deal of pressure during the process of chewing food.

Section through a temporomandibular joint

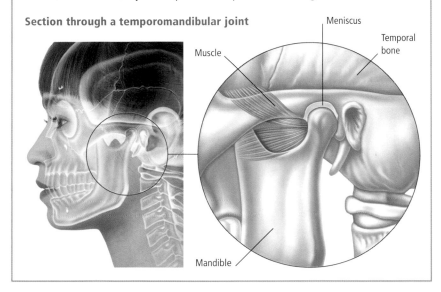

lems: a TMJ disc or joint; trigger points in a muscle (e.g. the temporalis), or trigger points resulting from another joint, such as in the cervical spine. Each require separate treatment. Trigger points can be treated by injection, acupuncture, self-stretching or by a combination of neuromuscular techniques that manipulate soft tissues.

Acupuncture

Trials comparing acupuncture with some rather ingenious placebo treatments have indicated that it is likely to be of substantial benefit in treating the pain of TMJ. Treatment is usually based on needling the tender points around the temporomandibular joint, and pain can be relieved for months and sometimes years after relatively few treatments. As with all painful conditions, four or five weekly acupuncture sessions will be enough to know whether this approach is likely to prove effective.

Mind–Body Therapies

BIOFEEDBACK AND COGNITIVE BEHAVIOURAL SKILLS TRAINING (CBST) may help counter any underlying stress that may be perpetuating symptoms, according to research. In 1977, a pioneering study showed that electromyographic (EMG) biofeedback could be effective in people with long-term pain related to the temporomandibular joint. The patients were trained to be aware of tension in the jaw. In 2000, a study assigned almost 100 patients with chronic TMJ to one of four groups for treatment: biofeedback, CBST, biofeedback and CBST, or a control. Results showed that the three treatment groups reported significantly decreased pain and improved mood. Patients in the biofeedback group were the most significantly improved of all when compared to the no-treatment group.

ments relieved both the pain and tenderness in the joint. Another beneficial effect of the supplements was to reduce the amount of painkillers needed.

In another study, 50 patients with osteoarthritis of the same joint took 3,200mg of glucosamine hydrochloride and 2,400mg of chondroitin sulphate each day, together with 2,000mg of vitamin C for three months. At the end of the study, 80 per cent of patients reported a decrease in both the noises coming from the joint, and the pain.

If you have TMJ, take 1,500–3,000mg of either glucosamine hydrochloride or glucos-amine sulphate with 1,200–2,400mg of chondroitin sulphate.

Physical Therapy

Temporomandibular joint disc displacement is the cause of many people's TMJ problems. A research study evaluated non-surgical treatments, such as splints to correct malocclusion, mobilisation of the jaw and pain medication. The results suggested that people with TMJ caused by anterior displacement of the disc are likely to improve with only minimal (i.e. non-surgical) treatment.

Another study showed that people with painful TMJ disc displacement made a greater improvement when they received physical therapy (mouth-opening exercises) and painkillers than if they received no treatment at all. At the same time, approximately 75 per cent of patients were successfully treated without painkillers and using only active and passive (i.e. assisted) jaw movement exercises, correction of body posture and relaxation techniques.

Bodywork Therapies

Where exercise and/or splint therapy fails to correct anterior disc displacement, active manipulation may be called for, followed by a splint, according to a Chinese study. Chiropractic manipulation of the temporomandibular joint and associated muscles has been shown to be a useful approach in correcting imbalances related to TMJ pain and dysfunction.

DEACTIVATION OF TRIGGER POINTS Muscular imbalances associated with TMJ disorder may involve the active presence of trigger points (*see p.55*), particularly in the temporalis muscles. However, the pain may be the result of three distinct prob-

PREVENTION PLAN

The following may help to prevent the development of TMJ disorder:

- Take dental advice about malocclusion.

- Try to stop clenching your jaw and grinding your teeth.

WHAT ARE THE SYMPTOMS?

Symptoms usually develop slowly over weeks or months and may include:

- Pain in the shoulder which is severe in the early stages and often worse at night
- Over time, decreasing pain but increasing stiffness and restricted movement of the joint
- Sometimes, pain extending down the arm to the elbow

WHY MIGHT I HAVE THIS?

PREDISPOSING FACTORS

- Poor posture
- Repetitive tasks, such as digging or painting walls
- Prolonged immobility of the shoulder
- Trigger points below collarbone
- Diabetes mellitus
- Diet rich in omega-6 and deficient in omega-3 fatty acids

TRIGGERS

- Injury to shoulder

TREATMENT PLAN

PRIMARY TREATMENTS

- Physiotherapy, chiropractic or osteopathy

BACK-UP TREATMENTS

- Pain-relieving drugs
- Homeopathy
- Nutritional therapy
- Alexander technique, Pilates, yoga and massage
- Acupuncture

For an explanation of how treatments are rated, see p.111.

FROZEN SHOULDER

Frozen shoulder is pain and stiffness in and around the shoulder joint that severely restricts movement. Often caused by injury to the shoulder, or following a bout of capsulitis (in which the joint is warm, tender and swollen), it occurs most frequently in people over 40 and is more common in women and in those with diabetes. It can last for up to two years. The integrated healing plan centres on manipulation therapies, which aim to stretch and strengthen shortened, weakened muscles. It also includes drugs to relieve pain and therapies such as yoga and the Alexander technique to improve posture and mobility.

WHY DOES IT OCCUR?

Frozen shoulder may result from an injury to the shoulder region that causes inflammation, or it may occur if the shoulder is immobilised for a long period of time. Often, the cause is unknown.

In many cases, frozen shoulder develops slowly over months or years. If your posture is slumped, with your head forwards and shoulders rounded, it puts the joints under stress (*see feature box, right*). Over time, especially if the muscles have to perform heavy, difficult or repetitive tasks (such as digging the garden, serving at tennis or painting walls) the shoulder may become inflamed. The inflammation could be restricted to the shoulder joint capsule itself or it may involve tissues just outside the capsule. If this happens, scar tissue which severely restricts movement of the shoulder may develop.

Sensitive areas in the muscles known as trigger points (*see p.55*) can create painful shortening of the muscles that control the shoulder joint (the rotator cuff group). This situation is more likely to occur when poor posture changes the relationship of the bones in the shoulder, causing increased mechanical stress on the rotator cuff group of muscles.

There are other situations in which the muscles, ligaments and tendons of the complex shoulder joint can become irritated, inflamed and restricted, resulting in frozen shoulder. These include nerve entrapment, muscle spasm, calcification of muscle attachments, activation of trigger points and partial dislocation of the shoulder joint due to injury or repetitive strain.

IMMEDIATE RELIEF

The following may help you to reduce the swelling and pain:
- Apply an ice pack to the area following the manufacturer's instructions, or wrap a bag of frozen vegetables in a hand towel and place on the painful area for 10 minutes once every hour.
- Alternatively, fill an empty soft-drink can with water, seal with tape and freeze. Roll the can over the painful area for 3–5 minutes every hour.
- Take analgesics for the pain.

TREATMENTS IN DETAIL

Conventional Medicine

If your symptoms seem to suggest that you have developed a frozen shoulder, consult your doctor who may arrange for your shoulder to be X-rayed in order to exclude an underlying disorder.

PAIN-RELIEVING DRUGS Your doctor may prescribe some pain-relieving drugs, such as non-steroidal anti-inflammatory drugs (NSAIDs) or a course of oral corticosteroids if your pain is particularly severe. Alternatively, a corticosteroid drug may be injected into your shoulder joint which may give relief from pain and stiffness – a treatment similar to the one that may be used for bursitis (*see illustration, p.285*).

> **CAUTION**
>
> NSAIDs may cause side-effects: ask your doctor to explain these to you.

HOW A FROZEN SHOULDER DEVELOPS

If you habitually hunch your shoulders and poke your head forwards, the socket into which your upper arm slots (glenoid fossa) will be further forwards than if your posture were upright. The rotator cuff muscles that link the shoulder joint to the humerus will need to work under immense mechanical stress. Over time, this may lead to the shoulder becoming inflamed, restricted and painful.

Inflammation of the shoulder

In frozen shoulder, the rotator cuff muscles (at the front and back of the shoulder) become strained, leading to a painful area just underneath the glenoid fossa (arm socket).

- Glenoid fossa
- Rotator cuff muscles
- Inflamed area
- Humerus
- Shoulder blade

Nutritional Therapy

OMEGA-3 AND OMEGA-6 FATTY ACIDS Excessive omega-6 fatty acids and a relative lack of omega-3 fatty acids seem to promote inflammation. Eating foods rich in omega-3 fatty acids can help reduce the inflammatory component of the condition. Omega-3 fatty acids are found in some nuts and seeds, and in oily fish. If you have repeated bouts of frozen shoulder, you may benefit from eating these foods regularly. Taking about 400mg of the omega-3 fatty acid EPA and about 300mg of DPA each day for at least two months may relieve inflammation and pain.

Homeopathy

Injections of the homeopathic preparation *Formica rufa* subcutaneously (i.e. under the skin, not into the joint as with steroid injections) often help frozen shoulder. The special injectable preparation must only be given by a qualified practitioner.

Several homeopathic medicines may be helpful for frozen shoulder, especially if given early, in the inflammatory stage. The most commonly suitable homeopathic medicine is *Rhus toxicodendron*. In people who respond to *Rhus tox.*, the pain is eased by gentle movement of the joint. Take two 6C pills three times a day.

Bodywork and Movement Therapies

PRIMARY TREATMENT **PHYSIOTHERAPY, CHIROPRACTIC OR OSTEOPATHY** is highly recommended for frozen shoulder. Once a shoulder has become very painful and movement significantly restricted, the healing process is often lengthy and needs careful and regular treatment, as well as self-treatment, to rehabilitate the joint. In some very severe cases, surgery may be necessary.

Visit a practitioner or a doctor who practises manual medicine as soon as your condition is diagnosed. As with most chronic joint problems, the process of arriving at a frozen shoulder starts with minor discomfort and mild restriction of movement. Do not neglect it at this stage as this will allow further gradual deterioration, increased irritation and inflammation, and ultimately the formation of scar tissue and severe restriction of movement.

Your treatment in the early stages is likely to include identifying muscular imbalances, stretching shortened muscles, toning and strengthening weakened muscles and deactivating trigger points. Your therapist will also probably advise on how to stand, sit and move, since poor posture can be a major cause of stress in the muscles, tendons and ligaments.

There are many cases recorded of spontaneous recovery of frozen shoulder, after approximately 30 months – evidence of the self-healing potential of the body.

ALEXANDER TECHNIQUE AND PILATES If poor posture contributes to the problem, try some lessons in the Alexander technique (*see p.62*). This may be useful in improving posture over a period of 6–12 months. A course of Pilates may also benefit your posture.

YOGA AND MASSAGE Yoga practice may help to relax you, relieve stress and stretch tight muscles. Massage also has this effect.

Acupuncture

Of five clinical studies, four support the use of acupuncture in treating shoulder pain. The fifth study gave negative results but it was poorly constructed.

Acupuncture should be used in the early stages of shoulder pain in order to prevent the development of a frozen shoulder. If frozen shoulder is established, acupuncture often offers pain relief after a substantial number of treatments, but physiotherapy is still required. Usually, a frozen shoulder needs weekly treatment for 10–12 weeks before significant improvement occurs.

PREVENTION PLAN

The following may help to prevent the development of frozen shoulder:

- Stretching and strengthening exercises to keep the shoulder strong and flexible.

WHAT ARE THE SYMPTOMS?

- Pain and swelling in the affected joint
- Restricted movement in the affected joint

WHY MIGHT I HAVE THIS?

PREDISPOSING FACTORS

- Overuse of a joint

TRIGGERS

- Injury
- Unaccustomed exercise
- Bacterial infection

TREATMENT PLAN

PRIMARY TREATMENTS

- Rest
- NSAIDs
- Fluid drainage and corticosteroid injections

BACK-UP TREATMENTS

- Antibiotics (for infective bursitis)
- Surgery (if the condition recurs)
- Acupuncture
- Bodywork therapies

WORTH CONSIDERING

- Homeopathy
- Nutritional therapy

For an explanation of how treatments are rated, see p.111.

BURSITIS

In bursitis, the fluid-filled sac (bursa) that surrounds a joint and cushions it against friction becomes inflamed, leading to tenderness and swelling. Movement of the joint may also be restricted. The knee is the most common site for bursitis (once called housemaid's knee), but the elbow and other joints, such as the hip, are also commonly affected. Treatment aims to reduce inflammation and so relieve pain.

WHY DOES IT OCCUR?

Points of pressure or friction may occur in a joint where a tendon or a muscle rubs against a bone or another muscle. The swelling and inflammation of bursitis may develop after an injury to a joint or following unaccustomed exercise. Some joint diseases, such as rheumatoid arthritis (*see p.293*) and gout (*see p.302*), can increase the risk of bursitis. Rarely, the condition may be due to a bacterial infection.

Overuse of the joint, or if the joint is put under prolonged or repeated stress, may also be involved. This is reflected in the traditional names for bursitis: housemaid's knee may be due to excessive kneeling; weaver's bottom (which affects the bursa overlying the pelvic bones, or ischia, that you sit upon) is named after weavers who shuffled up and down long benches as they worked their looms. The bursa of the knee is the most commonly affected, but the elbow and shoulder are also prone.

Bursitis usually improves on its own if you rest the affected joint, but this may take several weeks.

IMMEDIATE RELIEF

Try the following measures to help relieve the pain and discomfort of bursitis:

- Take plenty of rest. In particular, ischial bursitis is helped by sitting on either a foam rubber or an inflatable ring.
- Apply a cold compress. Wring out a double layer of cotton material in very cold water and wrap it round the joint. Immediately cover this with a layer or two of an insulating flannel or woollen material so that no damp edges protrude. The effect of this is to allow the cold cotton to become warm. Fix the compress in place with a safety pin and leave for 2–8 hours or overnight.

TREATMENTS IN DETAIL

Conventional Medicine

PRIMARY TREATMENT **REST AND DRUGS** Your doctor will examine the affected joint and will probably recommend that you rest the joint to allow the inflammation to settle. You may be prescribed NSAIDs to help this process. If the condition is caused by a bacterial infection, you will need to take antibiotics.

PRIMARY TREATMENT **INJECTIONS AND SURGERY** If symptoms persist, or are very severe, your doctor may drain the bursa of fluid and inject it with a corticosteroid to relieve the inflammation. In a few cases, if symptoms persist or the condition frequently recurs, the bursa may be removed.

> **CAUTION**
>
> Medication and surgery for bursitis may cause side-effects: ask your doctor to explain these to you.

Nutritional Therapy

OMEGA-3 FATTY ACIDS Studies have shown that taking omega-3 fatty acids reduces the inflammation and pain that are associated with bursitis. The omega-3 fatty acids eicosapentaenoic acid (EPA) and docosahexaenoic acid (DHA), given at doses of 378mg and 259mg respectively per day for two months or longer, have been found to reduce inflammation, and may therefore help people with bursitis.

Omega-3 fatty acids can be found in some nuts and seeds, especially walnuts and flaxseeds, but the main dietary source is oily fish, such as mackerel, trout, herring, salmon and sardines. Eating plenty of these

CORTICOSTEROIDS TO RELIEVE BURSITIS

An injection of corticosteroids, known as an infiltration, into the bursa of a joint is an effective way of relieving the pain and inflammation associated with bursitis. One of the advantages of such local injections is that, compared to oral administration of corticosteroids, there are fewer side-effects to the body as a whole. The knee and shoulder are two of the joints that benefit from corticosteroid injections.

Treating bursitis in the shoulder

The subacromial bursa is one of three regions of the shoulder that benefit from corticosteroid injections when it is inflamed.

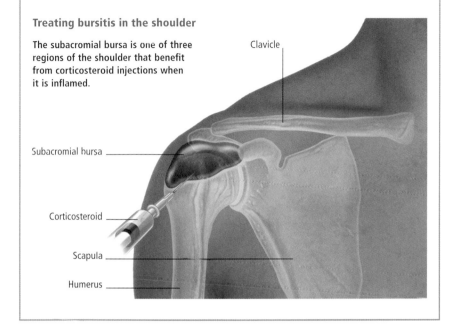

Clavicle

Subacromial bursa

Corticosteroid

Scapula

Humerus

---

foods may help to reduce the symptoms of bursitis. Another option you can try is to take 1,000mg of concentrated fish oil, once or twice a day.

> **CAUTION**
>
> Consult your doctor before taking either omega-3 fatty acids or fish oils with warfarin (*see p.46*).

Homeopathy

The following medicines should be taken in the 6C strength. Take two pills two or three times daily. *Ruta graveolens* can also be used as a cream.

APIS MELLIFICA is among the most important remedies for bursitis. It is a good illustration of the principle of homeopathy, as the symptoms of bursitis resemble those of a bee sting, from which *Apis* is made. The medicine is likely to help if the onset of bursitis was acute with much pain and swelling. The bursa is very

sensitive to pressure, but cold applications, such as ice packs, may relieve the pain.

RUTA GRAVEOLENS The most commonly suggested medicine for less acute situations is *Ruta grav.*, which is made from the herb rue. It is appropriate when the affected region feels weak and bruised, and there is some improvement from gentle movement.

STICTA is more commonly used for sinusitis, but is sometimes useful for knee bursitis.

Acupuncture

Painful conditions appear to respond very well to acupuncture, but there have been very few good-quality clinical trials that look specifically at bursitis. Some small studies or series of case reports indicate that acupuncture is immediately and rapidly effective in this condition: treatment is usually based on needling local tender painful areas and does not necessarily appear to require a traditional Chinese diagnosis. Acupuncture treatment can be safer and sometimes swifter than some of

the conventional treatment options that are available. As with all painful conditions, acupuncture treatment should be given on a weekly or twice-weekly basis. If there is no benefit after five or six sessions, acupuncture is unlikely to be effective.

Bodywork Therapies

DEACTIVATE TRIGGER POINTS At times, bursitis is accompanied by active trigger points (*see p.55*) in the area of the joint. For example, in subacromial bursitis in the shoulder joint the trigger points in the pectoralis or supraspinatus or teres major muscles often create more pain than the bursitis itself.

Manual methods, such as pressure and stretching, as well as acupuncture or a local anaesthetic injection can deactivate such trigger points and reduce the pain levels markedly. However, this may do little to change the actual bursitis.

PAIN RELIEF Treating the bursitis itself involves releasing any shortness or tightness in the muscles attached to the joint. At the same time, gentle pain-relieving strategies may be employed – hydrotherapy, ice packs and/or alternate hot and cold compresses can ease swelling and reduce discomfort. Lymphatic drainage massage (*see p.62*) will help to reduce fluid pressure around the joint.

HEEL PADS made of foam rubber or felt may be needed to treat bursitis of the heel joint (calcaneum). These elevate the heel, provide padding around the bursa and minimise shoe pressure. An orthotic (shock-absorbing foot support) to prevent abnormal heel motion may also be helpful.

GRADUATED EXERCISES, in which you gradually increase your effort or number of repetitions, are an important part of careful rehabilitation as the bursitis eases. These stretch short or tight muscles and tone weakened muscles.

> **PREVENTION PLAN**
>
> **The following may prevent bursitis:**
> - Avoid overuse of particular joints.

WHAT ARE THE SYMPTOMS?

The symptoms of RSI develop gradually and may only be present during the repeated activity at first. They may include:

- Pain, aching, tingling and restricted movement in the affected area
- In some cases, tissue swelling in the affected area

WHY MIGHT I HAVE THIS?

PREDISPOSING FACTORS

- Occupations that involve repetitive movements
- Poor posture
- Stress
- Low thyroid function
- Vitamin B6 deficiency

TREATMENT PLAN

PRIMARY TREATMENTS

- Ergonomic changes in work practices (*see Self-Help and Ergonomics*)
- Symptom relief with painkillers, non-steroidal anti-inflammatory drugs (NSAIDs) and physiotherapy

BACK-UP TREATMENTS

- Vitamin B6
- Bodywork and movement therapies
- Acupuncture
- Stress-management programme

WORTH CONSIDERING

- Homeopathy
- Nutritional therapy

For an explanation of how treatments are rated, see p.111.

REPETITIVE STRAIN INJURY

Prolonged, repeated movements of one part of the body can lead to so-called repetitive strain injury (RSI). It most commonly affects muscles and tendons in the arms (upper limb disorder is a better name since no injury is involved). RSI may be associated with stress at home or work. Treatment involves pain relief and reducing inflammation. Homeopathy, manipulation, acupuncture and ergonomics can all help.

WHY DOES IT OCCUR?

In repetitive strain injury, muscles or tendons become irritated over time due to movements that repeatedly subject them to strain and do not allow them sufficient time to recover. Tendinitis, tenosynovitis and carpal tunnel syndrome (*see p.152*) may cause symptoms similar to RSI.

People who carry out repeated movements on a daily basis, such as those who use a keyboard or work on a production line, are particularly at risk of developing RSI, as are musicians and athletes.

Skeletal muscles contain two types of fibre – Type 1 and Type 2 (*see p.51*). When the muscles, such as those in the arm, are overused repetitively, the Type 1 fibres shorten, while the Type 2 fibres weaken. Over time, an imbalance occurs in which muscles may not be able to perform their functions normally and other muscles are brought into action inappropriately. The end result is pain, cramp-like tension in the area and an inability to perform normal movements and actions.

Inflammation at the point where a tendon attaches to a bone, a condition known as enthesitis, may be part of RSI. Tennis elbow and golfer's elbow are the two common types of enthesitis affecting the arms. They affect the outer and inner sides of the elbow respectively.

IMPORTANT

Consult your doctor promptly if you develop the symptoms of RSI, because the condition is much more difficult to treat once it becomes long term.

SELF-HELP

PRIMARY TREATMENT If you have the symptoms of RSI or wish to prevent it, take the following steps:

- If your RSI is work-related, inform your employer and ask for an ergonomic assessment of your work (*see p.287*).
- Seek occupational health advice on relieving muscle and tendon strain.
- Take regular breaks from any repetitive activity with which you are involved.
- Learn a relaxation technique (*see p.99*).

TREATMENTS IN DETAIL

Conventional Medicine

Your doctor will examine you and ask whether you perform repetitive activities. Tests, such as X-rays, may be arranged to exclude an underlying condition.

PRIMARY TREATMENT **SYMPTOM RELIEF** Your doctor may recommend painkillers, NSAIDs or physiotherapy to help relieve the pain and inflammation.

CAUTION

NSAIDs may cause a range of side-effects: ask your doctor to explain them to you.

Nutritional Therapy

REDUCED THYROID FUNCTION If you are experiencing symptoms such as sensitivity to cold, cold hands and feet, dry skin and lethargy, your RSI may be related to a reduction in the function of your thyroid gland (*see Thyroid problems, p.319*).

VITAMIN B6 DEFICIENCY may, according to some doctors, be a major factor in the development of RSI. This vitamin, which is needed for normal function of nerve cells, reduces inflammatory reactions in soft tissues. Foods rich in vitamin B6 include lean meat, fish, poultry, eggs, dairy products, nuts, soya beans, brown rice, wholegrain cereals, potatoes and other vegetables.

Studies show that many people with RSI derive significant relief from taking B6 supplements. The recommended dosage would be to take 100mg of B6 3 times a day for three months, followed by a good B-complex supplement containing at least 25mg of B6 daily.

VITAMIN B2 can also be effective, even more so if you take it with vitamin B6, according to research. Take 100mg of vitamin B2 each day for three months, followed by a B-complex supplement containing at least 25mg of vitamin B2 each day.

BROMELAIN is an extract from pineapple which has natural anti inflammatory prop-erties and can be useful in the treatment of RSI, especially when taken in combination with vitamin B6. The recommended dose is 500mg of bromelain, taken 3 times a day on an empty stomach.

> **CAUTION**
>
> Consult your doctor before taking vitamin B6 with levodopa or phenobarbital, or bromelain with amoxicillin (*see p.46*).

Homeopathy

BRYONIA ALBA is the classical medicine for inflammation of tendons and the sheaths that surround them. People who respond to *Bryonia* typically have a sharp pain from particular movements, so that they may suddenly drop heavy objects. Pain, tenderness and sometimes visible swelling occurs along the course of the tendon.

People who respond to *Bryonia* find their symptoms are relieved by elasticated wrist support. They may have an associ-ated stiff neck with a headache, which is worse for sudden movements and jarring, but which is relieved by support, such as a soft collar. Thirst and a dry mouth may also be accompanying symptoms.

RUTA GRAVEOLENS is another homeo-pathic medicine that may help people who have RSI that affects the ligaments and ten-dons: they have a feeling of weakness, especially in the wrists. *Ruta grav.* is one of the most frequently indicated medicines for enthesitis.

CONSTITUTIONAL MEDICINES tailored to the constitution of particular individuals (*see p.73*) may be required for more com-plex and longstanding cases of RSI. The most common medicine is *Calcarea car-bonica*. Typically, those who respond to this medicine constantly strain their arms from slight overexertion. They easily get cramps in their hands and elsewhere. Often, their hands and feet are sweaty and they have low back pain.

Psychologically, people who respond to *Calc. carb.* are often fed up and jaded from long periods of overwork, and may become very anxious about their ability to cope with their workload. As workers, they are normally reliable and conscientious, if rather "plodding". Bad dreams and sweat-ing on the head at night are among their other associated symptoms.

Ergonomics

PRIMARY TREATMENT If you are experiencing RSI, it is most important that you review the ergonomics of the way you work. In other words, you need to examine your posture and activities, and look again at the design of the implements you use regularly, such as desks, chairs, shoes, key-boards or operating machinery, to assess the stress they place on your body. The most common causes of RSI are either overuse or the stressful use of computer keyboards and mice.

To prevent RSI you may need to re-design your work space. For example, your desk and chair should be at a height that is compatible with your particular measure-ments. You may also need to learn better ways of using instruments and tools – for example, typing with your hands and wrists at the correct angle.

REPETITIVE STRAIN INJURY IN THE FOREARM

The forearm is composed of various muscles, ligaments and tendons. It is particularly prone to RSI in people, such as those who use computer keyboards, who adopt a posture that puts stress on the wrist or who repeatedly use the same posture for prolonged periods without rest.

Muscles and tendons of the forearm

Carpal ligament of the wrist

Extensor muscle of the fingers

Trigger point

Biceps

Tendon of extensor muscle

Tendon

Elbow

Overuse of the muscles of the forearm can create soreness. This could be due to trigger points which may set off a continuous cycle of spasm and pain in the muscle fibres.

USING A COMPUTER SAFELY

A screen or a chair at the wrong height forces users to lean forward and hunch their shoulders. The muscles in the back, shoulders and neck stay contracted for long periods, which constricts blood flow and may in the long term contribute to RSI.

To avoid this, choose a chair with an adjustable back and seat, and use a computer stand if necessary to ensure the screen is at the correct height. Check that overhead lighting does not reflect on the screen and take a short break every hour.

A well-designed workstation

If you are correctly positioned, the keyboard will be at, or just below, elbow height and the top of the screen will be at eye level. Your wrists should be straight. Use a foot rest if your feet do not touch the ground.

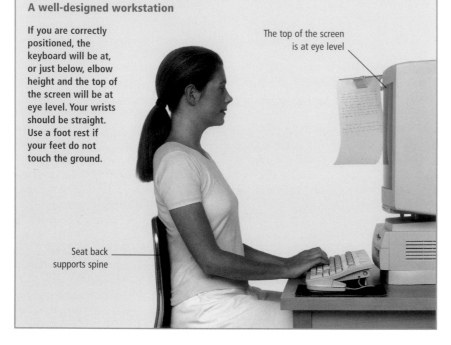

The top of the screen is at eye level

Seat back supports spine

Bodywork and Movement Therapies

The most effective approach to reversing the changes to Type 1 and Type 2 muscle fibres (*see p.51*) is to learn to perform whatever activities have caused the problem in a less stressful way. At the same time, you need to strengthen the muscles that have become weakened and simultaneously stretch and relax those muscles that have shortened.

THE ALEXANDER TECHNIQUE helps you learn to re-use your body in a better way. A qualified teacher will help you to undo your bad postural habits and show you how to stand, sit and move with the minimum of effort. You may only need lessons for a few weeks, although they can last up to a year (*see p.62*).

YOGA THERAPY may help to reverse many of the symptoms of RSI. A qualified yoga teacher will show you various exercises that

will stretch tight muscles and strengthen weak ones. For example, research revealed that the prayer position of the hands (*namaste – see p.153*), which gently extends and stretches the wrists and fingers, can significantly improve your grip strength and reduce pain.

DEACTIVATING TRIGGER POINTS Much RSI pain arises from active trigger points in overused muscles (*see p.55*). These can be treated by injection, acupuncture (using dry needling techniques known as intramuscular stimulation), self-stretching exercises or by a combination of soft-tissue manipulation methods known as neuromuscular techniques (*see p.61*).

FOOT AND ANKLE THERAPY Wearing inappropriate shoes can strain the the ligaments and muscles of your ankles. The resulting foot pain, which is a form of RSI, is very common, especially in women. Overuse, repetitive strain and minor, easily forgotten injuries can lead to chronic foot

and ankle pain. The correct diagnosis and efficient therapy should involve changing the type of footwear (and possibly adding orthotic supports), as well as the appropriate physiotherapy.

Acupuncture

Clinical experience suggests that acupuncture can be of real value in treating RSI. Sometimes, the acupuncturist will use electro-acupuncture and, occasionally, ear acupuncture. You will usually need six to eight weekly sessions. RSI can be a very persistent and difficult problem, so it is worth continuing with treatment for a reasonable period of time.

Mind-Body Therapies

STRESS MANAGEMENT Stress, both at home and in the workplace, can be a contributory factor in RSI. The pain you feel can affect you psychologically in a kind of vicious circle: pain leads to stress, which leads to more muscle tension and therefore more pain.

Often, there is a period of denial, in which the pain is ignored or not taken seriously. Yet the pain can be restricting and sometimes frightening. An inability to work fully can leave you frustrated and even more stressed. A psychologist, psychiatrist or clinical social worker may be able to give you guidance and help to reduce your levels of stress.

You may find that a stress-management programme (*see p.292*) is helpful, as well as relaxing and practising meditation on a regular basis (*see p.98*).

PREVENTION PLAN

To prevent RSI occurring, pay attention to the following:

- Improve the ergonomics of your work space by adjusting the height of your desk and chair, and using wrist supports for keyboards.

- Improve your posture while working.

- Take regular breaks from repetitive activities, such as working at a computer keyboard.

- Learn a relaxation technique.

OSTEOARTHRITIS

Osteoarthritis (OA) is the gradual degeneration of the cartilage that lines the joints, causing pain, swelling and restricted movement. It is more common in the large weight-bearing joints, such as the hips and knees, but the joints of the hands, feet, shoulders, neck and upper back may also be affected. Overall, women are twice as likely to be affected by osteoarthritis as men. The condition sometimes runs in families. Treatments focus on relieving pain and inflammation as well as reducing toxins and maintaining mobility.

WHAT ARE THE SYMPTOMS?

Symptoms are often mild initially and gradually worsen. They include:

- Pain and tenderness in the affected joint
- Swelling around the joint
- Stiffness after periods of inactivity
- Restricted movement in the affected joint
- Crackling of the affected joint (crepitus) when it is moved

WHY MIGHT I HAVE THIS?

PREDISPOSING FACTORS

- Repeated stress on joints
- Repeated injuries to joints
- Excess weight
- Hereditary factors
- Certain occupations

TRIGGERS

- Solanine containing foods

TREATMENT PLAN

PRIMARY TREATMENTS

- Lifestyle measures (*see also Self-Help*)
- Drugs, such as painkillers, NSAIDs and and corticosteroid injections
- Surgery in severe cases
- Glucosamine and chondroitin
- Arthritis Self-Management Program

BACK-UP TREATMENTS

- Nutritional therapy
- Homeopathy
- Western and Chinese herbal medicine
- Acupuncture
- Bodywork and movement therapies
- Mind–body therapies

For an explanation of how treatments are rated, see p.111.

WHY DOES IT OCCUR?

In osteoarthritis (OA), the cartilage that covers the ends of the bones in the joints gradually wears away. The bone around the affected joint thickens and bony growths, or osteophytes, form. Osteophytes on the last joint of the fingers are known as Heberden's nodes, while osteophytes on the middle joint of the fingers are called Bouchard's nodes. If the synovial tissue lining a joint capsule becomes inflamed, fluid may accumulate, causing swelling.

Risk factors for OA include repeated stress on joints or repeated minor injuries to joints. Athletes often develop it later in life. Some occupations are associated with an increased risk; those with certain demanding physical jobs, such as farming, may be susceptible to OA of the hip. Excessive weight also increases the risk of OA in weight-bearing joints because of the stress it puts on these joints.

Almost everyone develops OA to a certain degree by the age of 70, although it may not produce any obvious symptoms. However, OA may develop in younger people, usually as a result of joint injuries. Other joint diseases, such as gout (*see p.302*), may predispose to OA.

SELF-HELP

PRIMARY TREATMENT The following measures may help to reduce the pain of OA:

- Try a heat pad, warm baths or massage to ease pain.
- Lose any excess weight.
- Take gentle exercise within your limits.
- Wear shoes with rubber heels for support and use a walking stick if hips or knees are very painful.

TREATMENTS IN DETAIL

Conventional Medicine

Your doctor will probably be able to diagnose OA from your symptoms. There are no specific tests for detecting OA. X-rays may be taken, although they may not show signs of OA until the disease is quite severe.

PRIMARY TREATMENT **LIFESTYLE MEASURES** Your doctor will encourage you to take exercise, such as swimming, in order to strengthen the muscles around the joints. Try to reduce your weight if you need to. If OA restricts movement in your hands and you need help with everyday activities, an occupational therapist can give information about specially adapted cutlery and other equipment.

PRIMARY TREATMENT **DRUGS** Painkillers and NSAID gels and tablets may be given for short-term pain relief. Occasionally, corticosteroids may be injected into the affected joints to provide a longer period of pain relief.

PRIMARY TREATMENT **SURGERY** For severe OA, joint repair or replacement may be offered. For example, hip replacements are likely to be effective for at least ten years. For very severe pain, some joints, such as the wrist, can be fused so that they are rigid. This surgical procedure relieves the pain, but means the joint cannot subsequently be moved.

CAUTION

NSAIDs can cause side-effects: ask your doctor to explain these to you.

Nutritional Therapy

DIETARY CHANGES Avoid foods that can contribute to the build-up of acid and other residues. These include acid fruits and vegetables, such as oranges, grapefruit and other citrus fruits (except lemon, which has an alkaline effect in the body after digestion), strawberries, rhubarb, tomatoes, red meats and cheese. Wine may make symptoms worse. A diet rich in essential fatty acids, possibly supplemented by fish oils and evening primrose oil, is often beneficial.

ELIMINATING SOLANINE Those with OA may find their symptoms relieved if they avoid foods, such as tomatoes, peppers (capsicum), potatoes and aubergines, belonging to the nightshade (Solanaceae) family. They contain solanine, which may be involved in the processes that cause OA. Eliminating solanine from the diet may bring relief to about 50 per cent of people with OA. In practice, it often takes about six months before real benefit is seen.

PRIMARY TREATMENT | **GLUCOSAMINE AND CHON-DROITIN** Glucosamine is an essential constituent of cartilage and supplements have been shown to be effective in reducing the inflammation and pain associated with osteoarthritis. Reviews of double-blind clinical studies confirm that it is an effective treatment for the condition. It has been shown to control OA symptoms as well as ibuprofen, and without the same unwanted gastrointestinal side-effects that NSAIDs can produce. Two long-term studies show that it reduces joint space narrowing and thus not only treats the pain of OA but also slows down

the disease progression. The recommended dose of glucosamine sulphate is 500mg, to be taken 3 times daily. Once your symptoms have improved, you could reduce this dose to once or twice a day. Glucosamine hydrochloride supplements may also be taken in similar doses.

Chondroitin sulphate is often taken in conjunction with glucosamine sulphate. It seems to work by attracting fluid into the cartilage of the joint, thereby improving the spongy, shock-absorbing qualities of the cartilage and helping to bring essential nutrients to the area.

Many trials have shown that taking chondroitin sulphate supplements can reduce pain, increase joint mobility and/or bring about healing within the joints of people with OA. The normal recommended dose of chondroitin sulphate is 400mg, 3 times a day.

NIACINAMIDE (a form of vitamin B3) is a supplement that may also help people with OA. One 1996 study that compared the effects of taking niacinamide to taking a placebo, found that niacinamide improved joint flexibility and reduced inflammation, thus making a reduction in standard anti-inflammatory medications possible. A typical dose would be 250mg, taken 4–6 times a day, though larger doses may be needed for individuals with advanced OA. Results can take 12 weeks or more to become apparent.

> **CAUTION**
>
> Consult your doctor before taking vitamin B3 or niacinamide with HMG-CoA reductase inhibitors or oral diabetic drugs (*see p.46*).

Homeopathy

A systematic review of clinical trials published in 2001 concluded homeopathy seems to help people with OA, but more research is needed. The trials looked mostly at homeopathic complex medicines, including Zeel® which contains *Arnica, Dulcamara, Rhus toxicodendron* and *Sanguinaria*; SRL gel which contains *Symphytum, Rhus tox.* and *Ledum*; and another complex containing *Rhus tox., Causticum* and *Lac vaccinum.* In every case, symptoms improved.

Homeopaths most frequently prescribe *Rhus tox., Calcaraea carbonica, Calcarea fluorica, Ledum, Natrum sulphuricum* and *Causticum,* depending on a person's constitution (*see p.73*). However, for such a common and variable disease, this list is by no means comprehensive.

RHUS TOXICODENDRON One important symptom of people who respond to *Rhus tox.* is the rapid stiffening up of joints. They may say they cannot sit for half an hour without becoming stiff and achey; they get up from their seat, limber up and feel better for a while, only for the feeling to return and the process to be repeated. By the same token, they are woken, often several times in the night, feeling stiff and restless, and need to limber up before they can get back to sleep.

LEDUM is often appropriate for OA that starts in the feet. Unusually for chronic arthritis, the pain is often relieved by putting the affected joint in or against something cold, such as a cold bath or an ice pack.

CALCAREA FLUORICA is often appropriate when there are many osteophytes, including Heberden's and Bouchard's nodes on the fingers. Those who respond to the remedy often have lax connective tissues: when they were younger they may have been double-jointed, or had swayback knees or a tendency to develop hernias.

CALCAREA CARBONICA is given largely on constitutional grounds (*see p.73*). Those who respond to *Calc. carb.* tend to be overweight. Solid both physically and mentally, they are calm, hardworking and stubborn people. But beneath this solid exterior they may have many fears and anxieties, particularly about their health. They often sweat freely on the head and neck, especially in bed at night, without necessarily feeling hot. They may also suffer from arthritic pain in many regions, but particularly in the low back.

CAUSTICUM is one of the most commonly indicated medicines for OA of the hips, but it may also be used for other areas. Individuals who respond to it are very sensitive to damp: they are worse in damp weather, and "feel it in their bones" when it is going to rain.

> Drinking wine may make the symptoms of osteoarthritis worse

In a normal knee joint (*left*), the cartilage lining the ends of the femur and tibia prevent bone damage. In an osteoarthritic joint (*right*), the cartilage is damaged as the degenerative disease takes it course.

Western Herbal Medicine

Traditionally, Western herbalists consider joints to be potential bottlenecks in the circulatory flow, places where toxins from poor nutrition and waste metabolites can accumulate and, over time, cause stiffness, swelling and pain.

ELIMINATE WASTE PRODUCTS Gentle restorative remedies can improve liver function and the nutritive quality of blood, and can help remove waste material from joints and tissues. These include burdock (*Arctium lappa*) root and leaf, dandelion (*Taraxacum officinale*) root and leaf, blue flag (*Iris versicolor*), bladderwrack (*Fucus vesiculosus*) (particularly good for cold, sluggish conditions), yellow dock (*Rumex crispus*) root, figwort (*Scrophularia nodosa*) and sarsaparilla (*Smilax regelii*). These remedies work slowly over a period of weeks and months and are more effective if mixed together. They are best combined with remedies such as celery (*Apium graveolens*) seed, nettle (*Urtica dioica*) and juniper (*Juniperus communis*) berries, that encourage waste elimination through the kidneys and have a proven anti-inflammatory action.

ANTI-INFLAMMATORIES Some other antirheumatic remedies, such as birch (*Betula pendula*) leaves, meadowsweet (*Fil-ipendula ulmaria*), poplar (*Populus tremuloides*) bark and willow (*Salix alba*) bark, are rich in anti-inflammatory salicylates (the basis of aspirin) that can reduce joint swelling and pain. Birch and meadowsweet encourage the elimination of metabolic wastes via the kidneys.

Other well-known and well-researched anti-inflammatory remedies include devil's claw (*Harpogophytum procumbens*), which shows similar effects in back and knee pain to NSAIDs, and two oleo-gum resins used in Ayurvedic medicine – Indian olibanum tree (*Boswellia serrata*) and guggal (*Commiphora mukul*). Make sure you buy a purified extract from a reputable supplier.

TURMERIC (*Curcuma longa*) has been shown to have significant antioxidant and anti-inflammatory activity and is used throughout Asia to treat arthritis. In Chinese medicine, turmeric is also used to improve blood circulation. This is a useful strategy and if the pulse is frail, practitioners will use other circulatory stimulants, such as prickly ash (*Xanthoxylum americanum*) bark and ginger (*Zingiber officinale*), both of which have an anti-inflammatory effect.

EXTERNAL TREATMENTS Comfrey (*Symphytum officinale*) root poultices and ointment can be applied to help ease swollen painful joints and Heberden's nodes, as can kelp (seaweed) plasters.

Herbs can be effective at reducing swelling and inflammation, and improving joint mobility. Applying capsicum (*Capsicum annuum*) plasters and ointment to painful swollen joints (especially when the pain is aggravated by cold, damp weather conditions) invigorates local circulation, thereby imitating the body's natural inflammatory processes that herbalists see as an innate restorative response to disease. In the same way, foot and hand baths, which are made by boiling stinging nettles with celery, may also be effective.

Liniments (oily creams for soothing muscle pain) and embrocations (lotions for soothing a sore or pulled muscle) containing menthol, camphor and plant oils, such as wintergreen (*Gaultheria procumbens*), lavender (*Lavandula angustifolia*), St John's wort (*Hypericum perforatum*), cinnamon (*Cinnamomum zeylanicum*), pine (*Pinus spp.*), juniper, chamomile (*Matricaria recutita*) and rosemary (*Rosmarinus officinalis*), as well as extracts of calamus (*Acorus calamus*) root and arnica (*Arnica montana*) or daisy (*Bellis perennis*) can be massaged into affected joints and muscles. These invigorate local circulation, but should be avoided if the joints are seriously inflamed.

> **CAUTION**
>
> See p.69 before taking a herbal remedy. Considerable care and constant monitoring are needed if herbal and conventional medications are combined. Severe arthritic conditions need expert herbal care and are often unsuitable for self-medication.

Chinese Herbal Medicine

Traditional Chinese Medicine practitioners do not specifically differentiate between OA, rheumatoid arthritis (*see p.293*) or gout (*see p.302*), but see them as varieties of *Bi* (painful blockage) syndrome.

CLIMATIC FACTORS In *Bi* syndrome, two external "factors" (wind–cold–damp and wind–damp–heat) can invade the body, causing the flow of *Qi*, blood and body fluids to slow down and become blocked. Full movement of the body is lost and the joints become inflamed and painful.

AGEING *Bi* syndrome is more common as people age because their fundamental life force – called *Zheng* (upright) *Qi* – weakens, as do the liver and kidneys, which respectively sustain the tendons and bones.

TREATMENT OF BI SYNDROME depends on skillful diagnosis of the variable factors, based on symptoms as well as pulse and tongue diagnosis (*see p.83*).

> **CAUTION**
>
> Arthritic conditions need expert care. Consult a Chinese herbalist before taking a herbal remedy and see also p. 69.

Acupuncture

Acupuncture can diminish the need for painkilling drugs. Many clinical trials have established that it helps people with OA of the knee and, to a lesser extent, of the hip. Whether the benefit comes from treating particular acupuncture points, the process of receiving acupuncture or the specific effect of needling around a joint is unclear.

A series of treatments is probably much better than giving one or two. You will need to persist for at least six, or possibly eight, sessions on a weekly basis. If the condition is very acute, treatment may be given every day, or every other day.

Usually, when symptoms settle, more long-term constitutional acupuncture may be needed to avoid their recurrence, perhaps on a monthly basis. This involves identifying the underlying pathogens that trigger *Bi* syndrome (*see Chinese Herbal Medicine, above*).

Bodywork and Movement Therapies

It is important to realise that X-ray evidence of osteoarthritic changes in a joint does not necessarily mean that pain is the result of these changes. In fact, many arthritic joints can be virtually pain-free. It is essential to ensure that pain in the affected joint is attributable to osteoarthritis, and not to another cause. The joint pain may arise from neuropathies and/or trigger point activity (*see p.55*).

NON-DRUG THERAPIES The objective of manipulation therapy is to treat the symptoms of restriction and the pain. The best results come when non-drug therapies take the lead and painkillers and anti-inflammatory drugs play a secondary role. Non-drug approaches might include postural re-education (for example, learning good standing and sitting postures), joint protection (avoiding unnecessary stresses), hot and cold treatments (for example, hydrotherapy) and transcutaneous electrical nerve stimulation (TENS) to reduce pain.

The management of OA might usefully also include heat or cold therapy, and often-neglected measures, such as reducing chair height and using an orthotic (shock-absorbing foot support).

REHABILITATION EXERCISES taught by physiotherapists focus not only on the local joint problem, such as the knee, but also on the consequences of this problem, such as inactivity and awkward movements. Useful pain-relieving aids include patellar taping to support the kneecap, shoulder taping, wedged insoles for foot support and shock-absorbing insoles.

Regular rehabilitation exercises involving strength training can improve functional ability and reduce knee joint pain in people with OA. Indeed, general well-designed exercise programmes have been shown to increase the ability of people with OA of the knee to perform everyday tasks.

Therapeutic exercises, including warm-up exercises with range-of-motion, muscle strengthening and aerobic activity, such as swimming can benefit many patients. Furthermore, exercising by yourself may be just as effective as attending physiotherapy at a hospital or having hydrotherapy treatment under supervision.

MASSAGE The comprehensive treatment of OA joint dysfunction may at times include appropriate massage therapy and joint mobilisation (osteopathic or chiropractic). However, more research is needed to prove the efficacy and safety of these methods.

Mind–Body Therapies

PRIMARY TREATMENT **THE ARTHRITIS SELF-MANAGEMENT PROGRAM (ASMP)** was developed at the Stanford University School of Medicine in the US and is now presented at over 200 facilities worldwide. It has been highly successful and cost-effective in treating arthritis. The Arthritis Foundation now markets this course as the Arthritis Self-Care Program.

The programme features relaxation, guided imagery, other cognitive pain management techniques, communication skills, tips on handling the doctor–patient relationship and group support. Imagery and relaxation exercises play an important part in five of the six ASMP sessions.

People report that their health improves and they are more able to participate in everyday activities. They have less need for drugs and other types of healthcare. These benefits are the result of people being more in control of, and better able to manage, their condition.

GUIDED IMAGERY, RELAXATION AND SELF-HYPNOSIS have proved effective in a number of chronic pain conditions and clinical experience indicates that it is effective for arthritic pain. Guided imagery and relaxation are valuable skills for people with OA. As an adjunct therapy, a mind–body practice including relaxation and/or guided imagery can significantly increase an individual's well-being and ability to cope with daily life. It can also reduce excessive dependence on pain-relieving medications with their attendant side-effects.

> Pulsed electromagnetic fields may provide modest benefits for people with OA

> **PREVENTION PLAN**
>
> **Try these to prevent the onset of OA:**
>
> - Take regular exercise.
> - Lose weight if you need to.
> - If possible, avoid activities that put repetitive stress on the joints.

RHEUMATOID ARTHRITIS

Rheumatoid arthritis (RA) is an autoimmune disease in which joints become stiff and painful due to inflammation of the synovial membrane. Rheumatoid arthritis most commonly begins between the ages of 30 and 50 and is three times more common in women than men. The condition sometimes runs in families. Treatment involves relieving inflammation and pain, and maximising joint function and mobility through eliminating food sensitivities, taking pharmaceutical, homeopathic or herbal medicines and keeping environmental hazards to a minimum.

WHAT ARE THE SYMPTOMS?

RA usually develops slowly over weeks or months, although its onset can be abrupt over a few days. The main symptoms are:

- Stiffness and pain in the joints that may be worse in the morning and relieved by movement

Other symptoms may develop, including:

- Swelling of the affected joints
- Small, painless bumps (nodules) on areas of pressure, such as the elbows
- Wasting (thinning) of the muscles around the joints
- Restriction of movement
- Tiredness and depression

WHY MIGHT I HAVE THIS?

PREDISPOSING FACTORS

- Genetic factors
- Smoking
- Food sensitivity

WHY DOES IT OCCUR?

Rheumatoid arthritis (RA) is a disease that can affect many systems of the body. It mostly damages joints, causing pain, stiffness and deformity. It is an autoimmune disease, which means that, for some unknown reason, the body produces antibodies that attack its own tissues – in this case, the synovial membrane of a joint, which becomes inflamed. Eventually, the ends of the bones and the cartilage that covers the joint are damaged. In most cases, RA affects several joints and tends to appear in corresponding areas on both sides of the body.

AFFECTED AREAS OF THE BODY RA usually appears first in the small joints of the hands and feet, but it may develop in almost any joint. Sometimes, just one joint, in particular the shoulder or knee, is initially affected. Eventually, joint damage may lead to deformities, such as "ulnar deviation", in which the fingers slant (deviate) away from the thumb.

Other areas of the body that may be affected include the eyes, kidneys, lungs, heart and blood vessels. Raynaud's disease (*see p.264*) and carpal tunnel syndrome (*see p.152*) may develop.

COURSE OF THE DISEASE There is no single pattern. For example, it may halt after several years, leaving only slight damage, or progress rapidly over a few years. However, in most cases, RA is a chronic, persistent disease that usually occurs in episodes, lasting for several weeks or months.

GENETIC FACTORS A family history of RA is a predisposing factor and so genes may be an important influence in determining who develops RA and why. However, many people who never develop the disease share the genes that are thought to be associated with RA.

TREATMENT PLAN

PRIMARY TREATMENTS

- Drugs, including NSAIDs, anti-rheumatic drugs and corticosteroids
- Physiotherapy and occupational therapy

BACK-UP TREATMENTS

- Surgery, including joint replacement
- Food elimination diet
- Homeopathy
- Western and Chinese herbal medicine
- Bodywork and movement therapies

WORTH CONSIDERING

- Essential fatty acids
- Environmental health measures
- Acupuncture
- Mind–body therapies

For an explanation of how treatments are rated, see p.111.

SELF-HELP

To reduce the discomfort of RA:
- Take paracetamol or other painkillers.
- Try ointments that contain capsaicin, menthol, eucalyptus or salicylates – the latter have an aspirin-like effect.

Conventional Medicine

Your doctor will make a diagnosis mainly from a description of the symptoms and an examination. You will need to undergo tests, such as blood tests for signs of inflammation and X-rays to establish the extent of any damage.

Treatment aims to control the symptoms and halt or slow the progress of the disease. Your doctor will recommend rest during flare-ups.

PRIMARY TREATMENT **DRUGS** Your doctor may prescribe NSAIDs to relieve pain and stiffness. Painkillers may also provide some relief.

Disease-modifying antirheumatic drugs may be prescribed with the aim of reducing inflammation and helping to control symptoms. They may also slow the rate of joint damage. They include:

- *Sulfasalazine* About half of those with RA who are treated with sulfasalazine respond within six months.
- *Methotrexate* This drug can reduce inflammation and slow the damage to joints. It usually improves the symptoms within a few months.
- *Antimalarials* Inflammation can be reduced significantly when antimalarials are taken for up to 12 months.
- *Minocycline* This antibiotic may help to control the symptoms of RA.

Oral corticosteroids may be prescribed, since they can reduce joint inflammation and help to control the symptoms when given in low doses for a few weeks. They may also be given on an occasional basis as an injection into a muscle for particularly severe flare-ups. They may also provide relief when injected directly into affected joints, but this may be short term.

Some new immunosuppressants (drugs that suppress the immune response), such as etanercept and infliximab, may be given by injection. They have been found to improve symptoms and slow or even halt the damage in some cases. These drugs are only used after other disease-modifying, antirheumatic drugs have been tried.

PRIMARY TREATMENT **PHYSIOTHERAPY** is important for maximising joint movement and maintaining muscle strength.

Occupational therapists will also advise on how to cope with daily activities if mobility and dexterity are affected.

SURGERY may be performed to prevent worsening of joint damage and to relieve pain. This may be achieved by removing the inflamed tissue from a particular joint or by fusing the bones together so that there is no movement in the affected joint. Alternatively, the joint may be replaced when damage is severe.

> **CAUTION**
>
> - Some of the drugs used for treating RA have a range of serious side-effects: ask your doctor to explain these to you.
>
> - Some of the drugs should be avoided during pregnancy. Conception should be avoided when either partner is taking methotrexate and for a time afterwards.

HOW RHEUMATOID ARTHRITIS AFFECTS JOINTS

When a joint is affected by rheumatoid arthritis, the synovial membranes and the cartilage that lines the bones come under attack. As fluid accumulates, the joint swells and becomes inflamed, causing pain and restricting movement. Antibodies and molecules, such as enzymes and cytokines, damage and deform the membranes and cartilage. Eventually, the bones, ligaments and tendons are also affected.

A knee damaged by rheumatoid arthritis

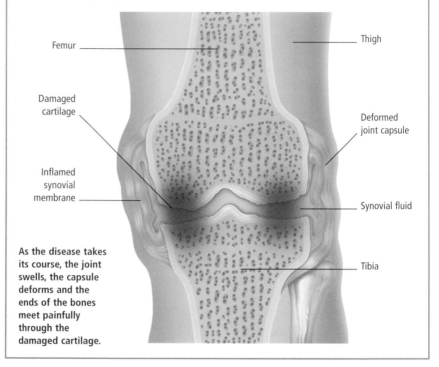

Femur

Damaged cartilage

Inflamed synovial membrane

Thigh

Deformed joint capsule

Synovial fluid

Tibia

As the disease takes its course, the joint swells, the capsule deforms and the ends of the bones meet painfully through the damaged cartilage.

Nutritional Therapy

FOOD ELIMINATION DIET Studies show that RA can be related to a food sensitivity, and that avoiding problem foods can improve symptoms. In one study, the worst offending foods were grains, milk, nuts, beef and eggs. (*For more information about elimination diets, see p.39.*)

ESSENTIAL FATTY ACIDS People with RA may benefit from eating foods that are rich in healthy essential fatty acids (EFAs). These foods include oily fish (mackerel, trout, sardines and salmon), extra-virgin olive oil and walnuts, as well as pumpkin, sunflower and sesame seeds.

There is some evidence that both omega-6 fatty acids (in the form of borage oil, blackcurrant seed oil and evening primrose oil) and omega-3 fatty acids (in the form of fish oil) can be effective in controlling the symptoms.

The effective daily doses appear to be about 1.5g of gamma-linolenic acid (GLA) and 10g of fish oil supplements (providing 3g per day of the fatty acids EPA and DHA). Both GLA and the fatty acids EPA and DHA are beneficial because the body uses them to make compounds that have an anti-inflammatory action.

A 2003 study suggests that fish oil is most beneficial as an anti-inflammatory agent in RA if it is taken while eating a diet low in arachidonic acid (an inflammatory omega-6 fatty acid found in eggs and meat, especially beef, liver and kidneys).

> **CAUTION**
>
> Consult your doctor before taking omega-3 fatty acids/fish oils with warfarin, or vitamin E with aspirin and warfarin (*see p.46*).

Homeopathy

RA is a serious and potentially crippling disease that needs treatment from a qualified and experienced homeopath. Clinical trials suggest that the complex homeopathic medicine *Rheumaselect* (not available in the UK), which contains *Bryonia, Rhus toxicodendron, Ledum, Berberis* and *Nux vomica* is effective in RA. Meta analysis of the clinical trials also suggest that homeopathy tailored to the individual is effective.

Among the homeopathic medicines that are most likely to benefit symptoms are *Apis mellifica* and *Rhus tox*. Constitutional medicines, which are prescribed almost entirely on whole-person characteristics rather than on the features of the illness, may act more deeply (*see p.73*). Among the most commonly indicated are *Lycopodium, Pulsatilla, Sepia* and *Causticum*.

APIS MELLIFICA is useful for hot, swollen and very tender joints, and also where the pain is relieved by cold, such as an ice pack, but made worse by pressure.

RHUS TOXICODENDRON helps people who are very stiff in the morning, and who become stiff and achey from even short periods of sitting or lying still; hence, they have restless nights. They are worse in cold, wet weather and feel better from warmth, such as from a heat pad or warm bath.

LYCOPODIUM may be appropriate when the feet are badly affected by RA. People who respond to *Lycopodium* can sometimes be recognised by the way they respond to questions: they will pause, then give a carefully considered reply.

Generally rather reserved, *Lycopodium* types may be socially inept, no good at small talk and at their best with small groups of old friends. A useful correlative symptom is that they frequently suffer from stomach trouble, particularly wind, and have a sweet tooth.

PULSATILLA A characteristic feature of people who respond to *Pulsatilla* is that the arthritis moves unpredictably from joint to joint. In women, it is often worse in the premenstrual period and may have started a few weeks or months after having a baby.

People who respond to *Pulsatilla* are typically gentle, soft spoken, indecisive and weepy – for instance, when they are talking about their illness.

SEPIA People who respond to *Sepia* may experience a low back pain – although RA does not usually affect the back, except for the upper neck – that particularly involves the sacroiliac joints where the spinal column meets the pelvis. In women, the onset of RA may have developed around the time of the menopause.

Typically, patients are depressed and emotionally flat, although they may appear lively and vivacious. But this is sometimes a "mask", and they do not like probing questions about how they feel. A common feature, unusual in this context, is that the symptoms are improved by exertion, such as dancing or working out.

CAUSTICUM People who respond to *Causticum* are often very sensitive to the weather – they are said to "feel it in their bones" well before it rains. Many homeopathic medicines for arthritis and rheumatism are associated with feeling worse in cold or wet weather.

People who respond to *Causticum* may experience the arthritis at unusual sites, such as the jaw joint, and tend to develop contractures (temporary shortening of ligaments) so they are unable to fully straighten their joints.

A characteristic feature of people who respond to *Causticum* is that they are very sympathetic to the sufferings of others – for example, they may find it too difficult to watch starving children on TV. They also often have "leakage" of urine when the bladder is full or during a sneeze or cough, as well as recurrent hoarseness.

Western Herbal Medicine

There are many theories to explain why the immune system becomes disrupted and causes RA. Some scientists see the trigger as a reaction to a long-term unresolved infection with a slow-acting virus, bacterium or fungus.

The traditional herbal view is that chronic toxic overload can trigger an attack of RA. (*For eliminating waste products, see Osteoarthritis, p.291.*) As with OA, successful treatment is only possible by analysing and treating each case individually. There is no standard herbal treatment for arthritis of any sort.

> ## The artist Renoir painted around 6,000 pictures despite having severe rheumatoid arthritis

ANTI-INFLAMMATORY HERBS During an acute attack of RA, the inflammation can be successfully doused with anti-inflammatory herbs. These include willow (*Salix alba*) bark, meadowsweet (*Filipendula ulmaria*), poplar (*Populus tremuloides*) bark and birch (*Betula pendula*) leaves, as well as devil's claw (*Harpogophytum procumbens*), borage (*Borago officinalis*), frankincense (*Boswellia spp.*), guggal (*Commiphora mukul*), sarsaparilla (*Smilax regelii*) and turmeric (*Curcuma longa*). (*See also Osteoarthritis, p.289.*)

Other anti-inflammatory remedies that may be effective include barberry (*Berberis vulgaris*) bark, centaury (*Centaurium erythrea*), bogbean (*Menyathes trifoliata*) and feverfew (*Tanacetum parthenium*).

Black cohosh (*Cimicifuga racemosa*) has a substantial folk reputation for treating inflammatory arthritis. It may be particularly appropriate for treating women with RA, especially menopausal women since it appears to have a weak oestrogenic action that reduces hot flushes and other menopausal symptoms.

Phytodolor is a German proprietary mixture that has been well researched and appears to be effective against RA.

Both liquorice (*Glycyrrhiza glabra*) and wild yam (*Dioscorea villosa*) contain steroidal saponins that can also rebalance female hormone levels and are anti-

Chinese Herbal Medicine

Traditional Chinese Medicine does not specifically distinguish between RA, OA and gout. (*For information about Chinese herbal treatments of arthritis, see p.291.*)

Environmental Health

There is ample evidence that environmental factors play an important role in the development of RA as well as in other autoimmune disorders. Studies of identical twins indicate that genetics play some part in the disease development, but the larger

Swedish study, it was found that people who were exposed to organic solvents (including spray painters, lacquer workers and hairdressers) had a higher than normal risk of developing RA. Farmers were also at higher risk, presumably due to organic dust or pesticide exposures, another potential trigger.

Another study revealed that occupational exposure to hydraulic oils doubles the risk of developing RA. Silica dust, which is frequently encountered among pottery and construction workers, has also been linked to the development of RA.

If exposure to these solvents and chemicals is a cause of RA, then all efforts to minimise exposure should be made, even if the disease process has already begun. Consequently, avoid freshly applied paints, thinners, varnishes and hydraulic oils. If you cannot avoid this exposure, then be sure to wear a respirator mask that is approved for organic vapours. Even exposure to common household solvents and chemicals, such as pesticides and fertilisers, should be limited.

INFECTIOUS AGENTS have been implicated in the development of autoimmune disease, such as RA. These include the Epstein-Barr virus (the cause of mononucleosis), parvoviruses and mycoplasma (the cause of "walking pneumonia"). However, the results are not consistent between studies and are thus difficult to interpret. There appears to be no link between vaccinations and the development of RA.

On average, about one person in a hundred develops rheumatoid arthritis

inflammatory. Liquorice is known to have a mild cortisone-like effect and is especially effective in treating hot and inflamed joints when combined with the unprocessed root of a Chinese herb called rehmannia (*Rehmannia glutinosa*).

IMMUNE-STRENGTHENING HERBS People with RA know it is a thoroughly debilitating disease which often renders them both exhausted and depressed. There are various herbs, such as astragalus (*Astragalus membranaceus*), ginseng (*Panax ginseng*) and Siberian ginseng (*Eleutheroccus senticosus*), that can improve their immune function as well as lift their spirits.

These herbs are best employed when the acute joint inflammation has been brought under control. Chinese angelica (*Angelica sinensis*), motherwort (*Leonurus cardiaca*) and nettle (*Urtica dioica*) can help to combat anaemia, which is a common complication of RA.

contribution seems to come from the environment. In fact, one study of over 37,000 twins in Denmark led to the conclusion that "genes are of minor importance in the development of rheumatoid arthritis".

AVOID SMOKING Many studies suggest that there is a link between smoking and RA. Smokers are twice as likely to develop the condition compared to non-smokers and this increased risk can persist for up to 20 years after stopping smoking. There are no controlled studies dealing with passive smoking, but if you have RA you should avoid smoky atmospheres.

ORAL CONTRACEPTIVE USE appears to confer some level of protection – women who take oral contraceptives are less likely to develop RA. Even ex-users seem to retain a somewhat lower, but measurable protection, although this disappears after several decades. Thus, it appears that the oral contraceptives may simply postpone the clinical development of RA. There has never been a clear explanation for the protective effect, nor are oral contraceptives recommended for this purpose in view of their possible detrimental effects as women age (including blood clots and stroke).

AVOID CHEMICAL SUBSTANCES Exposure to several chemical substances may increase the risk of developing RA. In a

Acupuncture

Acupuncture has often been employed in the treatment of RA – it may follow either an anti-inflammatory or a pain-relieving approach. Acupuncture appears to work as well as local steroid injections or many conventional anti-inflammatory medications. Moreover, adverse reactions to acupuncture are less likely.

ANTI-INFLAMMATORY EFFECTS One approach uses a Traditional Chinese Medicine diagnosis and focuses on the potential anti-inflammatory effects of acupuncture and therefore on the underlying disease process. It has not been adequately evaluated and its benefits are difficult to judge, particularly when RA can involve periods

> **CAUTION**
>
> • Herbal medication given to people with RA should be closely monitored and regular liver function tests are advisable.
>
> • Combining herbs with conventional drug therapy needs constant monitoring.
>
> • Severe arthritic conditions need expert care and are unsuitable for self-medication.

This X-ray of a hand severely affected by rheumatoid arthritis shows how the bones have become affected by the inflammation process. The fingers slant away from the thumb – a deformity known as ulnar deviation.

tolerate, active exercise can help maintain body function and well-being.

LOW-LEVEL LASER THERAPY (LLLT) has been used to treat the symptoms of RA for some years. A light source generates "pure" light of a single wavelength. It produces a photochemical reaction in the cells of the affected tissue. LLLT can be considered for short-term relief of pain and morning stiffness, particularly since it has few, if any, side-effects. LLLT is available at hospital rheumatology departments and from physiotherapists and pain clinics.

ULTRASOUND is a technique often used as a secondary therapy – in other words, together with another treatment, such as medication. It has both anti-inflammatory and pain-relieving properties. Ultrasound alone can be helpful in increasing grip strength. To a lesser extent it can relieve morning stiffness and reduce the number of both swollen and painful joints.

Mind–Body Therapies

Regular practice of mind–body therapies, such as yoga and relaxation, can have a beneficial effect on your pain levels. (*For information about general mind–body treatments of arthritis, see p.292.*)

THE PSYCHOSOCIAL ENVIRONMENT Many studies have linked the development of RA to major life stressors. One study of people with RA found many had marital problems about five years before the onset of RA symptoms and formal diagnosis. By comparison, control populations did not show significant increases in marital discord. If you have RA, you would be wise to reduce conflict and stress in your life, or at least to find a way to avoid the build-up of such emotions.

of both relapses and remissions. In general, 10 to 12 weekly sessions of acupuncture treatment will be needed while the disease is relatively stable, before it is clear whether or not the treatment is having a more fundamental effect.

Bodywork and Movement Therapies

BALNEOTHERAPY (also known as spa therapy or hydrotherapy) is one of the oldest forms of therapy for individuals with

> Women with RA who become pregnant may find their symptoms are temporarily relieved

PAIN RELIEF Acupuncture may be used to relieve pain, an approach supported by a number of clinical trials, which have shown that acupuncture can bring relief to inflamed joints or to joints that are damaged, mechanically disturbed or suffering from secondary osteoarthritis.

This approach is used in the treatment of either acute or chronic muscle and joint pain. Usually, six to eight sessions of acupuncture will be enough to benefit painful knees, hips or strained muscles. If they do not, you should consider carefully whether acupuncture will be of value in treating your pain.

arthritis. Its main aim is to soothe the pain and, as a consequence, to relieve suffering and improve well-being.

A 2003 review of the research into balneotherapy concluded that, although there were positive findings, "an answer about the efficacy of balneotherapy cannot be provided at this time". However, it is still worth trying.

AEROBIC EXERCISE is effective in increasing aerobic capacity and muscle strength, without making the disease or the pain worse. It is clear that, as long as you are exercising at a rate you can comfortably

PREVENTION PLAN

The following may help to prevent the development of RA:

- Avoid problem foods, which may include grains, milk, nuts and eggs.

- If you smoke, stop – and avoid smoky environments.

WHAT ARE THE SYMPTOMS?

The symptoms of fibromyalgia usually develop slowly over weeks and may include:

- Persistent connective tissue pain affecting almost any part of the body

- Fatigue, sleep disturbance and/or unrefreshing sleep

- Fibromyalgia is associated with other conditions, particularly migraine and irritable bowel syndrome – many people who have fibromyalgia also have these

- Fibromyalgia is often also associated with depression and anxiety

- Tenderness to pressure at 11 or more of 18 tender points (*see illustration opposite*).

Symptoms may become worse if stress levels increase.

WHY MIGHT I HAVE THIS?

PREDISPOSING FACTORS

- Physical, sexual or psychological abuse

- Stress

- Sleep deprivation

- Another disorder, such as rheumatoid arthritis, lupus or hypothyroidism

- Being sensitive to paint solvents and other chemicals

- Being sensitive to cleaning products, heavy metals, silicone

TRIGGERS

- Injury, trauma or major surgery

- Infection (bacterial or viral)

FIBROMYALGIA

Fibromyalgia, also known in the past as fibrositis, is a form of chronic rheumatism (a condition affecting the muscles, ligaments and other soft tissues). It is characterised by widespread pain, fatigue and sleep disturbance, and is surprisingly common and debilitating. People with fibromyalgia have tender areas of the connective tissues, particularly in the neck, spine, shoulders and hips. Fibromyalgia is much more common in women than in men. Treatment focuses on relieving pain, helping with sleep and depression, and reducing stress.

WHY DOES IT OCCUR?

Stress seems to be a predisposing factor and a number of triggers seem to be able to initiate fibromyalgia (*see left*). One 1997 study showed that a sub-group of fibromyalgia patients (estimated at around 15 per cent) have had an obvious traumatic injury – for example, a whiplash injury following a car accident.

People with fibromyalgia display a number of features that may help researchers to discover the underlying cause. One theory centres on the way the brain handles pain signals: reduced levels of serotonin cause an imbalance in the chemical substance P, which makes the brain register pain more readily than normal. Serotonin is also involved in the regulation of sleep and mood. Other studies have shown abnormalities of the metabolism in muscles.

The "tender points" in areas of muscle (*see right*), especially at the base of the skull and near the shoulder blades, are not specific to fibromyalgia. They may be also found in some people with chronic fatigue syndrome (*see p.474*) and other disorders. However, the formal diagnosis of fibromyalgia depends on the presence of quite large numbers of tender points in particular places.

TREATMENT PLAN

PRIMARY TREATMENTS

- Rehabilitation programme

- Homeopathy

- Mind–body therapies

BACK-UP TREATMENTS

- Nutritional therapy

- Acupuncture

- Aerobic exercise

- Breathing retraining

- Bodywork therapies

WORTH CONSIDERING

- Nutritional therapy

- Environmental health

For an explanation of how treatments are rated, see p.111.

SELF-HELP

The following may bring pain relief:
- Painkillers, such as paracetamol.
- Practising relaxation and meditation.
- Taking some exercise.

TREATMENTS IN DETAIL

Conventional Medicine

The description of the symptoms and an examination will usually enable a doctor to diagnose fibromyalgia. The doctor may arrange for you to have blood tests to exclude an underlying cause.

PRIMARY TREATMENT **REHABILITATION PROGRAMME** Your doctor will probably recommend a programme that involves you taking regular exercise, analgesics to relieve the pain (but not to be used continuously) and certain antidepressants, such as amitriptyline, in low doses to help improve your sleep and reduce pain.

TENDER POINTS

The medical diagnosis of fibromyalgia depends on the presence of tender points at particular locations on the body. The sites of the tender points are located in 9 symmetrical pairs on the body. For someone to have fibromyalgia, according to the strict definition, there should be tenderness to pressure in at least 11 of the 18 tender points. Diagnosis is made difficult because tenderness seems to vary from day to day.

Location of the 9 pairs of tender points

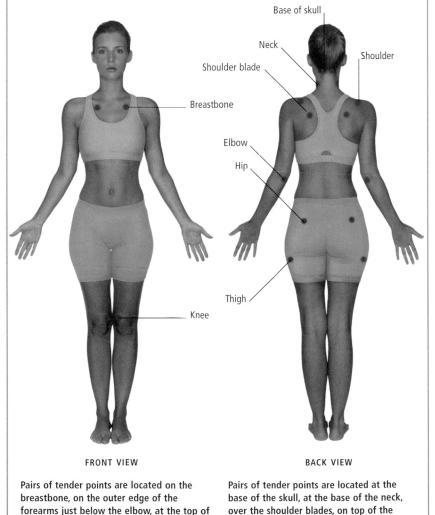

Base of skull

Neck

Shoulder blade

Shoulder

Breastbone

Elbow

Hip

Thigh

Knee

FRONT VIEW

BACK VIEW

Pairs of tender points are located on the breastbone, on the outer edge of the forearms just below the elbow, at the top of the hips and on the fat pad over the knees.

Pairs of tender points are located at the base of the skull, at the base of the neck, over the shoulder blades, on top of the shoulders and on the outside of the hips.

CAUTION

Drugs for fibromyalgia may cause side-effects: ask your doctor to explain these to you.

Nutritional Therapy

OMEGA-3 OILS FOR PERSISTENT MUSCLE PAIN associated with inflammation may be helped by supplementation with omega-3 fatty acids. Excessive consumption of omega-6 polyunsaturated fatty acids (found in vegetable oils and fast foods) and a relative lack of the omega-3 fatty acids EPA and DHA seem to promote inflammation and pain. Studies show that omega-3 fatty acid supplements reduce inflammatory processes and pain in the body. For example, taking a daily dose of 378mg EPA and 259mg DHA for at least two months may reduce inflammation.

Omega-3 fatty acids can be found in some nuts and seeds, especially walnuts and flaxseeds, and oily fish, such as mackerel, salmon and sardines. Including these foods in your diet and avoiding foods containing omega-6 fatty acids may help to control the pain. Taking 1–3g of concentrated fish oil is likely to help, too.

TRYPTOPHAN is an amino acid that is required for the release of beta-endorphin, one of the body's natural pain-relieving compounds. It is also needed for the production of serotonin, a brain chemical that may reduce a tendency to sense pain. Studies show that tryptophan supplements may be able to increase the body's pain threshold and reduce sensitivity to pain. Tryptophan can be found in foods such as meat, tofu, almonds, peanuts, pumpkin seeds, sesame seeds and tahini (a paste made from sesame seed).

Tryptophan supplements are not available over the counter in many countries, such as the UK and the US. However, 5-hydroxytryptophan (5-HTP), the substance tryptophan is converted into before it is made into serotonin, is a good alternative.

Research suggests that individuals with fibromyalgia may have low serotonin levels in their blood. Studies have shown that supplementation with 300mg per day of 5-HTP relieves some of the symptoms of fibromyalgia. For both persistent muscle pain and fibromyalgia, experts often recommend starting the 5-HTP dosages at 25–100mg a day and increasing to 300mg a day in small increments.

MAGNESIUM There is evidence to suggest that some individuals with fibromyalgia are deficient in magnesium. There is also evidence that the magnesium, in combination with malic acid, can relieve the symptoms of fibromyalgia. A daily intake of 300–600mg of magnesium, together with 1,200–2,400mg of malic acid, can help the production of ATP, the basic fuel source in the body's cells.

CAUTION

Consult your doctor before taking omega-3 fatty acids or fish oils with warfarin, or 5-HTP with zolpidem, venlafaxine, fluoxetine, fluvoxamine, sumatriptan or paroxetine (*see p.46*).

Homeopathy

PRIMARY TREATMENT — There is quite strong evidence from clinical trials of the effectiveness of homeopathy in treating fibromyalgia. See p.77 for guidelines on how to take the following medicines.

RHUS TOXICODENDRON is the most frequently used medicine. The most important characteristic of syndromes which respond to this medicine is restlessness and rapid stiffening up.

Typically, people who respond to *Rhus tox.* wake up two or three times a night (because they are physically restless, not because they need to go to the toilet), and cannot sit and watch TV, or drive for more than 30–45 minutes without becoming very stiff and achey, and needing to limber up. They may also get a lot of pins and needles and have a tendency to itchy, blistery rashes that may be triggered by contact – for instance, with certain plants or drugs.

IGNATIA is usually thought of as a treatment for emotional shocks, but can be very helpful in fibromyalgia. *Ignatia* is likely to help when the pains are erratic and unpredictable, or when they are severe but short-lived in any one spot. There is often a lot of muscle twitching, and a sensation as if something was stuck in the throat. The problem may have been triggered, or aggravated by, an emotional shock, such as a bereavement or the break-up of a relationship.

CALCAREA CARBONICA is another homeopathic medicine frequently used for fibromyalgia. It is a constitutional medicine, prescribed more for a particular type of person than a disease. Such people may have many of the features of fibromyalgia, including widespread pain, particularly in the low back and knees, and irritable bowel syndrome, often with constipation. Commonly, the cause is a long period of stress, particularly work stress, which has left the person exhausted.

People who respond to *Calc. carb.* tend to be well-built, solid, conscientious people, but often with a phobia and anxiety, particularly about their own health. They may conceal these feelings, but if asked will say they are on the verge of cracking up. Their sleep is poor and they have bad dreams and typically sweat a lot on the head, particularly in bed.

CAUSTICUM may also be useful for fibromyalgia. One of its typical symptoms is a great sensitivity to the weather – those who respond to *Causticum* may be able to predict rain (unlike people who respond to *Rhus tox.*, who feel worse when the weather is cold and wet, but cannot predict the weather). The strongest mental characteristic of people who respond to *Causticum* is their great sympathy for the sufferings of others. For instance, they cannot bear to watch images of starving children on TV – they have to turn it off or leave the room.

Environmental Health

Some of the possible environmental triggers of persistent pain or fibromyalgia include paint solvents and other chemicals, cleaning products, heavy metals and silicone. The complexities and difficulties in investigating these areas for connections to symptoms underscore the importance of obtaining a detailed environmental and occupational history, perhaps from an environmental health expert who can look for relevant environmental exposures (*to find a therapist, see p.93*). The next step often involves various prevention strategies, removing the offending triggers from your life or, if that is not possible, just decreasing overall exposure.

Some individuals are particularly sensitive to certain environmental chemicals or they have a genetic predisposition that causes them to react to the chemicals and develop symptoms of fibromyalgia or other related syndromes. These reactions can occur at low chemical concentrations that are otherwise considered safe and well below toxic level.

SICK BUILDING SYNDROME An example of a reaction that occurs at a low concentration is what has been termed the "sick building syndrome". This is a set of general symptoms that result from exposure to various compounds in new offices. Though no single cause has been determined, it is postulated that some people react to the release of compounds in building materials. The problem is compounded by well-sealed, energy-efficient construction methods.

Sick building syndrome may cause fibromyalgia, in addition to such symptoms as headaches, asthma or skin reactions, including dermatitis.

SILICONE BREAST IMPLANTS have been controversially implicated in causing symptoms of fibromyalgia and chronic fatigue syndrome. Some authors have reviewed the data and conclude that there is no connection with implants and diseases or conditions. Others point out that some studies seem to indicate that not all women can tolerate breast implants, developing symptoms similar to chronic fatigue syndrome or fibromyalgia.

Consult your doctor about the risks and benefits of having breast implants in your specific situation.

DETOXIFICATION Some experts advocate detoxification programmes as a way of treating chronic health problems, such as fibromyalgia, especially if a toxic environmental cause is suspected. Removing possible environmental toxins from the

> Fibromyalgia can affect children, sometimes as young as eight years old

body involves a special diet, such as a low allergenic diet, or taking liver-tonifying herbs. Taking supplements, such as vitamin C, vitamin E, selenium, green tea or mixed carotenoids, can improve the detoxification process in the liver or the function of the intestinal tract.

Bodywork Therapies

CHIROPRACTIC, OSTEOPATHY AND PHYSIOTHERAPY aim to normalise the spinal areas that may be contributing to pain, to remove associated myofascial trigger points (*see p.55*) and to rehabilitate muscles following disuse.

Many people with fibromyalgia have other pain-inducing conditions, including active trigger points in their muscles and restrictions in spinal and other joints. Many of these conditions can be improved or corrected by a chiropractor, osteopath, physiotherapist or suitably trained massage therapist. Any reduction in the overall amount of pain experienced makes coping with the primary condition less difficult.

HYDROTHERAPY, including the use of seawater baths in balneotherapy, can benefit some fibromyalgia patients.

> **CAUTION**
>
> Tissue repair is slow in fibromyalgia patients, so any manual therapy must be moderate and gentle to avoid strong reactions, increased pain and a delayed recovery. Make sure that your therapist is familiar with the manual treatment of fibromyalgia. Over-enthusiastic, deep-tissue treatment is inappropriate.

Aerobic Exercise

If you have fibromyalgia, take some gentle exercise, such as walking, cycling or swimming, for 20 minutes a day. Numerous studies show that aerobic exercise helps fibromyalgia in several ways. First, when non-stressful, moderate, aerobic exercise is carried out regularly (for not less than 20 minutes at least three times weekly), it improves both cardiovascular and muscular conditioning. Second, regular exercise reduces pain and other symptoms. Finally, it stimulates growth hormone production, which fibromyalgia patients usually have in short supply.

Breathing Retraining

Clinical experience suggests that people with fibromyalgia have breathing patterns that are abnormal. Upper-chest, rapid-rate breathing is common and often linked to feelings of anxiety. Sometimes, anxiety and breathing pattern disorders are a response to the distress of being in pain, and so are not actually a cause. However, they are nevertheless frequent contributors to many of the additional, secondary symptoms of fibromyalgia. (*For more on breathing pattern disorders, see p.57*)

Retraining exercises can help to reduce feelings of anxiety and to ease pain, especially when they are accompanied by appropriate manual therapy to relax and normalise the breathing mechanism structures (*see p.62*).

Acupuncture

Two very good clinical trials have examined the application of acupuncture in the treatment of fibromyalgia. The acupuncture was directed towards the tender points (*see illustration, p.299*) and sometimes included the use of intramuscular stimulation, which involves deep and sometimes painful needling (one of the studies used a technique called electroacupuncture). Both studies reported a significant reduction in the amount of pain experienced.

However, it is important to realise that a more traditional Chinese approach to the treatment of fibromyalgia is one that has been largely untested and may ultimately prove to be equally effective to the approaches involving repeated needling of tender points.

Acupuncture may be able to bring about immediate relief from pain, but because fibromyalgia is a chronic illness it requires repeated treatment. If no effect emerges after six treatments, then it is probably not worth continuing. However, if benefit is apparent, then long-term treatment will frequently be required.

Mind–Body Therapies

PRIMARY TREATMENT | **PAIN CONTROL** Results strongly indicate that practising mind–body therapies, combined with regular physical exercise, can help to alleviate the pain associated with chronic fibromyalgia. The therapies include meditation or breathing retraining (either at home, with a practitioner or both).

A 1993 study discovered that a stress-reduction programme which is based on meditation can be effective for people with fibromyalgia. Five years later, further research into the use of mind–body therapies revealed that three treatment regimes – clinical biofeedback with relaxation, exercise and a programme that combined both – all helped people with fibromyalgia to control their experience of pain, cope with their discomfort and improve their levels of physical activity.

However, in 2000, a review of the studies into the effectiveness of mind–body therapies for fibromyalgia revealed some evidence for improving quality of life, but

Restless legs syndrome (RLS) may occur in 50 per cent of fibromyalgia patients

also showed that there was inconclusive evidence for improving certain aspects of fibromyalgia, such as pain.

There is strong evidence that moderate/high intensity exercise (*see Aerobic exercise, left*) is more effective than most of the mind–body therapies for both pain and improvement in overall, daily functions. Long-term results, however, show that people benefit most from mind–body therapies and exercise. From this review, it is evident that mind–body practices in combination with exercise and/or antidepressants can alleviate fibromyalgia.

GUIDED IMAGERY Concentrating on pleasant imagery may help to relieve the pain of fibromyalgia, according to research. A 2002 study explored the effectiveness of guided imagery (*see p.99*), which was either attention-distracting or attention-focusing, on the pain of fibromyalgia. The study also examined the effect of the antidepressant amitriptyline and found that pleasant imagery reduced the pain, but amitriptyline was no better than a placebo.

> **PREVENTION PLAN**
>
> The following may help to prevent fibromyalgia:
>
> - Avoid environmental hazards.
> - Take regular exercise.

GOUT

Gout is a metabolic disorder that causes a severely painful type of arthritis. The joint at the base of the big toe is frequently affected, but gout can occur in any joint. The condition is about ten times more common in men than in women and sometimes runs in families, suggesting genetic factors may be involved. Gout rarely affects women before the menopause. Treatment involves reducing the pain, swelling, and inflammation, as well as lowering the uric acid levels in the blood by increasing its excretion and inhibiting its production.

WHAT ARE THE SYMPTOMS?

- Severe pain in the affected joint
- Redness, tenderness, warmth and swelling in the affected joint
- Fever

WHY MIGHT I HAVE THIS?

PREDISPOSING FACTORS

- Being a middle-aged man
- Being a post-menopausal woman
- Drinking excessive quantities of alcohol, particularly beer
- Eating large amounts of foods containing purines (e.g. red meats and shellfish)
- High-protein diet
- Obesity
- Hereditary factors
- Insulin resistance syndrome
- Long-term use of diuretics

TREATMENT PLAN

PRIMARY TREATMENTS

- Lifestyle measures (*see Self-Help*) including restriction of refined starches and sugars

For acute attacks:
- Non-steroidal anti-inflammatory drugs (NSAIDs), colchicine or corticosteroid injections

For recurrent gout:
- Drugs that reduce uric acid levels
- Nutritional therapy

BACK-UP TREATMENTS

- Homeopathy
- Western and Chinese herbal medicine

For an explanation of how treatments are rated, see p.111.

WHY DOES IT OCCUR?

People with high blood levels of uric acid are prone to gout. Uric acid is a substance produced in the body when proteins and chemicals called purines are broken down. It can accumulate in the blood when the body produces too much uric acid and/or the kidneys do not excrete enough.

The uric acid is deposited as sharp crystals in a joint where they accumulate and cause inflammation and severe, sometimes excruciating, pain. The joint at the base of the big toe is most commonly affected. The first attack of gout usually comes without warning and often wakes the individual early in the morning.

People who eat a high-protein diet may have high uric acid levels, as may those who are obese or who drink excessive amounts of alcohol, particularly beer. Uric acid excretion by the kidneys may be impaired for a variety of reasons, including long-term use of diuretics.

People who have gout over a long period of time may develop deposits of uric acid crystals in the earlobes and soft tissues of the hands, where they form small lumps known as tophi. People with gout may also develop kidney stones that are composed of uric acid.

SELF-HELP

PRIMARY TREATMENT If you have gout, it is important to make the following changes to your diet:
- Reduce your alcohol intake.
- Follow a weight-reducing diet if needed.
- Avoiding purine-rich foods may help.
- Cut down on refined and starchy foods, such as bread.

TREATMENTS IN DETAIL

Conventional Medicine

Your symptoms and an examination will usually enable the doctor to diagnose gout, but the levels of uric acid in the blood may need to be measured. In some cases, fluid is withdrawn from the affected joint and tested for the presence of uric acid crystals.

PRIMARY TREATMENT **DRUGS** Acute attacks of gout tend to subside after a few days without any treatment. However, you may be prescribed non-steroidal anti-inflammatory drugs (NSAIDs), such as naproxen, to relieve the pain and reduce the swelling. Aspirin is not used to relieve the pain of gout because it slows down the elimination of uric acid from the blood.

Alternatively, you may be prescribed colchicine to relieve the pain. This traditional remedy has been used for gout since the 18th century and is usually taken at the first sign of symptoms. Corticosteroids may be injected into a muscle or directly into the affected joint.

Recurrent gout may be controlled with uricosuric drugs, which act upon the kidneys to reduce the levels of uric acid in the blood. The uricosuric drug most commonly used is allopurinol, which not only prevents the production of uric acid but also rapidly reduces the levels of uric acid in the blood. Alternative drugs include probenecid and sulfinpyrazone.

> **CAUTION**
>
> The drugs used for treating gout have a range of side-effects: ask your doctor to explain them to you.

Uric acid crystals are shaped like tiny needles. When the level of uric acid in the bloodstream rises, the crystals may be deposited in certain joints, where they accumulate. Their sharpness can cause excruciating pain.

Homeopathy

Gout is a metabolic disorder whose main manifestation is joint pain and inflammation, but it can affect other organs, especially the kidneys. For this reason, treating the inflamed joint alone may not be sufficient. The homeopathic medicines most frequently suggested for gout are *Benzoic acid*, *Ledum* and *Lycopodium*.

BENZOIC ACID is appropriate for gout that occurs in the big toe. There may also be pain in the Achilles tendon at the back of the ankle, and small lumps (tophi) elsewhere in the body. However, the most characteristic feature of people who respond to *Benzoic acid* is that their urine smells very strongly.

LEDUM PALUSTRE is appropriate for gout in the base of the big toe which is swollen and tender, yet sometimes unusually pale rather than red. The most characteristic feature of the type of gout that responds to *Ledum* is the great relief that cold brings – putting the affected foot in cold water, or walking barefoot on a cold floor eases the pain, although the patient often feels generally chilly. People who respond to *Ledum* are sometimes heavy drinkers and their faces tend to be both red and pimply.

LYCOPODIUM is prescribed for gout mostly on constitutional grounds (*see p.73*). One indication that *Lycopodium* may be appropriate is when the gout affects joints on the right side of the body, or has

Nutritional Therapy

PRIMARY TREATMENT **AVOID PURINE-RICH FOODS** Uric acid is an end product of the metabolism of dietary elements known as purines. Foods rich in purines include meat (including organ meats and meat extracts), fish, seafood, yeast and yeast extracts, peas, beans, lentils, asparagus, spinach and mushrooms. Beer and other alcoholic drinks are also rich in purines.

Traditionally, sufferers of gout are advised to limit purine-rich foods. However, this approach is believed to have limited effectiveness, which may relate to the fact that the majority of purines in the bloodstream do not come from the diet, but are made naturally within the body.

ALCOHOL consumption has long been closely associated with high uric acid levels and gout. Limiting alcohol consumption may therefore be effective in the treatment and prevention of gout, although this is far from proven.

INSULIN RESISTANCE SYNDROME There is evidence to suggest that high uric acid levels in the blood and gout are often related to a condition known as insulin resistance syndrome (IRS). Believed to be a potential precursor of both heart disease and diabetes, IRS is characterised by a range of factors including excess weight (typically concentrated around the middle of the body), raised levels of total cholesterol and triglycerides in the body, low levels of "healthy" HDL cholesterol and high blood pressure (*see p.244*).

IRS is likely to have a number of underlying factors, one of which seems to be the over-consumption of sugar and refined carbohydrates. In one study, the potential benefits of a carbohydrate-restriction diet was tested in a group of middle-aged men with gout. The men were instructed to minimise their intake of bread, potatoes, rice and pasta and eat plenty of healthy fats in the form of olive oil, nuts and oily fish such as salmon, trout and sardines.

Following this diet for 16 weeks brought about significant lowering of uric acid and cholesterol levels, and a reduction in weight and the number of gout attacks. Consequently, restricting carbohydrates, especially refined sugar and starches, may be an effective strategy in combating IRS and gout in the long term.

Cruelly referred to as the disease of kings, gout is in fact not a sign of overindulgence

first affected the right foot and then the left. People who respond to *Lycopodium* are often thoughtful and reserved, and may be anxious and depressed. They often have stomach trouble. Their "eyes are bigger than their stomachs" – in other words, they feel hungry when they start eating, but quickly become satisfied. This feature is accompanied by a bloated feeling. They may crave sweet food and they tend to feel at their worst during the late afternoon.

Western Herbal Medicine

The treatment of gout needs to be considered in two phases: during acute attacks and when gout is in remission. Treatment in the acute phase has to be fast and effective because an attack of gout is usually very painful. It is sensible to use conventional drugs, such as NSAIDs or colchicine – an alkaloid found in the autumn crocus (*Colchicum autumnale*) – which can bring pain relief within a few hours.

Once the levels of uric acid have fallen and the pain has gone, herbal medicines come into their own. Like conventional drugs, plant medicines can increase the excretion of uric acid or prevent its synthesis. They can significantly reduce the inflammation, too.

DIURETICS AND ANTI-INFLAMMATORIES Burdock (*Arctium lappa*) root is a favoured gout remedy that is said to have a diuretic and "blood cleansing" action, while research supports its anti-inflammatory properties. Another study indicates that it can help to eliminate kidney stones formed from uric acid.

Celery (*Apium graveolens*) seed is another well-known gout remedy with anti-inflammatory, diuretic and anti-arthritic actions. Nettle (*Urtica dioica*) tea is a diuretic and

anthocyanidins and proanthocyanidins in cherries, which give them their dark, red-blue colour.

Other fruits, such as strawberries (*Fragaria spp.*), blackcurrants (*Ribes nigrum*) and cranberries (*Vaccinium macrocarpon*) may be effective for people with gout because of the anti-inflammatory polyphenol flavonoids they contain.

Conventional medicines, such as allopurinol, inhibit xanthine oxidase, a key enzyme in the synthesis of uric acid in the body. Studies show that several herbs, such as milk thistle (*Silybum marianum*), centaury (*Centaurium erythrea*), turmeric (*Curcuma longa*) and liquorice (*Glycyrrhiza glabra*), have the same inhibitory effect on xanthine oxidase.

Foods, such as strawberries, that are rich in folic acid may also help to relieve the symptoms of gout. Studies show that folic acid is not only an inhibitor of xanthine oxidase, but may also be several times more potent than allopurinol.

Drinking tea (*Camellia sinensis*) on a regular basis may well reduce attacks of gout as the polyphenol catechins and flavones in tea are also inhibitors of xanthine oxidase.

Studies show that silymarin, found in the fruits of milk thistle, is an inhibitor of xanthine oxidase, too. Similar claims are

Chinese Herbal Medicine

Practitioners of Traditional Chinese Medicine treat gout as *Bi* syndrome (*see Osteoarthritis, p.291*), rather than as a separate ailment. *Bi* means "painful blockage".

Of the many well-known Chinese herbal medicines for treating arthritic conditions, 122 have been investigated for their ability to inhibit xanthine oxidase. Over half (69) have been extracted in alcohol and shown to have a significant effect. Cinnamon (*Cinnamomum cassia*), wild chrysanthemum (*Chrysanthemum indica*) and shiny bugleweed (*Lycopus lucidum*) were the most effective. Those herbal medicines that were extracted in water showed a somewhat lower rate of inhibiting xanthine oxidase. *Hu zhang* (*Polygonum cuspidatum*) was the most potent.

Studies have shown that purple-leafed perilla (*Perilla fructescens*) is also a potent xanthine oxidase inhibitor and may help to control uric acid levels. One active component was shown to be as potent as the conventional drug allopurinol.

Gout is most common in people between the ages of 30 and 60

detoxifier; one study indicated that it enhanced the effect of the NSAID diclofenac in treating rheumatic conditions. There is also research to prove the diuretic and anti-inflammatory actions of sarsaparilla (*Smilax regelii*), yarrow (*Achillea millefolium*) and dandelion (*Taraxacum officinale*) root and leaf.

REDUCING URIC ACID LEVELS Many herbal remedies can reduce the levels of uric acid in the blood. Studies confirm anecdotal accounts of the effectiveness of cherries (*Prunus spp.*) in lowering the levels of uric acid and preventing gout. This action is probably due to the antioxidant and anti-inflammatory properties of the

made for the antioxidant properties of the polyphenols in centaury, which is the basis of the famous Portland Powder remedy for gout, as well as for the phenolic constituents of liquorice.

Turmeric contains curcumin, which appears to have a powerful inhibitory action on xanthine oxidase and has anti-inflammatory properties, too.

EXTERNAL TREATMENTS include a poultice of fresh cabbage (*Brassica spp.*) leaves, a vinegar compress and a footbath of natrum sulphate or magnesium sulphate with chopped celery and watercress (*Nasturtium officinale*). These may help to reduce swelling and inflammation.

PREVENTION PLAN

The following may help to prevent an increase in blood levels of uric acid:

- Avoid excess alcohol, proteins and purines in your diet.
- Restrict your intake of refined starches and sugars.

ANKYLOSING SPONDYLITIS

Ankylosing spondylitis is a chronic, progressive inflammation and stiffness of the joints, usually in the spine and pelvis. The disorder is about three times more common in men than women and mainly affects young white men, usually under the age of 45. The condition may run in families. Treatment involves easing the inflammation with NSAIDs, steroid injections, a diet rich in omega-3 fatty acids and vitamin D. Exercise, manipulation and homeopathy can help to ease the pain and maintain range of motion and muscle tone.

WHAT ARE THE SYMPTOMS?

- Pain in the low back, which may radiate into the buttocks and thighs
- Stiffness in the low back, which is worse in the morning and better with exercise
- Pain in other joints, such as the hips, knees and shoulders
- Pain in the ribcage and a limited ability to expand the chest
- Without treatment, curvature of the spine and weakening of the back muscles may eventually develop

Other possible features include:
- Uveitis (inflammation of the eye), which may need urgent treatment

WHY MIGHT I HAVE THIS?

PREDISPOSING FACTORS

- Genetic factors, such as having HLA-B27
- Inflammatory diet
- Vitamin D deficiency

WHY DOES IT OCCUR?

The symptoms of ankylosing spondylitis usually appear in late adolescence or early adulthood. They develop gradually over a period of months or years, with periods that are symptom free between episodes of inflammation. As well as the spine and pelvis, the ribcage and other joints around the body may also be affected. Walking and movement become awkward and other, non-inflamed joints and muscles become painful and stiff. Eventually the disease affects joints between the ribs and mid-spine, reducing chest expansion.

If left untreated, ankylosing spondylitis can result in curvature of the spine. If the spine is severely affected, new bone may start to grow between the vertebrae, which eventually fuse together.

Ankylosing spondylitis is a reactive spondarthropathy, a family of diseases that includes psoriasis (*see p.172*), inflammatory bowel disease and Reiter's syndrome. Its cause is unknown. However, about 90 per cent of people affected share a common factor – they have human leukocyte antigen B27 (HLA-B27). These antigens are proteins present on the surface of most cells in the body. They enable the body's immune system to differentiate body cells from foreign cells, such as bacteria, that it needs to attack. There are many different human leukocyte antigens: individuals inherit their own set from their parents. Not everyone who has HLA-B27 develops ankylosing spondylitis.

What triggers the ankylosing spondylitis in certain individuals is unknown, although some practitioners think that dietary factors and vitamin D deficiency are involved.

IMMEDIATE RELIEF

Acupuncture may bring relief from the back and hip pain and the homeopathic medicine *Rhus toxicodendron* may relieve the symptoms.

TREATMENT PLAN

PRIMARY TREATMENTS

- Exercises
- Drugs such as NSAIDs and steroid injections

BACK-UP TREATMENTS

- Nutritional therapy
- Homeopathy
- Bodywork and movement therapies
- Acupuncture

For an explanation of how treatments are rated, see p.111.

IMPORTANT

Consult a doctor immediately if you develop eye pain, redness, blurred vision or are bothered by bright lights. These symptoms may indicate that uveitis is present.

Conventional Medicine

To help make a diagnosis your doctor will arrange various tests, including X-rays, to look for changes that may occur in ankylosing spondylitis.

PRIMARY TREATMENT **EXERCISES** Early diagnosis is important so that you can start a regime of morning physiotherapy exercises to maintain mobility and help prevent deformities of the spine.

PRIMARY TREATMENT **DRUGS** During episodes of inflammation, your doctor may prescribe non-steroidal anti-inflammatory drugs (NSAIDs) to reduce the pain and stiffness, and to enable you to continue with the physiotherapy exercises. A doctor may also inject steroids into inflamed joints.

> **CAUTION**
>
> NSAIDs and steroids may cause side-effects: ask your doctor to explain these to you.

Nutritional Therapy

OMEGA-3 FATTY ACIDS Eating foods that are rich in omega-3 fatty acids (*see p.34*) should help to reduce inflammation and its associated pain. They can be found in some nuts and seeds, especially walnuts and flaxseeds, and oily fish, such as mackerel, salmon and sardines. One study has shown that taking the omega-3 fatty acids EPA (378mg) and DHA (259mg) each day for at least two months can help to reduce inflammation.

Conversely, excessive omega-6 polyunsaturated fatty acids (found in vegetable oils) and a relative lack of omega-3 fatty acids seems to promote inflammation.

VITAMIN D Studies reveal that ankylosing spondylitis patients have very low levels of the chemical resulting from vitamin D metabolism. Research also shows that low levels of vitamin D may accelerate the inflammation associated with the condition. Taking a dose of 500 IU of vitamin D supplements each day may help to reduce the inflammation and may also reduce the risk of any associated osteoporosis.

> **CAUTION**
>
> Consult your doctor before taking omega-3 oil or fish oils with warfarin or vitamin D with verapamil (*see p.46*).

Homeopathy

RHUS TOXICODENDRON Although there is little formal research to support them, homeopaths claim that their treatments

---

QUAD STRETCH FOR ANKYLOSING SPONDYLITIS

Stretching the major muscle groups every day and putting joints through their range of motion can ease pain. Practise this exercise once or twice a day. Always stretch slowly and gently and stop if it hurts.

1.Stand to the side of a sturdy chair and hold the back with your right hand. Stand tall, keeping your spine as straight as possible.

2. Keeping your head and neck in alignment with your spine, bend your right knee and place it on the seat of the chair.

3. Place your left foot as far forward as you can. You should feel a slight stretch in your right thigh.

can often help to relieve the symptoms of ankylosing spondylitis, most commonly with *Rhus tox.*, a medicine that is prepared from poison ivy.

A key feature of the rheumatic conditions that respond to this medicine is the way a patient's joints rapidly stiffen up. Typically, patients report that they are woken two or three times every night by pain and stiffness; after they get out of bed and "limber up" they feel much better and are able to sleep again for a couple of hours, before the process repeats itself. Similarly, they get stiff and achey from sitting still for about 30 minutes. Such symptoms may be masked if the person with ankylosing spondylitis is taking anti-inflammatory drugs.

Other features that suggest *Rhus tox.* may be appropriate include symptoms that are worse in cold and wet weather, and a tendency to having itchy rashes consisting of fine blisters.

4. To increase the the intensity, bend your left knee, while still keeping your back and neck aligned and relaxed. Hold for 10 seconds. Repeat twice and then turn round to stretch the opposite leg.

DEEPER-ACTING TREATMENTS If the condition is deep-seated, you will need to consult a well-trained homeopath who may prescribe a remedy, such as bowel nosodes, that acts at a more profound level. Bowel nosodes are prepared from bacteria that may be found in human intestines, although they are not part of the healthy intestinal flora.

Bowel nosodes may be helpful when the ankylosing spondylitis seems to be triggered by a "cross-reaction" – the body's immune system attacks invading bacteria and then turns its attention to the body's tissues, because they are of a similar type to the bacteria.

Bodywork and Movement Therapies

As a result of the inflammation that develops in the spinal joints, walking and movement becomes awkward and other, non-inflamed, joints and muscles become painful and stiff.

The objective of the manipulation therapies and exercises is to help you maintain your range of motion (the normal extent that joints can be moved in certain directions) and the tone of your muscles, and to ease the pain.

PHYSIOTHERAPY, OSTEOPATHY, CHIROPRACTIC AND THERAPEUTIC MASSAGE are all manipulation therapies that may be able to help you ease the pain and restrictions of your condition. They may also assist the circulation in muscles and joints that are affected by the pain and by altered movement patterns. The Alexander technique (*see p.62*) may also help you to improve your posture.

PRIMARY TREATMENT **EXERCISE** Try gently stretching and toning, every other day, those muscles and joints that are not actually inflamed, but which are affected by the pain and restriction of the disorder. Experience has also shown that it is important to put joints through gentle range-of-motion movements every day, even when the inflammation has flared up. Practising yoga can be an effective way of achieving this.

Exercise conducted in water may be easier to perform than out of it, as this allows greater flexibility and ease of movement because of the buoyancy. Many physiotherapy departments are equipped with warm-water pools where you can have exercise sessions under supervision.

Research shows that exercise (whether physiotherapy, exercising in water or exercising at home) brings benefits as long as it is maintained.

ANTI-AROUSAL BREATHING METHODS may help you to cope with chronic pain, according to research. Pursed-lip breathing exercises, for example, may improve both the mechanics and efficiency of breathing. Breathe in slowly through your nose and then, pursing your lips as if blowing up a balloon, exhale slowly (taking 4–6 seconds) through your mouth. Try practising anti-arousal breathing methods for a few minutes each morning after you have finished your exercises.

> **CAUTION**
>
> Manual treatment needs to be extremely gentle when joints are inflamed, to avoid aggravating the tissues.

Acupuncture

There are no direct clinical trials involving the use of acupuncture and ankylosing spondylitis as such, but evidence suggests that it helps back and hip pain which is a feature of the condition. Acupuncture does not alter the natural progression of ankylosing spondylitis, but it may provide prolonged periods of pain relief after relatively few treatments.

Usually, treatment is given weekly with the expectation that some benefit will begin to emerge after four to six treatments, and treatments should continue until no further clinical improvement occurs.

> **PREVENTION PLAN**
>
> **The following may help to slow the progress of ankylosing spondylitis:**
>
> ● Follow a daily exercise routine or take up yoga.
>
> ● Learn the Alexander technique to help improve posture.

OSTEOPOROSIS

Osteoporosis is characterised by a loss of bone tissue that is greater than normal and an increased susceptibility to fractures. Common in men and women over the age of 50, osteoporosis is more prevalent in white and Asian people. Certain factors predispose to developing osteoporosis. These include a family history of the condition, being thin and not taking enough exercise. Treatments are aimed at slowing the rate of bone loss, building up bone density and reducing the risks of developing the disease.

WHAT ARE THE SYMPTOMS?

- For many people, the first sign is a fractured bone following a minor injury

Other symptoms may include:

- A gradual loss of height and rounding of the back, both due to vertebral fractures

WHY MIGHT I HAVE THIS?

PREDISPOSING FACTORS

- Smoking
- Alcoholism
- Genetic factors
- Being underweight
- Lack of regular exercise
- Insufficient calcium in the diet, particularly during childhood and adolescence
- Ageing
- Early menopause
- Long-term use of corticosteroids
- Joint conditions, such as rheumatoid arthritis
- Other conditions, such as an overactive thyroid gland

WHY DOES IT OCCUR?

Bone is a living tissue that is continually being broken down and rebuilt by the body. From the age of about 25 when peak bone mass is reached, there is a gradual loss of bone tissue as bone breakdown occurs more rapidly than bone formation. However, in many people, bone mass remains within an acceptable range even in old age. In osteoporosis, the bone mass is below this acceptable range and the risk of fractures is markedly increased.

In both men and women, the sex hormones play a part in bone replacement. In women, there is a rapid decrease in bone density in the ten years following the menopause. An early menopause (*see p.339*) increases the risk of osteoporosis, as do other conditions in which there is reduced production of sex hormones, such as anorexia nervosa (*see p.441*).

People who have certain joint disorders, such as rheumatoid arthritis (*see p.293*), and hormone disorders, such as an overactive thyroid gland (*see p.319*), are also more prone to developing osteoporosis. Osteoporosis can develop as a complication of taking certain drugs, including long-term corticosteroids. Other risk factors include poor nutrition in childhood, smoking and chronic alcohol abuse.

TREATMENT PLAN

PRIMARY TREATMENTS

- Lifestyle measures
- Drugs, such as biphosphonates, calcitonin, HRT, raloxifene
- Calcium and vitamin D

BACK-UP TREATMENTS

- Nutritional therapy
- Weight-bearing exercise and t'ai chi
- Environmental health measures

WORTH CONSIDERING

- Acupuncture

For an explanation of how treatments are rated, see p.111.

TREATMENTS IN DETAIL

Conventional Medicine

If your doctor suspects osteoporosis, the diagnosis may be confirmed and the severity of the disease measured by bone densitometry of the spinal column or hip. This test uses low-dose X-rays to measure bone density. Further investigations may be arranged to look for a possible underlying cause.

PRIMARY TREATMENT **LIFESTYLE MEASURES** For those with a slightly low bone mass, lifestyle factors, such as stopping smoking, will be recommended with a follow-up assessment of bone density a few years later (*see also Prevention, below*).

PRIMARY TREATMENT **DRUGS** In more severe cases and where osteoporosis is confirmed, drugs may also be prescribed. This is particularly the case where fractures have occurred as a result of minor injuries.

Drug treatments include biphosphonates, such as risedronate, which reduce the rate of bone breakdown and increase bone density, and calcitonin, which also reduces the rate of bone breakdown and can help to prevent and treat osteoporosis after the menopause. Your doctor may recommend calcium supplements (*see Nutritional therapy, below*).

Hormone replacement therapy taken for 5–10 years reduces bone loss after the

the amount of calcium in the diet in later life (including calcium from dairy products) has little or no bearing on bone health and risk of fracture.

PRIMARY TREATMENT **VITAMIN D** The effect of calcium supplementation on bone health may be more effective if it is combined with vitamin D supplementa-

VITAMIN D AND CALCIUM
The table shows the recommended adequate intakes (AIs) of vitamin D for adults, calculated in 1998 (Source: US National Institutes of Health), and the recommended daily allowance (RDA) of calcium for various ages and for pregnant and breastfeeding women.

One in 3 women and 1 in 12 men over the age of 50 will develop osteoporosis

menopause and so reduces the risk of osteoporosis. HRT is no longer a first-line treatment because of it potential risks. It may be used when other first-line treatments are not effective or tolerated. The drug raloxifene is sometimes used to treat or prevent the osteoporosis that occurs in post-menopausal women.

All of these treatments have been shown to increase bone density; some, such as biphosphonates and HRT, have also been found to reduce the risk of fractures. Regular follow-up is needed to monitor the progress of treatment.

CAUTION

Drugs for osteoporosis may have side-effects: ask your doctor to explain these to you.

Nutritional Therapy

PRIMARY TREATMENT **CALCIUM SUPPLEMENTS** Most studies show that calcium, either as a regular supplement or as a significant dietary ingredient, is important at a young age in order to reach a good peak bone mass (at around the age of 25). This intake of calcium may protect against the development of osteoporosis in later life. A daily dose of 600–1,000mg of calcium before the age of 25 is thought to help optimum bone mass. (*See table, right, and Environmental health, p.311.*)

However, the evidence regarding calcium supplementation in later life (especially in post- menopausal women) in order to prevent osteoporosis and fractures is controversial. A 2003 study suggests that

tion. Vitamin D plays an important role in calcium balance in the body by aiding the absorption of calcium from food. It may also help to reduce the loss of bone tissue after the menopause.

Many studies show that taking vitamin D (20mcg/800 IU daily) in combination with calcium (at about 1,000mg daily) reduces the rates of fracture and numbers of falls in the elderly. One study and a meta-analysis shows that vitamin D alone may be beneficial in reducing fracture risk. The normal recommended daily dose is 20mcg/800 IU of vitamin D.

FRUIT AND VEGETABLES A number of studies have suggested that there is a clear, positive link between fruit and vegetable consumption and bone health. This probably reflects the fact that eating fruit and vegetables helps to increase alkalinity in the body, which plays a role in preventing calcium loss from bone. Findings in other studies have demonstrated that women with the lowest intakes of potassium, magnesium, fibre, vitamin C and beta-carotene had significantly lower bone mineral densities and higher bone loss than other women. Nutrients, such as potassium and lutein, which are abundant in fruit and vegetables also seem to be associated with better bone mass in men.

OMEGA-3 FATTY ACIDS There is a certain amount of evidence to suggest that eating a diet that is rich in eicosapentaenoic acid (EPA) and docosahexaenoic acid (DHA) may also be useful in preventing osteoporosis. These omega 3-fatty acids (*see p.34*) can be found in oily fish, such as

VITAMIN D	
Age	**AI**
	IU
51–69	400 IU
over 70	600 IU
CALCIUM	
Age	**RDA**
0–6 months	210mg
7–12 months	270mg
19–50	1,000mg
over 50	1,200mg
Pregnant women	
under 18	1,300mg
over 18	1,000mg
Breast-feeding women	
under 18	1,300mg
over 18	1,000mg

mackerel, salmon and sardines. In one study, elderly women with osteoporosis were given 4g of fish oil daily for 16 weeks. Giving fish-oil supplementation was found to bring about biochemical changes that can be detected in the serum part of blood. These changes include an increase in the levels of calcium, osteocalcin and collagen and a reduction in the levels of alkaline phosphatase – all of which are signs of improved bone health.

Eating a diet that is rich in the omega-3 fatty acids EPA and DHA may also reduce the risk of osteoporosis by inhibiting the production of eicosanoids in the body. These inflammatory and hormone-like substances are believed to be involved in the process of bone loss.

Normal bone (*above left*) features struts that are both light and strong. In osteoporosis (*above right*), the fabric of spongy bone tissue becomes thinner, reducing bone mass and making the bones more brittle.

PHYTOESTROGENS are plant-derived substances that have a similar action to the hormone oestrogen in the body. However, this action is much weaker than that of oestrogen. Studies suggest that including soy foods, such as soy milk, tofu and soy flour, and other sources of phytoestrogens, such as beans, lentils, chickpeas and flaxseeds, in the diet may be beneficial in protecting the bones against osteoporosis, especially in post-menopausal women.

MAGNESIUM appears to be an important nutrient for bone health as it helps to encourage the incorporation of calcium into bone. In one study, eating plenty of magnesium was associated with higher bone mass. Research also shows that taking magnesium supplements and eating a diet that is rich in the mineral can help to reduce biochemical signs of bone loss.

In a 1993 study, most of the people who took 250–750mg of magnesium in supplement form over a two-year period stopped losing bone or else increased their bone density. Nuts, seeds, pulses, beans and whole grains are good sources of magnesium and should be included in the diet of individuals wishing to maximise bone

health. Taking a supplement that contains 500mg of magnesium each day may also be beneficial to bone health.

MULTIVITAMIN AND MINERAL SUPPLEMENTS Research suggests that zinc, copper, potassium, vitamin K, vitamin C, silicon and manganese may be important to bone health. Taking a multivitamin and mineral supplement regularly may benefit the health of your bones.

AVOID CAFFEINE AND FIZZY DRINKS A high intake of caffeine and carbonated drinks has been linked to reduced bone mass and an increased risk of fracture. These drinks contain phosphoric acid, which leaches (removes) calcium from the bones. Try to limit your intake of these foodstuffs in your diet.

> **CAUTION**
>
> Consult your doctor before taking vitamin D with verapamil; omega-3 fatty acids/fish oils with warfarin; magnesium with ciproflaxin, iron, warfarin or spironolactone; calcium with antibiotics, beta-blockers or thyroxine (*see p.46*).

Exercise

Exercise and movement techniques, such as t'ai chi, may reduce bone loss, increase bone density, improve strength, balance and coordination, and reduce the chances of falling and fracturing fragile bones.

PHYSICAL EXERCISE increases bone mineral density (BMD) in healthy young adults and slows the rate of bone loss in later life. One study also shows that progressive low-impact exercise is a potentially effective method of increasing BMD in people with Crohn's disease (*see p.216*), Because of intestinal inflammation, these people absorb nutrients poorly and bone loss is a very real risk. If the exercise is sustained, the increases in bone mass should reduce the risk of osteoporotic fracture.

WEIGHT-TRAINING AND WEIGHT-BEARING EXERCISE The objectives of treatment and exercise change with age. One study found that structured weight-training and weight-bearing exercise in the middle adult years may generate small increases in bone mass. The aim in older adults, particularly those who have osteoporosis, is to combine physiotherapy treatment and exercise to conserve bone mass, improve mobility and function, encourage extended posture and reduce pain. Walking is a recommended weight-bearing exercise.

Italian research has shown that physical exercise combined with thermal mud packs increases bone density and is more effective than exercise alone.

REDUCING THE RISK OF FALLING is important for people with osteoporosis, not least because they become increasingly unsteady with age and more likely to fracture a bone, most commonly the hip. Approximately 95 per cent of hip fractures result from falls. Suggestions for ways to reduce falls include wearing footwear that promotes stability and protective hip pads that reduce the risk of fracture if and when falls do occur.

T'AI CHI A number of studies confirm that movement techniques, such as t'ai chi, can help to restore some sense of balance. A three-month study of older women living in a retirement community who attended twice-weekly, 30-minute t'ai chi classes found that they had significant improvements in balance and mobility, and so were less likely to fear falling.

Another study demonstrated that elderly people who regularly practised t'ai chi developed a postural stability in challenging conditions, such as maintaining balance on an unstable surface when they had their eyes closed, which made them less likely to have falls.

Acupuncture

Acupuncture cannot treat the bone demineralisation that occurs in osteoporosis, but it can relieve the pain, particularly pain from the stress fractures that may occur in the spine. Acupuncture will probably need to be provided on a weekly basis until the pain settles. Benefit should be apparent within the first six to eight treatment sessions, and if there is no obvious pain relief then discontinue treatment.

Environmental Health

VITAMINS AND MINERALS Osteoporosis prevention and treatment depend upon environmental factors to a large extent. If

Cod liver oil is an easy way to supplement your diet with vitamin D, but take it in moderation or else you may inadvertently consume too much of another fat-soluble vitamin – vitamin A – which can weaken bones. Recent research warns that the retinol form of vitamin A (not the carotene form) is associated with frail bones and clinical fractures.

As well as consuming enough vitamin D, you need sunlight to transform the inactive dietary form of vitamin D into the bio-active vitamin D necessary for calcium absorption and bone formation.

If possible, try to receive at least 10–15 minutes a day of unfiltered sunlight – this is sunlight that is not filtered through clouds, pollution, sunscreens, clothing or glass windows – to ensure that your skin is exposed to enough UV radiation to transform your vitamin D into the form necessary to combat osteoporosis.

CADMIUM Studies have shown that the more cadmium is present in the body the less dense the bones are likely to be. Since cadmium can persist in your tissues for several decades, make sure your children also limit their cadmium exposures.

In the UK, the risk of exposure to cadmium should be declining since the country adopted the Protocol on Heavy Metals in 1998. This aims to reduce the amount of cadmium, lead and mercury in airborne emissions and to regulate stationary sources of cadmium in order to minimise its release into the environment. Targeted sources include the iron and steel industries, power generators, road transport and waste incinerators.

PSYCHOLOGICAL STRESS that raises your body's production of the stress hormone cortisol can, theoretically, contribute to worsening osteoporosis. This is because cortisol and the related steroid, cortisone, are notorious for inducing and exacerbating osteoporosis.

DRUGS AND OTHER SUBSTANCES that seem to be detrimental to bone health include blood thinners, anticonvulsants, lithium, antacids containing aluminium, chemotherapy and certain antibiotics.

FLUORIDE is commonly added to public supplies of drinking water to help reduce dental decay. Fluoride has also been used as a treatment for osteoporosis because it encourages osteoblasts to generate new bone tissue and increase the bone mineral density. Although fluoride may make bones thicker, it also makes them more brittle and more vulnerable to fractures.

A diet low in dairy products may be low in calcium, predisposing you to osteoporosis

you live in northern latitudes, or your access to sunlight is otherwise impeded (due to air pollution or style of dress, or because you wear sunscreen that is SPF 8 or greater), you may also be putting yourself at risk for osteoporosis. This is because you may not be receiving enough sunlight on your skin and therefore not producing enough vitamin D, or getting enough calcium in your diet (*see also Nutritional Therapy, p.309*).

It is important to make sure that you consume enough, but not too much, calcium in order to build strong bones (*see table in Nutritional therapy, p.309*). Be aware, however, of the source of your calcium supplement, since bone meal and other sources of medical or supplemental calcium can be laden with toxic heavy metals, especially lead.

You will markedly elevate your intake of cadmium by smoking cigarettes or by working in zinc-refining areas, or in a nickel/cadmium battery manufacturing plant or with metal soldering. If you have osteoporosis or are at risk from it, you need to stop smoking and avoid exposure to occupational sources of cadmium in the air or in the soil near sites that produce cadmium-polluted air.

Most foods have small amounts of cadmium, but certain vegetables, shellfish (but not regular fish), liver and kidney meats tend to have higher concentrations.

Unfortunately, there is no compelling evidence at the present time to support the use of chelation therapy (in which cadmium is bound and filtered from the bloodstream by chemical means) from a clinical point of view.

PREVENTION PLAN

The following may help to prevent the development of osteoporosis:

- Eat plenty of calcium-containing foods, particularly in childhood and adolescence, to help achieve good bone mass.

- Avoid becoming too thin.

- Take vitamin D supplements to help you absorb calcium.

- Take regular weight-bearing exercise, such as walking.

- Do not smoke, and avoid caffeine and carbonated drinks.

- Stay within the recommended limits for alcohol consumption (14 units weekly for women and 21 for men).

Hormonal System

A complex chemical communication system flows via the bloodstream and modifies the way we function on every level. Drug treatments are often effective in hormonal disorders, and nutritional controls are vital in diabetes. However, using herbs and other more subtle therapies can also enhance the function of these delicate systems.

DIABETES MELLITUS

In diabetes mellitus, the pancreas does not produce sufficient amounts of insulin, or body cells become resistant to its effects. In some cases, both abnormalities are present. The hormone insulin enables the body's cells to absorb the sugar glucose from the bloodstream, which provides the cells with energy. Treatment aims to keep the amount of glucose in the blood within normal levels. This may be achieved through dietary measures, drug treatment or insulin injections, depending on the individual circumstances. Exercise and relaxation also help.

WHY DOES IT OCCUR?

TYPES There are two types of diabetes mellitus. In type 1, the pancreas produces little or no insulin. The disorder usually develops suddenly in childhood or adolescence, and a genetic tendency to diabetes is thought to be involved. In type 2 diabetes, which is much more common than type 1, the body cells become resistant to the effects of insulin, and there may also be a lack of insulin (but to a much lesser degree than occurs in type 1 diabetes). Type 2 develops slowly and may go unnoticed for many years. Like type 1 diabetes, type 2 may be due in part to a genetic tendency.

CAUSES Type 1 diabetes is usually caused by an autoimmune response in which the body produces antibodies against its own tissues, in this case the insulin-secreting cells of the pancreas. Although genes are thought to contribute to the development of type 1 diabetes, the actual triggers of the abnormal immune reaction are unknown. It may be that viruses play a role.

Why type 2 diabetes develops is also not fully understood, but genes and obesity are important factors. Type 2 diabetes is a growing problem in affluent societies where food intake is excessive and increasing numbers of people, including children, are very overweight. The sedentary lifestyle led by many is also thought to be a major factor. Type 2 diabetes, which was once considered a disease of middle and old age, is now occurring in adolescents.

Diabetes mellitus sometimes develops temporarily during pregnancy, when it is known as gestational diabetes. Urine tests are done regularly at antenatal visits to check for the development of this kind of diabetes, which can usually be treated with dietary measures alone. Gestational diabetes usually resolves after the baby is born.

In a few cases, diabetes mellitus results from another disorder, such as cirrhosis (in which the liver becomes damaged, often as a result of chronic alcohol abuse) or long-term inflammation of the pancreas.

KETOACIDOSIS If individuals with type 1 diabetes miss their insulin or have another illness, such as an infection, that disrupts their blood-sugar control, unused glucose

NORMAL REGULATION OF BLOOD GLUCOSE

The amount of glucose (a simple sugar) in the blood is kept within a fairly narrow range by the body. The mechanism for keeping blood-glucose within these relatively narrow limits is complex and involves the liver and the pancreas. If blood-glucose levels are high, the pancreas produces insulin to enable the transport of glucose into body cells. If blood-glucose levels are low, the pancreas produces the hormone glucagon, which enables release of glucose stores from the liver into the bloodstream.

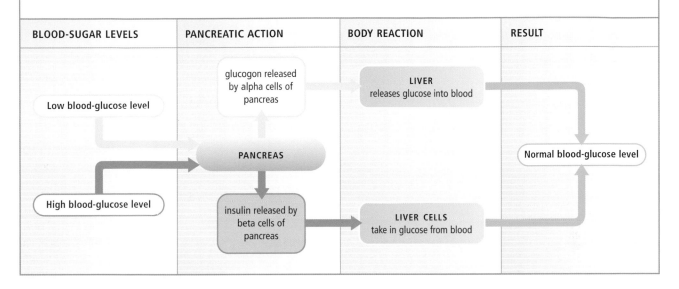

BLOOD-SUGAR LEVELS	PANCREATIC ACTION	BODY REACTION	RESULT

builds up in the blood and a condition known as diabetic ketoacidosis may arise. In this condition, the body begins to use its fat cells for energy, causing ketones (toxic substances) to be released into the blood. Ketoacidosis may lead to coma within a few hours if it is not treated promptly.

HYPOGLYCAEMIA Hypoglycaemia is a condition in which the level of blood sugar falls too low in a person with diabetes. The usual cause of hypoglycaemia is too much insulin in the bloodstream, which may be caused by too high a dose or an incorrect diet. Hypoglycaemia may also result from certain medications taken for type 2 diabetes (*see p.316*). Symptoms include irritability, sweating, tremor and drowsiness. If blood-sugar levels continue to fall, the person may lose consciousness or have a seizure.

LONG-TERM COMPLICATIONS The possible long-term complications of diabetes include coronary artery disease (*see p.252*), peripheral vascular disease (in which the blood supply to the limbs, hands and feet is impaired) and stroke (*see p.148*). In addition, the retina (the light-sensitive layer at the back of the eye) may be damaged, kidney damage may occur and neuropathy (*see p.127*) may develop, symptoms of which

may include tingling, burning pain, numbness of the feet and impotence. These complications come about because diabetes damages blood vessels throughout the body, especially if poorly controlled. Why damage occurs is not understood.

TREATMENTS IN DETAIL

Conventional Medicine

PRIMARY TREATMENT MONITORING Diabetes mellitus is usually diagnosed by measuring blood-glucose levels. People with diabetes must monitor their blood-sugar levels carefully and regularly.

In both type 1 and type 2 diabetes, regular check-ups are needed, not only to check blood-glucose control but also to look for evidence of complications; for example the eyes are examined to look for disease of the retina. Peripheral vascular disease in diabetes mellitus makes the feet vulnerable to

disease. They need to be looked after carefully and checked for signs of injury. This is because individuals may be unaware of damage to their feet as a result of loss of sensation, and so minor injuries may become serious without appropriate care.

PRIMARY TREATMENT LIFESTYLE MODIFICATIONS are recommended for people with both types of diabetes mellitus, including following a diabetic diet, taking regular exercise (as advised by the doctor), moderating alcohol intake and not smoking. The latter is important because smoking causes atherosclerosis (accumulation of fatty deposits in the arteries; *see p.252*) and can cause complications to occur earlier and make them more serious.

An Egyptian papyrus from 1552 BC noted frequent urination as a symptom of diabetes

PRIMARY TREATMENT INSULIN People with type 1 diabetes need insulin injections to control the amount of glucose in the bloodstream. There are various types of insulin preparations available.

The types of insulin given and frequency of injections vary according to the needs of the individual. The dose of insulin may need to be changed according to the blood-glucose levels.

Insulin is injected under the skin; common sites for injection are the wall of the abdomen and the outer thighs. The drug may be delivered by a needle and syringe or a pen device. Less commonly, pumps are used that can deliver insulin as a continuous trickle under the skin. The site of insulin injections should be changed regularly to avoid the development of fatty lumps in the area, which can affect insulin absorption.

PRIMARY TREATMENT **ANTIDIABETIC DRUGS** For type 2 diabetes the doctor may prescribe one or more drugs. These might include sulphonylurea drugs, such as tolbutamide and gliclazide, which stimulate the pancreas to produce insulin.

These drugs tend to be associated with weight increase and are therefore not usually given to people who are overweight. There is a small risk of hypoglycaemia occurring with these drugs.

The drug metformin may also be prescribed. It tends to be used less now due to its possible side-effects (which include a

small risk of hypoglycaemia); however, unlike the sulphonylurea drugs, it is not associated with weight increase. It is thought to work by increasing the sensitivity of the tissues to insulin and so promoting glucose uptake.

Thiazolidinediones (also known as glitazones), such as rosiglitazone, may be prescribed. These are newer drugs that also increase the sensitivity of the tissues to insulin. They are used in combination with sulphonylureas or metformin. They may also be associated with weight gain and there is a small risk of hypoglycaemia.

Other fairly new drugs known as meglitinides, such as repaglinide, may also be prescribed for some people. These drugs stimulate insulin production and are taken before meals. Side-effects are relatively

uncommon with these drugs but there is a small risk of hypoglycaemia.

Finally, a group of drugs known as alpha-glucosidase inhibitors, such as acarbose, may be prescribed. These work by delaying the absorption of glucose in the small intestine, thus regulating blood glucose.

> **CAUTION**
>
> Drugs for diabetes mellitus can cause a range of possible side-effects: ask your doctor to explain these to you.

Nutritional Therapy

PRIMARY TREATMENT **DIETARY CHANGES** Whatever the precise nature and cause of diabetes, eating a diet that helps to keep blood-sugar levels steady is important. Eating regular meals with an emphasis on low glycaemic index (GI) foods is the cornerstone of this approach. See p.44 for more details about how to do this.

Most people who have type 2 diabetes are overweight or obese. Excess weight around the middle of the body (abdominal fat) is believed to increase the risk of the body becoming resistant to the effects of insulin,

which is a central feature in the development of type 2 diabetes. Many studies show that type 2 diabetes improves when people follow a weight-reducing diet.

FISH OIL People who have type 2 diabetes may benefit from eating more oily fish (such as salmon, trout, mackerel, herring and sardines). Those who eat fish regularly seem to be protected against the development of blood-sugar related problems, and some studies suggest that fish oil supplements can improve blood-sugar control in type 2 diabetes. If you have type 2 diabetes, try taking 1g of concentrated fish oil, once or twice a day, and eat more oily fish.

SUPPLEMENTS The definitive clinical trials on the effectiveness of supplementation in

diabetes have yet to be done. Therefore, these suggestions are based on some clues derived from clinical research.

VITAMIN E Some studies indicate that taking vitamin E supplements improves blood-sugar control in people with type 2 diabetes, although benefits may not be apparent for three or more months. Vitamin E has also been shown to reduce a process known as glycosylation in diabetes. Glycosylation, when sugar binds to and damages protein molecules in the body, is thought to be an important cause of many of the complications of diabetes. If you have type 2 diabetes, take 400–800IU vitamin E daily.

Recent large trials of vitamin E supplements failed to show any benefit in preventing cardiovascular disease in people with diabetes. However, the supplemental dose used was quite low at 450mg per day.

VITAMIN C Individuals with both types of diabetes appear to have low vitamin C levels. Taking vitamin C supplements may help to correct this and can perhaps reduce glycosylation. In type 2 diabetes, vitamin C may also improve glucose tolerance. If you have type 2 diabetes, try taking 1–2g of vitamin C per day.

B VITAMINS Many people with diabetes have low blood levels of vitamin B6. Vitamin B6 supplementation may improve blood-sugar control. If you have diabetes, try taking 50–100mg of vitamin B6 per day.

The B vitamin niacinamide (vitamin B3) at a dose of 500mg daily for one month, followed by 250mg daily, has been shown to help some individuals with type 2 diabetes reduce blood-sugar levels. If you have type 2 diabetes, try taking a supplement of niacinamide at these doses.

CHROMIUM This mineral in the form of chromium picolinate appears to help improve glucose control in people with both types of diabetes. In type 2 diabetes chromium may increase insulin sensitivity and normalise blood-sugar levels. If you have diabetes, try taking 250–500mcg of chromium picolinate daily.

MAGNESIUM Levels of magnesium are often low in people with diabetes and research shows taking magnesium supplements can improve insulin production in

The effect of diet on diabetes was first noticed during the siege of Paris in the early 1870s

type 2 diabetes. Some research suggests that insulin requirements are lower in people with type 1 diabetes who supplement with magnesium. If you have diabetes, take 300–400mg of magnesium daily.

Homeopathy

There is no substitute for good control of blood sugar in treating diabetes, but homeopathy can help in borderline type 2 diabetes and with certain complications. An individualised diagnosis from a skilled practitioner is essential. Medicines that may be helpful for diabetes and its complications include *Phosphoric acid*, *Phosphorus*, *Lycopodium*, *Arsenicum album* and *Secale*.

PHOSPHORIC ACID may be useful in the early stages of the illness, particularly if the diabetes may have been precipitated by an acute illness or emotional upset. Typically the patient feels absolutely exhausted, especially mentally, with a very weak memory and poor concentration. There is profuse urination and there may also be diarrhoea.

PHOSPHORUS People who respond to *Phosphorus* typically feel run down and tired but are briefly better from rest, and so feel better first thing in the morning. There is a general tendency to easy bleeding, including nosebleeds and easy bruising of the skin. Other associated symptoms include recurrent laryngitis and vertigo, especially in older people. There may be pancreas or liver problems, such as pancreatitis. People who respond to *Phosphorus* tend to be slim and sensitive both to the human and physical environment. They may be phobic of things such as storms or being alone in the dark.

LYCOPODIUM would usually be prescribed on "constitutional" grounds (*see p.73*). It is typically appropriate for rather reserved, intellectual people with digestive problems. When this medicine is indicated there tends to be right-sided pain or pain that starts on the right, before moving to the left. These people tend to feel worse between 4 and 8 pm.

ARSENICUM ALBUM AND SECALE may be indicated for the circulatory problems associated with diabetes. When these homeopathic medicines are indicated the person's extremities are usually very cold. *Arsenicum*

album is often helpful for skin ulcers associated with severe, burning pain.

Environmental Health

BREAST-FEEDING Many studies strongly indicate that early exposure to cow's milk may increase the likelihood of developing type 1 diabetes. Breast-fed babies may have a lower risk of diabetes later in life.

TOXINS Possible environmental triggers for diabetes include nitrosamines, dioxins and dioxin-like compounds (DLCs), nitrates, arsenic and smoking.

NITROSAMINE compounds, most prevalent in cured and smoked meats, have been proven to cause damage to the pancreas and hasten the onset of diabetes. You should try to avoid these products, especially if you have other risk factors for diabetes.

DIOXINS AND DLCS are highly toxic environmental contaminants and by-products of certain industries. They may be implicated in diabetes because they compete for receptors with the body's natural hormones. It is estimated that 90 per cent of human exposure to dioxins occurs through the food supply. Although the relationship between

dioxin exposure and diabetes is speculative, you can decrease your dioxin exposure by trimming fat from meat, consuming low-fat dairy products and cooking food as simply as possible. Avoid eating predatory fish from rivers or lakes known to be contaminated with dioxins or close to industrial centres.

NITRATES AND ARSENIC are both threats to the water supply and have been associated with increased prevalence of diabetes. Nitrates are toxic to the pancreas, while arsenic disrupts the insulin receptor and glucose transport mechanisms in the body.

The primary sources of nitrates include human sewage and livestock manure and fertilisers. Arsenic, a naturally occurring element, is a component of many pesticides.

To reduce the risk of nitrate and arsenic exposure, you should be aware of your community's water quality and have your tap water checked.

VACOR A final example of a toxin that may lead to diabetes is the rodenticide Vacor. This N-nitroso compound was clearly shown to induce diabetes because of its toxic effects on the beta cells of the pancreas. Although Vacor was removed from the commercial market in the late 1970s, if it was used to treat your home or work environment traces of it may still be present. Check with your local environmental health officer if you are concerned.

Acupuncture

The overall control of diabetes lies firmly within the sphere of diet, exercise and appropriate medication to normalise blood-sugar levels. However, frequently people with diabetes develop neurological and circulatory disorders associated with the slow degeneration of the blood supply to various organs and tissues. Acupuncture may help stave off these complications by directly improving local micro-circulation. Studies indicate that long-term acupuncture may help diabetic neuropathy and improve

Insulin was discovered at the University of Toronto in 1921

digestive function. There is also some evidence that it may affect the autonomic nervous system and create vasodilatation, which can maximise blood flow to organs that are potentially affected by diabetes. While not definitely proven, this is probably the mechanism through which acupuncture may help in conditions such as diabetic retinopathy and intermittent claudication (damage to leg arteries).

Massage

Stress levels seem strongly to influence both the progression and seriousness of type 2 diabetes. Stress appears to affect blood-sugar levels, causing them to rise, and may also make individuals more susceptible to unhealthy habits, such as smoking. Massage has been shown to reduce stress levels and to allow better control of blood-sugar levels. Research was done to see what effect there would be when parents were taught to give massages regularly to their children with type 1 diabetes. Twenty-four children, aged between five and eight years, were either taught to use progressive muscular relaxation methods (which was carried out under supervision by a parent just before bedtime) or were given a daily 15-minute massage by a parent just before bedtime.

> ## Type 2 diabetes is becoming increasingly common in children and adolescents

Both groups improved, but both parents and children in the massage group showed greater reduction in stress and anxiety. The children showed behavioural improvements as well. The outcome at the end of the month was "blood-glucose levels decreased significantly toward the normal range [in the massage group]".

Exercise

Regular exercise has a positive effect on many aspects of type 2 diabetes, including better functioning of insulin and improved metabolism of glucose and fats. Exercise can also be a powerful preventive measure if you think you may be predisposed to developing type 2 diabetes.

The best exercise for diabetes is aerobic exercise, although yoga (*see below*) can be beneficial for stress levels. Brisk walking, done for 20–30 minutes at least five times a week, is a good way to start. Begin any exercise regime gradually and, if you have diabetes, check with your doctor first.

If you have type 1 diabetes, you may need to monitor your blood-glucose levels before, during and after any strenuous exercise to determine how the activity affects your need for insulin and food.

Yoga

Practising yoga regularly can help to lower stress levels, which affect blood-sugar levels (*see Mind–Body Therapies, below*). The

slower, gentler forms of yoga are the most suitable for this purpose. Yoga that emphasises slow, abdominal breathing is especially good for reducing stress.

Mind–Body Therapies

STRESS AND BLOOD SUGAR Stress affects blood sugar both directly and indirectly. It can cause chronic overproduction of stress hormones, such as adrenaline and cortisol, which makes blood-sugar levels rise. In addition, people under stress tend to adopt unhealthy habits, such as eating a poor diet, not exercising, smoking and drinking alcohol. These can all have a negative impact on blood-sugar levels.

Studies demonstrate a strong physiological relationship between stress and blood-sugar levels in people with diabetes. For example, researchers in Japan studied the health effects of the 1995 Kobe Earthquake on diabetic patients. Compared to diabetics in the city of Osaka, where little earthquake damage occurred, Kobe residents with diabetes found it harder to manage their blood sugar. Research also suggests that stress can increase insulin resistance, making it harder for people to manage their condition.

IMPROVING COMPLIANCE Many people with diabetes find their dietary restrictions and medication programmes burdensome and frustrating. Anxiety and depression may develop. These things may lead some people with diabetes to ignore dietary restrictions some or much of the time, and to neglect drug treatment. Failure of patients to comply with dietary measures and drug treatment to control diabetes is the biggest cause of diabetic complications, which include kidney failure, blindness (due to diabetic retinopathy), amputation (due to peripheral vascular problems) and heart disease.

However, when depression and anxiety can be alleviated using mind–body techniques, compliance with diet and drug treatment regimes tends to improve, leading

to a better quality of life for people with diabetes, as well as fewer short- and long-term complications from the condition.

RELAXATION AND SELF-HYPNOSIS Mood improvement techniques are a vital component of diabetes management, especially in type 2 diabetes, where they appear to lower blood-glucose levels directly. Researchers at the Medical College of Ohio, for example, found that depression and anxiety, which can have a negative impact on blood-sugar levels, could be partially relieved through relaxation and self-hypnosis.

GUIDED IMAGERY Nurse researchers at the University of Wisconsin-Green Bay in the US found that a group of diabetes patients who listened to guided imagery tapes took better care of themselves and complied more closely with their care regimes.

STRESS-MANAGEMENT PROGRAMMES In a randomised trial at Duke University Medical Center in the US, patients with type 2 diabetes who participated in a five-session stress-management programme (including training in relaxation, imagery and other techniques) showed significant reductions in blood-glucose levels.

SELF-HELP TECHNIQUES If you have diabetes, try practising mind–body techniques such as relaxation and guided imagery regularly (*see p.99*). This may be especially beneficial if you have type 2 diabetes. These techniques may enable you to manage stress more effectively and thereby have better control over your blood-glucose levels and your diabetes in general.

> ### PREVENTION PLAN
>
> **The following may help to prevent the onset of type 2 diabetes:**
>
> - Breast-feed babies to give them the best start in life.
> - Lose weight if you need to.
> - Follow a blood-sugar stabilising diet.
> - Take regular exercise.
> - Avoid environmental toxins.
> - Do relaxation and guided imagery exercises to reduce stress levels.

THYROID PROBLEMS

The thyroid gland is situated in the neck and produces two types of hormone, both of which help to control the body's metabolism, which is the rate at which it burns fuel. The most common thyroid disorders are hyperthyroidism, in which excessive amounts of thyroid hormones are produced, and hypothyroidism, in which the thyroid gland does not produce sufficient hormones. Treatment aims to restore a normal balance of thyroid hormones in the body. Hormonal and other drugs are usually tried first, depending on the individual situation.

WHAT ARE THE SYMPTOMS?

Symptoms of hyperthyroidism include:
- Weight loss, despite increased appetite
- Palpitations
- Trembling of the hands (tremor)
- Lowered tolerance to heat
- Excessive sweating
- Anxiety and insomnia
- Swelling in the neck (goitre)
- Frequent bowel movements
- Muscle weakness
- Irregular menstruation
- Protruding eyes (exophthalmos) in Graves' disease

Symptoms of hypothyroidism include:
- Tiredness
- Poor memory
- Weight gain
- Constipation
- Deepened voice
- Swelling In the neck
- Lowered tolerance to cold
- Puffy eyes and dry, thickened skin
- Generalised thinning of the hair
- Heavy or less frequent menstrual periods
- Weakness and aching of muscles
- Joint pains

WHY MIGHT I HAVE THIS?

PREDISPOSING FACTORS

For hyperthyroidism:
- Genetic predisposition

For hypothyroidism:
- Previous radioiodine treatment or surgery for hyperthyroidism
- Autoimmune problems

IMPORTANT

Rarely, hyperthyroidism gets worse very rapidly. Symptoms may include a high temperature and agitation. If this happens, seek medical help urgently.

WHY DOES IT OCCUR?

Hyperthyroidism (an over-active thyroid gland) may have several causes, the most common of which is Graves' disease, an autoimmune disorder in which antibodies attack the thyroid gland, causing it to produce excess hormones. Graves' disease appears to have a genetic component. Hypothyroidism (an under-active thyroid) may also have a variety of causes, the most common being atrophic thyroiditis, in which antibodies are produced that result in shrinkage of and damage to thyroid tissue. Radioactive iodine or surgery to treat hyperthyroidism (by destroying or removing part of the thyroid gland) can also result in permanent hypothyroidism, for which thyroid hormone supplements must be taken. Insufficient iodine in the diet can also cause hypothyroidism, but this is rare in developed countries. Only a minute quantity of iodine is required each day and it is normally obtained through vegetables, iodised salt and seafood.

Thyroid disorders are common, but their onset is usually gradual and they may not be diagnosed for months or even years. In both hyper- and hypothyroidism, there may be swelling in the neck due to an enlarged thyroid gland (goitre). Both conditions are more common in women.

TREATMENT PLAN

PRIMARY TREATMENTS

For hyperthyroidism:
- Antithyroid drugs
- Radioiodine

For hypothyroidism:
- Thyroid hormone replacement

BACK-UP TREATMENTS

- Surgery to remove part of the thyroid gland (for hyperthyroidism)
- Iodine and other nutritional supplements

WORTH CONSIDERING

- Thyroid glandulars
- Avoiding toxic chemicals
- Acupuncture
- Manual lymphatic drainage (after surgery)

For an explanation of how treatments are rated, see p.111.

TREATMENTS IN DETAIL

Conventional Medicine

Your doctor will arrange blood tests to check the levels of thyroid hormones and the level of thyroid-stimulating hormone (TSH), which is produced by the pituitary gland (a small gland at the base of the brain) and controls the production of thyroid hormones. He or she will also examine the thyroid to see if it is enlarged.

PRIMARY TREATMENT **TREATMENT FOR HYPERTHYROIDISM** If hyperthyroidism is diagnosed, there are three treatment options: drugs, radioiodine and surgery.

The first option is antithyroid drugs, such as carbimazole and propylthiouracil,

THYROID FUNCTION

The body has a complex system for regulating the function of the thyroid gland, which is situated in the neck just below the Adam's apple. The hypothalamus secretes thyrotropin-releasing hormone (TRH), which causes the pituitary gland to release thyroid-stimulating hormone (TSH).

This hormone causes the thyroid gland to produce thyroid hormones (T3 and T4). When levels of thyroid hormones in the blood reach a certain level, the pituitary gland produces less TSH. If the levels of thyroid hormones drop too low, the pituitary gland produces more TSH.

Thyroid hormone feedback mechanism

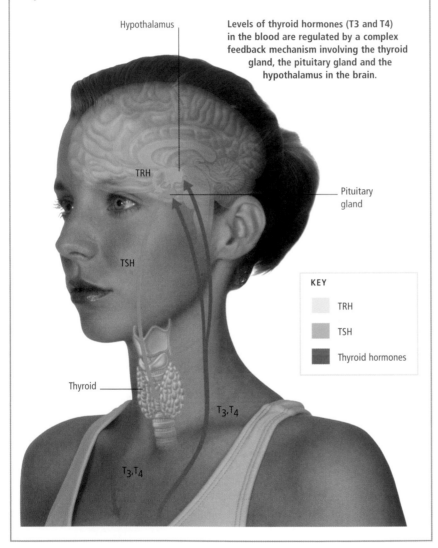

Hypothalamus

Levels of thyroid hormones (T3 and T4) in the blood are regulated by a complex feedback mechanism involving the thyroid gland, the pituitary gland and the hypothalamus in the brain.

TRH

TSH

Pituitary gland

KEY

	TRH
	TSH
	Thyroid hormones

Thyroid

T_3, T_4

T_3, T_4

The third treatment option is surgery to remove part of the thyroid gland. Possible side-effects include damage to the nerve supplying the voice box, resulting in hoarseness, and hypothyroidism.

PRIMARY TREATMENT **TREATMENT FOR HYPOTHYROIDISM** Thyroid hormone replacement is needed for hypothyroidism. The drug is taken in tablet form. Levels of thyroid hormones are monitored by blood tests and supplements may be increased or decreased. It may take up to six months for symptoms to be brought under control and treatment is likely to be life-long.

> **CAUTION**
>
> Drugs for hyperthyroidism and hypothyroidism can cause a range of possible side-effects. Ask your doctor to explain these to you.

Nutritional Therapy

The thyroid is essentially the body's thermostat, determining its temperature and the speed at which it burns fuel. If, for any reason, thyroid function is disrupted, all the cells in the body tend not to function as well as they should. There are many tests to measure how efficiently the thyroid gland is working and whether it is over- or underproducing hormones (*see above and p.43*).

SUPPLEMENTS If mild hypothyroidism is the problem, several herbs and nutrients may help, including iodine, selenium, vitamin A and the amino acid L-tyrosine. Some practitioners recommend supplements containing actual thyroid tissue. These extracts, often referred to as "thyroid glandulars", are usually made from cow or pig thyroid and should only be taken under the supervision of a doctor experienced in their use. (*For more information on nutritional approaches to thyroid problems, see p.43.*)

FOODS TO AVOID Brassica vegetables (such as broccoli, cabbage, Brussels sprouts and cauliflower) contain glucosinolates, which can impair the uptake of iodine and may impair thyroid function. For this reason, vegetables from the brassica family are best avoided by anyone with thyroid problems.

which prevent the production of the thyroid hormones. With these drugs, symptoms may take up to three weeks to improve, and a course of beta-blockers may be prescribed to help control them. Antithyroid drugs may need to be taken for up two years, or longer in some cases. Hyperthyroidism recurs in about half of people treated.

There is a second option which is treatment with radioiodine to destroy some of the thyroid tissue. This involves taking a capsule containing radioactive iodine, which accumulates in the thyroid. Thyroid hormone levels usually take up to three months to return to normal following treatment. There is a risk of developing hypothyroidism after this treatment.

Homeopathy

Homeopathy may be useful alongside conventional drugs in alleviating the symptoms of an over-active thyroid. The most useful medicines are *Iodum*, *Lachesis*, *Lycopus* and *Natrum muriaticum*.

> The Dublin physician Dr Robert Graves first described hyperthyroidism with goitre in 1835

IODUM This medicine is useful if exophthalmos (protruding eyes) is present. The patient may be very thin, although the appetite is good. He or she may feel hot most of the time and want to be in the open air. These patients feel worse for being in a warm room and better for eating and after strenuous exercise.

OTHER MEDICINES These should be used only under the supervision of an experienced homeopath and in collaboration with your doctor. Under- or over-active thyroid, unless very mild, always require conventional investigation and treatment.

Environmental Health

Thyroid function can be altered by many substances in the environment, including herbicides, pesticides, fungicides, organohalogen compounds (such as polyhalogenated aromatic hydrocarbons (PHAHs), polychlorinated biphenyls (PCBs), and chemicals in cigarette smoke. These agents can all disrupt the delicate working of the body's hormones, including those involved in thyroid function.

HERBICIDES AND PESTICIDES You should limit the use of these products around your work and home environments, especially when there are small children present. Any substances that affect thyroid function can be particularly disruptive for children, given the importance of thyroid hormones in foetal and childhood development. Try to choose organic foods as much as possible. These foods, when certified by a reputable regulatory body, are free of herbicides, pesticides, fungicides, fertilisers and other contaminants.

PCBS AND PHAHS Polychlorinated biphenyl compounds (PCBs) and polyhalogenated aromatic hydrocarbons (PHAHs) are human-made compounds that are used in plastics, transformers and in other industries. They can disrupt the body's hormonal system.

The two PHAHs which are most commonly implicated in thyroid problems are polychlorinated biphenyl compounds (PCBs) and dioxins. They share a similar structure with natural thyroid hormones and may interfere with thyroid function by imitating the natural hormones, rendering actual thyroid hormones inactive.

PCBs and PHAHs are common environmental contaminants, despite recent efforts to remove them. The production of PCBs was banned in the US in 1977, but people can still be exposed to them through contact with old transformers, capacitors, fluorescent lighting fixtures and old electrical devices and appliances. The most common source of exposure for people is from contaminated food, such as predatory fish that have been caught in contaminated waterways.

Dioxins are found everywhere in the environment, and most people are exposed to very small background levels of dioxins from the air, food or milk, or have skin contact with dioxin-contaminated materials. For the general population, more than 90 per cent of the daily intake of dioxins comes from food, mainly meat and dairy products and fish.

PHAHs require a long time to degrade in the environment and become concentrated in higher levels of the food chain (bioaccumulation), especially in the fatty tissues of animals. Bioaccumulation occurs when PHAHs enter the soil or water and contaminate plants which are then eaten by animals, which in turn are eaten, until even the largest predators are affected.

To reduce exposure to PHAHs, you should choose low-fat meat products and trim excess fat off meat. Also, limit or avoid eating predatory fish or fish from sources known to be contaminated with PHAHs. An environmental health expert can provide individual advice.

Acupuncture

Thyroid disease, whether due to an under- or over-active thyroid, always needs conventional diagnosis and treatment. Acupuncture may occasionally be used for the treatment of some of the symptoms but it is not a treatment for thyroid disease itself. It may be able to help with generalised aches and pains, lack of energy in people receiving appropriate thyroid treatment and sometimes the relief of symptoms that may be caused by thyroid eye disease.

Depending on how severe and acute the thyroid problem is, it will probably take between four and six weekly treatment sessions, based on a traditional Chinese approach, for treatment to work. If no benefit is apparent after this time, discuss this with your acupuncturist.

Bodywork Therapies

Evidence suggests spa therapies and massage may help in the treatment of thyroid conditions. Russian research, for example, suggests that spa treatment (involving mud and electrotherapy) for children with cardiac conditions produced general health benefits including "a positive trend in… thyroid conditions".

MANUAL LYMPHATIC DRAINAGE Surgery for thyroid conditions can sometimes result in local swelling and fluid retention (oedema). A study evaluated the benefits of massage to encourage normal circulation and drainage in such situations. A gentle massage technique known as manual lymphatic drainage was found to eliminate swelling and oedema completely in approximately half of cases after ten days of daily massage. The researchers conclude: "We consider it mandatory that massotherapy of the neck be instituted in all those patients who have undergone surgery to the thyroid."

> **CAUTION**
> Do not have neck massage or manipulation if you have an enlarged thyroid (goitre).

Women's Health

Many women's health issues are linked to monthly changes in hormones. They often respond well to drugs, and dietary changes or supplements. Talking therapies can be useful in managing emotional fluctuations and their effects, while the gentle influence of herbs and other complementary therapies also helps to keep hormones in balance.

WHAT ARE THE SYMPTOMS?

- Tenderness and/or lumpiness of the breasts
- A feeling of being bloated, caused by fluid retention
- Mood changes, including irritability, depression and anxiety
- Feeling tired
- Difficulty concentrating and making decisions
- Headaches, including migraines
- Backache and muscle stiffness
- Disrupted sleep
- Unusual food cravings

WHY MIGHT I HAVE THIS?

PREDISPOSING FACTORS

- High-sugar diet
- Caffeine
- Genetic tendency

PREMENSTRUAL SYNDROME

The term premenstrual syndrome (PMS) is used to describe a varying combination of symptoms that begin about two weeks or so before menstruation and stop by the end of the period. The condition affects as many as one woman in three, and in one woman in 20 PMS is severe enough to disrupt her life. Treatment for PMS usually depends on the symptoms and their severity, but it might involve hormonal and other drugs and dietary changes. Manipulation therapy, exercise, acupuncture and relaxation can also be beneficial.

WHY DOES IT OCCUR?

The cause of PMS is not known, but it is thought that the symptoms are triggered by the action of the female sex hormones, particularly progesterone, in the weeks or days before menstruation begins.

Sugar, caffeine and stress may make PMS worse, and women are more likely to experience the condition if close female relatives also have had similar problems, suggesting that genetic factors may also be involved.

SELF-HELP

In the weeks before menstruation:
- Reduce or eliminate your intake of tea, coffee, cola and other caffeinated drinks.

- Avoid sugary foods and snacks, such as chocolate, and try to keep your blood-sugar levels stable (*see p.42*).
- Take regular, moderate exercise.
- Practise relaxation exercises, yoga or meditation each day.

TREATMENTS IN DETAIL

Conventional Medicine

There are many possible treatments for premenstrual syndrome, ranging from dietary supplements and exercise to hormonal drugs. Vitamin B6 supplements may help to relieve the symptoms, as may regular aerobic exercise. Relaxation techniques may be helpful and may also be recommended (*see p.327*).

TREATMENT PLAN

PRIMARY TREATMENTS
- Combined oral contraceptive pill
- Non-steroidal anti-inflammatory drugs for headaches and backache
- Chaste berry

BACK-UP TREATMENTS
- Other hormonal medicines
- Diuretics for fluid retention
- Magnesium
- Elimination of caffeine and sugar
- Antidepressants

WORTH CONSIDERING
- Vitamin B6 and other supplements
- Evening primrose oil and other Western herbs
- Indivdualised homeopathy
- Bodywork therapies
- Exercise
- Acupuncture
- Mind–body therapies

For an explanation of how treatments are rated, see p.111.

PRIMARY TREATMENT

FIRST-LINE TREATMENTS Non-steroidal anti-inflammatory drugs (NSAIDs), such as ibuprofen, may help to relieve headaches and backache. The combined oral contraceptive pill can be helpful in relieving PMS symptoms.

PRIMARY TREATMENT

TREATMENTS FOR SEVERE SYMPTOMS If symptoms are persistent and troublesome, certain other drugs may be suggested.

The antidepressants known as SSRIs (selective serotonin reuptake inhibitors), such as fluoxetine, have been shown to relieve premenstrual symptoms.

The drug danazol prevents ovulation and reduces PMS symptoms. However, side-effects associated with long-term use, such as hirsutism (increased body hair), acne and deepening of the voice, mean it is only given for relatively short periods.

Certain drugs known as gonadotrophin-releasing hormone (GnRH) analogues inhibit the release of the sex hormones oestrogen and progesterone and reduce PMS symptoms. However, they cannot be used for more than six months as they may cause osteoporosis.

DRUGS FOR SPECIFIC SYMPTOMS Studies have shown that the diuretic spironolactone improves symptoms of PMS associated with fluid retention, such as breast tenderness and bloating. Bromo-criptine is a drug that acts on the pituitary gland (the tiny gland at the base of the brain); it also relieves breast tenderness.

CAUTION

Drugs for PMS can cause a range of possible side-effects: ask your doctor to explain these to you.

Nutritional Therapy

CAFFEINE AND SUGAR If you are prone to PMS, it is wise to avoid caffeine and sugar as in clinical practice these both seem to increase the risk of PMS. A number of scientific studies note that women who eat more sugary foods appear to have an increased risk of PMS. Studies also show that consumption of caffeine-containing beverages is associated with increases in the prevalence and severity of PMS.

MULTIVITAMIN SUPPLEMENTS A daily multivitamin and mineral supplement may be one of the simplest ways to help reduce symptoms. There is evidence that this can bring positive benefits for women with PMS.

VITAMIN B6 There is good evidence from a number of studies to support taking vitamin B6 for PMS. It can help control a variety of premenstrual symptoms, including depression, irritability, tension, poor coordination, violence, breast tenderness, bloating, headache and acne. The effective dose for most women seems to be 100mg vitamin B6 per day. If you experience PMS symptoms on a regular basis, try taking it at this dosage.

MAGNESIUM Studies show that women with PMS are often deficient in the mineral magnesium and that supplementation may reduce symptoms. In a double-blind trial, a daily supplement of 200mg magnesium per day over a two-month period produced significant improvement in women with PMS, resulting in reduced fluid retention, breast tenderness and abdominal bloating. Magnesium may also relieve menstrual migraine. A reasonable dose to try would be 200–400mg per day for two to three months.

CALCIUM Taking calcium supplements appears to relieve the symptoms of PMS. Women who include a lot of calcium in their diets experience less PMS, and, when they do have it, the symptoms are less severe. In a large, double-blind trial over three menstrual cycles, women who took 1,200mg of calcium per day had a 48 per cent reduction in PMS symptoms, compared to a 30 per cent reduction in the placebo (sham treatment) group. Other double-blind trials have also shown that taking 1,000mg of calcium per day relieves PMS symptoms.

ZINC It is possible that some women who experience PMS have lower levels of zinc in their bodies, particularly during certain times in their ovulatory cycle. Taking 50mg of zinc per day may be useful for women with PMS. If you take zinc supplements, you should take 1mg of copper for every 15mg of supplemental zinc because zinc supplements can induce copper deficiency.

CAUTION

Consult your doctor before taking zinc, magnesium or calcium supplements. These can reduce the effectiveness of certain drugs, including some antibiotics, beta-blockers and blood-thinning drugs, such as warfarin. (*For more information, see p.46.*)

Homeopathy

A clinical trial showed that individualised homeopathy is effective in PMS. Five homeopathic medicines were used: *Lachesis*, *Natrum muriaticum*, *Nux vomica*, *Pulsatilla* and *Sepia*.

LACHESIS is a useful remedy for women whose PMS symptoms improve soon after bleeding begins. These women cannot tolerate tight clothes and collars and may have a sensation of constriction at the throat. They may have hot flushes and find

Women who have had more children tend to get more severe PMS symptoms

it difficult to breathe lying down. They tend to sleep on their right side and most of their menstrual pain is on the left side of the body. There may be dark clots in the menstrual blood. These women tend to have a jealous or suspicious disposition, and this may become much worse during the premenstrual period.

NATRUM MURIATICUM is prescribed when women with PMS have a taste for salty things. They often have headaches, which tend to start in the morning and are caused or made worse by the sun. These women tend also to be sad and averse to consolation; they are reserved, closed and prefer to be alone.

NUX VOMICA may be useful for women who have constipation, in which there is urge but no result, as part of their PMS symptoms. These women are generally tense and irritable and are very sensitive to cold, noise and smells.

PULSATILLA is useful for women whose periods stop at night and in whom the menstrual flow is generally intermittent. These women tend to feel worse in closed rooms. They weep easily, but their moods change rapidly. They dislike being alone.

SEPIA may be used when women have much vaginal discharge that is greenish in colour. Their sexual drive is low and they may feel pressure or heaviness in the lower abdomen. In these women menstruation usually starts in the morning. They feel detached especially towards their families.

> **CAUTION**
>
> Avoid coffee if taking *Nux vomica*.

Western Herbal Medicine

A herbalist selects a range of plant medicines to relieve PMS symptoms. For example, cramp bark (*Viburnum opulus*) and wild yam (*Dioscorea villosa*) can provide relief from period cramps and, in the longer term, help to restore menstrual regularity and hormonal balance.

example, chaste berry (*Vitex agnus-castus*) inhibits secretion of several hormones including prolactin. Chaste berry is the most frequently used herb for PMS, helping to regulate the menstrual cycle and improve hormone balance. Clinical studies involving over 5000 women have found it has positive benefits in PMS (and to a lesser extent in breast pain).

There are also other herbs with a hormonal action that may be prescribed. For example, helonias (*Chamaelirium lutea*) helps to improve ovarian function.

RELAXING HERBS As well as advising women to take exercise and get plenty of rest, a herbalist, where appropriate, will prescribe relaxant and adaptogenic herbs (which help the body to adapt to stress), such as withania (*Withania somnifera*). If there is emotional disturbance, such as nervous irritability, sedative, relaxant or stimulant herbs such as St John's wort (*Hypericum perforatum*) will be given. Other herbs used to treat emotional disturbance, especially irritability, include skullcap (*Scutellaria laterifolia*), vervain (*Verbena officinalis*) and lime flowers (*Tilia cordata*).

EVENING PRIMROSE OIL Results are contradictory when it comes to the value of taking evening primrose (*Oenothera biennis*) oil. However, the oil is a rich source of gamma-linolenic acid (GLA), and there is some evidence that women with PMS have trouble metabolising linoleic acid, which is

Acupuncture

There are several small and limited studies of a traditional Chinese medicine-based approach to treating premenstrual syndrome, and all the evidence suggests that acupuncture is an effective treatment for the symptoms of PMS.

Clinical experience suggests that acupuncture has a long-term effect on PMS; it prevents symptoms from recurring in menstrual cycles after treatment has been completed. Ideally, women should have several treatment sessions over two to three months.

Bodywork Therapies

A review of pooled research evidence to support the use of manual therapies such as massage, reflexology and chiropractic in the treatment of PMS concluded: "Despite some positive findings, the evidence was not compelling for any of these therapies, with most trials suffering from various methodological limitations. On the basis of current evidence, no complementary/alternative therapy can be recommended as a treatment for premenstrual syndrome."

However, among the "positive findings" discounted in this overview are some studies that seem to strongly suggest that there are indeed benefits to be gained in using methods such as massage, reflexology, chiropractic, aerobic exercise and acupressure in treating PMS.

MASSAGE AND RELAXATION In one study, 24 women with a history of severe PMS were divided into two groups, one to receive massage (twice weekly for 30 minutes for five weeks) with the other group given instruction in the use of progressive muscle relaxation methods, to be followed for 30 minutes, twice weekly for five weeks. The results showed that those women in the massage group had significantly reduced anxiety levels and improved mood, along with reduction in pain and fluid retention levels, when compared with the women in the relaxation group.

REFLEXOLOGY may also be beneficial for women who regularly experience PMS. In a study of 32 women with PMS, half had treatment to specific reflexology points on the feet, hands and ears and the other half

Premenstrual syndrome was first recognised as a medical disorder by Dr T. Frank in 1931

DETOXIFICATION Herbs such as dandelion root (*Taraxacum officinale*) may be given to stimulate liver and colon function. They promote detoxification and elimination, clearing oestrogens from the body. Improved liver metabolism also leads to a reduced load on the kidneys.

PRIMARY TREATMENT **CHASTE BERRY** A herbalist will suggest hormone-balancing herbs, which act on the pituitary gland. These help to correct imbalances in hormone release by the pituitary gland. For

converted in the body to GLA. Therefore, extra GLA should be helpful in PMS. If you want to try using evening primrose oil to ease PMS symptoms, take 3–4g per day for several menstrual cycles. It may be particularly helpful if you have breast tenderness or fibrocystic disease.

> **CAUTION**
>
> See p.69 before taking a herbal remedy and, if you are already taking prescribed medication, consult a medical herbalist first.

REFLEXOLOGY FOR PREMENSTRUAL SYNDROME

Reflexology, in which points on the feet (and sometimes on the hands and ears) are pressed to influence health in corresponding parts of the body, may be effective in relieving both the physical and psychological symptoms of PMS. You can visit a reflexologist, or you can perform reflexology for yourself. The most relevant point on the feet for relieving PMS and menstrual pain is shown in the picture below. For PMS, you should work the

uterus reflex area every day throughout the month. For menstrual pain, work the uterus reflex area three or four times a day until the pain subsides. Do one foot at a time, giving each foot equal treatment.

Using your thumb, press firmly on the uterus reflex area just above the inside of the heel (shown below). You can also press on this area while rotating the ankle, first clockwise, then anti-clockwise.

Rotation of foot

Firm pressure from thumb

Uterus reflex area

---

had "placebo" reflexology (i.e. gentle massage to these general areas). Symptom records were kept daily for the week prior to the next period. The results are described in the study as follows: "At the end of the study the reflexology group reported a 45 per cent decrease in both somatic (bodily) and psychological symptoms, compared with a 20 per cent reduction in the placebo group."

Exercise

The effects of aerobic exercise and strength training on premenstrual symptoms were evaluated in 23 women. Results showed that while participation in both forms of exercise was associated with an improvement of many premenstrual symptoms, the symptoms of those women in the aerobic group (especially their premenstrual depression) improved more markedly.

If you experience PMS on a regular basis, you could try doing some mild aerobic exercise, such as fast walking, for at least 20 minutes, three times a week. Try to exercise is the open air if possible.

Regular exercise of the abdomen and pelvis, such as occurs in Egyptian belly dancing, is also worthwhile. It may be particularly helpful in relieving PMS and menstrual cramps.

Yoga

Practising yoga may help to reduce stress in the weeks leading up to menstruation. Some practitioners also believe that practising yoga on a regular basis can help to regulate hormone levels in the body. In this way, doing yoga may help to reduce the severity of PMS symptoms.

Yoga for easing PMS symptoms should be gentle, incorporating plenty of floor poses. Poses that work the low back, such as the bridge and the cobra, may influence the kidneys and adrenal glands and relieve fatigue. These poses have the added advantage of easing any muscle tension and stiffness in the low back.

Yoga that incorporates side stretches helps to tone the muscles as well as improve flexibility. Poses that open the chest, such as the fish, can also help to

reduce stress levels and, done regularly, may promote calmness and clarity.

If you have not done yoga or stretching exercises before or have not done them for some time and would like to try yoga, be sure to start gradually. Make sure you listen to your body and do not try to do too much too soon.

Mind–Body Therapies

RELAXATION AND GUIDED IMAGERY If you experience PMS regularly, you could try doing 20 to 30 minutes of relaxation exercises or meditation daily throughout the month. (*For a sequence of relaxation exercises, see p.99.*) You could also try using a relaxation or guided imagery tape, or a tape of soothing music or sounds.

Regular relaxation has proven effective in dealing with both the physical and emotional symptoms of PMS, according to a number of studies. One study looking at biofeedback, for example, found "a significant positive correlation" between frontalis muscle tension (which is felt in the forehead) and the psychological symptoms of PMS. If the tension can be relieved, the psychological symptoms may also be eased. In another study, women who took part in a regular relaxation programme reported a quite significant improvement of 58 per cent in their premenstrual symptoms.

Using relaxation and guided imagery to reduce the severity of PMS can lead to less stress, increased comfort and lower absenteeism, without the cost and potential side-effects of some medications.

PREVENTION PLAN

The following may help if you are prone to PMS:

- Avoid caffeine and sugar, at least in the weeks leading up to menstruation.

- Take a multivitamin daily.

- Eat nutritious snacks regularly to help keep your blood-sugar level stable.

- Take regular aerobic exercise.

- Practise relaxation exercises on a regular basis throughout the month.

MENSTRUAL PAIN

Menstrual pain, or dysmenorrhoea, affects about 75 per cent of women at some time. Doctors identify two types: primary dysmenorrhoea, for which no cause can be found; and secondary dysmenorrhoea, which has an identifiable cause. About 15 per cent of women have menstrual pain severe enough to disrupt normal life. Treatment depends to some extent on severity of symptoms and might include painkillers and other drugs. Dietary changes, homeopathy, manipulation therapy, relaxation, yoga and acupuncture may all bring relief.

WHAT ARE THE SYMPTOMS?

- Cramping lower abdominal pain that comes in waves and may radiate to the lower back and down the legs
- Dragging sensation in the pelvis

The pain may be accompanied by other symptoms, such as bloating and headache.

WHY MIGHT I HAVE THIS?

PREDISPOSING FACTORS

- Stress
- Genetic tendency
- Endometriosis or fibroids
- Pelvic inflammatory disease

IMPORTANT

Consult a doctor if you begin to experience period pain that is substantially worse than usual.

WHY DOES IT OCCUR?

Primary dysmenorrhoea (where periods have always been painful) is thought to result from excessive production of prostaglandins, hormone-like substances that make the uterine wall contract before and during menstruation. It is not known why it occurs but women with close female relatives who have had primary dysmenorrhoea are more likely to experience it, suggesting genetic factors may be involved.

TREATMENT PLAN

PRIMARY TREATMENTS

- Painkillers and NSAIDs
- Drugs that suppress ovulation
- Treatment of underlying cause (secondary dysmenorrhoea)
- Magnesium and calcium supplements

BACK-UP TREATMENTS

- Niacin, vitamin E and fish oil supplements
- Osteopathy and chiropractic
- Trigger point deactivation

WORTH CONSIDERING

- Acupuncture
- Massage and yoga
- Homeopathy
- Relaxation and guided imagery

For an explanation of how treatments are rated, see p.111.

Primary dysmenorrhoea often begins soon after the onset of menstruation. Unlike primary dysmenorrhoea, secondary dysmenorrhoea usually starts later in a woman's reproductive life and has identifiable causes. These include endometriosis (*see p.334*), in which fragments of the tissue that normally lines the uterus are found elsewhere in the pelvis. Secondary dysmenorrhoea may also be caused by fibroids, benign tumours that grow in the wall of the uterus, and pelvic inflammatory disease, in which the female reproductive organs become inflamed as a result of bacterial infection.

IMMEDIATE RELIEF

- Take an over-the-counter painkiller such as paracetamol.
- Relax with a hot-water bottle or take a warm bath.
- Take the homeopathic remedies *Magnesia phosphoricum*, *Chamomilla* or *Nux vomica*.

TREATMENTS IN DETAIL

Conventional Medicine

Your doctor may arrange investigations, such as ultrasound scanning of the pelvis, to look for an underlying cause.

PRIMARY TREATMENT **PRIMARY DYSMENORRHOEA** may be relieved by simple painkillers, such as paracetamol or codeine, or by certain non-steroidal anti-inflammatory drugs (NSAIDs), including ibuprofen. Suppressing ovulation, often by using the combined oral contraceptive pill, may be recommended if pain persists.

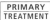

PRIMARY TREATMENT **REMEDIES FOR SECONDARY DYSMENORRHOEA** This is relieved by treating the underlying cause wherever possible. For endometriosis, treatment may involve drugs, such as the oral contraceptive pill, or surgery (*see p.334*), often involving diathermy (heat treatment). If the cause is fibroids (*see p.332*), these benign tumours of the uterine wall may have to be reduced surgically.

> **CAUTION**
>
> Drugs used to treat primary and secondary dysmenorrhoea can cause a range of possible side-effects: ask your doctor to explain these to you.

Nutritional Therapy

PRIMARY TREATMENT **CALCIUM AND MAGNESIUM** Although there are no clinical trials to support it, clinical experience suggests that 1,000mg of calcium and 500mg of magnesium should be taken each day to help alleviate menstrual pain. During the period itself, you could try taking about 250mg of calcium and 100mg of magnesium every four hours, which often helps to relieve symptoms.

NIACIN Fifty years ago a research study showed that niacin (a form of vitamin B3) appears to have the ability to relieve menstrual cramps. In the study, 40 women were given 200mg of niacin per day, and up to 100mg every two or three hours on the days when they experienced cramping. Eighty-seven per cent of the women studied reported relief on this regime in the uncontrolled trial. Unfortunately, no further research appears to have been done since. However it may be worth taking this vitamin in the above dosages.

VITAMIN E also seems to be effective in relieving menstrual pain. In one study, taking 150mg of vitamin E daily improved the condition of 68 per cent of patients. In another study, 500IU (350mg) of vitamin E per day, given two days before the beginning of menstruation and for the first three days of bleeding, was effective in relieving pain. If you have menstrual pain regularly, try adding these supplements to your diet at these doses.

FISH OILS There is growing evidence to suggest a role for fish oil supplementation (omega-3 fatty acids) in relieving menstrual pain. One research study found that supplementation with fish oil providing 1,080mg EPA and 720mg DHA for two months caused a significant reduction in menstrual pain. In addition to including oily fish (such as salmon, trout, mackerel, herring and sardines) in the diet, taking supplements of concentrated fish oils (2–3g per day) may help to control period-related pain.

> **CAUTION**
>
> Consult your doctor before taking vitamins B3 and E, magnesium and calcium, or fish oil supplements. These supplements can affect the action of certain drugs. (*See also p.46.*)

Homeopathy

As is often the case with homeopathy, menstrual pain can be tackled on different levels: there are several medicines that you could try for yourself, based on your symptoms. If they do not help or only partly relieve the problem, it may be worth trying "constitutional" homeopathic treatment (*see p.73*), for which you need to consult a trained homeopath. *Chamomilla*, *Magnesia phosphoricum* and *Nux vomica*

are some of the most common homeopathic medicines that are suggested for menstrual pain.

CHAMOMILLA AND NUX VOMICA have some similarities: women who respond to these medicines tend to be irritable with the pain of menstruation. Women who respond to *Chamomilla* tend to get relief from vigorous activity (such as brisk walking), while women who respond to *Nux vomica* can be bad-tempered and impatient, particularly over minor frustrations or inefficiency. Symptoms tend to be worst first thing in the morning.

MAGNESIA PHOSPHORICA Women who respond to this medicine have quite a different character. Their pains are severe and cramping, but they feel exhausted and washed out rather than bad-tempered. They may find relief from heat over the lower abdomen (from a hot-water bottle or a heat pad).

OTHER MEDICINES For more complicated problems and especially for secondary dysmenorrhoea, other homeopathic remedies may help. These include *Viburnum opulus*. Women who respond to this medicine have light periods and, perhaps strangely, the pains seem worst when the bleeding is at its lightest. By contrast, women who respond to *Cactus grandiflorus* have pain associated with passing clots of blood.

In women who respond to *Kalium carbonicum*, the pains are felt particularly in the low back and women usually feel weak and run-down and also tend to perspire quite easily. They often have a tendency to chest trouble and may be prone to getting bronchitis that is typically slow to clear up. An unusual but typical feature of people who respond to this medicine is that they are worse at around 3–4 a.m., when they may be woken up from sleep by period pains or fits of coughing.

Of the major "constitutional" medicines, the most commonly indicated is *Pulsatilla*. In women who respond to it, periods are

Prostaglandins, which make the uterus contract, may be responsible for menstrual pain

irregular and unpredictable, as are the pains. These women are typically gentle, soft-spoken and indecisive. They may weep easily, but respond to human warmth and quickly cheer up.

Acupuncture

The evidence from clinical trials is limited, but acupuncture and acupressure have frequently been used to treat menstrual pain. There are many reports of cases in which they have helped in both the short and long term, with possibly some preventative effect in subsequent cycles after the end of treatment. A traditional Chinese diagnosis is usually required before embarking on treatment, and several treatments are likely to be needed, over two to three months. Commonly, a diagnosis of blockage and blood stagnation is made and the spleen channel (which runs down the inside of the leg) may be needled.

Bodywork Therapies

OSTEOPATHY AND CHIROPRACTIC Clinical experience suggests that the painful symptoms of primary dysmenorrhoea are often significantly reduced following either osteopathic or chiropractic manipulation to those regions of the spine from which the nerve supply to the pelvic region emerges.

Spinal manipulation has recently been shown, in a full-scale clinical trial, to reduce pain as well as the levels of prostaglandins, the hormone-like substances that induce the uterine contractions. In osteopathic research, tests following manipulation showed a marked reduction in prostaglandins. This finding coincided with reports from the 12 patients being studied that menstrual cramping was much reduced, as well as low back discomfort. In one chiropractic study, close to 90 per cent of women with menstrual pain reported that their symptoms were significantly relieved following treatment of the low back.

MASSAGE Massage therapy during and before the menstrual period that specifically relaxes the spinal and abdominal muscles (as well as providing general relaxation) has produced marked relief for women suffering from the symptoms of premenstrual syndrome, as well as from the pain of menstruation itself.

TRIGGER POINT DEACTIVATION Research into the effects of trigger points (sensitive areas in muscles) on chronic pain report that trigger points in the abdominal muscles (lower rectus abdominis) can initiate period pain. Earlier research suggested that menstrual pain may involve irritation and tension in the lower abdominal muscles. Trigger points may be released by appropriate manual therapy such as physiotherapy (*see p.55*).

YOGA FOR MENSTRUAL PAIN

Gentle bending and stretching exercises can often help to ease menstrual pain. Some yoga positions, such as the Cat pose (shown below), are especially beneficial because they gently stretch the abdominal area and the low back. These areas are often the sites of pain and cramping during menstruation. Exercise increases blood flow to these areas and helps to loosen muscles that may have become tense due to pain. (Avoid this exercise if you have severe back problems.)

The Cat exercise

Arched back

Straight legs

Hands shoulder width apart

Kneel on the floor and place your hands below your shoulders. Tucking your pelvis down, arch your back. Pull your stomach in. Slowly release. Repeat 10 times.

Yoga

Certain yoga positions that stretch the muscles of the abdomen and lower back can help to ease menstrual aches and cramping (*see above*). Try to practise some gentle yoga positions daily throughout your menstrual period.

Mind-Body Therapies

RELAXATION AND GUIDED IMAGERY If you experience menstrual pain on a regular basis, try doing a series of relaxation exercises for 20 minutes to half an hour each day (*see p.99*). Alternatively, try meditation or listen to a guided imagery tape for the same amount of time.

Studies support the use of psychological therapies, such as relaxation and guided imagery, for menstrual pain. One study demonstrated that relaxation training, either alone or combined with imagery, was effective in reducing the amount of time women with spasmodic dysmenorrhea needed to rest.

Relaxation not only helps menstrual pain and discomfort but is also effective in reducing absenteeism due to them. These effects have been shown to last as long as 18 months. While psychological strategies can relieve menstrual distress, they can also affect the length of the menstrual cycle: women in a guided imagery study were able to lengthen their cycles.

PREVENTION PLAN

The following may help:

- Eat a balanced diet that is high in calcium, magnesium and B vitamins.
- Do relaxation exercises every day.
- Take some daily exercise.

HEAVY PERIODS

The amount of menstrual flow varies from woman to woman and may also vary from period to period. Unusually heavy bleeding on a regular basis, known as menorrhagia, may lead to iron-deficiency anaemia, which in turn may cause faintness and fatigue. About one woman in 20 has heavy periods. The condition is more common in overweight women and in those approaching menopause. Treatment aims to reduce blood loss and might involve drugs or surgery. Homeopathy, supplements and acupuncture may also help to relieve symptoms.

WHAT ARE THE SYMPTOMS?

- Unusually heavy and often prolonged bleeding during menstruation

WHY MIGHT I HAVE THIS?

PREDISPOSING FACTORS

- Fibroids
- Uterine polyps
- Endometriosis (see p.334)
- Underactive thyroid (see p.319)
- IUD use
- Being overweight
- Approaching the menopause

TREATMENT PLAN

PRIMARY TREATMENTS

- Treatment for any underlying cause
- Hormonal and non-hormonal drugs

BACK-UP TREATMENTS

- Surgery

WORTH CONSIDERING

- Iron therapy; vitamins A and D; flavonoids
- Homeopathy
- Herbal treatment
- Acupuncture
- Exercise

For an explanation of how treatments are rated, see p.111.

WHY DOES IT OCCUR?

In some cases, there is no apparent cause for heavy periods and if a woman's periods have always been heavy, there may be no cause for concern. However, it is always best to consult a doctor in order to rule out any underlying disorder.

Heavy menstrual bleeding may be a symptom of certain disorders of the uterus, including fibroids (benign swellings that can arise from the muscle of the uterine wall – see p.332) or uterine polyps (non-cancerous swellings in the uterus). Both these conditions increase the surface area of the endometrium (the lining of the uterus) and so can cause increased blood loss during menstruation. Cancer of the endometrium can also cause heavy periods. Endometriosis (see p.334) and persistent pelvic infections are other possible causes. A single late, heavy period may be an early miscarriage. Heavy periods may also occur as a side-effect of using the intrauterine contraceptive device (the coil or IUD). They may also be due to a more general medical disorder, such as hypothyroidism (see Thyroid Problems, p.319). Finally, heavy periods sometimes occur in women who are approaching the menopause (see p.339) because the uterine lining becomes thicker than normal.

IMPORTANT

If you begin to experience periods that are heavier or more prolonged than is usual for you, see your doctor without delay. In some cases heavy periods may have a serious underlying cause.

TREATMENTS IN DETAIL

Conventional Medicine

PRIMARY TREATMENT **TREATING THE CAUSE** The doctor will make a diagnosis from a description of the symptoms. Investigations may include blood tests to look for anaemia and sometimes for an underactive thyroid (hypothyroidism). Other tests to look for an underlying cause may include an endometrial biopsy (taking a sample of the lining of the uterus for analysis). This is particularly likely to be necessary in women over the age of 40. It may be performed during a hysteroscopy, in which a thin, flexible viewing instrument is passed into the uterus through the vagina. Pelvic ultrasound scanning may be arranged. This procedure can detect certain conditions such as fibroids. A laparoscopy, in which a small viewing instrument is inserted into the abdomen, may be arranged to look for evidence of endometriosis or of a pelvic infection.

The underlying cause will be treated where possible; for example, fibroids may be removed surgically (myomectomy). However, often no cause for heavy bleeding can be found, in which case it may be treated with non-hormonal or hormonal drugs and, in some cases, with surgery.

PRIMARY TREATMENT **NON-HORMONAL DRUGS** Non-hormonal treatments include the drug tranexamic acid, which is taken during periods. It prevents the breakdown of blood clots and has been shown to reduce the blood loss of heavy periods. Studies have also shown that non-steroidal anti-inflammatory drugs (NSAIDs), such as mefenamic acid, can reduce blood loss.

DEVELOPMENT OF FIBROIDS

Fibroids, which are a very common cause of heavy periods, affect about one woman in five over the age of 35. They are non-cancerous tumours that grow in the uterus and can be as small as a pea or as large as a grapefruit. The most common variety are intramural fibroids which grow within the muscular wall of the uterus. Subserosal fibroids grow just under the surface of the outer uterine wall and submucosal fibroids grow under the endometrium. A pedunculated fibroid can protrude into the cervix.

Types of fibroid

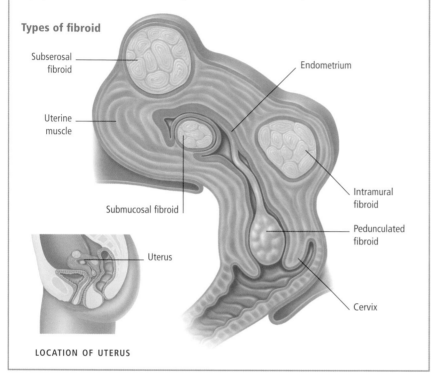

Subserosal fibroid

Uterine muscle

Submucosal fibroid

Endometrium

Intramural fibroid

Pedunculated fibroid

Uterus

Cervix

LOCATION OF UTERUS

PRIMARY TREATMENT **HORMONAL DRUGS** Hormonal treatments include the combined oral contraceptive pill, which suppresses ovulation and therefore can reduce bleeding. Progestogen tablets, such as norethisterone, are sometimes prescribed. An intrauterine device containing progesterone is also available, which often makes periods become light or even absent, although initially there may be spotting or prolonged periods. The drug danazol may reduce bleeding and in higher doses it stops bleeding altogether. It is only used in very severe cases and then only for short periods due to the side effects of long-term use; these include hirsutism, acne and deepening of the voice. You must use contraception while taking danazol because it can adversely affect the developing foetus.

SURGERY Surgical options for treating heavy periods include endometrial ablation, in which laser or diathermy (heat treatment) may be used to destroy most of the tissue lining the uterus. This may result in lighter or even absent periods. Possible complications of this procedure include perforation of the uterus. In some severe cases of heavy periods, hysterectomy (removal of the uterus) may be performed where a woman does not wish to conceive.

CAUTION

Drugs and surgery for heavy periods can cause a range of possible side-effects. Ask your doctor to explain these to you.

Nutritional Medicine

Clinical experience suggests that low thyroid function (hypothyroidism) is quite a common cause of heavy periods. (*For details about the diagnosis and treatment of low thyroid function, see p.319.*)

VITAMIN A One nutrient that seems to be very effective in treating heavy periods is vitamin A. A study showed that 25,000 IU of vitamin A taken twice a day for 15 days brought about a significant reduction of menstrual flow in more than 90 per cent of women. You can also try eating foods rich in vitamin A; these include oily fish, butter, apricots and carrots.

IRON Another useful nutrient in treating heavy periods is the mineral iron. It is well known that iron deficiency is a common consequence of heavy periods. However, it is less well known that iron can sometimes treat the problem. It appears to help blood vessels contract, which is important if the body is to bring an end to the bleeding from the uterus. The best way to have the levels of iron in the body checked is with a blood test to determine the amount of ferritin in the blood. If iron levels are found to be low, iron supplements may help improve heavy periods.

VITAMIN C AND BIOFLAVONOIDS Vitamin C and bioflavonoids, both of which are found abundantly in citrus fruits, may be useful for heavy periods. Both help to protect capillaries (small blood vessels) from becoming damaged and may help to protect against the excessive blood loss during menstruation. One study found that taking 200mg of vitamin C and 200mg of bioflavonoids three times per day helped reduce symptoms of heavy periods.

CAUTION

Vitamin A should not be taken in doses exceeding 10,000 IU per day by women who are pregnant or trying to conceive. Consult your doctor before taking vitamin C with blood-thinning drugs such as warfarin. (*For more information, see p.46.*)

Homeopathy

A number of medicines may help with heavy periods (*for dosages see p.77*). These include the *Phosphorus* family, particularly *Phosphorus* and *Calcarea phosphorica*, and the *Carbonica* family, especially *Calcarea carbonica* and *Kali carbonica*. Other helpful homeopathic medicines include *Natrum muriaticum* and *Sabina*.

PHOSPHORUS AND CALCAREA PHOSPHO-RICA Women who respond to medicines of the *Phosphorus* group tend to be slim and sensitive. They tire quickly and may have a general tendency to bleeding and easy bruising. *Calc. phos.* is often useful for heavy periods in teenage girls who have just had a growth spurt and complain of joint aches and pains. It may be best to have a constitutional medicine prescribed for you (*see p.73*).

CARBORUNDUM People who respond to medicines of the *Carbonica* group are more stocky and solid but feel "worn out", have frequent backaches and a tendency to sweat freely. *Kali carb.* patients are often "chesty", they get bronchitis at least once every winter.

NATRUM MURIATICUM The clue to *Natrum muriaticum* patients is in their mental make-up: they are "copers" who take care of everybody else but never discuss their own feelings and they may be quite depressed. There are other constitutional features that also suggest this medicine (*see p.73*).

SABINA This homeopathic remedy is useful for women whose periods are heavy with a lot of clots and there is pain that passes around the pelvis to the back; the pain may resemble labour pains. A "rare, strange and peculiar" symptoms of this medicine is that women who respond to it may be irritated by hearing music.

Western Herbal Medicine

SEAWEED Trace minerals, such as iodine, can be important in helping to curb excessive blood flow during a period. They improve the health of the thyroid gland, which plays a major role in regulating menstrual flow. These trace minerals are found in abundance in seaweed of all types. Try milder-tasting seaweed, such as hizike or dulse. Kelp, while beneficial, can have a very strong flavour that does not appeal to everyone. You can include seaweed in your cooking by adding it to soups, salads and casserole dishes.

TRADITIONAL REMEDIES Cinnamon (*Cinnamomum cassia*) is a traditional remedy for various menstrual problems, including heavy periods. You can include cinnamon in cooking, or you can add it to beverages. The herb black horehound (*Ballota nigra*) is another traditional remedy for heavy periods, but its effectiveness has not been studied scientifically. There is some research on the anti-haemorrhagic effect of avens (*Geum urbanum*). Many Western herbalists use the aerial part of the plant, but the research, such as it is, is on the root (known as burnet). Burnet is also widely used in Traditional Chinese Medicine to treat heavy periods.

Astringent herbs, including cranesbill (*Geranium maculatum*), witch hazel (*Hamamelis virginia*) and periwinkle (*Vinca minor*) are also traditionally given for heavy periods. They contain tannin, which decreases menstrual discharge. Rasperry (*Rubus idaeus*), alfalfa (*Medicago sativa*) and nettle (*Urtica dioica*) leaves and yarrow (*Achillea millefolium*) have the same effect. You can make a tea with these herbs using two parts raspberry leaf, two parts nettle leaf, one part alfalfa leaf, and one-half part yarrow leaf. Put four to six tablespoons of the mixed herbs in a jug and cover with a a litre of boiling water. Cover the jug and let the herbs infuse for 20 minutes. Drink two or three cups of this tea every day. You can keep the leftover tea and drink it later on, either at room temperature or heated up.

> **CAUTION**
>
> See p.69 before taking a herbal remedy and, if you are taking prescribed medication, consult your doctor first. The iodine content in seaweed may interfere with treatment for thyroid problems: ask your doctor for advice.

> The loss of blood during persistent heavy periods may lead to anaemia and tiredness

Acupuncture

The effectiveness of acupuncture for heavy periods is unproven by randomised controlled trials, but its usefulness has been borne out by acupuncturists. It can also help with problems associated with polycystic ovary syndrome (*see p.337*) and the associated hormone imbalance.

In order to treat heavy periods effectively, a traditional Chinese diagnosis is required. The usual diagnoses are *Qi* deficiency, which leads to an inability to keep blood in vessels; excess heat, which leads to heavy bleeding; deficiency of heat, which may be due to long-term emotional stress or excessive sexual activity; or blood stasis, which may be due to depression.

Ideally treatment should be given over three to four cycles, perhaps involving six to nine treatments. If this fails to prove effective, then it is unlikely that acupuncture will be helpful in the longer term.

Exercise

Being overweight can be a factor in heavy periods. In women who are overweight, regular exercise, such as walking, cycling or swimming, aids weight loss and also helps to to keep weight at a steady healthy level once an ideal weight has been reached. Brisk walking for 30 minutes five times a week is a good way to start, gradually working up to more strenuous activity. Swimming and cycling are other beneficial activities. If you have not exercised for some time, make sure you begin slowly and avoid doing too much too soon. If you have any pre-existing medical conditions, check with your doctor before beginning an exercise programme.

> **PREVENTION PLAN**
>
> **The following measures can help to prevent heavy periods:**
>
> - Keep to a normal weight.
> - Choose a different method of contraception than the IUD (coil), which can cause heavy periods.
> - If you have an underactive thyroid, follow your treatment plan carefully.

WHAT ARE THE SYMPTOMS?

- Pain in the lower abdomen, which is often most severe before and during menstruation
- Irregular periods
- Heavy periods
- Pain during sex

WHY MIGHT I HAVE THIS?

PREDISPOSING FACTORS

- Not having children

TREATMENT PLAN

PRIMARY TREATMENTS

- Hormonal drugs (e.g. oral contraceptive pill)

BACK-UP TREATMENTS

- Surgery (if symptoms are severe)

WORTH CONSIDERING

- Nutritional therapy
- Western and Chinese herbs
- Homeopathy
- Bodywork therapies
- Acupuncture
- Psychological therapy

For an explanation of how treatments are rated, see p.111.

ENDOMETRIOSIS

In endometriosis, pieces of the tissue that lines the uterus (known as the endometrium) are found attached to other areas within the pelvis, such as the ovaries. These pieces of tissue respond to the hormones of the menstrual cycle and bleed during menstruation. The blood, which cannot escape, irritates the surrounding tissues, causing pain and eventually scarring and cysts. Treatment depends on the severity of the symptoms and usually involves drugs or, less commonly, surgery. Dietary changes, homeopathy and other therapies can also help.

WHY DOES IT OCCUR?

The exact cause of endometriosis is not known, but there are many theories as to why it occurs. One theory is that fragments of the uterine lining that are shed during menstruation do not leave the body through the vagina as normal, but travel along the fallopian tubes and into the pelvis, where they attach themselves to nearby organs. These patches of endometrial tissue are usually found in the pelvic cavity, but in rare instances pieces of endometrial tissue are found in other parts of the body, such as the lungs and the kidneys. Tissue may arrive at such sites via the circulatory or lymphatic systems. The condition only affects women of childbearing age and is found particularly in women in their 30s and early 40s.

Endometriosis may not produce any symptoms. If severe symptoms are present, they do not necessarily indicate severe endometriosis, and conversely a woman who has severe endometriosis may have few symptoms or none at all.

If symptoms do develop, they may vary depending on which organs are affected. Occasionally, a cyst formed from blood released by the misplaced endometrial tissue bursts, leaking its contents and causing severe pain. Rarely, there may be blood in the urine or stools if the bladder or rectum is affected. Endometriosis may also cause fertility problems (*see p.346*).

The condition tends to resolve during pregnancy and around the menopause. Women who do not have children are more at risk of developing the condition, probably because they do not experience the hormonal changes that take place during pregnancy.

TREATMENTS IN DETAIL

Conventional Medicine

Your doctor may suspect endometriosis from a description of your symptoms, and will refer you to a gynaecologist for further examination. Endometriosis may be diagnosed during a laparoscopy, in which a viewing instrument is passed through a small incision made in the abdominal wall. (The procedure is done under a general anaesthetic, usually as a day case.)

If endometriosis is discovered incidentally during tests or surgery for another condition, treatment may not be needed if there are no symptoms. Otherwise, the condition may be treated with either drugs or surgery.

All drugs used for endometriosis are likely to reduce pain that is associated with the condition. However, the symptoms tend to return once the drugs are stopped. Also, if infertility is a problem, drug treatment is unlikely to improve it. The options include the drugs described below.

PRIMARY TREATMENT **ORAL CONTRACEPTIVES** The combined oral contraceptive pill may be prescribed because it induces a pregnancy-like state. In other cases, progestogens alone, such as medroxyprogesterone, may be prescribed. These drugs also induce a pregnancy-like state.

DANAZOL The drug danazol is another treatment option. It has similar effects to the hormone testosterone (androgenic effects) and also counteracts the effects of oestrogens. You must use contraception while taking danazol because it can have adverse effects on a developing foetus.

ORGANS COMMONLY AFFECTED BY ENDOMETRIOSIS

The abdominal organs are most often affected by endometriosis, in which fragments of endometrial tissue travel from the uterus and attach themselves to other organs. The most commonly affected organs include the ovaries, fallopian tubes, ileum (lower part of the small bowel), large bowel, rectum, appendix and bladder. Symptoms of endometriosis may depend on which organs are affected. However, some women with endometriosis experience few symptoms or none at all.

Endometriosis in the abdominal cavity

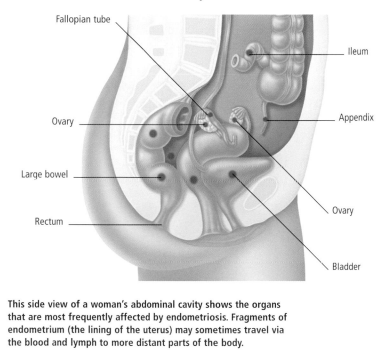

Fallopian tube

Ileum

Ovary

Appendix

Large bowel

Rectum

Ovary

Bladder

This side view of a woman's abdominal cavity shows the organs that are most frequently affected by endometriosis. Fragments of endometrium (the lining of the uterus) may sometimes travel via the blood and lymph to more distant parts of the body.

GNRH ANALOGUES Gonadotrophin-releasing hormone (GnRH) analogues may be prescribed. They mimic the hormones that trigger the pituitary gland (the tiny gland at the base of the brain) to release follicle-stimulating hormone (FSH) and luteinizing hormone (LH). (These gonadotrophin hormones act with oestrogens and progesterone to regulate the menstrual cycle.) These drugs prevent the ovaries from producing oestrogens and induce a state that is similar to the menopause.

GESTRINONE Another drug that may be used to treat endometriosis is called gestrinone. Like GnRH analogues described above, this drug also acts on the pituitary gland. Along with danazol, it is androgenic (i.e. it acts like a male hormone) and so can cause acne, hot flushes, fluid retention and hirsutism.

SURGERY If surgical treatment is appropriate, laser treatment or diathermy (heat treatment) performed during a laparoscopy may be used to destroy the patches of endometrial tissue. Alternatively, adhesions (fibrous tissue that forms between tissues and organs due to inflammation) may be cut and cysts removed.

These surgical methods may provide a longer-lasting improvement in the symptoms than drug treatments and may also improve fertility. Occasionally, for very severe pain and in cases where a woman does not wish to conceive, the uterus, ovaries and fallopian tubes are removed, inducing menopause.

> **CAUTION**
>
> Drugs for endometriosis can cause a range of possible side-effects: ask your doctor to explain these to you.

Nutritional Therapy

DIETARY CHANGES There is some evidence that endometriosis is related to an excess of, or extra sensitivity to, the female hormone oestrogen. Improving liver function may help to reduce oestrogen levels by enhancing its breakdown in the liver. More details about improving liver function can be found in the section starting on p.32.

NUTRITIONAL SUPPLEMENTS Fish oils (omega-3 fatty acids) may help in the management of endometriosis. Fish oils appear to increase the production of substances called eicosanoids, which may reduce the inflammation and pain associated with the condition. In addition to eating plenty of foods rich in omega-3 fatty acids (such as oily fish), taking supplements of concentrated fish oils at a dose of 1g, once or twice a day, may also help.

> **CAUTION**
>
> Consult your doctor before taking fish-oil supplements with anticoagulant drugs, such as warfarin. (*For more information, see p.46.*)

Homeopathy

Successful homeopathic treatment of endometriosis is likely to need a consultation, and probably a course of treatment, with a skilled homeopathic practitioner.

A case series has suggested that the condition responds well to homeopathy. In the studies, several medicines were often required, with some being given to relieve pain and other being appropriate on "constitutional" grounds (*see p.73*). The homeopathic medicine *Lachesis* was the most frequently helpful; other helpful medicines included *Graphites*, *Nux vomica* and *Oophorinum*.

LACHESIS is useful for endometriosis, particularly affecting the left side. In women who respond to this, the symptoms are made worse by pressure (as caused by tight clothes and so forth) and heat and are worst in the premenstrual period.

GRAPHITES Women who respond to *Graphites* often have bowel problems, particularly constipation before or during the period. They may also have skin problems, particularly eczema that tends to crack and weep. This eczema often appears behind the ears or on the nipples or genitalia.

NUX VOMICA is useful when great irritability is part of the picture. Women who respond to this medicine may also have bowel or bladder problems, particularly tenesmus (the urge to empty the bowel or bladder again just after doing so).

OOPHORINUM (which is made from healthy ovary tissue) was used in the studies as a general supportive medicine, particularly when infertility was also part of the problem.

OTHER REMEDIES including *Pulsatilla*, *Sepia* and *Sulphur*, may also be helpful for some patients when prescribed on an individual basis (*see p.73*).

Western Herbal Medicine

Whatever the initial cause for endometriosis, oestrogen affects its growth. Reducing oestrogen levels in the body and regulating hormonal production are both key aims of herbal treatment.

The liver is the organ that is responsible for turning oestrogen into a substance known as oestriol. This a particular form of oestrogen that does not cause endometrial tissue to proliferate. For this reason, improving liver function can be an important factor in treating endometriosis. By improving liver function and thereby increasing the ratio of oestriol to oestrogen in the body, the growth of endometrial

officinale), milk thistle (*Silibum marianum*), and burdock (*Arctium lappa*). Drinking tea made using 3 parts dandelion root, 3 parts wild yam root, 1 part chaste berry, 2 parts burdock and half a part dong quai three or four times a day may be helpful in easing endometriosis symptoms.

> **CAUTION**
>
> See p.69 before taking a herbal remedy.

Chinese Herbal Medicine

In Traditional Chinese Medicine, the mechanism that causes endometriosis is known as Blood Stasis. The objective of treatment is to invigorate the blood and remove stasis, and to this end both acupuncture (*see below*) and Chinese herbal medicine are used.

HERBS FOR BLOOD STASIS The herbs most often prescribed for dispersing blood stasis are *Dan Shen* (salvia), *Chi Shao* (red peony root), *Tao Ren* (persica seed), *Hong Hua* (safflower) and *San Leng* (bur-reed rhizome) Endometriosis may also involve Cold, Heat, Deficiency or Excess patterns, which are determined from a patient's signs and symptoms. Various decoctions may be prescribed based on the diagnosis.

> **CAUTION**
>
> Do not attempt to self-treat for endometriosis using traditional Chinese herbs. Seek advice from a qualified Chinese herbalist. See also p.69.

acupuncture may be effective in managing the pain of endometriosis. The clinical experience of many acupuncturists is, however, that acupuncture does appear to be very successful in the treatment of this particular condition.

Further research into the use of acupuncture for endometriosis is required. More detailed clinical trials are particularly important for us to understand exactly how effective acupuncture actually is and what its mechanisms might be.

If you would like to try acupuncture for endometriosis, treatment should initially be given on a weekly basis, which will usually trigger a positive response within the first four to six treatments. If acupuncture is beneficial, treatment should continue until no further benefit is apparent. After this, maintenance treatments should be considered on a monthly or three-monthly basis.

Bodywork Therapies

A significant number of women with chronic pelvic pain have been shown to have myofascial trigger points (sensitive points in the muscles) in the structures of the lower abdomen and pelvis, close to surgical incision scar-tissue sites, following hysterectomy to remove endometrial tissues or as a result of endometrial adhesions. These trigger points are partially or totally responsible for the pain. They may be deactivated by acupuncture, or, in some cases, by manual pressure and stretching techniques, as used by osteopaths, massage therapists (particularly those with a neuromuscular therapy training) and some physiotherapists and chiropractors. Self-treatment (massage) of tense tissues has been found to be a useful addition to treatment.

Psychological Therapy

GROUP THERAPY Preliminary reports suggest that support groups for women with endometriosis may help them to cope better with the psychological and emotional issues associated with this condition, which may include depression and anxiety.

A pilot study showed that simply discussing treatments and problems with other women added to women's satisfaction with their overall care.

> ## In most women with endometriosis, the condition is mild and does not impair fertility

tissue may be limited and, therefore, the symptoms of endometriosis may be lessened, although they may not resolve.

HERBS FOR ENDOMETRIOSIS The most important herbs for treating endometriosis are chasteberry (*Vitex agnus-castus*), dong quai (*Angelica sinensis*), wild yam (*Dioscorea villosa*), dandelion (*Taraxacum*

Acupuncture

Acupuncture is widely used to treat pelvic pain, such as occurs in endometriosis. Usually, a traditional Chinese diagnosis (*see above*) is required. There have been one or two series of case studies published in the acupuncture literature (which are not available on Medline) suggesting that

POLYCYSTIC OVARY SYNDROME

In polycystic ovary syndrome (PCOS), multiple, small, fluid-filled cysts on the ovaries are accompanied by an imbalance of sex hormones, including higher than normal levels of the sex hormone testosterone. In some cases multiple cysts are present but there is no hormonal imbalance, in which case the women are simply said to have polycystic ovaries. Various measures, such as weight loss and drug treatment, may bring about an improvement. Dietary changes, homeopathy, herbal medicines and acupuncture may also help.

WHAT ARE THE SYMPTOMS?

The symptoms of PCOS vary from woman to woman. In some cases there are no symptoms. Typical symptoms include:

- Infrequent or absent periods
- Obesity
- Acne
- Excessive hair growth (hirsutism)

WHY MIGHT I HAVE THIS?

PREDISPOSING FACTORS

- Genetic tendency
- Blood-sugar instability (possibly)

TREATMENT PLAN

PRIMARY TREATMENTS

- Weight loss (if necessary)
- Antidiabetic drugs
- Combined oral contraceptive pill
- Ovulation-inducing drugs and/or assisted conception techniques (for women who wish to conceive)
- Blood-sugar stabilising diet

BACK-UP TREATMENTS

- Surgery
- Acupuncture

WORTH CONSIDERING

- Nutritional supplements
- Individualised homeopathy
- Western herbal medicine

For an explanation of how treatments are rated, see p.111.

WHY DOES IT OCCUR?

How polycystic ovary syndrome develops is not fully understood but tissue resistance to insulin, a hormone produced by the pancreas that enables cells to absorb the sugar glucose from the bloodstream, is thought to play a key role. To compensate for this resistance, the pancreas produces large amounts of insulin, which is thought to cause excess production of male sex hormones (androgens), such as testosterone. These male hormones disrupt the normal functioning of the ovaries and, as a result, ovulation may be absent or irregular. It is not known why some women develop PCOS, but genetic factors are thought to be involved.

Around 5 per cent of women of childbearing age are affected by PCOS. The condition is associated with infertility if ovulation does not occur, but this can often be successfully treated.

Women who have PCOS are at increased risk of developing diabetes mellitus (*see p.314*) because their tissues are resistant to insulin. They may also be at increased risk of developing high blood pressure (*see p.244*), coronary artery disease (*see p.252*) and cancer of the endometrium (uterine lining).

TREATMENTS IN DETAIL

Conventional Medicine

If your doctor suspects that you may have PCOS, he will arrange investigations, such as blood tests to check hormone levels and ultrasound scans, which may show cysts on the ovaries. If PCOS is diagnosed, various treatment options are available.

PRIMARY TREATMENT **WEIGHT LOSS** Your doctor will suggest losing weight if you are overweight or obese. This may reduce insulin resistance and so correct the hormonal imbalance, restoring ovulation and regulating periods.

PRIMARY TREATMENT **DRUGS** Drugs that induce ovulation, such as clomiphene, may be prescribed if fertility is affected and a woman wishes to become pregnant. Clomiphene is taken at the beginning of the menstrual cycle and can be taken for up to six months. If clomiphene does not induce ovulation, gonadotropins may then be tried. With all of these drugs there is a risk of multiple pregnancy.

Women who do not wish to conceive may take the combined oral contraceptive pill to regulate periods and reduce the risk of endometrial cancer. A pill containing the antiandrogen drug cyproterone acetate may be prescribed if acne and hirsutism are particular problems. However, this treatment may make periods irregular and the symptoms will return after the treatment is stopped.

Recent evidence suggests that certain antidiabetic drugs (such as metformin), which increase the sensitivity of the tissues to insulin, may be beneficial for PCOS in terms of reducing insulin levels in the blood and so reducing excess androgen levels. Such drugs may therefore restore ovulation and regulate menstruation.

SURGERY If drugs are unsuccessful, the ovaries may be treated surgically using a technique known as laparoscopic ovarian diathermy (LOD), often called "ovarian drilling". In this procedure, diathermy (a form of heat treatment) is used to make several small holes in each ovary during

be distributed around the middle of the body. Women with PCOS tend carry excess weight around the middle of their bodies. High levels of insulin are also associated with insulin resistance, which is strongly implicated in PCOS. Women with PCOS seem to be at greater risk of

and be constipated. These women may be depressed and "flat", uninterested in their families or partners. Symptoms may improve with vigorous exertion.

PULSATILLA In women who respond to *Pulsatilla*, menstrual periods are completely irregular and unpredictable; they are frequently completely absent. There may be breast swelling and tenderness.

Polycystic ovary syndrome is one of the leading causes of infertility

laparoscopy (in which a viewing instrument is introduced through a small incision in the abdominal wall under a general anaesthetic). This surgery is usually performed as a day case.

Ovarian drilling can restore regular ovulation or make the ovaries more sensitive to ovulation-stimulating drugs, such as clomiphene, if a woman wishes to conceive. It is not known why it has this effect. Multiple pregnancy rates tend to be lower in women who received ovarian drilling compared to those who received treatment with gonadotrophins.

ASSISTED CONCEPTION If the drugs and surgery described above are unsuccessful in inducing ovulation, assisted conception methods, such as in vitro fertilisation or gamete intrafallopian transfer (GIFT), may be considered (*see p.346*).

> **CAUTION**
>
> Drugs to treat PCOS can cause a range of possible side-effects: ask your doctor to explain these to you.

Nutritional Therapy

PRIMARY TREATMENT **BLOOD-SUGAR STABILISING DIET** There is evidence that some women with PCOS have a problem with blood-sugar regulation. It may be that surges of sugar into the bloodstream stimulate the secretion of large amounts of the hormone insulin, which may in turn stimulate the secretion of male hormones (androgens).

High insulin levels can also make weight gain more likely and cause excess weight to

having problems tolerating sugar in their systems (impaired glucose tolerance), especially if they are overweight.

The best diet for women with PCOS seems to be one that ensures stable levels of blood sugar and lower insulin levels. See p.32 for more details and the specific nutrients that help this condition (such as chromium, magnesium and vitamin B3).

Homeopathy

In a study, 40 women were treated with individualised homeopathy for ovarian cysts, of whom 14 had PCOS. When ultrasound examination of the ovaries was repeated after nine months of homeopathic treatment, the cysts had resolved in all but three women.

The homeopathic medicines most frequently associated with a good result in this study were *Calcarea carbonica*, *Sepia* and *Pulsatilla*.

CALCAREA CARBONICA In women who respond to *Calcarea carbonica*, menstrual periods are irregular, although when they do occur they are often heavy and prolonged. These women tend to be stout and phlegmatic, although they may have many anxieties and fear that they are suffering from a severe or incurable condition. They feel run down and may experience other problems, including polyps at various sites (such as the uterus), hives (urticaria) and low back pain. A particularly characteristic feature is easy sweating.

SEPIA Women who respond to *Sepia* have low back and pelvic pain, typically of a dragging character, and usually loss of sex drive. They may also have haemorrhoids

Western Herbal Medicine

Several key remedies are available for PCOS that promote hormonal balance and ovarian function, and at the same time reduce the severity and frequency of symptoms. A diet low in refined carbohydrates is essential, with attention to eating foods low on the glycaemic index (*see p.43*).

CHASTE BERRY (*Vitex agnus-castus*) is almost invariably used to treat PCOS, as it inhibits androgen release and raises progesterone levels.

OTHER HERBS for PCOS include saw palmetto (*Serenoa repens*) and nettle root (*Urtica dioica*). Liquorice (*Glycyrrhiza glabra*) and white peony (*Paeonia lactiflora*) may also be used. A Japanese study showed that these lower androgen levels and normalise pituitary hormone balance.

> **CAUTION**
>
> Consult a herbalist for treatment for PCOS and see p.69 before taking a herbal remedy.

Acupuncture

Acupuncture has well-documented and fundamental effects on the hormonal system in PCOS. In a study, women with PCOS who were receiving acupuncture demonstrated a decrease in male hormone levels combined with a more normal pattern of ovulation. PCOS is a chronic condition that usually requires weekly treatment with acupuncture over a period of a couple of months before any sustained benefit begins to emerge. If you are planning to try using acupuncture to treat PCOS, you should be prepared to persist with it for a reasonably lengthy period of time to see if it works for you.

MENOPAUSAL PROBLEMS

The end of a woman's childbearing years, when the ovaries stop releasing eggs and produce less of the female sex hormones oestrogen and progesterone, is known as the menopause. It is said to have occurred when a woman has not had a menstrual period for a year. Many women feel well throughout the menopausal transition, but some have distressing symptoms, such as hot flushes and mood swings, which may be eased with drugs, dietary measures, homeopathy, relaxation exercises and other treatments.

WHAT ARE THE SYMPTOMS?

- Irregular periods, when the menstrual cycle has previously been regular
- Heavier than normal periods
- Hot flushes, in which the face, chest, and arms become red and hot
- Heavy sweating, often at night
- Mood swings
- Poor concentration
- Feelings of anxiety, panic or depression
- Vaginal atrophy (thinning of the vaginal tissues that may be accompanied by discomfort)
- Painful intercourse
- Reduced libido
- Dry skin and thinning hair
- Bladder weakness and urinary tract infections

TREATMENT PLAN

PRIMARY TREATMENTS

- Black cohosh
- Self-help measures

BACK-UP TREATMENTS

- HRT, tibolone and other drugs
- Isoflavone-rich foods
- Vitamin E
- Western herbal medicine
- Breathing retraining

WORTH CONSIDERING

- Homeopathy
- Massage and reflexology
- Exercise, yoga and t'ai chi
- Acupuncture
- `Mind–body therapies

For an explanation of how treatments are rated, see p.111.

WHY DOES IT OCCUR?

As women approach the menopause – usually between the ages of 45 and 55 – ovarian production of the sex hormones oestrogen and progesterone becomes erratic. During the menopausal transition, levels of these hormones may vary between higher than normal levels and lower than normal levels. This happens because as levels of oestrogen in the body decline, the pituitary gland in the brain secretes more follicle-stimulating hormone (FSH) to try to stimulate the failing ovaries. Eventually, the hormones stabilise at a new level.

Symptoms associated with higher than normal levels of hormones (such as heavy periods and breast tenderness) are always resolved by menopause. Symptoms associated with lower hormone levels (such as hot flushes and vaginal dryness) may persist for months or years. Most of the symptoms of menopause result from the increased levels of FSH and decreased levels of oestrogen in the body. Menopausal symptoms tend to be more severe when menopause takes place prematurely or abruptly, for instance if the ovaries are removed surgically or are damaged by chemotherapy or radiation therapy. The menopause process usually lasts between one and five years, after which most symptoms disappear.

The decline in oestrogen levels affects the body in other ways than simply preventing ovulation and menstruation. In particular, the gradual loss of bone tissue that normally occurs with age is accelerated during the ten years after the menopause as a result of the lack of oestrogen. This may increase a woman's risk of developing osteoporosis (*see p.308*), in which the bones become brittle and prone to fracture. Oestrogen also appears to have a preventative effect against high blood pressure and coronary artery disease, which is why premenopausal women are at less risk of coronary artery disease than men. The protective effect of oestrogen wears off by about the age of 60, after which the risk of developing heart disease is the same for men and women.

In the years leading up to menopause, many women's menstrual cycles become irregular and other menopausal symptoms related to the changing hormone levels, such as mood swings and hot flushes, may also develop.

A tendency to have an early or late menopause may sometimes run in families, suggesting that genetic factors may play a part. Smoking may lower the age at which menopause occurs. Many women have no bothersome symptoms during the menopausal transition. No symptoms of the menopause require treatment unless they are troublesome.

SELF-HELP

PRIMARY TREATMENT You can reduce the discomfort of menopausal symptoms with the following self-help measures:

- Maintain a healthy weight (making sure that you are not underweight, as well as overweight) and include flaxseeds and plenty of soya-rich foods, such as tofu, in your diet.
- Don't smoke.
- Take regular daily exercise.
- Use yoga, relaxation, deep breathing (*see p.99*) and other techniques to deal with underlying stress.

COMPLEMENTARY THERAPIES FOR MENOPAUSE

Many of the problems that arise during the menopausal years can be addressed successfully with complementary therapies. While some of these therapies carry a lower risk of side-effects than many of the drug treatments that are available to treat menopausal problems, many of them have not been subjected to rigorous or long-term testing. Approaches that incorporate yoga and meditation are likely to benefit well-being on the whole and can be combined with conventional treatments.

SYMPTOMS	CAUSE	TRY THE FOLLOWING
Hot flushes, night sweats	Sudden drop in oestrogen	• Soya, black cohosh, evening primrose, dong quai, vitamin E, homeopathy • Avoid caffeine, alcohol, stress, spicy foods, hot environments
Mood disturbances, depression, anxiety	Less oestrogen	• St. John's wort, valerian, ginseng, counselling, exercise, acupuncture • Avoid tea, coffee, sugar
Loss of libido, vaginal dryness	Low hormone levels making vaginal walls thinner. Less natural lubrication	• Water-soluble lubricant, homeopathy, soya, chasteberry, ginseng
Menstrual disorders, heavy periods	Fluctuating hormones	• Wild yam
Increased coronary artery disease risk	Less oestrogen (which protects the heart)	• Soya, flax seeds and oil, fish oil
Increased osteoporosis risk	Less oestrogen (which aids calcium uptake)	• Ipriflavone (a soya extract), calcium, magnesium, vitamin C, weight-bearing exercise • Avoid fizzy drinks, which contain phosphoric acid that depletes the body of calcium

- If you have hot flushes, avoid alcohol, caffeine and spicy foods and wear layers that you can easily remove.
- Maintain regular sexual activity.

TREATMENTS IN DETAIL

Conventional Medicine

HORMONE REPLACEMENT THERAPY Hormone replacement therapy (HRT) may be prescribed for the short-term relief of menopausal symptoms. It may also be taken for the prevention of osteoporosis, but it is only considered for this purpose when other treatments are not suitable, because the risks of long-term therapy (*see below*) are thought to outweigh the benefits.

HRT usually comprises both oestrogens and progestogens. Giving oestrogens alone can increase the risk of cancer of the endometrium (uterine lining), but progestogens are given at the same time to counteract this effect. Oestrogen alone can be taken by women who have had a hysterectomy. Progestogens may be taken alone, as studies have shown that, on their own, they may improve hot flushes and night sweats.

HRT is available in various forms, including tablets, patches, gels and implants (which are inserted beneath the skin under local anaesthetic). When gels, implants and some patches are used, oral progestogens must also be taken.

HRT is also available as tablets and rings that can be placed in the vagina on a short-term basis to relieve vaginal atrophy. If they are used over the long term instead, oral progestogens may be needed in order to counteract the possible increased risk of uterine cancer.

LONG-TERM USE OF HRT The recommendations for prescribing HRT have changed to take into account the evidence that long-term use of HRT is associated with an increased risk of breast, endometrial and ovarian cancer.

HRT may also increase a woman's risk of a heart attack or stroke, or of a blood clot forming in a vein, usually in the leg. However, HRT has been shown to offer some protection against bowel cancer. It is important that you discuss the benefits and risks of HRT for your individual situation with your doctor before making a decision on whether to use it.

OTHER MEASURES The drug tibolone combines the effects of oestrogens and progesterones as well as having a mild testosterone-type (male hormone-like) effect. It not only reduces hot flushes and night sweats, but may also improve libido in women whose libido is reduced.

Other drugs may be prescribed for specific problems, such as antibiotics for urinary tract infections.

EMOTIONAL ASPECTS For some women during the menopause, anxiety and depression may be a problem. As depression may be related to coming to terms with the end of the fertile phase of life, emotional support and, for some women, counselling may be beneficial (*see p.104*). In some cases, antidepressants may also be appropriate.

> **CAUTION**
>
> HRT and other drugs for menopause can cause a range of possible side-effects: ask your doctor to explain these to you.

Nutritional Therapy

ISOFLAVONE-RICH FOODS Women from Eastern countries, such as Japan, seem to have relatively few problems with the menopause. The low rate of menopausal symptoms, especially hot flushes, may be related to the consumption of significant quantities of soya-based foods, including tofu and soya milk.

Soya and flaxseed contain substances called isoflavones (also known as phytoestrogens), which can mimic the effect of oestrogen in the body. They are thought to "lock-on" to oestrogenic receptor sites and compensate for the drop in oestrogen levels that occurs naturally at the menopause.

In one double-blind study of menopausal women receiving either soya protein or placebo, the soya protein was found to be significantly superior compared to the placebo in reducing the number of hot flushes after four, eight and 12 weeks of treatment.

Other double-blind research has also reported a reduction in the number of hot flushes menopausal women experience with soya-product supplementation.

ANTIOXIDANTS Phytoestrogenic foods also have antioxidant and anti-inflammatory actions and are thought to help prevent osteoporosis and coronary disease. Flaxseed (the ground seed taken fresh) is particularly useful because it contains unusually high levels of omega-3 oils. If you are experiencing menopausal symptoms, include flaxseed and soya products (such as tofu, soya milk and soya flour) in your diet.

VITAMIN E Several studies done in the 1940s showed that vitamin E supplements can also be very effective in relieving hot flushes and vaginal dryness in menopausal women. Unfortunately there are no recent studies to guide us.

However, recent research does suggest that a diet rich in vitamin E (although not vitamin E supplements) can decrease the normally increased risk of cardiovascular disease after the menopause. A recent six-day study of 54 women discovered that when vitamin E is absorbed from food, it acts as an antioxidant, reducing the effect on blood vessels of LDL cholesterol, which can lead to atherosclerosis (*see* p.252).

Good food sources of vitamin E include nuts, vegetable oils and cereals, in particular wheat germ.

> **CAUTION**
>
> Ask your doctor for advice before taking vitamin E with drug warfarin (*see also p.46*). Women on thyroid medication should avoid eating soya products within three hours of taking their medication.

About 75 per cent of women experience troublesome symptoms during menopause

Homeopathy

Menopausal symptoms, especially hot flushes, tend to respond quite well to homeopathic treatment. It is best to consult a homeopath who can prescribe the most suitable medicine for you. The homeopathic medicines that most frequently give good results are *Amyl nitrosum, Calcarea carbonica, Lachesis, Natrum muriaticum, Pulsatilla* and *Sepia*.

REMEDIES FOR HOT FLUSHES *Amyl nitrosum* is specific for hot flushes when there is a sensation of blood surging to the head, sometimes with a throbbing headache, followed by profuse sweat and chilliness. The other medicines mentioned below are more deep acting and may help with a number of menopausal problems as well as hot flushes.

LACHESIS is the most frequently prescribed medicine for the menopause. It is appropriate when there are frequent hot flushes and the woman feels too hot much of the time. Other features that suggest this medicine are migraines (particularly left-sided), intolerance of tight clothes, (particularly collars, but also tight belts and bras) and easy bruising.

CALCAREA CARBONICA may be useful when sweating is particularly marked on the head and neck at night. Women whom it helps are often anxious and tend to "niggle" over little things, they may be woken up by bad dreams. They are tired and run down and may suffer from other problems, such as skin trouble including hives, polyps in the nose and low back pain.

NATRUM MURIATICUM AND SEPIA *Natrum muriaticum* may be prescribed for women who are depressed, but keep it well-hidden. They often have vaginal dryness and recurrent cold sores on the lips. Women who respond to *Sepia* may also have these. However, *Sepia* women may have become bad-tempered and less affectionate to their families since menopausal symptoms began.

PULSATILLA may be given to women who show great changeability, both in mood and in symptoms. These women are typically soft-spoken and easily moved to tears.

GRAPHITES is another medicine which may help with menopausal symptoms; it has some similarities with *Pulsatilla*, but the woman who responds to *Graphites* is typically weepy over sentimental films and sad music, rather than as a result of depression. Strangely, women who respond to *Graphites* may become pale during a hot flush. They may also have skin trouble, particularly cracked eczema, which easily exudes a sticky fluid. Constipation is also quite common in these women.

Western Herbal Medicine

A herbal approach to ill health at the menopause seeks to look wider than the narrow focus of hormone levels. Menopausal symptoms can result from long-term stress and chronic ill health, and these are factors which in turn make it harder for the body to adapt and establish a new (post-menopausal) hormonal balance. Advice on diet, exercise and relaxation is central, but practitioners will also prescribe herbs to support hormonal function, relieve menopausal symptoms and promote emotional balance.

PRIMARY TREATMENT **BLACK COHOSH** (*Cimicifuga racemosa*) is a traditional Native American remedy for women's health problems, which has gained a reputation as a helpful alternative remedy for the menopause. Black cohosh is especially useful for hot flushes, sweating, sleep disorders and nervous irritability. Where nervous exhaustion or depression is also a feature, it combines well with St John's wort (*Hypericum perforatum*).

Black cohosh is commonly recommended as an alternative to HRT and a 1998 review of eight clinical trials concluded that black cohosh extract might be a safe and effective alternative where HRT was contraindicated or rejected.

Extrapolating from Japanese research into other species of herbs related to black cohosh, it has also been proposed that this herb might inhibit the loss of calcium from bone and thus protect against osteoporosis in menopausal women.

SAGE AND ALFA-ALFA may also be useful for menopausal symptoms. A small clinical trial investigated the efficacy of a sage (*Salvia officinalis*) and alfa-alfa (*Medicago sativa*) combination in relieving hot flushes and night sweats. It found significant improvement in symptoms, with all the women experiencing reduced symptoms and most finding that hot flushes and night sweats completely disappeared.

RED CLOVER A systematic review published in the journal *Menopause* suggested the herb red clover (*Trifolium pratense*) might benefit women suffering with severe menopausal problems.

OTHER HERBS Many other herbal medicines have long been used to treat menopausal symptoms. Liquorice (*Glycyrrhiza glabra*) and fenugreek (*Trigonella foenum-graecum*), for example, are both valuable for treating dry skin, vaginal dryness and lowered libido. Chaste berry (*Vitex agnus-castus*), which has a progesterogenic action, is most commonly used for problems in the phase of a woman's life leading up to menopause.

> **CAUTION**
>
> See p.69 before taking a herbal remedy.

Acupuncture

Acupuncture can be used to treat certain symptoms, such as hot flushes. There is some evidence that a course of four to six acupuncture treatments will have a beneficial effect on hot flushes for three months or longer. Other menopausal symptoms, such as tiredness, muscular aches and joint pains, may also be improved by treatment with acupuncture.

A traditional Chinese diagnosis is required and treatment may need to be carried out intermittently throughout the menopausal period. Usually treatment focuses on the prevailing symptoms at the time, so the traditional Chinese diagnosis may vary depending on the exact symptoms. If symptoms are acute (sudden and short-lived), weekly treatment is recommended, and if it appears to be effective then it is probably worthwhile having acupuncture every month or two as a preventative measure.

Bodywork Therapies

Manual therapies such as massage may promote restful sleep and relieve symptoms. A survey of 886 women aged 45–65 years was carried out in Washington state, USA. Of the women surveyed, 31.6 per cent had consulted a chiropractor, while 29.5 per cent had had massage therapy. More than 89 per cent of the women reported that they had found the treatment "somewhat or very" helpful, particularly in improving sleep. The researchers concluded that "the use of alternative therapies for menopause symptoms is common, and women who use them generally find them to be beneficial."

CHIROPRACTIC Chiropractic manipulation of the upper back and neck has been shown in one study to decrease the frequency of hot flushes by up to 90 per cent.

REFLEXOLOGY AND FOOT MASSAGE When the benefits of treating specific reflexology points on the foot were compared with the effects of general foot massage in easing some symptoms of menopause, it was found that both methods were equally effective. Symptoms that improved with these treatments included anxiety, depression, hot flushes and night sweats.

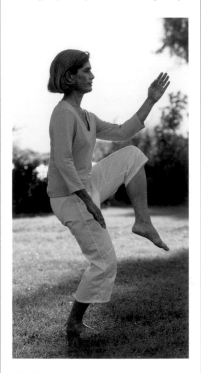

> ## T'AI CHI
>
> The slow, gentle, focused movements of t'ai chi can help you to relax, which may help you to cope better with menopausal changes. As a form of exercise, t'ai chi does not put undue stress on the joints and promotes flexibility and suppleness. As a form of meditation, t'ai chi may help to lessen anxiety, especially if it is done regularly.
>
> T'ai chi is an easy and inexpensive way to take gentle exercise. It can be done outdoors and does not require special clothing or equipment.

Since the reduction in symptoms associated with the menopause after foot massage seem to derive from reduced feelings of anxiety, it is worth considering trying other treatments (such as general massage, yoga, t'ai chi and regular use of breathing exercise – *see below and opposite*), which also have calming effects. See also Anxiety and Panic Disorder, p.414.

Exercise

AEROBIC EXERCISE Physical exercise can reduce anxiety levels and hot flushes and maintain bone density. For these reasons, women should be sure to exercise regularly in the years around the menopause. The use of exercise programmes during these years has been shown to increase bone density by a significant amount. Many experts say that doing some aerobic, weight-bearing exercise, such as fast walking or slow jogging, for about 30 minutes every other day can be very beneficial.

However, while there is evidence that mild but regular exercise, such as walking, can slow down bone loss, "there is no suggestion that exercise can provide an alternative to some type of hormone replacement therapy treatment in preventing bone loss in the early years of menopause". (*See also Osteoporosis, p.308.*)

T'AI CHI Performing t'ai chi (*see opposite*) can help improve mood and preserve flexibility and physical strength during menopause. The gentle, flowing movements of t'ai chi do not put stress on joints, while the stretching and deep breathing it incorporates help maintain suppleness and encourage relaxation. Since t'ai chi demands focus, it is also a form of meditation, which can help to relieve anxiety and bring about a sense of calm.

Breathing Retraining

BREATHING FOR PANIC ATTACKS Learning to control the breath and avoiding shallow, rapid breathing can be very helpful in controlling stress, anxiety and panic attacks, which some women find accompany the menopause. See p.62 for more information on how to do this.

BREATHING FOR HOT FLUSHES Abdominal breathing has been found to help relieve menopausal hot flushes. Studies show that the frequency of hot flushes can be reduced by about 50 per cent by regularly using slow, abdominal breathing. Robert Freeman, a professor of psychiatry and behavioural neurosciences at at Wayne State University in Detroit, Michigan, says that women can prevent or shorten the duration of hot flushes by slowing their breathing to a rate of seven or eight breaths a minute.

If you are experiencing hot flushes, try doing abdominal breathing (*see p.62*) regularly, and try to avoid shallow breathing, particularly if you are feeling tense or under stress.

Yoga

Practising yoga can help during the period around the menopause and during the menopause. Yoga can reduce stress and foster a positive attitude to the changes that menopause involves.

Some practitioners believe that yoga can also help to regulate hormone levels in the body. In this way, doing yoga regularly may help to reduce the frequency of menopausal symptoms such as hot flushes and mood swings.

> ### During menopause, production of oestrogen drops by as much as 90 per cent in a few years

The best yoga for menopause is slow and gentle, with an emphasis on floor poses. Poses that work the low back, such as the bridge and the cobra, may influence the kidneys and adrenal glands and relieve fatigue. These poses have the added advantage of easing muscle tension and stiffness in the low back.

Side stretches can help to tone the muscles and improve flexibility. Poses that open the chest, such as the fish, can help to reduce stress and induce a state of calmness and clarity.

If you have not done yoga or stretching exercises before or have not done them for some time and would like to try yoga, be sure to start gradually. Make sure you listen to your body and do not try to do too much too soon.

Mind–Body Therapies

RELAXATION Regular relaxation has been found to be effective in reducing the frequency and intensity of hot flushes, decreasing tension and anxiety and improving mood in women going through the menopause.

Researchers in Detroit found that women who were taught to slow their breathing rate had fewer hot flushes than those who did not (*see Breathing Retraining, above*). Doing daily relaxation exercises was also found to help to reduce the intensity of hot flushes as well as many depressive symptoms.

GUIDED IMAGERY Simply sitting quietly and listening to a guided imagery tape, which helps you to imagine that you are in a soothing and pleasant place, may help you to relax and may relieve anxiety during menopause.

BIOFEEDBACK Learning to control your body's responses to certain signals using biofeedback (*see p.94*) can also help you to relax during menopause. Once you have learned to relax your body at will, you can also use the technique to help you cope with anxiety and panic attacks, if these things are an issue for you.

If you are experiencing symptoms of the menopause, try a programme of daily relaxation exercises (*see p.99*), which may increase your ability to cope with this stage of your life. You could also try guided imagery or learn biofeedback. Following a relaxation programme may mean that you have less need of medication for menopausal symptoms.

SOCIAL SUPPORT Social support is very important in the menopausal period, since women may feel isolated and may experience "empty nest syndrome" as grown children leave home. Women at this stage of life may need help in redefining their roles, and counselling may provide this.

PREVENTION PLAN

As the menopause approaches, try the following to minimise problems:

- Eat a balanced diet.
- Avoid having too much caffeine or alcohol.
- Take regular, weight-bearing exercise.
- Do relaxation exercises regularly.
- If you smoke, stop.

VAGINAL THRUSH

The condition known as vaginal thrush occurs when there is increased growth of the yeast *Candida albicans*, which is often present naturally in the vagina. The condition is not serious but can cause uncomfortable symptoms. Vaginal thrush affects many women at some point in their lives, often during their childbearing years, and once it occurs it may recur regularly. There are several ways to treat vaginal thrush and prevent its recurrence, including antifungal drugs, dietary changes and supplements, homeopathic medicines and stress-relieving techniques.

WHAT ARE THE SYMPTOMS?

- Intense irritation and itchiness in the area around the opening of the vagina (the vulva) and inside the vagina
- Vaginal discharge, which may be thick and white, cheesy or watery in appearance
- Redness of the vulva

WHY MIGHT I HAVE THIS?

PREDISPOSING FACTORS

- Pregnancy
- Diabetes mellitus (*see p.314*)
- Oral contraceptives
- Menstruation

TRIGGERS

- Perfumed bath products
- Spermicides
- Antibiotics
- Stress

TREATMENT PLAN

PRIMARY TREATMENTS

- Vaginal or oral antifungal preparations
- Probiotics and probiotic pessaries

BACK-UP TREATMENTS

- Anti-candida diet

WORTH CONSIDERING

- Homeopathy
- Relaxation and meditation

For an explanation of how treatments are rated, see p.111.

WHY DOES IT OCCUR?

The candida fungus is naturally present in the vagina of many women and does not usually cause problems because its growth is suppressed by the immune system and bacteria that normally live in the vagina. If these harmless bacteria are destroyed, for example by certain antibiotics or spermicides, the candida fungus may multiply. Changes in the levels of a woman's sex hormones, which can occur as a result of pregnancy, menstruation or oral contraceptives, can also result in fewer protective bacteria and allow the condition to become established.

Stress may trigger the condition, as may perfumed bath products and spermicides, both of which can interfere with body's natural defenses against candida. Infection with *C. albicans* can also occur in other areas of the body, such as the mouth (*see* Oral thrush, *p.383*).

Occasionally, male sexual partners can catch thrush. Symptoms of thrush in men include redness, itchiness and soreness of the foreskin and the head of the penis. If these symptoms are present, men should see their doctor for treatment.

SELF-HELP

If you have had thrush before and are confident that your symptoms are due to a recurrence, you can ask your pharmacist for over-the-counter antifungal drugs and pessaries. You can also:
- Try using probiotic supplement capsules as pessaries.
- Be sure to eat a pot of plain, live yoghurt every day.
- Follow an anti-candida diet (*see p.40*).

TREATMENTS IN DETAIL

Conventional Medicine

The doctor may take a swab from your vagina, which will be sent to a laboratory and tested for the fungus. If vaginal thrush is diagnosed, he or she may then prescribe the following treatments. Your doctor will also be able to advise you on self-help measures you can follow.

PRIMARY TREATMENT **PESSARIES AND CREAMS** Studies have shown that vaginal pessaries or creams containing imidazole antifungal drugs, such as clotrimazole, are helpful in relieving the symptoms of thrush.

The antifungal drug nystatin used vaginally may also help. Both of these vaginal treatments are safe to use during pregnancy, when thrush sometimes occurs.

PRIMARY TREATMENT **ORAL DRUGS** Alternatively, oral treatment with a triazole antifungal drug, such as itraconazole, may be preferred. Women who experience recurrent thrush may be treated using long-term antifungal therapy. In some instances women may be given oral drugs to take as well as pessaries or creams to use along with them.

Some vaginal and oral treatments for vaginal thrush are now available over the counter; ask your pharmacist for advice.

CAUTION

Drugs to treat vaginal thrush can cause a range of possible side-effects: ask your doctor or pharmacist to explain these to you.

This light micrograph shows infection with *Candida albicans*. Fungal hyphae (purple strands), by which fungi feed and grow, and spores (small purple dots), by which fungi spread, are visible.

KREOSOTUM The remedy *Kreosotum* may well help if vaginal thrush is accompanied by irritation and soreness of the vulva and if the discharge it causes seems to burn and smells foul.

TREATMENT FOR RECURRENT THRUSH Individualised constitutional treatment by a qualified homeopath may be necessary if thrush is chronic or recurrent. Important medicines that may be used include *Pulsatilla*, *Sepia* and *Thuja*; deciding which of these to use is based on woman's constitutional features (*see p.73*).

Mind–Body Therapies

RELAXATION AND MEDITATION Most women experience at least one episode of vaginal thrush at some time in their adult lives. Since stress is known to be a trigger for attacks of vaginal thrush, it stands to reason that taking steps to reduce stress may help to reduce the frequency of attacks. Chronic stress is known to lower immunity and make the body more vulnerable infection.

If you have recurrent bouts of vaginal thrush, it may be worth keeping a diary recording them to see whether they coincide with periods of stress. If they do, you could try practising a sequence of relaxation exercises every day (*see p.99*). Alternatively, you could try meditating for 20 minutes daily or taking up a mind-body therapy such as yoga.

Nutritional Therapy

The source of *C. albicans* in the body is the digestive tract, which is why treating only the vaginal source of the infection with pessaries and creams often fails to bring lasting relief. The candida fungus may be transferred from the anal area to the vagina when wiping after using the toilet, and it is important to wipe from front to back to help prevent this from occurring.

To treat vaginal thrush efficiently, it is usually necessary to combat the overgrowth of *C. albicans* in the digestive tract. See p.40 for details of how to follow an anti-candida diet.

PRIMARY TREATMENT **PROBIOTICS** If you have recurrent vaginal thrush, try eating 225ml (8oz) of unsweetened live yoghurt every day. This approach is backed up by research.

A study assessed whether daily ingestion of probiotic ("live") yoghurt containing the bacterium *Lactobacillus acidophilus* could prevent vaginal candida infection. A group of women who had recurrent vaginal candida infection ate a yoghurt-free diet for six months and a diet containing yoghurt for six months. A threefold decrease in vaginal candida infections was seen when they ate yoghurt containing *Lactobacillus acidophilus*. Eating 225ml (8oz) of yoghurt containing *Lactobacillus acidophilus* decreased both candidal colonisation of the bowel and infection of the vagina.

PROBIOTIC PESSARIES The use of probiotic supplement capsules inserted vaginally (as a pessary) can often be helpful too. Increasing the number of healthy bacteria in and around the vagina seems to help to keep thrush at bay.

Homeopathy

ISOPATHY A clinical trial indicated that isopathy (treatment of a disease with a homeopathic preparation of the agent that causes the disease) may be effective in alleviating vaginal thrush. To this end, Nelsons in the UK market a homeopathic preparation for vaginal thrush under the name Candida. This preparation is widely available in pharmacies, health food stores and nutrition centres.

HELONIAS Although *Helonias* is not a widely used homeopathic remedy, it is important for vaginal thrush when the discharge is lumpy, like curdled milk. The discharge may be accompanied by low back pain.

PREVENTION PLAN

Try the following if you are prone to vaginal thrush:

- Avoid perfumed bath products and soaps when bathing.
- Do not use vaginal deodorants or scented tampons.
- Wear cotton underwear, or underwear with a cotton gusset.
- Avoid tight jeans or trousers.
- Wipe from front to back when using the toilet.
- Include live yoghurt in your daily diet.

WHAT ARE THE SYMPTOMS?

- Inability to become pregnant after about a year of regular intercourse

WHY MIGHT I HAVE THIS?

PREDISPOSING FACTORS

- Polycystic ovary syndrome (see p.337)
- Endometriosis (see p.334)
- Previous pelvic infection
- Previous abdominal surgery
- Fibroids
- Low thyroid function
- Caffeine
- Smoking
- Nutritional deficiency
- Stress and anxiety
- Being significantly underweight or overweight

TREATMENT PLAN

PRIMARY TREATMENTS

- Treatment of underlying cause (e.g. low thyroid function) where possible

BACK-UP TREATMENTS

- Stimulation of ovulation
- Assisted conception techniques

WORTH CONSIDERING

- Caffeine elimination
- Nutritional supplements
- Western herbal medicine
- Homeopathy
- Avoiding toxic chemicals
- Acupuncture
- Breathing retraining
- Relaxation and group counselling

For an explanation of how treatments are rated, see p.111.

INFERTILITY IN WOMEN

Many couples begin to feel anxious if they have been trying to conceive for several months without success. If they are under about 35, most couples will be advised to keep trying for a year before seeking medical treatment. On average, 80 per cent of couples trying to conceive will be successful within a year, and 90 per cent will be successful within two years. If conception does not occur naturally, there are a number of measures that might help, ranging from dietary changes and psychological therapies to drugs and assisted conception techniques.

WHY DOES IT OCCUR?

For conception to occur naturally, at least one of a woman's two ovaries must be capable of releasing a mature egg; and if fertilisation occurs, the fertilised egg must travel down the fallopian tube and implant in the uterine lining. If any stage in the process is interrupted, natural conception cannot take place. Conception also relies on production of enough healthy sperm by the man to make fertilisation possible, and delivery of this sperm into the vagina. Problems with male fertility and treatment options are described on p.373.

There are various factors that can cause infertility in women.

PROBLEMS WITH OVULATION (the release of a mature egg by an ovary) are a common cause of infertility. Ovulation is controlled by a complex hormonal interaction in the body, and if there is a hormonal imbalance it may not take place regularly or at all. Polycystic ovary syndrome (see p.337) is a common cause of hormonal imbalance. Underactivity of the thyroid gland (see p.319) may also disrupt hormonal balance and affect fertility. In some cases, if women have been taking the contraceptive pill for many years or have used the contraceptive injection, it may take time to re-establish a normal hormonal cycle and pattern of ovulation. Other factors that can disrupt hormone levels and affect fertility include stress, excessive exercise and being significantly underweight or overweight.

PROBLEMS WITH SPERM DELIVERY can also cause infertility. In some women, it may not be possible for the man's sperm to reach the egg, because the cervix produces mucus containing antibodies that destroy the sperm.

DAMAGED FALLOPIAN TUBES may prevent conception. Once an egg has been fertilised, it needs to travel down one of the fallopian tubes to reach the uterus. Damage to the tubes may prevent this and is a common cause of infertility. The fallopian tubes may be damaged by pelvic infections, endometriosis (see p.334) or previous abdominal surgery.

PROBLEMS WITH THE UTERUS may prevent a fertilised egg from implanting and result in infertility. Damage to the uterine lining by an infection such as gonorrhoea is one such problem. Fibroids (benign swellings in the muscle of the uterine wall – see p.332) are another. In rare cases, structural abnormalities of the uterus can cause problems with implantation.

AGE may be a factor in some cases. Fertility in women decreases with age and is significantly lower in women over 35. This is partly due to lower egg quality in older women and partly due to hormonal changes. Fertility also tends to decrease in men as they age, since sperm tend to become less mobile and less robust.

IMPORTANT

If you have been trying to conceive for several months unsuccessfully and you are concerned, go as a couple to see your doctor. This is especially important if one or both partners are over 35.

To increase the chances of conceiving both partners should do the following:

- Avoid smoking or drinking alcohol.
- Eliminate caffeine from the diet.
- Get enough rest and relaxation.
- Eat well and keep to a healthy weight.
- Take adequate, but not excessive, exercise.
- Have sex regularly – particularly halfway through the menstrual cycle (a woman's most fertile time).

TREATMENTS IN DETAIL

Conventional Medicine

TIMING OF INTERCOURSE If both members of a couple are under 35 and have been trying to conceive for a year or less, they may be advised to try timing intercourse so that it occurs about halfway through the woman's menstrual cycle. If this does not help, various other measures may be taken (*see below*).

TESTS Various tests may be arranged to look for underlying causes of fertility problems. If investigations are needed to discover whether there is a problem conceiving, it is important that both the man and the woman are examined. In about half of all cases, the problem lies with the woman and in about a third of all cases, the problem lies with the man. In some couples, no problem can be found, and their infertility is unexplained.

In the first instance, investigations are likely to include blood tests for the woman, to assess hormone levels and whether ovulation is likely to be taking place, as well as semen analysis for the man. If the results of these are normal, a couple may decide to continue trying to conceive for an agreed period of time.

Otherwise, further tests may be arranged. For example, ultrasound scanning may be used to check a woman's pelvic organs. The fallopian tubes may be assessed using a procedure known as hysterosalpingography, in which radio-opaque dye is introduced into the uterus through the cervix and a series of X-rays is taken as the dye passes along the tubes. Alternatively, the passage of dye along the tubes may be monitored during a laparoscopy, in

In this hysterosalpingogram (reproductive contrast X-ray), the woman's right fallopian tube (left on image) cannot be seen because a blockage near the uterus has prevented the contrast medium from reaching it.

which a viewing instrument is passed through a small incision in the wall of the abdomen under a general anaesthetic.

PRIMARY TREATMENT **UNDERLYING CAUSES** If an underlying cause is identified, it will be treated where possible. For example, the hormone supplement thyroxine may be prescribed for an underactive thyroid gland (hypothyroidism). In some cases, it may be possible to repair damaged fallopian tubes with keyhole surgery.

STIMULATING OVULATION Impaired ovulation, as occurs in polycystic ovary syndrome (*see p.337*), may be treated with the drug clomiphene, which stimulates ovulation. There is a risk of multiple pregnancy with this treatment. Clomiphene is taken at the beginning of the cycle and can be continued for up to six months.

ASSISTED CONCEPTION TECHNIQUES If a cause for infertility cannot be found (unexplained infertility) or the cause cannot be treated, various techniques that aim to improve the chances of conception may be considered.

Intrauterine insemination (IUI) may be tried, in which sperm are introduced into the uterus through the cervix via a thin, soft tube. This may be used in cases of unexplained infertility and is only suitable if the fallopian tubes are normal. Drugs may be given to ensure ovulation.

In-vitro fertilisation (IVF) involves removing eggs from the ovaries, adding sperm outside the body and then, if fertilisation occurs, introducing the eggs into the uterus. It is sometimes used for women who have damaged tubes, as well as in cases of unexplained infertility.

Gamete intrafallopian transfer (GIFT) involves removing eggs from the ovaries and introducing them and the sperm into the outer end of the fallopian tube through a fine tube. The egg and sperm can then mix and fertilisation may occur. This may be used for unexplained infertility.

Both IVF and GIFT require a number of fertility drugs to be given to stimulate the ovaries to produce eggs. The ovaries are monitored regularly by ultrasound until the eggs are ready to be removed.

Other methods, such as intracytoplasmic sperm injection (ICSI), are used when there is a problem with the sperm (*see p.373*). Success rates for all treatments depend on the individual couple as well to a certain extent on the clinic they attend.

COUNSELLING Having fertility treatment can affect couples both emotionally and in some cases financially. Support and understanding is needed for both partners during what, for most couples, is a very difficult time. To help couples undergoing treatment, fertility clinics offer counselling. Other psychological treatments, such as group therapy, may also help.

> **CAUTION**
>
> Drugs given to treat infertility can cause a range of possible side-effects: ask your doctor to explain these to you.

Nutritional Therapy

Infertility in women may occasionally be related to low thyroid function (hypothyroidism; see p.319).

Infertility affects about 10 per cent of the population who are of reproductive age

---

ELIMINATING CAFFEINE Caffeine consumption appears to reduce fertility and to increase the length of time it takes to conceive. Just one to one and a half cups of coffee per day is associated with delayed conception and may reduce fertility by half. If you are trying to conceive, you may benefit from giving up coffee, tea and cola.

NUTRITIONAL SUPPLEMENTS Infertility may be related to nutrient deficiencies. A study found that taking a general multivitamin and mineral supplement increased fertility. The multivitamin-mineral supplement appeared to make female ovulatory cycles more regular.

Having said this, a healthy, balanced diet based on fruits, vegetables, nuts, fish, wholegrains and unprocessed foods is very important. However, additional supplementation with a good multivitamin and mineral preparation may help.

Homeopathy

Although there is no published research, many homeopaths report success in treating infertility and repeated miscarriage in the first three months of pregnancy, especially when no organic cause can be found.

SEPIA The most commonly used homeopathic medicine for infertility in women is *Sepia*, which has been found particularly helpful in "post-pill" infertility (trouble conceiving after being on the contraceptive pill). However, it may also be effective in other circumstances.

Women who respond to *Sepia* are said to be depressed, emotionally "flat" and lacking in sex drive; they have low back pain on a regular basis and are often chilly. Yet some women who respond to *Sepia* appear to be happy and vivacious. This is sometimes a mask: these women don't easily "open-up" and discuss their feelings. They feel better from exercise, especially done to music. The normal dose would be *Sepia* 30, two pills weekly for two or three menstrual cycles.

OTHER MEDICINES Other medicines that may be helpful include *Aristolochia*, when the periods are light, irregular or even completely absent. Some doctors use the homeopathic medicines *Oophorinum* and *Folliculinum* (made from human ovary and ovarian follicle respectively) at particular points in the menstrual cycle to stimulate ovulation. This treatment requires specialist advice.

Some women conceive but suffer recurrent early miscarriage in the first three months of pregnancy. Many early miscarriages are due to foetal abnormalities, and it is best to let nature take its course. This problem should not be treated unless it has happened repeatedly. Among the homeopathic medicines recommended for recurrent miscarriage are *Sepia* and *Kalium carbonicum*. *Caulophyllum* and *Helonias* may be appropriate when there is lack of cervical tone.

Western Herbal Medicine

Within certain limits, herbal medicine (Chinese as well as Western) can prove very effective in increasing fertility. It may be useful where the woman is in moderate to good general health, particularly if she is over 35.

However, herbal medicine will not overcome physical factors that impair fertility, such as a blocked fallopian tube, which should have first been excluded before herbal treatment is undertaken. Neither can herbal treatment compensate for very disordered pituitary and ovarian hormone levels. These should be within normal range or only moderately imbalanced before considering herbal treatment.

OBJECTIVES OF TREATMENT Establishing regular ovulation and menstruation is often the first objective of treatment and may involve treatment of an underlying hormonal imbalance. Relevant hormone levels should be monitored. Other factors that may require treatment and are amenable to herbal medicine include heavy menstrual blood loss and anaemia (*see p.331*), endometriosis (*see p.334*), anxiety and stress (*see p.414*), mild thyroid dysfunction (*see p.319*) and problems when the woman's mucus contains antibodies that attack the sperm.

POSSIBLE HERBS A herbalist will prescribe a mix of herbs to treat infertility. He or she will select from a variety of hormonally active remedies, such as the progesterogenic chaste berry (*Vitex agnus-castus*) and the oestrogenic black cohosh (*Cimicifuga racemosa*), helonias (*Chamaelirium luteum*) and wild yam (*Dioscorea villosa*). Circulatory stimulants, such as cayenne pepper (*Capsicum annuum*) and prickly ash (*Zanthoxylum americanum*), and menstrual tonics, such as dong quai (*Angelica sinensis*) and motherwort (*Leonurus cardiaca*), which improve blood flow to the pelvis, may also be chosen. Bitters and liver tonics, which improve nutritional status, may be given as well.

> **CAUTION**
>
> See p.69 before taking a herbal remedy and, if already taking prescribed medication, consult a medical herbalist first.

Environmental Health

Exposure to compounds that may be toxic to egg development or parts of the reproductive tract may affect fertility in women. Women who have problems with fertility or menstruation should consider possible exposure to chemicals at home or work and take measures to decrease it. It may be useful to speak to an environmental health expert to assist with this.

LEAD AND SOLVENTS Lead exposure at high levels may cause spontaneous abortions. Also, exposure to solvents, such as those used in laboratory work or paints, increased spontaneous abortions by two- to four-fold in one research study, and led to infertility and menstrual disorders in other studies.

SMOKING Research has shown that exposure to cigarette smoke may cause infertility or increase the time it takes to conceive. Women should not smoke in pregnancy because exposing a female foetus to cigarette smoke can affect the baby's egg development and future fertility.

CHEMICALS AND ALCOHOL Compounds such as perchloroethylene (used in the dry-cleaning industry), chlorinated hydrocarbons (such as the pesticide DDT, or PCBs), or ethylene oxide (a chemical used in medical and dental clinics) may increase the possibility of spontaneous abortion. Exposure to toluene (a chemical used in some colour-printing businesses) may increase the time it takes for a woman to conceive. Regular alcohol consumption may have a similar effect.

XENOHORMONES Xenohormones are compounds that have a hormonal effect on the human body. Examples include the pesticide DDT and other pesticides, dyes and paints, and bisphenol A, which is a common lining in cans and tins. Some studies show that these compounds may increase spontaneous abortion, although this remains controversial.

Acupuncture

Many infertile couples, and particularly women with infertility, visit acupuncturists. The main aim of the acupuncturist in this situation is to make a clear diagnosis of the underlying energy imbalances that a woman may be experiencing, and then to treat the appropriate organs and pathogens. The aim, within a traditional Chinese context, is to maximise appropriate energy flow around the body and improve the chances of conception.

While there are no hard data, many women report that apparently unexplained infertility resolves after a period of acupuncture. This usually involves two to four treatments a month, taken over a three or four month period.

There is some preliminary work that has been carried out in conditions such as polycystic ovary disease (*see p.337*) that

> ## Many couples with one to three years of unexplained infertility conceive spontaneously

suggests that acupuncture may help to normalise hormone levels in the body. This mechanism may help to explain the positive affect acupuncture may have in treating infertility.

Breathing Retraining

Anxiety is widely considered to contribute to infertility in some instances. It is certainly a common reaction to intensive, high-technology infertility treatments. Anxiety symptoms can usually be helped by practising anti-anxiety breathing exercises or having massage. For a description of suitable breathing methods, see p.62.

Mind–Body Therapies

There is increasing evidence that psychological approaches may be effective in treating the emotional aspects of infertility and may lead to higher conception rates.

RELAXATION TRAINING A study looked at the "relaxation response" in a group of women trying to conceive. As a result of the practice of this well-documented psychological technique the participating women showed significant decreases in anxiety, depression and fatigue and had increased energy levels. In addition, 34 per cent of these women became pregnant within six months of completing the programme. The study further suggested that behavioural treatment should be considered for couples with infertility before and/or in conjunction with reproductive technologies such as intrauterine insemination (IUI), in vitro fertilisation (IVF) and gamete intrafallopian transfer (GIFT).

PSYCHOTHERAPY In a different study, the same research team found infertile women had much higher levels of distress than fertile women and became most distressed between the second and third years of infertility. Overall, participants in the study showed significant psychological improvement after both six and 12 months compared with a control group. Generally, the women who received cognitive behavioural therapy experienced the greatest positive change.

Another study was done to determine the effectiveness of two different group therapies on conception rates in women with infertility of less than two years' duration. The women joined a ten-session cognitive behavioural group, a standard support group or a control group who received no therapy. Group therapies appeared to lead to increased pregnancy rates in women with infertility.

If you are experiencing infertility, you may want to try cognitive behavioural or group therapy.

PREVENTION PLAN

The following may help to maintain fertility:

- Avoid smoking, caffeine and alcohol.
- Maintain a healthy weight.
- Avoid toxic chemicals.
- Make time to relax every day.

WHAT ARE THE SYMPTOMS?

- Lack of interest in sex
- Inability to enjoy sex
- Pain during sex

WHY MIGHT I HAVE THIS?

PREDISPOSING FACTORS

- Anxiety and stress
- Depression
- Relationship difficulties
- Fatigue
- Hormonal changes
- Certain drugs, including oral contraceptives and some antidepressants
- Previous traumatic sexual experience
- Sexual inhibitions
- Poor sexual technique of partner
- Poor communication between couples
- Pregnancy, postpartum or menopause

TREATMENT PLAN

PRIMARY TREATMENTS

- Treatment of any underlying physical cause
- Couple therapy and/or psychotherapy

BACK-UP TREATMENTS

- Arginine and vitamin B6
- Western and Chinese herbal medicine

WORTH CONSIDERING

- Homeopathy
- Manipulation therapies
- Acupuncture

For an explanation of how treatments are rated, see p.111.

SEXUAL PROBLEMS IN WOMEN

Many women experience a sexual problem of some kind during their lives. Some of the most common include a lack of or decrease in sex drive, failure to achieve orgasm and painful intercourse. If an underlying physical cause can be identified, it will usually be treated as a first course of action. Since many sexual problems involve mental as well as physical factors, psychological therapies are often an important part of treatment. Nutritional supplements, homeopathy, herbal treatments, acupuncture and manipulation therapy may also help.

WHY DOES IT OCCUR?

Sexual difficulties are usually the result of psychological or physical problems, or may be a combination of the two. Upbringing and attitudes to sex may play a role.

PROBLEMS WITH SEX DRIVE A decrease in sex drive is more common with increasing age and may be seen as part of the ageing process. As sex drive varies among individuals, a woman's sex drive should only be judged in comparison with her own usual behaviour, not in comparison to the claims of other people. Many women find that their interest in sex declines after childbirth, and some women lose interest in sex during pregnancy. This is usually temporary, as is the case with women who report a decline in interest in sex around and after the menopause. In all of these cases, hormonal changes are likely to play a role. Low thyroid function (*see p.319*) and low adrenal gland function can also be responsible.

Psychological conditions, such as anxiety disorders, depression and stress, can also have an adverse effect on a woman's sex drive. Tiredness is a common factor. Relationship difficulties are also likely to reduce sexual desire and arousal, perhaps more in a woman than a man. Some drugs, including oral contraceptives and some antidepressant drugs (such as paroxetine), can also cause a decrease in sex drive.

PROBLEMS WITH ORGASM Failure to achieve orgasm is a common problem in women and is usually due to psychological factors, including anxiety about sexual performance, a previous unpleasant sexual experience or sexual inhibitions. The latter may be due to a strict upbringing regarding sex or physical, emotional or sexual abuse in childhood.

Poor sexual technique between partners is also a common contributing factor in failure to achieve orgasm; often insufficient time is allowed for a woman to become fully aroused. Sexual inexperience or lack of communication between partners can also make orgasm difficult. Certain physical disorders, such as chronic constipation, can in rare cases affect a woman's ability to reach orgasm. Probably around half of women achieve orgasm through clitoral stimulation rather than penetrative sex and many couples are happy with this.

PAINFUL INTERCOURSE Painful intercourse (dyspareunia) may have either a psychological or physical cause. Superficial dyspareunia is felt around the entrance to the vagina and in the lower part of the vagina. This may be due to psychological factors, such as anxiety, guilt or fear of sexual penetration. These factors can also lead to vaginismus (*see below*). Physical causes of painful intercourse include infection or vaginal atrophy (thinning of the vaginal

IMPORTANT

If you experience persistent pelvic pain or painful intercourse, see your doctor as soon as possible to rule out any serious underlying causes, such as pelvic inflammatory disease.

tissue), which occurs after the menopause; genital tract infections; and poor vaginal lubrication, which may be related to psychological factors or insufficient arousal or may accompany vaginal atrophy.

Pain that is felt higher in the vagina and deep within the pelvis during intercourse (known as deep pareunia) may be due to a disorder of the pelvic cavity, such as a pelvic infection or endometriosis (*see p.334*).

VAGINISMUS This condition, in which the pelvic floor muscles go into spasm before or during intercourse, is usually due to psychological factors and often occurs in women who believe that penetration will be painful. This belief may be due to a previous traumatic sexual experience, sexual abuse or painful vaginal examination. Another cause of vaginismus is fear of pregnancy. Anxiety and guilt about sex can be a contributing factors.

TREATMENTS IN DETAIL

Conventional Medicine

A doctor will take a careful history to look for evidence of physical and psychological causes. He or she will aim to treat the underlying cause where possible.

PRIMARY TREATMENT **PHYSICAL CAUSES** Management of physical causes may include changing prescribed medication, laxatives for chronic constipation or antibiotics for genital tract infections. Vaginal atrophy may be relieved by lubrication or hormone replacement cream (*see p.339*), which may be used locally in the vagina. Poor lubrication may be improved by allowing time to achieve adequate arousal during foreplay and using lubricating jelly if needed.

PRIMARY TREATMENT **PSYCHOLOGICAL FACTORS** Various options are available to address psychological factors that contribute to sexual problems. For example, relaxation techniques may help with stress. Depression may be treated with drugs and psychotherapy as appropriate. Psychotherapy may also be used to help with anxiety and sex therapy may be needed to address attitudes to sex, which may be deeply entrenched. Your doctor may refer you to a specialist for this. Sex therapy can also

focus on key issues such as communication between partners and sexual technique (*see Psychological Therapy, below*).

Nutritional Therapy

ARGININE Sexual function and responsiveness, in both men and women, is to a degree dependent on the supply of blood to the genital organs. Dilation of blood vessels, allowing increased blood flow, depends on a substance called nitric oxide. The amino acid arginine is essential for the formation of nitric oxide in the body and many studies have shown that it improves male sexual function (*see p.376*).

One study assessed the effect of a supplement called containing arginine in combination with herbs, vitamin and minerals in a group of women. After four weeks, more than 70 per cent of the group taking the supplement reported greater satisfaction with their sex lives, compared with only 42 per cent of women taking a placebo (inactive medication). Notable improvements were observed in sexual desire, increased vaginal lubrication, frequency of sexual intercourse and orgasm, and clitoral sensation.

VITAMIN B6 Women taking oral contraceptives may have low levels of vitamin B6, and this has been linked to decreased sex drive in some women. Vitamin B6 is needed in the formation of many brain chemicals involved in pleasure, sensation and mood (such as dopamine, serotonin and acetylcholine). Although no studies support this, vitamin B6 supplements may improve sex drive in women who are deficient in this nutrient. Taking 25–50mg of vitamin B6 daily may help.

CAUTION

Ask your doctor for advice before taking vitamin B6 supplements with certain drugs, such as levodopa and phenobarbital. (*For more information, see p.46.*)

Homeopathy

For decreased sex drive, perhaps relating to depression or age, the most commonly used medicines are *Causticum* and *Sepia*.

A number of studies have looked at homeopathic treatment of childhood sexual abuse and its consequences. Several homeopathic medicines are reported to be helpful where sexual problems in adult life are a result of childhood abuse, including *Sepia*, *Platina*, *Phosphoric acid* and *Staphysagria*.

CAUSTICUM Women likely to respond to *Causticum* are often quite depressed as a result of a long period of stress, but this often manifests itself in strong feelings about injustice. These women are often campaigners for human or animal rights. A very characteristic feature is that they find it too painful to watch images of human suffering. Other features include urge or stress incontinence (leakage of urine when the bladder is full or if they sneeze or cough), recurrent hoarseness or a tickling cough coming from the throat, and localised paralyses, for instance of the face (Bell's Palsy).

Causticum and *Staphysagria* are medicines that are often used together, with *Causticum* often being used after *Staphysagria* as a follow-up treatment.

Up to 70 per cent of couples experience problems with sex at some time

STAPHYSAGRIA In the context of sexual problems, *Staphysagria* is an important medicine; its keynote is said to be suppressed indignation.

Women who respond to *Staphysagria* may have suffered sexual assault or an abusive relationship as an adult and are tremendously angry about what has been done to them. However, this anger may be suppressed and expressed through physical symptoms, particularly recurrent bladder problems (*see p.238*) that have no identifiable cause. Sometimes the anger is expressed, in which case these patients can often be prickly, sensitive and generally difficult to deal with.

SEPIA Women who respond to *Sepia* are flat and are often indifferent to others. They are depressed and irritable, particularly with their families, and have no interest in sex. They often suffer from low back pain and a range of menstrual or menopausal problems.

PLATINA Women who respond to *Platina* often have either a sensation of numbness or the opposite, with excessive sensitivity or itching of the genitalia that is made worse by sexual activity and prevents intercourse. They may "put on airs" and appear haughty, but this may be a defensive mechanism to hide their sense of shame. They may be very depressed and fear violence, especially from their partners. *Platina* patients (and *Staphysagria* patients, *see above*) may also have other psychosexual problems, apart from loss of sex drive. These may include such things as promiscuity and sexual perversion.

PHOSPHORIC ACID Patients who respond to *Phosphoric acid* are quite similar to *Sepia* patients, being emotionally flat and worn out, with no interest in sex. Symptoms that suggest *Phosphoric acid* might be suitable, rather than *Sepia*, include weak memory and poor concentration, along with diarrhoea or loose bowels.

Western Herbal Medicine

Western herbal medicine can be used to treat sexual problems when they are related to problems with circulation, mild hormonal imbalances or depression and anxiety. If problems are longstanding, it is probably best to consult a trained herbal practitioner for help with treatment.

HERBS TO IMPROVE CIRCULATION Ginkgo (*Ginkgo biloba*) helps to increase peripheral circulation and may therefore improve circulation to the sexual organs. This herb should be taken at a dose of 50–100g per day to see whether sexual responsiveness improves.

Other herbs that may be used to stimulate the circulation include hawthorn (*Crataegus monogyna*), ginger root (*Zingiber officinalis*), rosemary (*Rosmarinus officinalis*) and prickly ash (*Zanthoxylum clavaherculis*). These herbs may be used alone or in combination. Three cups of tea per day, or 20–30 drops of tincture taken three times each day, is the usual dose.

IMPROVING HORMONAL BALANCE Mild hormonal imbalances may be treated with various herbs, of which the most important is probably chaste berry (*Vitex agnus-castus*). However, this herb must be taken over a relatively long period of time (12–18 months) before its effects are seen.

Damiana (*Turnera diffusa*) appears to support testosterone levels, which may be too low in women with reduced or absent sex drive. Milk thistle (*Silybum marianum*), vervain (*Verbena officinalis*) and dandelion root (*Taraxacum officinale*) are all valuable for supporting the liver and restoring hormonal balance. They may be used in combination to make a tea (or a tincture), of which one cup (or 15–20 drops) should be taken before each meal. Saw palmetto (*Serenoa repens*) may also help to restore hormonal balance.

HERBS FOR DEPRESSION-RELATED PROBLEMS St John's wort (*Hypericum perforatum*) may be used to alleviate depression, as may kava kava (*Piper methysticum*), lemon balm (*Melissa officinalis*), gotu kola (*Centella asiatica*), skullcap (*Scutellaria lateriflora*) and passionflower (*Passiflora incarnata*). These herbs may be combined equally to make a tea (or a tincture), which should be taken one cup (or 20–30 drops) two times each day. It may take up to two months before results are apparent.

> **CAUTION**
>
> See p.69 before taking a herbal remedy and, if you are already taking prescribed medication, consult a medical herbalist first.

Chinese Herbal Medicine

Traditional Chinese herbalists may treat sexual problems using herbs that strengthen the adrenal glands and improve muscle strength. These herbs may be combined with blood-strengthening and moistening herbs, which act to reduce stress and increase sexual fluids.

ADRENAL TONICS Herbs that act on the adrenal glands are especially important for women, whose sexual problems are often related to fatigue and/or hormonal imbalances. Nettle (*Urtica dioica*) is important for women who have long-term exhaustion, which may be coupled with autoimmune problems and allergies. Other important adrenal tonics include clove (*Syzygium aromaticum*), sage (*Salvia officinalis*) and fenugreek (*Trigonella foenum-graecum*).

> ### Women between the ages of 35 and 65 are more likely to experience problems with sex

GINSENG Traditional Chinese herbalists have used ginseng (*Panax ginseng*) to treat sexual problems for many centuries. It is believed to improve hormonal function. A study at Yale University School of Medicine showed that ginseng stimulates nitric oxide, which assists the body in a number of circulatory functions, improving blood vessel dilation and blood pressure regulation. Ginseng may be combined with Solomon's seal (*Polygonatum multiflorum*) to balance its stimulating effects.

> **CAUTION**
>
> Do not take ginseng if you have high blood pressure. See also p.69.

Acupuncture

Acupuncture may be useful in treating sexual problems, particularly when it is combined with other therapies such as herbal treatments, psychological therapies and massage or manipulation therapies. Case studies have shown that women with loss of libido and a history of prior sexual abuse have responded well to acupuncture, although it was recommended that they persist with psychological therapies to help them come to terms with their past

CHIROPRACTIC TREATMENT FOR SEXUAL PROBLEMS

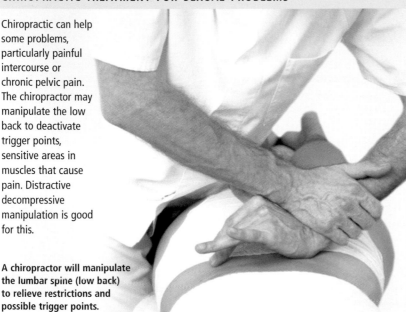

Chiropractic can help some problems, particularly painful intercourse or chronic pelvic pain. The chiropractor may manipulate the low back to deactivate trigger points, sensitive areas in muscles that cause pain. Distractive decompressive manipulation is good for this.

A chiropractor will manipulate the lumbar spine (low back) to relieve restrictions and possible trigger points.

trauma. An initial course of 3–4 treatments is likely to be given. If the response is good, treatment may be given once or twice weekly for two months, with maintenance treatment twice yearly after that.

Bodywork Therapies

Sexual dysfunction that develops because of painful intercourse or chronic pelvic pain can sometimes be eased or treated by appropriate chiropractic or osteopathic manipulation, or by deactivation of active trigger points that produce pain in the pelvic organs. Trigger points can be deactivated by acupuncture, as well as by manual pressure and stretching techniques as used by osteopaths and chiropractors.

A particular form of chiropractic treatment, using a technique known as distractive decompressive manipulation of the lumbar spine (this is the low back, from where the nerves that supply the pelvic organs emerge), has been shown in suitable individuals to be especially effective in relieving the cause (commonly pain) of some women's sexual dysfunction.

Psychological Therapies

Female sexual disorders can generally be divided into four main categories: low sexual desire, difficulties in sexual arousal,

difficulties in achievement of orgasm and pain (and related anxiety) associated with sexual activity.

PRIMARY TREATMENT **COUPLE THERAPY** is used to treat sexual dysfunction and is perhaps the most eclectic of the talking therapies, in that it combines a variety of approaches, including cognitive-behavioural therapy (CBT) and psychodynamic ideas. A woman with sexual problems is usually treated with her partner on the assumption that their relationship is stable enough to enable clear communication to take place. If the relationship is not stable, couple or marital therapy may be more appropriate, because some of the sexual difficulties may be an expression of a troubled relationship.

PRIMARY TREATMENT **SEX THERAPY** Pioneered by Masters and Johnson in 1970, sex therapy normally follows a series of stages. An initial assessment is followed by a formulation or plan of therapy. This is usually followed by counselling, which may have psychodynamic and CBT components. This stage is usually accompanied by "homework" tasks and simple sex education. The couple may be asked to examine their attitudes to sex and how these ideas were formed earlier in their life. Then they may be asked to try out new

ways of touching each other without focusing on each other's genitals (known as non-genital sensate focus) before moving into more overt genital contact (genital sensate focus). Masturbation exercises may also be encouraged, particularly for women who have difficulty in achieving orgasm. Other methods such as gradual introduction of the penis into the vagina with the woman in control can be used for problems such as vaginismus.

RESEARCH A number of studies support the use of sex therapy for treating sexual problems. For low sexual desire, researchers worked with 32 couples and found that nearly 70 per cent of the women said they had totally or partially regained interest in sex. Another study examined the effect of working with couple and women-only treatment. They found that both methods achieved significant results. Researchers also examined the use of CBT for both women and men and found it effective in increasing positive attitudes towards sex.

The treatment of women who have difficulty in achieving orgasm has been studied by a number of researchers. They found that the Masters and Johnson method was effective in helping women achieve orgasm, although in one study this was achieved mainly through masturbation. The treatment of vaginismus has also been positive. In a study of 30 couples in which the women had vaginismus, researchers found that the problem was totally or largely resolved in 80 per cent of the women.

PREVENTION PLAN

The following measures can help prevent sexual problems:

- Try to get adequate rest so that you do not become over-tired. This is especially important after the birth of a baby, or if you have young children.

- Practise relaxation exercises or yoga regularly to reduce levels of stress and anxiety.

- Do pelvic floor exercises regularly, and every day if possible.

- Eat a healthy, balanced diet and maintain a normal weight.

Pregnancy
& Childbirth

During pregnancy and childbirth the body undergoes immense changes, which can be stressful, both physically and emotionally. Conventional medicine plays a vital role in protecting the health of mother and child, but supportive complementary therapies should not be underestimated, particularly as pregnancy is a time when many drugs should be avoided.

MORNING SICKNESS

The nausea known as morning sickness is one of the most common complaints of early pregnancy. Its name is misleading as it is not always confined to the morning but may also be present during the day and the evening. However, it usually clears up by the 14th to 16th week of pregnancy and, although it is unpleasant, it is not usually dangerous. Dietary changes and other measures such as acupressure can relieve morning sickness, but a pregnant woman should not take any remedies for nausea without first consulting her doctor.

WHAT ARE THE SYMPTOMS?

- A feeling of nausea, which may be worse on awakening
- Vomiting
- Sensitivity to strong smells, such as garlic

WHY MIGHT I HAVE THIS?

TRIGGERS

- Exposure to strong smells
- Fatty foods
- Large, infrequent meals

TREATMENT PLAN

PRIMARY TREATMENTS

- Small, frequent meals (*see Self-help*)
- Ginger
- Acupressure
- Acupuncture

BACK-UP TREATMENTS

- Intravenous fluids and drugs (for hyperemesis gravidarum)
- Nutritional therapy

WORTH CONSIDERING

- Homeopathy
- Chamomile and slippery elm
- Osteopathy and reflexology

For an explanation of how treatments are rated, see p.111.

WHY DOES IT OCCUR?

It is not known why morning sickness occurs. Some women do not develop it at all, while others may feel sick most of the time during their pregnancies. It is thought that the rapidly increasing levels of certain hormones, perhaps human chorionic gonadotrophin (a hormone produced by the placenta), during early pregnancy are at least partially responsible for the condition. Although a woman with morning sickness may not feel well for much of the time, she should continue to eat and gain weight. Morning sickness is not dangerous for either the mother or the baby unless vomiting becomes so severe that no fluids or food can be kept down at all. This is known as hyperemesis gravidarum and may cause dehydration, chemical imbalances and weight loss. This requires hospital admission for intravenous fluids and possibly antihistamines or antivomiting drugs.

SELF-HELP

- Eat small, frequent meals high in protein.
- Nibble dry biscuits and crackers.
- Sip chamomile tea.
- Eat ginger or drink it as a tea.
- Drink plenty of water.
- Press the P6 point (*see Acupressure*).

IMPORTANT

Consult your doctor before taking any remedies (conventional or herbal) for morning sickness. If vomiting becomes severe and you are unable to keep down any fluid or food, see your doctor urgently.

TREATMENTS IN DETAIL

Conventional Medicine

No medical treatment is usually required for mild nausea and occasional vomiting in pregnancy. More persistent vomiting may require tests to look for a possible underlying cause, such as a urinary tract infection, and admission to hospital may be necessary, where intravenous fluids may be given.

In hyperemesis gravidarum, antihistamines such as promethazine or the antivomiting drug metoclopramide may be prescribed. However, these treatments are only rarely needed. Although there is no evidence to suggest that they cause harm in pregnancy, they are used only when absolutely necessary. If vomiting is persistent, vitamin supplements, particularly vitamin B6, may be necessary (*see below*).

CAUTION

Drugs for hyperemesis gravidarum can cause a range of possible side-effects.: ask your doctor to explain these to you.

Nutritional Therapy

PRIMARY TREATMENT **DIETARY CHANGES** Nausea in pregnancy has been associated with a poor diet and with eating large, infrequent meals. In practice, morning sickness appear to be worse on an empty stomach. Symptoms may be relieved by eating small, frequent meals, to help keep blood-sugar levels stable. Foods that are low in fat are particularly important, since fatty foods, such as red meat, dairy products and fried foods, tend to make nauseous feelings worse. Improving digestion by chewing food thoroughly and not drinking too much fluid with meals can also help.

NUTRITIONAL SUPPLEMENTS Vitamin B6 may be beneficial in relieving nausea and vomiting in pregnancy. One 1990s study found that pyridoxine (a form of vitamin B6) at 30mg per day was effective in relieving the severity of nausea in early pregnancy. There is evidence that vitamin C taken together with vitamin K may be very useful in relieving the symptoms of morning sickness. In one uncontrolled study, women who received 5mg of vitamin K and 25mg of vitamin C per day reported the complete disappearance of morning sickness within three days. It might be worth trying a multivitamin and mineral supplement to control morning sickness.

> **CAUTION**
>
> Women who are pregnant, trying to conceive or breastfeeding should not take a supplement containing more than 2,000IU of vitamin A without their doctor's advice.

Homeopathy

IPECACUANHA The most commonly used homeopathic medicine for morning sickness is *Ipecacuanha* (also known as *Ipecac*). Women who respond to it have severe and constant nausea, retching and vomiting, and vomiting does not relieve the nausea. The vomiting may be accompanied by nosebleeds and/or coughing. It should be taken in the 12C strength, two pills four times daily, or more frequently if required.

NUX VOMICA Other commonly suggested medicines for morning sickness include *Nux vomica*. It is indicated for women who have nausea that is much worse in the morning, often waking them early. There is often severe nausea and a lot of retching, but relatively little vomiting. All the senses seem oversensitive, with every smell making the nausea worse, noises seeming too loud and bright lights hurting the eyes.

COCCULUS AND SEPIA Women who respond to *Cocculus* have dizziness and are sensitive to movement. Travelling makes the nausea much worse. Those who respond to *Sepia* have nausea that is made much worse by the smell of food, especially frying food. These women may crave sharp, acidic foods (such as pickles or lemons), which may temporarily relieve the sickness. There is often a heavy low back pain; these women may feel very tired and emotionally "flat".

Western Herbalism

SAFETY ISSUES As a rule, herbal remedies (in common with all medicines) should not be taken during the first three months of pregnancy, and some herbs should be avoided throughout pregnancy. That said, appropriate herbal treatment may be a safe and effective option for pregnancy problems such as morning sickness. There are some foods, such as ginger (*Zingiber officinale*), that have medicinal properties and in general it is this category of herbal medicines that can be safely used during pregnancy.

Many herbs are traditional remedies for morning sickness, such as ginger, chamomile (*Matricaria recutita*) and slippery elm (*Ulmus rubra*). With the exception of ginger, little research has been undertaken.

PRIMARY TREATMENT **GINGER** Over the last 20 years, research into ginger has slowly gathered pace, establishing that the dried root has powerful anti-inflammatory and anti-emetic activity. A number of clinical trials have shown ginger to be as effective as conventional treatments in preventing travel sickness and post-operative nausea in patients undergoing surgery. In one 1990 double-blind, randomised, crossover trial 30 pregnant women with morning sickness took four 250mg capsules of dried ginger a day. It significantly helped to relieve symptoms.

CHAMOMILE AND SLIPPERY ELM Tea made with chamomile is a useful, safe treatment for morning sickness: its ability to soothe and relieve nausea and indigestion is well established. Slippery elm capsules can help settle the digestion – the powder may also be taken mixed with water, though its sticky consistency is often off-putting.

PROFESSIONAL ADVICE There is a range of other herbs, some with hormonal activity, which are commonly prescribed by practitioners. If self-medication with ginger, chamomile or slippery elm is unsuccessful, it is worth consulting a herbalist.

Acupuncture

PRIMARY TREATMENT Acupuncture is particularly useful for morning sickness, since ailments that occur in early pregnancy are problematic to treat with medicines because of the risk of side-effects. There is absolutely no doubt that acupuncture provides a safe treatment for morning sickness. A number of clinical trials have examined applying pressure to the P6 acupuncture point (*see below*), which helps even quite severe morning sickness. Vickers produced a systematic review of a large number of clinical trials looking at acupuncture and nausea. Clinical trials carried out subsequently confirmed its positive effect. Some of the studies include using acupressure on the P6 acupuncture point.

Bodywork Therapies

PRIMARY TREATMENT **ACUPRESSURE AND REFLEXOLOGY** A number of research studies have confirmed that pressure applied to the Pericardium acupoint 6 on the forearm (known in Chinese medicine as *Neiguan*), can significantly reduce the morning sickness and nausea. This point lies about two of your own thumb widths above the front wrist crease, in line with the ring finger (*see p.154*). Find a tender area on one wrist, by careful probing, and then press this firmly for five to 10 minutes. Treat yourself in this way as often as needed. You can also buy special wrist straps ("sea-bands") which can be worn to produce a constant pressure on this point. Reflexology has also been shown to be useful.

OSTEOPATHY Experience suggests that osteopathic treatment that alleviates spinal imbalances and restrictions can improve morning sickness. However, no studies as yet confirm this.

> **PREVENTION PLAN**
>
> The following measures may help:
> - Eat little and often.
> - Avoid fried, fatty or spicy foods.
> - Eat something bland, such as crackers, before getting up in the morning.

TREATMENT PLAN

PRIMARY TREATMENTS

For pain relief:
- Abdominal breathing techniques
- Relaxation and self-hypnosis
- Drug-free methods, e.g. TENS
- Entonox and other drugs for pain
- Epidural analgesia

To accelerate labour:
- Oxytocin injections

BACK-UP TREATMENTS

- Active labour
- Massage and birthing pool
- Forceps or ventouse delivery
- Caesarean section

WORTH CONSIDERING

- Homeopathy
- Intradermal water blocks
- Acupuncture
- Mind–body therapies

For an explanation of how treatments are rated,
see p.111.

LABOUR

The process of childbirth, known as labour, usually begins around the 40th week of pregnancy. Labour has three distinct stages: the first, when the uterus contracts and the cervix widens; the second, when the baby passes through the birth canal; and the third, when the placenta is delivered. Many things can be done to make labour a more comfortable process, including taking pain-relieving drugs and having a birthing partner present to give psychological support. Techniques such as massage, acupuncture, relaxation and self-hypnosis can also help.

HOW DOES IT OCCUR?

STAGE ONE The trigger for labour to begin is not known, but it may be a surge of the hormone oxytocin, which causes the uterus to contract. The first signs of labour are usually strong and mildly painful contractions of the uterus. The plug of mucus that has been blocking the cervix during pregnancy usually comes away at this time or some time up to 10 days before, and is known as the "show". A small amount of blood and mucus is passed from the vagina when this happens, but many women are unaware of it. Additionally, the amniotic sac that has been surrounding the baby usually ruptures either shortly before or during the first stage of labour and is often referred to as the waters breaking. If a woman's waters break before labour is established she usually notices it, but if it happens during the first stage of labour it may go unnoticed. Contractions become stronger and more painful as labour progresses and the cervix becomes wider (dilates).

STAGE TWO The second stage of labour begins when the cervix is fully dilated to 10cm (4in). At this stage the baby passes from the uterus through the vagina and is born. The second stage is much quicker than the first stage and usually lasts between one and two hours. The baby's head presses on the pelvic floor, causing an overwhelming urge in the mother to bear down, or push. When the baby's head is visible at the opening of the vagina, the birth is imminent.

STAGE THREE The third stage of labour takes place shortly after the baby is born. The placenta, which has been nourishing the baby during the pregnancy, separates from the inner surface of the uterus, which resumes contracting to expel it. Blood vessels in the uterus also contract to stop the bleeding.

DIFFERENT EXPERIENCES OF LABOUR The length of each stage of labour varies and may partly depend on the number of times a woman has given birth previously – second and subsequent labours tend to be shorter than the first.

The contractions women experience during labour are painful, and the birth of the baby is also painful and may be exhausting if it takes a long time. Many pregnant women are understandably concerned about the length of labour and pain. However, different women have different pain tolerance, so the experience of labour and birth is not the same for every woman. Becoming familiar with the process of labour can help women know what to expect at each stage and to approach the birth and pain relief with an open mind.

SELF-HELP

The following suggestions may help to make your labour more comfortable:
- Attend antenatal classes regularly and discuss any worries with your midwife.
- Make sure you have a birth partner who will support you in having the type of birth you want.
- Practise guided imagery and relaxation during pregnancy (see p.99).
- Make a birth plan beforehand but be prepared to change it during the labour.
- Take regular, gentle exercise during pregnancy – get advice from your midwife or doctor about what is appropriate.

Conventional Medicine

CHOICES IN LABOUR There are various options for pain relief during labour. Some women choose to avoid medication and rely on breathing techniques and relaxation methods instead (*see below*). Many women choose a combination of natural methods and drugs. The help and encouragement of a supportive birthing partner can be invaluable. Attending antenatal classes can also be helpful in making prospective mothers and their partners aware of what may happen and the many options available to enable them to cope with labour.

PRIMARY TREATMENT | **DRUG-FREE METHODS** Taking up different positions during labour may help relieve discomfort. TENS (transcutaneous electrical nerve stimulation) is sometimes helpful, particularly in the early stages. TENS can help to relieve pain by delivering tiny electrical impulses through electrodes on the back. Why this helps is not fully understood.

USING TENS IN LABOUR

A transcutaneous electrical nerve stimulation (TENS) machine is a pain-relieving device that delivers small electrical impulses through electrodes on the skin. The wearer can control the intensity and timing of the impulses.

PRIMARY TREATMENT | **ENTONOX AND OTHER DRUGS** Entonox is a mixture of nitrous oxide and oxygen, commonly known as "gas and air", which is delivered through a mask or a mouthpiece. It is a relatively mild analgesic but its effects come on rapidly. However, not all women find entonox helpful and it may cause nausea and dizziness.

The drug pethidine may be given as an injection into the muscle. It has a mild analgesic effect and may cause women to feel drowsy and confused. Antinausea medication is usually given with it. Pethidine may also cause sedation in the newborn, which is reversed by another drug, naloxone.

Some women choose to have an epidural, which is an injection of local anaesthetic into the epidural space (the space surrounding the membranes that envelop the spinal cord) in the low back. The anaesthetic can either be given continuously or individual doses can be given intermittently as needed. An epidural can give complete pain relief; in fact all sensation from the top of the abdomen down is usually lost, although women can still feel pressure. Once the epidural is set up, movement is limited and regular monitoring of pulse rate and blood pressure is required. Troublesome side-effects are relatively uncommon, but may include severe headaches.

PRIMARY TREATMENT | **DRUGS AND OTHER METHODS** may assist labour. Measures may be taken to speed up the first and second stages of labour. In the first stage, if the cervix is dilating too slowly, a doctor or midwife may break the membranes if this has not occurred. This may speed up the process. The drug oxytocin may be given by intravenous infusion to increase the frequency, strength and duration of contractions. Careful monitoring is needed and the dose is adjusted accordingly, as oxytocin may cause various side-effects. Eventually a Caesarean section may be

> # The length of a full-term pregnancy may be anywhere between 37 and 43 weeks

recommended if there has been little or no progress and the baby's well-being is considered to be at risk.

If the second stage of labour is prolonged, oxytocin may again be given. If the baby is still not delivered, an assisted delivery using forceps or a ventouse (suction device) may be advised.

Oxytocin may also be given routinely in combination with ergometrine, which also stimulates the muscles of the uterus to contract, in preparation for the third stage of labour. These drugs help the uterus expel the placenta and reduce the bleeding from the uterine surface.

CAUTION

Drugs and procedures to assist labour have a range of possible side-effects: ask your midwife or doctor to explain these to you.

Homeopathy

CAULOPHYLLUM There is evidence from clinical trials in the 1990s that homeopathic treatment decreased the duration of labour and reduced the number of Caesarean sections required.

The main medicine used in the trials was *Caulophyllum*. It is given for delay in labour, when the cervix is rigid, preventing it from fully dilating. It can also be used in preparation for labour, when it should be taken in the 6C strength twice daily, starting between the 34th and 36th weeks of pregnancy, with an additional three doses at half-hourly intervals when labour starts.

OTHER MEDICINES A number of other homeopathic medicines may help with labour problems, but these should be used only on the advice of a midwife or other health professional trained in homeopathy. One of the most frequently suggested is *Actea racemosa* (also known as *Cimicifuga racemosa*). It is appropriate when the contractions are weak and irregular, although

MASSAGE FOR BACK PAIN IN LABOUR

Many women experience pain in the low back during labour. This can be helped greatly by simple massage techniques, which can be done by a carer or a birthing partner. Diluted essential oils of lavender and/or rose help the hands glide over the skin and may also heighten the relaxing effect of massage for the mother.

Massaging the low back during labour can help relieve pain in this area, which may be caused by the baby's head pressing on nerves as it passes through the pelvis.

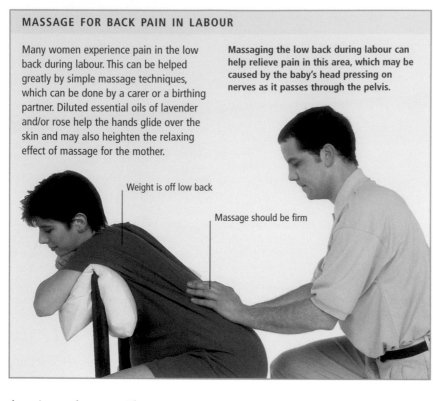

Weight is off low back

Massage should be firm

the pain may be severe. The woman may become almost hysterical, as well as very loquacious.

Other homeopathic medicines that your practitioner may use include *Pulsatilla*, when the contractions are irregular and the woman feels faint with them. Typically she feels better for a breeze or being fanned. She may be weepy and emotional.

Chamomilla and *Magnesia phosphoricum* have a reputation for helping with labour pains. Women who respond to *Chamomilla* are typically very angry, responding to the pain by shouting and swearing. Strangely perhaps, the only thing that seems to help these women is moving around quite vigorously.

Women who respond to *Magnesia phosphoricum* have quite a different character. By contrast, they are exhausted rather than bad-tempered from the pain, which is severe and of a cramping character. Warmth over the lower abdomen (from a hot-water bottle or heating pad) provides some pain relief.

Acupuncture

Acupuncture may be used both to induce labour in cases where this is necessary, and to relieve pain during it.

ACUPUNCTURE TO INDUCE LABOUR Acupuncture has commonly been used to induce ripening of the cervix and indeed full normal labour. However, a review of the research available in 2003 failed to show that acupuncture helped ripen the cervix or induce labour. It is quite possible that acupuncture will induce cervical ripening and consequent labour, but better-designed randomised controlled trials are needed to evaluate the role of this treatment in labour.

Usually two or three daily sessions of acupuncture are required and needles are applied to specific points. It is usual to give electroacupuncture to induce labour, which involves electrical stimulation of the needles.

ACUPUNCTURE FOR BREECH PRESENTATION Traditional Chinese Medicine uses moxibustion (burning herbs to stimulate acupuncture points) of acupoint BL67 (located beside the outer corner of the fifth toenail) to promote turning of babies in breech presentation. Its effect may be through increasing activity of the baby in the uterus. A randomised controlled trial published in 1998 evaluated the efficacy of this therapy for breech presentations and showed it produced good results.

ACUPUNCTURE FOR PAIN RELIEF Acupuncture has been used extensively to alleviate pain during labour, and there are a number of clinical trials indicating that it may have both a substantial and immediate effect.

A study involving 46 women in labour compared the pain intensity, degree of relaxation and delivery outcomes of those who had acupuncture with those who did not. Acupuncture during labour significantly reduced the need for epidural pain relief and allowed the women who had it a greater degree of relaxation than the women who did not receive acupuncture.

Acupuncture had no negative effects and so it could be a good alternative for women seeking an alternative to drugs for pain relief during childbirth. Further trials with a large number of women are needed to clarify whether the main effect of acupuncture during labour is pain relief or relaxation.

Both body and ear acupuncture have been used to alleviate labour pain: the advantage of the latter technique is that it can be controlled by the mother during labour and delivery. Acupuncture-related techniques, such as TENS (transcutaneous electrical nerve stimulation, see p.359), have also proved to be helpful in reducing pain in labour.

Bodywork Therapies

The value of five non-drug methods for relieving pain in labour – continuous labour support, baths, touch and massage, maternal movement and positioning, and intradermal water blocks – were evaluated in a review of research evidence. All five methods were researched in controlled studies and were found to be effective in reducing labour pain and improving other obstetric outcomes. They are all considered safe when used appropriately.

LABOUR SUPPORT Continuous labour support means having a birth partner who can provide physical comforting, touch and massage, assistance with positioning, bathing and grooming, hot-water bottles or ice-packs as required, and emotional support and information. The latter includes non-medical advice and acting as a mediator between the woman and her medical staff.

LABOURING IN WATER Simple baths are " … safe and most effective if the water temperature does not exceed body temperature and if the bath is withheld until after 5-cm cervical dilation". Research published in 2004 involved 99 first-time mothers in spontaneous, active labour and at low risk of complications who were making slow progress during childbirth. Labouring in water under midwifery care may be an effective option for treating slow progress in labour, as it reduced the need for obstetric intervention and was an alternative to giving drugs.

TOUCH AND MASSAGE According to research, "Reassuring touch (in the form of hand-holding, stroking, caressing, embracing, or patting, which communicates caring and reassurance) by a nurse, and massage (the intentional and systematic manipulation of the soft tissues) during labour may relieve pain, reduce anxiety, and enhance labour progress with no identified risks."

MOVEMENT AND POSITIONING Maternal movement and positioning, such as "upright positions in stage I and squatting during stage II, may speed labour and increase maternal comfort".

ACTIVE LABOUR Recent research proposes that movement is a central aspect of normal labour. Given the choice, women change position an average of seven times in the course of normal labour. Yet bed-bound labours and birth with women semi-lying is still the norm in many hospitals despite the benefits of "active birth" being recognised since the 1970s.

In active birthing, women are encouraged to move and position themselves freely throughout labour and to give birth in more upright positions.

Active birth centres teach antenatal yoga classes to help build stamina and flexibility. A review of 18 randomised controlled trials suggests that active birth tends to result in more effective contractions and shorter labours with less fetal distress and fewer medical interventions.

INTRADERMAL WATER BLOCKS may help to relieve severe, continuous back pain, which is experienced by up to one-third of women during labour. Intradermal water blocks entail injections of only 0.1ml of sterile water into the skin of the low back in four different locations (corresponding approximately to the borders of the sacrum). The reason why these blocks relieve back pain in labour is not known, but numerous research studies confirm that women receiving the sterile water blocks get better pain relief than do women who have had placebo (sham) injections.

> Women with good support from a birth partner are less likely to require medical interventions

CRANIAL MANIPULATION AND OSTEOPATHY Clinical experience suggests that the use of very gentle cranial manipulation (such as cranial osteopathy, craniosacral therapy and sacro-occipital technique), as well as osteopathic treatment of the pelvic structures, can enhance the efficiency of the delivery process.

Mind–Body Therapies

PRIMARY TREATMENT **SELF-HYPNOSIS** Although the programmes of Lamaze and Dick-Read are the most widely used forms of childbirth preparation in the US, psychological and educational preparation with self-hypnosis (also known as guided imagery) has proven effective in several studies. Self-hypnosis combines deep relaxation with positive suggestion for a normal, comfortable birth.

In a recent study of pregnant teenagers in Florida, 22 women who had learned self-hypnosis before labour had shorter hospital stays and fewer surgical interventions than other women.

In another study, half of a group of 60 pregnant women received hypnotic suggestions for an enjoyable childbirth, deep relaxation and glove anaesthesia. Their first stages of labour progressed more quickly than those of the other women, they reported less pain during the birth, they needed less medication, and their babies had higher Apgar scores (in which a midwife "scores" the baby from one to 10 on breathing, movement and colour) at one and five minutes after birth.

PRIMARY TREATMENT **RELAXATION** Relaxation techniques, imagery and self-hypnosis are also effective in reducing complications. For example, the researcher Mehl at Beth Israel Hospital in New York taught guided imagery to 100 women with a baby in breech (feet first) position, comparing them to another group of women who also had breech babies. In the hypnosis group, 81 per cent of the breech babies spontaneously converted to a normal (head first) presentation, compared to 48 per cent of the babies who were in the comparison group.

TYPES OF PROGRAMMES In some preparation programmes for labour using hypnosis, few mothers use the techniques once labour starts, making the programmes less effective.

More effective programmes use continuous play tapes that mothers can listen to all the way through labour, for optimum relaxation and comfort. The use of taped lessons, instead of live therapists, makes the programme less costly and much more flexible, and workbooks can provide valuable educational material about the childbirth process.

MIND–BODY PRACTICES From these and other studies, as well as clinical experience, it is clear that relaxation and/or guided imagery incorporating childbirth education can increase pregnant women's feelings of control and confidence in the labour process.

Pregnant women should seek their doctors' or midwives' advice in finding a suitable programme that teaches self-hypnosis and relaxation for labour. Such techniques can also significantly reduce perception of pain and help women handle any complications that might arise; overall they might help to reduce the likelihood of a lengthy hospital stay or a major surgical intervention, such as a Caesarean section.

POSTNATAL DEPRESSION

Many mothers experience mild depression and mood swings in the first weeks following the birth of their baby. These "baby blues" usually resolve on their own within a few weeks. However, if depression persists or symptoms are severe, a new mother could have postnatal depression, which may require medical attention. Treatment for postnatal depression involves emotional support, and counselling usually plays a central role in this. Antidepressant drugs are necessary in some cases. Dietary changes, relaxation and acupuncture may also be of benefit.

WHAT ARE THE SYMPTOMS?

The symptoms of postnatal depression may develop up to six months after the birth of a baby and may include:

- Sadness
- Feeling constantly exhausted
- Having little or no interest in the new baby
- Feeling inadequate and overwhelmed by responsibilities
- Feeling guilty
- Having difficulty sleeping
- Loss of appetite

WHY MIGHT I HAVE THIS?

PREDISPOSING FACTORS

- Isolation
- Lack of emotional support
- Difficult labour
- Problems with partner
- Single motherhood
- Past history of depression
- Family history of postnatal depression

TREATMENT PLAN

PRIMARY TREATMENTS

- Emotional support and, if depression is severe, psychiatric support
- Counselling and other psychological therapies
- Antidepressants if appropriate

BACK-UP TREATMENTS

- Nutritional therapy
- Homeopathy
- Mind–body therapies

WORTH CONSIDERING

- Acupuncture

For an explanation of how treatments are rated, see p.111.

WHY DOES IT OCCUR?

Hormonal changes following the birth of a baby may be at least partially responsible for postnatal depression. Tiredness and lifestyle changes associated with having a new baby may also be contributory factors. Some women who experience postnatal depression have been depressed previously in their lives, and some come from families in which other women have also had the condition.

Certain other factors, such as isolation, feelings of inadequacy and doubts about being able to cope with motherhood, can all contribute to feelings of depression. Women who have had difficult labours or a history of depression may be at greater risk of developing postnatal depression, along with women who are having relationship difficulties with partners or who are on their own.

TREATMENTS IN DETAIL

Conventional Medicine

PRIMARY TREATMENT **PSYCHOTHERAPY AND ANTI-DEPRESSANTS** Women with postnatal depression need emotional and practical support from friends and family as

IMPORTANT

If you are a new mother and experience depression or mood swings that are extreme or last beyond the first few weeks after the birth, see your doctor or health visitor. Pregnant or breast-feeding women should not take any over-the-counter drugs, herbal remedies or nutritional supplements without consulting their doctor first.

well as care from their doctor. It is very important to get medical help if the depression is more than mild. Psychological therapies are likely to be recommended (*see below*) and antidepressants may also be prescribed (*see Depression, p.436*).

Nutritional Therapy

ESSENTIAL FATTY ACIDS The omega-3 fatty acids such as eicosapentaenoic acid (EPA) and docosahexaenoic acid (DHA) seem to play an important role in mood maintenance (*see Depression, p.436*). During pregnancy, mothers transfer DHA to the foetus to support development of the brain. Low levels of DHA in the diet increase the risk of the mother becoming depleted of this important nutrient, which in turn may increase the risk of postnatal depression.

One study found that higher concentrations of DHA in mothers' milk (a sign that that DHA had not been depleted during pregnancy) and greater seafood consumption (during and after pregnancy) were associated with lower risk of postnatal depression. These findings suggest that having adequate intake of omega-3 fatty acids before, during and after pregnancy might help prevent postnatal depression. Pregnant mothers should try to ensure good oily fish consumption (at least two portions a week). Some species of oily fish (such as tuna, marlin, swordfish) tend to be contaminated with mercury, and there is some thought that this might interfere with the neurological development of the foetus. Oily fish that tend not to be contaminated with mercury include salmon, trout, mackerel, herring and sardine. It considered safer for women to consume these types of oily fish during pregnancy and breastfeeding. However,

THE "BABY BLUES" AND POSTNATAL DEPRESSION

Postnatal depression is not the same as the "baby blues", the short period of sadness or moodiness that many women experience a few days after giving birth. The baby blues are not serious and are probably due to tiredness and fluctuating hormone levels. Most women recover in a few weeks. Postnatal depression is a more serious condition in which a woman may feel a deeper and more prolonged sense of inadequacy and despondency, which requires professional help.

BABY BLUES	POSTNATAL DEPRESSION
• Mood swings, from happy to weepy	• Sadness that persists for weeks on end
• More irritable than usual on occasion	• Lack of interest in the outside world
• Difficulty concentrating	• Profound and persistent tiredness
• Difficulty resting when baby is asleep	• Feelings of guilt and inadequacy
• Diminished appetite	• Insomnia
• Feeling overwhelmed by responsibility	• Anxiety and panic attacks
• May affect up to 50 per cent of mothers	• Feelings of negativity towards the baby

recent US research showed that farmed Scottish salmon may be contaminated with high concentrations of certain chemicals. Pregnant and breastfeeding women might also take a supplement of 1–2g of concentrated fish oils each day.

FOLIC ACID Low levels of folic acid have also been found to be associated with depression, and there is some evidence that they may play a part in postnatal depression. Pregnancy tends to deplete the body of folic acid. Also, women with postnatal depression tend to have lower levels of folic acid compared to postnatal women who are not depressed. Supplementing with 400mcg of folic acid per day is often advised for women with postnatal depression.

5-HYDROXYTRYPTOPHAN Women with postnatal depression also seem to have low tryptophan levels. Tryptophan is an amino acid found in foods such as meat, tofu, almonds, peanuts, pumpkin seeds, sesame seeds and tahini (sesame seed paste). Tryptophan is an essential building block for the manufacture of serotonin, a brain chemical that helps maintain mood.

Unfortunately, tryptophan is not available as an over-the-counter supplement in many countries, including the UK and the US. However, 5-hydroxytryptophan (5-HTP), the substance tryptophan is converted into

before it is made into serotonin, is an alternative that is available in the UK and the US. The normal recommended dose is 50mg of 5 HTP, taken two or three times a day.

> **CAUTION**
>
> Ask your doctor for advice before taking fish oil supplements with anticoagulant drugs such as warfarin. (*See also p.46.*)

Homeopathy

Homeopathy may help depression following childbirth, but if symptoms are severe or persistent (lasting more than two to three weeks), a woman should consult her doctor without delay.

IGNATIA This medicine is appropriate if the woman feels upset and tense; grief may be a component of her emotions, sometimes due to a difficult birth or one that did not go as she had planned.

ARSENICUM ALBUM Women who respond to this medicine feel insecure; they may be very restless, yet seem incapable.

CIMICIFUGA This medicine is indicated when the woman feels anxious and may perceive, probably falsely, that everything

in her life is going wrong. Significantly in terms of postnatal depression, she may also doubt her capabilities as a mother.

CALCAREA CARBONICA Women who respond to this medicine may feel weak and be very tired in general. They are easily fatigued by exercise and may also have anxiety, insomnia and nightmares.

AURUM METALLICUM Women who respond to this medicine may feel worthless. Dark days and bad weather make them worse, and they may also feel worse at night time. Women who had depression before often respond well to this medicine.

NATRUM MURIATICUM This medicine is appropriate when a woman feels sensitive and emotional; she may cry frequently. She may have trouble getting along with other members of the family and doubt her ability to cope with the baby.

SEPIA Women who respond to *Sepia* may feel exhausted to the point of indifference. They may feel resentful. Physical symptoms may include a weak pelvic floor.

PULSATILLA Women who respond to *Pulsatilla* are extremely insecure and may require almost constant emotional reassurance. They feel better in the open air and worse in warm, stuffy rooms.

Acupuncture

Acupuncture has been used to treat depression that has many different causes, including postnatal depression. There is some clear evidence that acupuncture can help with depression. Two clinical trials were done comparing electro-acupuncture with conventional antidepressants in the treatment of depression (*see p.436*). It is probable that acupuncture has an effect on the chemical messengers within the brain and may act to "balance" processes and reactions. Although there are no clinical trials that have been done to look at postnatal depression specifically, it is very likely that acupuncture can help with this condition.

Deciding on whether acupuncture treatment is appropriate in a particular case depends on the severity of the depression. If it is very severe, verging on psychotic or suicidal, then it is unwise to use a relatively untested treatment such as acupuncture. However, if the depression is mild, acupuncture could offer a very safe and effective treatment, perhaps alongside counselling or mind–body therapy. This is particularly true for breastfeeding mothers, since no chemical medication is involved.

A traditional Chinese diagnosis and treatment would probably be the best approach for postnatal depression. Treatment should usually be given two or three times a week, and you would usually expect to see a response within four to six treatments. If there is a response, continue with treatment, but if not, abandon this approach after six to eight sessions.

Mind–Body Therapies

RELAXATION AND GUIDED IMAGERY A 1995 study on the effects of these therapies showed that women with depression who used them had less anxiety and greater self-esteem than women who did not.

diagnosed with postnatal depression. There are a variety of approaches that are effective. Methods from the supportive/experiential group, from the CBT group, interpersonal psychotherapy, group and couple therapy have all been researched.

Most of these therapies can be used individually or with the inclusion of the mother's partner. One study suggests the inclusion of the partner can help with parenting skills and increase support for the mother. This study reported a reduction in the couples' depressive symptoms and a general improvement in their health.

SUPPORTIVE AND EXPERIENTIAL GROUP THERAPY Using this method, the practitioner gives the woman an opportunity to explore ways of becoming more self-reliant, which can help with well-being. Sometimes this technique allows women to focus on ways to address and resolve specific problems. Supportive/experiential group therapy may also enable them to make decisions

depressive symptoms in women during the postnatal period. These brief types of treatment can be as effective as antidepressants in treating mild to moderate depression in new mothers.

Unlike antidepressants, CBT also leaves clients with reusable skills should they become depressed again in the future. CBT has been done successfully over the telephone, which is particularly useful when the mother is in an isolated position.

PRIMARY TREATMENT | **INTERPERSONAL THERAPY** The interpersonal therapy approach focuses on how the mother relates to others, such as her partner, her relatives and her baby. It also focuses on how she might relate to herself. An important aspect of this form of therapy is the focus on her relationship with her own mother to examine how parenting skills have been learned and passed down a generation. This form of "talking therapy" helps her to relate problematical aspects of these relationships to her current depression. Interpersonal therapy has been shown to significantly reduce symptoms of postnatal depression.

PRIMARY TREATMENT | **TREATMENTS FOCUSED ON INTERACTION** The way in which a mother relates to her new baby may also affect the level of her depression. Women who have not bonded well with their babies may feel less satisfaction with motherhood and less effective as mothers than women who have bonded well with their babies. Some studies have focused on teaching the mother different ways of relating to her baby and have found that an improved mother–baby bond has helped relieve the mother's depression.

> # Between 10 and 15 per cent of women develop postnatal depression lasting over two weeks

OTHER TREATMENTS Approximately 13 per cent of women experience postnatal depression. In 2001 a meta-analysis updated the findings of an earlier meta-analysis of postnatal depression risk factors. Thirteen significant predictors or predisposing factors were revealed, which ranged from prenatal depression and low self-esteem to a lack of family support, difficulties in the family relationship, history of previous depression, being a single mother and an unplanned pregnancy. Although there is little actual research into mind–body treatments for postnatal depression, many of these predisposing factors may be helped by therapies such as yoga, guided imagery or relaxation. If you have any of the risk factors, a mind–body therapy during pregnancy may help to ward off depression after the birth.

Psychological Therapies

A number of studies indicate that talking therapies can be effective, significantly reducing depressive symptoms in women

and to improve their ways of coping with crises, working through conflict, or improving relationships with others.

PRIMARY TREATMENT | **SUPPORTIVE TALKING THERAPIES** Other studies have shown the benefit of supportive talking therapies when provided by health professionals who have been trained in the method. The treatment is brief, around six to eight sessions, and has been shown to be effective in reducing postnatal depression.

PRIMARY TREATMENT | **COGNITIVE-BEHAVIOURAL APPROACHES** Several studies support the use of CBT for postnatal depression. Women are encouraged to become more aware of unhelpful thoughts and their consequent behaviour as a result of them. They are then encouraged to generate alternative thoughts and ways of behaving using problem-solving techniques.

CBT is often a brief course of treatment, involving eight to twelve sessions, and studies have shown that it is effective in reducing

PREVENTION PLAN

The following may help:

- Avoid becoming isolated.
- Make sure you get adequate rest and some time to yourself every day.
- Let relatives and friends know when you feel you need help or support.
- Practise yoga or relaxation during pregnancy.

WHAT ARE THE SYMPTOMS?

Symptoms of engorgement include:
- Hard, swollen, painful breasts

Symptoms of cracked nipples include:
- Red, sore patches on the nipples
- Fine cracks on the nipples

Symptoms of mastitis include:
- A red, sore patch on the breast that may feel hot
- Sometimes, flu-like symptoms such as muscle aches and fever

WHY MIGHT I HAVE THIS?

PREDISPOSING FACTORS

For engorgement:
- Not feeding regularly

For cracked nipples:
- Not positioning the baby correctly on the nipple during feeding
- Not drying the nipples after feeding

For mastitis:
- Cracked nipples
- Engorgement

IMPORTANT

Untreated mastitis may develop into a breast abscess (a collection of pus in the breast tissue), which requires urgent treatment. If you think you are developing mastitis, see your doctor.

BREAST-FEEDING PROBLEMS

Although breast-feeding is a natural process, it isn't always an easy one. Problems can arise before and even after feeding is established. These include engorged breasts, cracked nipples, and mastitis, which is an infection of the milk ducts in a breast. Treatment for breast-feeding problems depends on what is wrong, but might include expressing milk and using creams to soothe cracked nipples. Homeopathy, hot and cold cloths and manual therapies can all help to ease engorgement and related pain. If mastitis develops, antibiotics may be necessary.

WHY DOES IT OCCUR?

Breast engorgement may occur when a mother's milk first comes in during the first few days after the birth, or it may occur if a baby's feeding routine is interrupted for some reason, such as illness.

Cracked nipples are usually caused by a baby not "latching on" properly to the mother's breast. To feed correctly, a baby must take the whole nipple and most of the areola (the darker area that surrounds the nipple) into his or her mouth, so that the lips form an air-tight seal on the breast (*see p.366*).

TREATMENT PLAN

PRIMARY TREATMENTS
- Position the baby correctly and other self-help measures (*see right*)
- Express excess milk (for engorgement)

BACK-UP TREATMENTS
- Antibiotics (for mastitis)

OTHER OPTIONS
- Homeopathy
- Trigger point deactivation
- Lymphatic drainage
- Mind–body therapies

For an explanation of how treatments are rated, see p.111.

Mastitis results from infection of a milk duct in the breast with a bacterium, usually *Staphylococcus aureus*. The bacterium may enter the skin through a cracked nipple. Mastitis tends to occur when the breasts have have become engorged.

SELF-HELP

PRIMARY TREATMENT The following will help you avoid problems:
- Wear a firm, supportive bra.
- Make sure the baby is positioned on the nipple correctly (*see p.366*).
- Dry the nipples after each feed.
- Try to relax as much as possible.
- Drink plenty of fluids.
- Take a painkiller (such as paracetamol if breastfeeding) for any discomfort.
- Saturate a piece of woollen material (towelling will do, but is not as effective) in hot water, wring it out and place it on the breasts. After five minutes, remove and replace with a cool, damp cloth for a few seconds, while the hot material is rewarmed, wrung out and replaced. Repeat this process two or three times.

TREATMENTS IN DETAIL

Conventional Medicine

PRIMARY TREATMENT **AVOIDING ENGORGEMENT** Women who are not intending to breast-feed should avoid expressing milk, since this is likely to stimulate further milk production. The engorgement should settle within a few days. Paracetamol and/or ice packs may help to relieve the discomfort.

CORRECT BREAST-FEEDING TECHNIQUE

In order to feed properly, a baby must be correctly "latched on" to her mother's breast. When this happens, the baby's mouth forms an airtight seal around the nipple and most or all of the areola, the darker area of skin around the nipple. If a baby is not latched on correctly, the mother's nipple will soon become irritated and sore; in time, it may even crack and bleed. To remove a baby from the breast once she has finished feeding, or to switch to the other breast, gently insert a finger between the baby's mouth and the breast to break the seal. Pulling the baby away from the breast without doing this first will also irritate the nipple.

Latching on

Removing the baby from the breast

The baby's mouth must form an airtight seal around the nipple and areola in order for the baby to feed effectively and without irritating the mother's nipple.

Gently inserting a finger between the baby's mouth and the nipple breaks the airtight seal and allows the baby to be removed from the breast without irritating the nipple.

Occasionally, drugs such as bromocriptine are prescribed. Bromocriptine stops the pituitary gland (a tiny gland at the base of the brain) from releasing the hormone prolactin, which stimulates milk production by the breasts.

A woman who does wish to breast-feed and whose breasts become engorged may gently express the excess milk until the baby's feeding pattern has become established and the breasts are producing the correct amount of milk to meet the baby's needs. When women decide to stop breast-feeding, they should gradually replace one feed at a time with a formula feed with the aim of avoiding engorgement.

PRIMARY TREATMENT **AVOIDING CRACKED NIPPLES** Carefully drying the nipples after feeding should help prevent cracked nipples. Women should also seek advice on the positioning of the baby from their mid-wife or breast-feeding counsellor. If you do develop cracked nipples, the problem should settle over a few days. Creams bought over the counter probably will not help, so seek medical advice if the problem persists. An infection may be present that requires treatment with antibiotics.

PRIMARY TREATMENT **HELP FOR MASTITIS** If you develop mastitis you should continue breast-feeding and express any milk left after feeding if possible. Paracetamol may help relieve the pain, as may warmth applied to the affected area. This may also help the milk flow. (*See Self-Help, above.*) It is important to keep drinking plenty of fluids.

See your doctor if you develop mastitis, since antibiotics might be necessary to prevent an abscess from developing. The doctor may send a sample of the milk for analysis to identify the infection and ensure the appropriate antibiotic is prescribed.

If an abscess develops, you should not feed from the affected side, but you should express the milk. Like mastitis, an abscess is treated with antibiotics, but the pus may need to be drained with a needle and syringe under local anaesthetic.

> **CAUTION**
>
> Drugs to treat breast-feeding problems can cause a range of possible side-effects: ask your doctor to explain these to you.

Homeopathy

Homeopathy can help with a number of breast-feeding problems. The homeopathic medicine *Graphites* may be used to treat cracked nipples, while a number of homeopathic medicines may be used for mastitis. The three most common are *Belladonna*, *Bryonia* and *Phytolacca*.

GRAPHITES The remedy *Graphites* (made from graphite, a form of carbon) taken by mouth is the classical homeopathic treatment for cracked nipples.

Suck two *Graphites* pills, in the 6C strength, three or four times daily. This medicine is available from many chemists and health food shops and can be used in conjunction with creams to help soothe and heal the nipples.

BELLADONNA The sort of mastitis that responds to *Belladonna* is usually of sudden onset and the breast is hot, red and very tender, with throbbing pain. The woman herself may be flushed and feverish and the pupils of her eyes may be dilated.

BRYONIA The type of condition that responds to *Bryonia* is also usually quite acute. The breast is hard and the pain is typically stitching in character and is made

muscular therapy training) and some physiotherapists and chiropractors.

LYMPHATIC DRAINAGE Because some of the main lymph drainage channels pass through, in front of, and around the pectoralis major muscles, if these tissues are tense and shortened (or contain trigger points) lymph will not be able to flow as easily and congestion in the breast tissues becomes likely.

time during pregnancy and/or during labour and delivery took longer to arrive than in other women.

If you feel anxious that your milk is not coming in as quickly as it should, try practising relaxation techniques (*see p.99*) and make sure you are getting adequate rest.

MIND–BODY TECHNIQUES Despite the importance of this problem and the clear indication that stress interferes with lactation and breast-feeding, there are few studies to date of the potential effectiveness of mind–body methods to alleviate this stress and promote healthy, timely lactation for the benefit of the mother and baby.

Virtually all women can breast-feed if given the proper instruction and support

worse by any movement or jarring. The support of a well-fitting bra is helpful. The woman's mouth is often dry and she may be thirsty; she may also have sharp pains elsewhere, including in the neck and head.

PHYTOLACCA When *Phytolacca* is indicated, the breast is hard and there may be an excessive milk flow, with pains that seem to shoot from the breast all over the body. This type of mastitis may be associated with a sore throat and rheumatic aches and pains in the back, legs and elsewhere.

Bodywork Therapies

TRIGGER POINT DEACTIVATION Trigger points (sensitive spots) in the pectoral and serratus anterior muscles in the chest can cause extreme discomfort and pain in the breasts and nipples (these symptoms have been reported in both men and women). These symptoms may be accompanied by a sense of engorgement of the breast tissue, related to sluggish lymphatic drainage. If this occurs during breast-feeding, the woman may find it impossible to continue breast-feeding.

It has been reported that deactivation of trigger points, particularly those found in the pectoralis major muscle (located near the armpit) rapidly eases symptoms of pain and congestion.

Trigger points can usually be deactivated by acupuncture, by injections of procaine and by manual pressure and stretching techniques, as used by osteopaths, massage therapists (particularly those with a neuro-

Lymphatic drainage massage (or, if appropriate, trigger point deactivation) can usually ease this restriction of normal lymph flow, and so the congestion.

Mind–Body Therapies

STRESS AND BREAST-FEEDING Although the precise connection between emotional stress and breast-feeding difficulties is not clear, experimental studies of breast-feeding women have shown that acute physical and mental stress can impair the milk ejection reflex by reducing the release of the hormone oxytocin during a feed. If this occurs repeatedly, it can reduce milk production by preventing proper emptying of the breast.

Having a stressful labour and delivery may be a factor in many breast-feeding difficulties. Studies indicate that urgent Caesarean sections or long duration of labour in vaginal deliveries are associated with delayed onset of breast-feeding. Mothers who experience high levels of stress during and after childbirth should receive additional breast-feeding guidance from their midwife or breast-feeding counsellor.

DELAYED ONSET OF LACTATION Usually milk comes into the breast during the first few days after the birth. If there is a delay beyond these few days, it can affect a woman's confidence and therefore her ability to breast-feed.

One recent study examined the onset of lactation in a group of 136 Guatemalan women. Researchers found that the breast milk of the women who had had a stressful

However, one such study looked at mothers separated from premature babies in intensive care units. Understandably, these mothers often find it difficult to keep up production of breast milk, despite expressing milk using a pump. Research showed that periods of holding their babies skin-to-skin increased the milk supply.

Breast-feeding mothers obviously need rest and time to establish the relationship with their babies needed to make milk flow, and experience certainly suggests that a protected rest day spent in intimate, quiet contact with the new baby will encourage more frequent feeds and therefore greater milk production.

Stress and fatigue tend to turn off the let-down reflex, which causes milk to flow. In a research trial, mothers whose babies were in a premature care unit listened to a relaxation and guided imagery tape. They showed a 60 per cent increase in milk production afterwards.

In light of these findings, it seems very likely that relaxation techniques could play an effective part in helping women to overcome breast-feeding difficulties, in conjunction with good breast-feeding education and support.

PREVENTION PLAN

Try the following:

- Get advice on positioning and technique early from a midwife or breast-feeding counsellor.

- Use stress-reduction techniques if you feel tense.

Men's Health

Men may find it difficult to accept problems with their reproductive and sexual ability. An integrated approach acknowledges that sexual function is closely linked with the emotions so relaxation techniques, stress reduction, and talking therapies may all appropriate, as well as conventional drugs. Herbs and homeopathy can also be effective.

BENIGN PROSTATIC HYPERTROPHY

Benign prostatic hypertrophy (BPH) is an enlargement of the prostate gland. The majority of men over the age of 50 have some degree of prostate enlargement. Among older men the disease is practically universal; it is found in around 90 per cent of men over 85 years old. It is not cancerous and is different from prostate cancer. Treatment aims to shrink the prostate tissue and control the flow of urine.

WHAT ARE THE SYMPTOMS?

- Frequent urination, during both the day and night
- Delay in beginning to urinate, especially at night or when the bladder is full
- Weak and intermittent urine flow
- Dribbling of urine at the end of urination
- A feeling that the bladder has not emptied completely

WHY MIGHT I HAVE THIS?

PREDISPOSING FACTORS

- Being male and over 50

TREATMENT PLAN

PRIMARY TREATMENTS

- Restricting fluid intake in the evening (for mild symptoms)
- Drugs
- Surgery (for severe symptoms)
- Saw palmetto

BACK-UP TREATMENTS

- Essential fatty acids
- Zinc supplements, pumpkin seeds and linseed oil
- Isoflavones
- Herbs containing beta-sitosterol

WORTH CONSIDERING

- Lycopene
- Chinese herbal medicine
- Exercise
- Acupuncture

For an explanation of how treatments are rated, see p.111.

WHY DOES IT OCCUR?

The cause of benign prostatic hypertrophy (BPH) is not known, but the male hormone testosterone plays a role. If the prostate gland is only slightly enlarged in a middle-aged man, it may be seen as a normal part of the ageing process. It only becomes a problem if the gland encroaches on the urethra, the tube that carries urine from the bladder to the outside.

This encroachment can restrict urination, which may lead to various complications. For example, if the bladder is not emptied fully, it may enlarge and cause the abdomen to become distended. Urine may also collect in the bladder and stagnate, which may make urinary tract infections more likely and increase the risk of bladder stone formation. Rarely, backward pressure from retained urine in the bladder causes kidney damage. If an enlarged prostate gland suddenly blocks the flow of urine completely, emergency medical treatment is required.

BPH symptoms may be worse in cold weather or after drinking large amounts of fluid, especially alcoholic beverages. Drugs such as diuretics that increase urine production, can also make symptoms worse.

IMPORTANT

- If you cannot urinate despite having the urge to do so, seek medical help at once.
- Prostate cancer can cause similar symptoms to BPH (although it is much less common).
- Men with symptoms of BPH should consult their doctor as soon as possible so that prostate cancer can be excluded.

TREATMENTS IN DETAIL

Conventional Medicine

The doctor will give you a digital rectal examination and may recommend tests to find out whether your prostate gland has become significantly enlarged. These tests include monitoring the rate of urine flow and ultrasound scanning to measure the amount of urine left in the bladder after you have urinated.

Particular treatments are recommended on the basis of several factors, including general health, the severity of the symptoms and the size of the prostate gland.

PRIMARY TREATMENT **RESTRICTING FLUID INTAKE** If your symptoms are mild, you may not need treatment. Your doctor may simply recommend restricting fluid intake in the evening and may change existing medication.

PRIMARY TREATMENT **DRUGS** If your symptoms are more severe, your doctor may prescribe alpha-blocker drugs, such as alfuzosin or indoramin, which relax the smooth muscle around the urethra to improve the flow of urine and help reduce the symptoms.

Alternatively, your doctor may prescribe anti-androgen drugs, such as finasteride, which prevent the activation of testosterone in the prostate gland with the aim of shrinking the swollen tissue. This may have the effect of improving the symptoms and reducing complications.

PRIMARY TREATMENT **SURGERY** Prostate gland tissue that reduces the flow of urine may be removed with an instrument

The walnut-sized prostate gland surrounds, and secretes fluid into the urethra during ejaculation. In BPH, excessive cell division in the centre of the gland causes it to expand and press on the base of bladder so that it does not empty completely.

inserted along the urethra. In transurethral resection, the instrument cuts the tissue. In transurethral microwave thermotherapy, the instrument applies heat to the tissue. If the prostate gland has become very enlarged, the surgeon may need to remove the tissue through an incision made in the lower abdomen.

> **CAUTION**
>
> Alpha-blockers and anti-androgens have side-effects and surgery may involve certain risks. Ask your doctor to explain these to you.

Nutritional Therapy

DIET Studies show that eating more fruit and vegetables appears to protect the prostate gland and may reduce the risk of enlargement. Studies also reveal that butter, milk, margarine and meat seem to be associated with an increased risk of prostate enlargement.

ESSENTIAL FATTY ACIDS (EFAS) seem to play an important role in maintaining the health of the prostate gland. Research suggests that they may improve the symptoms of prostatic enlargement. EFAs, such as omega-3 fatty acids, can be found in raw nuts and seeds, oily fish such as salmon, trout, mackerel and herring, as well as extra-virgin olive oil. Eating an abundance of these foods, together with plenty of fruit and vegetables, is likely to help maintain the health of the prostate gland and may possibly reduce the risk of enlargement.

LINSEED OIL In addition, take one tablespoon of linseed oil, which is rich in omega-3 fatty acids, each day for several months. Then reduce the dose to 1–2 teaspoons a day. Take 200 IU of vitamin E daily with the linseed oil to protect the oil from oxidation damage in the body.

PUMPKIN SEEDS Try to include pumpkin seeds in your diet. They are rich in zinc and vitamin E, both of which are known to be important for the health of the prostate gland. They also contain beta-sitosterol (see Western Herbal Medicine, below). In a German study, pumpkin seed extract was tested on over 2,000 men with mild to moderate BPH and over 40 per cent experienced significant improvement.

ZINC SUPPLEMENTS The prostate gland contains a very high concentration of zinc. Supplementation with zinc, especially in conjunction with linseed oil, may help to reduce prostatic enlargement. Zinc can be found in fish, seafood (especially oysters) and seeds. In practice, taking 30–60mg of zinc supplements a day is often useful. Long-term consumption of zinc supplements can deplete the body of copper, so take 1mg of copper for every 15mg of zinc.

LYCOPENE Regular intake of lycopene, which is present in tomatoes, watermelon, pink grapefruit and chillies, appears to confer protection against prostate cancer. Researchers suggest that lycopene might also have a general therapeutic effect on the prostate gland. Eating cooked tomatoes and olive oil, as in the Mediterranean diet, is recommended because the absorption of lycopene by the body requires the presence of fats or oils.

> **CAUTION**
>
> Consult your doctor before taking zinc with antibiotics (see p.46).

Western Herbal Medicine

As men age, the level of testosterone in their blood falls as the level of dihydrotesterone (DHT), a derivative of testosterone, increases. Under normal circumstances, the enzyme 5-alpha-reductase converts testosterone to DHT and stimulates growth of the prostate gland. There is evidence that 5-alpha-reductase activity is higher in cells affected by BPH than in normal prostate gland tissue.

Herbal medicines offer excellent outcomes in preventing and treating mild to moderate BPH. Plant medicines have been used to treat BPH in Germany, France and Italy for the last 20 years. Several have been shown to inhibit 5-alpha-reductase, thereby reducing the size of an enlarged prostate. They also have an anti-inflammatory effect on the gland.

PRIMARY TREATMENT **SAW PALMETTO** (*Serenoa repens*) is an effective herbal treatment for the early stages of BPH. In the 1960s, researchers discovered that saw palmetto berries contained fatty acids (liposterols) that inhibit 5-alpha-reductase. One study revealed that the plant also relaxed smooth muscle within the wall of the urethra, thereby increasing the output of urine. It also reduces swelling and inflammation of the prostate gland. You can safely take saw palmetto – try 2–4g of berries a day, or 160mg of a standardised extract twice a day.

BETA-SITOSTEROL Meta-analyses showed that beta-sitosterol displayed significant improvements in relieving the symptoms of BPH and in increasing urine flow.

The bark of the evergreeen pygeum tree (*Pygeum africanum*) is rich in beta-sitosterol, which also inhibits the enzyme 5-alpha-reductase. However, in a double-blind study that compared pygeum with saw palmetto, the latter produced a greater reduction in BPH symptoms. Pygeum has been widely used in Germany and France, but the pressure to provide medicine for prostatic treatment has endangered the plant in its native African habitat.

Other plants containing beta-sitosterol include the African potato (*Hypoxis hemerocallidea*) and species of both pine (*Pinus spp.*) and spruce (*Picea spp.*). These plants are an effective option for treating BPH.

ISOFLAVONES Plants that have isoflavones can help patients with BPH. Evidence suggests that the isoflavones in legumes are related to lower rates of BPH and prostate cancer among Asian men. Men concerned about their prostate health should consider incorporating soya (*Glycine max*) into their diet.

Red clover (*Trifolium pratense*), which is available in tablet form, is another rich source of isoflavones. An Australian study showed that isoflavones derived from red clover had a significant effect on prostatic growth apparently by acting as an anti-androgenic agent.

OTHER PLANTS that show promise for the treatment of BPH include willowherb

(*Epilobium spp.*) and golden rod (*Solidago virgaurea*). Nettle (*Urtica dioica*) root contains phytosterols that can relieve the symptoms of BPH and is often combined with saw palmetto to good effect.

CAUTION

See p.69 before taking a herbal remedy and, if you are already taking prescribed medication, consult a medical herbalist first.

Chinese Herbal Medicine

Benign prostatic hypertrophy occurs in older men. Practitioners of Traditional Chinese Medicine (TCM) generally consider it to be due to a waning of kidney *Qi* that can be complicated with "damp heat" and "stagnation of the blood". In general, they recognise four main BPH syndromes.

DEFICIENCY OF KIDNEY YIN First, BPH may occur against a background of "deficient kidney *Yin*". The patient complains of an aching back, weak legs and knees, insomnia and dream-disturbed sleep. The urine flow is unsteady, dark and possibly burning. The treatment aim is to nourish kidney *Yin* and clear damp heat from the bladder. Treatment is based on Anemarrhena and Phellodendron Rehmannia Six Ingredient Pill (*Zhi Bai Di Huang Wan*).

DEFICIENCY OF KIDNEY YANG is another common pattern of BPH. The patient has frequent urination and/or retention of urine, is tired and cold, especially in the lower back, legs and knees. Treatment is based on The Golden Chest Kidney Pill (*Jin Gui Shen Qi Wan*). In the UK, aconite (*Aconitum carmichaely*) is replaced with either red ginseng (*Panax ginseng*) or dried ginger (*Zingiber officinale*).

"DAMP HEAT" A damp-heat presentation of BPH occurs when the man's urination is hesitant, dribbling yet burning, and the urine is dark with a strong smell. The prescription is usually based on a variation of the Eight Herb Powder for Rectification (*Ba Zheng San*). In the UK, *Mu Tong* and rhubarb root are replaced by juncus (*Juncus effusus*), seven-lobed yam (*Dioscorea hypoglauca*) and the rhizome of sweet flag (*Acorus gramineus*).

BLOOD STAGNATION The fourth pattern of BPH appears because of "blood stagnation" in which urination becomes difficult and may even cease in severe cases. There is distending pain in the low back, loin perineum and lower abdomen. The prescription is based on Resolve Resistance Decoction (*Dai Di Dang Tang*). In the UK, non-plant products are replaced with vaccaria (*Vaccaria segetalis*) seed, zedoary (*Curcuma zedoaria*) and burreed (*Sparganium stoloniferum*) tuber.

CAUTION

See p.69 before taking a herbal remedy and, if you are already taking prescribed medication, consult a medical herbalist first.

Exercise

A 1998 research study showed that exercise and physical activity reduce the chances of a man developing prostate problems. Take regular exercise three to four times a week.

Acupuncture

Acupuncture may help some symptoms of BPH. Relief may only be transitory if the enlarged prostate is not managed appropriately with conventional and nutritional treatments. Initial treatment should be on a weekly basis. If there is improvement, which should be noticeable within the first five or six treatments, continue until no further benefit is apparent. Treatments every one to three months may be needed, particularly if symptoms tend to recur.

PREVENTION PLAN

The following may help to prevent the development of BPH:

- Eat plenty of oily fish, extra-virgin olive oil, soya, nuts, pumpkin seeds, fruit and vegetables.
- Keep your intake of butter, milk, margarine and meat to a minimum.
- Take zinc supplements.
- Take linseed oil each day.
- Take regular exercise.

MALE INFERTILITY

Many couples feel anxious if they have been trying to conceive for several months without success. Statistically, 80 per cent of couples trying to conceive will be successful within a year, and 90 per cent will be successful within two years. Older couples may be advised to start having investigations earlier as fertility declines with age, particularly in women. Treatment focuses on resolving any underlying cause, boosting sperm viability and function, assisted conception, relieving anxiety and avoiding exposure to potentially harmful environmental toxins.

WHAT ARE THE SYMPTOMS?

- Non-conception after about a year of regular intercourse

WHY MIGHT I HAVE THIS?

PREDISPOSING FACTORS

- Low sperm count
- Production of abnormal sperm
- Poor sperm motility
- Higher than normal scrotal temperature
- Long-term illnesses
- Certain infections, such as mumps
- Treatments, such as chemotherapy and radiation, for testicular cancer
- Disorder of the pituitary gland
- Chromosomal disorder
- Consuming too much alcohol
- Sexually transmitted disease
- Prostate surgery
- Exposure to xenoestrogens
- Exposure to environmental toxins, such as lead, phthalates and glycol ethers
- Erectile problems
- Abnormalities of bladder or testicles

IMPORTANT

If you have been trying to conceive for several months unsuccessfully and you are concerned, go as a couple to see your doctor. This is especially important if one or both partners are over 35.

WHY DOES IT OCCUR?

Male fertility depends partly on producing enough normal sperm to fertilise an egg, and partly on the ability to deliver the sperm into the vagina during intercourse. If there are problems with either of these, fertilisation of an egg may not be possible.

The cause of infertility is identifiable in only about a third of men investigated. In about half of all couples with fertility problems, the problem lies with the woman (*see Infertility in women, p.346*) and in about a third, the problem lies with the man. In some couples, no problem can be found.

TREATMENT PLAN

PRIMARY TREATMENT

- Treatment for underlying cause wherever possible

BACK-UP TREATMENTS

- Assisted conception techniques
- Supplements, such as vitamins C and E, selenium and zinc
- Homeopathic medicines
- Environmental health measures, such as avoiding toxic exposures, avoiding xenoestrogens and stopping smoking

WORTH CONSIDERING

- Stress management
- Western herbal medicine

For an explanation of how treatments are rated, see p.111.

LOW SPERM COUNT Semen analysis is one of the first tests and various measurements are made. There should be more than 20 million sperm per millilitre of semen. More than 50 per cent should have good motility (ability to swim along) and at least 30 per cent should be a completely normal shape.

An abnormal sperm count may have various causes. Because of their position in the scrotum, the testes have a temperature that is about 2°C (3.6°F) lower than the rest of the body. Anything that raises this temperature, such as tight underwear, may have an adverse effect on sperm production.

Sperm production can also be affected by long-term illnesses, such as chronic renal failure, by mumps (*see p.395*) if it occurs after puberty and by medical treatments, including surgery, chemotherapy and radiation therapy for disorders, such as testicular cancer.

Occasionally, a low sperm count may be due to low levels of testosterone, sometimes caused by a disorder of the pituitary gland (the tiny gland at the base of the brain which controls testosterone production by the testes) or, rarely, by a chromosomal abnormality. Lifestyle factors, such as drinking excessive alcohol, smoking and using certain prescription or recreational drugs, may also affect sperm production.

In most cases, the cause of a low sperm count cannot be identified, and the condition is known as idiopathic oligospermia.

POOR SPERM DELIVERY Many factors can cause problems with delivery of sperm into the vagina. The most easily identified is erectile dysfunction (*see p.376*). Other less obvious factors are damage to the epididymides (the tightly coiled tubes that lie above and behind each testes where sperm

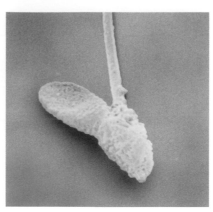

A healthy human sperm cell (above left) is composed of a rounded head, which contains the male DNA, and a tail that enables the cell to swim. An abnormal sperm cell (above right) would be infertile.

are stored and mature) and the vasa deferentia (the tubes that transport sperm away from the epididymides towards the urethra). Damage is often due to a sexually transmitted disease, such as gonorrhoea.

Sperm delivery is also affected by retrograde ejaculation, when semen flows back into the bladder from the urethra. This occurs if the valves at the outlet of the bladder fail to close properly and may be caused by prostate surgery.

SELF-HELP

The following measures may improve your chances of producing normal sperm:
- Have sex regularly.
- Don't smoke or take recreational drugs.
- Don't drink alcohol excessively.
- Eat organic food and drink filtered water to reduce exposure to toxins.
- Avoid hot baths.
- Avoid wearing tight underpants. If you sit for long periods, stand up and stretch or walk briefly on a regular basis.

TREATMENTS IN DETAIL

Conventional Medicine

PRIMARY TREATMENT **UNDERLYING CAUSES** A doctor will give you a physical examination, ask about your sex life and recommend tests to assess your sperm count and sperm motility. If these are low, the underlying cause is treated if possible. For example, hormone injections may be given if testosterone levels are low. Erectile dysfunction may be treated with the drug sildenafil (Viagra), or one of various other treatment options and psychological therapies may be recommended, including sex therapy (see p.379).

ASSISTED CONCEPTION If it is not possible to identify or to treat the cause of male infertility, measures may be taken to try to increase a couple's chances of conceiving.

If there are few or no sperm in the ejaculate, some couples choose to use donor sperm. If the sperm count is very low or sperm motility is poor, a single sperm selected from a semen sample may be injected into an egg removed from the ovaries (this process is called intracytoplasmic sperm injection, or ICSI). If an embryo starts to develop, it is introduced into the uterus, where it may become embedded in the wall and grow. ICSI may still be possible even if the ejaculate contains no sperm. In such cases, sperm may be removed directly from the testes or epididymides. Sperm removed in this way may also be introduced into the uterus through a soft plastic tube passed through the cervix (intrauterine insemination).

If the sperm count is only slightly low, in-vitro fertilisation (IVF) may be an option. In this technique, a sample of sperm is added to eggs collected from the ovaries in the hope that fertilisation will occur.

Nutritional Therapy

VITAMIN C SUPPLEMENTS Low or deficient vitamin C levels have been associated with low sperm count, increased numbers of abnormal sperm, reduced motility and agglutination (when sperm stick together). In one study into the effect of vitamin C on smokers, as much as 1,000mg of vitamin C per day improved sperm viability, motility and agglutination, and reduced the percentage of abnormal sperm. The authors of the study concluded that 1,000mg a day of vitamin C is reasonable to give to any infertile man because it seems to improve sperm function and viability. Taking 500mg of vitamin C, twice a day may help.

VITAMIN E SUPPLEMENTS Vitamin E also seems to be important to maintain sperm function. In one study, in which sperm samples were taken from infertile men, the more motile sperm contained greater vitamin E concentrations. The authors suggest that the vitamin E may help protect sperm against free radical damage. Other studies show that supplementation with vitamin E increases the quality of sperm and fertilisation rates. The recommended dose is 200–400 IU of vitamin E each day.

SELENIUM SUPPLEMENTS Selenium seems to be important for normal sperm structure and function. One study showed that selenium supplementation in sub-fertile men who lacked this mineral improved sperm motility and the chance of successful conception. The recommended dose is 100–200mcg of selenium per day.

ZINC SUPPLEMENTS Zinc plays an important role in normal testicular development, sperm production and sperm motility. In one study, infertile men had significantly lower serum and semen zinc levels compared to fertile men.

For men with low testosterone levels, zinc supplements raise testosterone levels and increase fertility. In men with low semen zinc levels, zinc supplements can increase sperm count and fertility. The recommended dose is 50mg per day for several months. Long-term consumption of zinc supplements can deplete the body of copper, so take 1mg of copper for every 15mg of zinc.

CAUTION

Consult your doctor before taking vitamin E with blood thinners, or vitamin C with antibiotics or warfarin, or zinc with antibiotics (see p.46).

Homeopathy

In a 2002 clinical study of men with fertility problems, individualised homeopathy helped improve sperm count and sperm motility, and in some cases their wives became pregnant. The most commonly used medicines are *Sulphur*, *Natrum muriaticum*, *Lycopodium* and *Calcarea carbonica*.

SULPHUR Men who respond to *Sulphur* are often "larger than life" characters: sociable, outgoing, flamboyant and untidy. They are generally strong-willed, to the point sometimes of being argumentative or garrulous. Their feet are especially hot and may be smelly – they kick off their shoes at every opportunity and may stick their feet out of the bed at night. They frequently have skin trouble, with a rash that is often very itchy. They are very thirsty and enjoy rich and spicy food.

NATRUM MURIATICUM The type of man who responds to *Nat. mur.* often has a masked depression – he is very depressed, but does not like to talk about it. He may have had an upsetting experience, such as a bereavement or relationship break-up, that he has never discussed. These men may have other problems, such as migraine, various skin problems, including dry, crusty skin rashes, hives (*see p.176*) and recurrent cold sores on the lips. They often crave salty food, such as savoury snacks.

LYCOPODIUM Men who respond to *Lycopodium* are often serious people in responsible, demanding jobs, yet they may lack self-confidence. They may be socially rather inept, no good at small talk, yet they do not like being alone; they are at their best with small groups of old friends. They often have stomach trouble as their "eyes are bigger than their stomachs".

Lycopodium men feel hungry when they sit down to eat, but quickly become full up. They suffer from an excess of wind and bloating, and their favourite flavour is sweet. Their worst time of day is 4–8pm, or after lunch, when they feel very drowsy.

CALCAREA CARBONICA The type of man who responds to *Calc. carb.* is stocky and solidly built, with a tendency to be overweight. He is phlegmatic – solid, stubborn and hard-working. His calm exterior may conceal many anxieties and fears and he may have bad dreams. He tends to sweat a great deal, especially on the head and neck.

Western Herbal Medicine

Herbal treatment for infertility may be useful when a man is in general good health. Low sperm count or low sperm motility can sometimes successfully be treated with remedies such as ginseng (*Panax ginseng*), ashwagandha (*Withania somnifera*) and ginger (*Zingiber officinale*).

> **CAUTION**
>
> See p.46 before taking a herbal remedy and, if you are already taking prescribed medication, consult a medical herbalist first.

Environmental Health

Environmental medicine aims to help men avoid exposure to compounds that may be toxic to sperm development or to parts of the reproductive tract. A lack of convincing scientific evidence, combined with problems applying animal studies to humans, means that it is not always possible to establish beyond doubt that a chemical or toxic exposure leads to infertility. Nonetheless, there are many compounds that seem to have negative effects on male fertility.

If you have problems with libido, sperm counts, sperm quality or overall fertility, look for possible exposures in the home or workplace. If there are offending chemicals, make changes to reduce your exposure.

AVOID TOXIC EXPOSURES A high level of lead exposure may lower sperm counts, increase the proportion of abnormal sperm and decrease overall fertility. Glycol ethers, which are solvents used in the manufacture of paints, dyes, inks, cleaners and soaps, seem to damage testicular function, lower sperm counts and possibly cause infertility.

Researchers examining the decline in sperm quality over the past few decades indicate that environmental agents, even in low concentrations, might be involved. For example, exposure to phthalates may be related to the decline in semen quality. Phthalates are extremely common compounds, found in food, consumer products (plasticisers or spreading agents) and medical devices. Certain phthalates may be more toxic to sperm than others.

Exposure to different types of solvent cause sperm to be abnormal and decrease libido. Research has shown that exposure to manganese, in steel manufacturing, mining and dry-alkaline battery production plants, can cause impotence, reduced fertility and decreased libido.

STOP SMOKING Some studies have found a connection between boys born to women who smoked during pregnancy and low sperm counts years later, perhaps through an adverse effect on sperm development. Other studies have shown that exposure to cigarette smoke decreases semen volume and overall male fertility.

XENOESTROGENS may play a part in falling sperm counts by mimicking the action of female hormones and/or blocking the effect of androgens (male hormones). Agrochemicals, plastic bottles, food wrappings and tap water are thought to be the main sources. Examples are DDT and other pesticides, dyes and paints, such as phenol red, or bisphenol A, which comes from the degradation of plastics.

Avoiding xenoestrogens altogether is probably unrealistic, though eating organic food as much as possible and drinking mineral water from glass bottles will help to reduce exposure. Animal studies and some human studies show an effect of these compounds on male libido, sperm counts and sperm quality, though the exact association is unclear.

Stress Management

Anxiety contributes to infertility in some instances and its symptoms can usually be eased by regularly practising anti-anxiety breathing exercises (*see Anxiety, p.414*).

> **PREVENTION PLAN**
>
> **The following may improve fertility:**
> - Avoid alcohol and give up smoking.
> - Ensure your diet is rich in zinc, selenium, vitamins C and E.
> - Avoid exposure to environmental hazards.

ERECTILE DYSFUNCTION

Erectile dysfunction, which used to be called impotence, is the inability to achieve or sustain an erection. Occasional problems with erection are normal and affect most men at some time, becoming more common with increasing age. Persistent, long-term difficulties may cause distress, both to a man and to his partner. Despite this, only about 10 per cent of men experiencing long-term erectile dysfunction seek help for it. Treatment is aimed at relieving the underlying cause, either by increasing blood flow to the penis or helping men to relax and feel less anxious.

WHAT ARE THE SYMPTOMS?

- The inability to achieve or sustain an erection

WHY MIGHT I HAVE THIS?

PREDISPOSING FACTORS

- Stress
- Anxiety about sex
- Depression
- Relationship problems
- Overwork
- Tiredness
- Drinking alcohol excessively
- Smoking
- Drugs, such as certain antidepressants and antihypertensives
- Surgery
- Vascular disease (especially in diabetes)
- Chronic illness

WHY DOES IT OCCUR?

Erectile dysfunction (ED) can be caused by either psychological or physical factors. Sometimes, erectile dysfunction is due to a combination of the two. In general, if the condition is intermittent it is usually the result of a psychological cause, such as an anxiety disorder (*see p.414*) and depression (*see p.436*). Other psychological factors may include stress (*see p.408*), anxiety about sexual performance or relationship difficulties. Erectile dysfunction may be prolonged by the fact that many men are reluctant to discuss it, even in private with their doctor.

Erectile dysfunction that develops gradually and becomes persistent tends to be the result of physical causes. These include drugs, such as certain antidepressants and antihypertensives (drugs used to treat high blood pressure), poorly controlled diabetes, surgery that may affect the nerves supplying the penis and chronic illness.

In middle-aged and older men, erectile dysfunction may be due to vascular disease (disease of the blood vessels), commonly caused by atherosclerosis (in which fatty deposits on the lining of arteries cause progressive narrowing) that reduces the blood supply to the penis. Lifestyle factors, such as heavy drinking, smoking or overwork, can also increase the risk.

TREATMENT PLAN

PRIMARY TREATMENTS

- Treatment of any underlying cause
- Lifestyle changes, such as avoiding heavy drinking, overwork
- Better communication (*see Self-Help*)
- Counselling and sex therapy
- Drugs, such as sildenafil (Viagra)
- Ginseng

BACK-UP TREATMENTS

- Other drugs
- Devices and prostheses
- Arginine supplements
- Homeopathy
- Western herbal medicine
- Osteopathy and chiropractic

WORTH CONSIDERING

- Chinese herbal medicine
- Breathing retraining
- Acupuncture
- Vitamin B12 supplements

For an explanation of how treatments are rated, see p.111.

SELF-HELP

PRIMARY TREATMENT You can reduce your anxiety about sex and improve your relationship with your partner through communicating. When you discuss your problem with your partner, remember to:

- Choose your words and timing carefully – you need to be positive and open, not hostile and critical.
- Make practical suggestions about what you would like to do and how you would like to improve your sex life.
- Listen carefully to your partner's replies.
- Devise a plan that suits both your needs.

TREATMENTS IN DETAIL

Conventional Medicine

PRIMARY TREATMENT **UNDERLYING CAUSE** The doctor will discuss lifestyle, medical and psychological factors with you to look for an underlying cause. In some cases, treatment may involve replacing a medication that is causing the erectile dysfunction and sometimes psychological therapy may be recommended.

PRIMARY TREATMENT **DRUGS** Some approaches aim to treat the erectile dysfunction directly. For example, the drug sildenafil (Viagra) relaxes the muscles in the penis and in the walls of the blood vessels supplying it, thereby increasing the flow of blood. Alprostadil may be either injected into the penis or introduced into the urethra.

DEVICES AND PROSTHESES In some circumstances, a vacuum device may be suggested to draw blood into the penis to make it erect. A special rubber band is then placed around the base of the penis to maintain the erection.

An alternative is a prosthesis that can be inserted into the penis to keep it stiff. The position of the penis can be altered. Other implants can be inflated by a pump to erect and deflate the penis as required.

> **CAUTION**
>
> The drugs sildenafil (Viagra) and alprostadil may have side-effects: ask your doctor to explain these to you.

Nutritional Therapy

ARGININE SUPPLEMENTS A man's ability to attain and maintain an erection is, to a certain degree, dependent on the blood supply to the penis. The dilation of the blood vessels (allowing increased blood flow) that is necessary to achieve an erection depends on the presence of a substance called nitric oxide. The amino acid arginine is essential for the formation of nitric oxide.

A 1994 study found that some men with erectile dysfunction, after taking 2,800mg of arginine every day for two weeks, experienced improved erections and were able to achieve better vaginal penetration.

In 1999, a larger, double-blind, placebo-controlled study showed that a third of men with confirmed erectile dysfunction benefited from taking 5,000mg of arginine each day for six weeks. They reported improvement and satisfaction in their sexual performance.

In a 1998 study of men who experienced mild to moderate erectile dysfunction, a formulation with a principal constituent of 2,800mg of arginine helped many of the participants. It improved their ability to maintain an erection during sexual intercourse and enhanced their satisfaction in their sex lives.

In general, at least some men with erectile dysfunction may be helped by taking 2,800–5,000mg of arginine each day.

VITAMIN B12 SUPPLEMENTS There is some evidence to suggest that erectile dysfunction can sometimes be the result of vitamin B12 deficiency and that taking 1,500mcg per day of the methylcobalamin form of vitamin B12 may help.

> **CAUTION**
>
> Consult your doctor before taking arginine if you have a herpes infection (*see p.46*).

Homeopathy

PHOSPHORIC ACID In case reports in which the homeopathic treatment of erectile dysfunction was successful, the medicine that is most frequently suggested is *Phosphoric acid*.

AGNUS CASTUS is another important medicine that may be recommended by a homeopath when a man's erectile dysfunction is accompanied by depression, with anxiety about health, and itching – particularly of the eyes.

CONIUM may be appropriate for older men whose erectile dysfunction accompanies the start of a new relationship after a long period without sex. The man may experience a dizziness that is made worse by lying down.

LYCOPODIUM is a constitutional medicine (*see p.73*), which is prescribed more for the person than the complaint. Men who respond to *Lycopodium* are typically rather reserved; they dislike large gatherings. They are often conscientious people who worry in advance of important occasions and may be quite depressed, because they take their responsibilities very seriously. They often have stomach trouble, especially wind, and tend to be at their worst in the afternoon.

Western Herbal Medicine

Various plants have the reputation of being able to treat erectile dysfunction, but some have only a placebo effect. Not only is reliable evidence scarce, but some remedies, such as yohimbe (*Pausinystalia yohimbe*), may have significant and dangerous side-effects or else they may interact with conventional medicines.

TRADITIONAL HERBS The following herbs have traditionally been used to treat erectile dysfunction. Ashwagandha (*Withania*

About 10 per cent of men in the UK experience erectile dysfunction on a recurrent basis

It is appropriate for men who have lost their libido (sex drive) and it often helps when the problem has started after a prolonged period of emotional stress or, sometimes, an acute illness. There is accompanying weakness of memory and loss of concentration; there may be diarrhoea or looseness of the bowels.

somnifera), cowhage (*Mucuna pruriens*), catuaba (*Erythroxylum catuaba*), red kwao krua (*Butea superba*), damiana (*Turnera diffusa*), ginseng (*Panax ginseng*), garlic (*Allium sativum*), ginkgo (*Ginkgo biloba*), maca (*Lepidium meyenii*).

Other traditional herbs include muira puama (*Ptychopetalum olacoides*) and its close relative with the same Brazilian common name (*Liriosma ovata*), sarsaparilla (*Smilax officinalis*), suma (*Pfaffia paniculata*), tribulus (*Tribulus terrestris*), saw palmetto (*Seronoa serrulata*) and Siberian ginseng (*Eleutherococcus senticosus*).

Only a few of these remedies have reliable research data to justify this traditional use and safety data is scanty in many cases. For this reason, it is unwise to attempt self-medication for erectile dysfunction. Professional herbalists will be able to assess the cause of erectile dysfunction in each case before recommending treatment. There is no one magic formula to remedy this condition.

Plant medicines are at their best when they are prescribed by a practitioner who can take health problems as a whole into account rather than focusing narrowly on the mechanisms of erection.

PRIMARY TREATMENT **GINSENG** provides perhaps the best-known herb for treating erectile dysfunction. Famed throughout China as a *Qi* (energy) tonic, accumulated research has confirmed its adaptogenic (restoring balance within the body) and tonic properties.

The root of ginseng contains steroidal saponins called ginsenosides, which are generally thought to enhance the action of the adrenal hormones through an indirect effect on the pituitary gland.

Taking ginseng on a long-term basis is said to increase overall well-being, and

GINKGO leaves may be effective in treating erectile dysfunction that is due to a lack of blood flow to erectile tissue. This may be due to ginkgo's ability to increase blood flow through arteries and veins without a rise in blood pressure However, gingko probably needs to be used for several months before results can be expected.

RED KWAO KRUA The tubers of red kwao krua constitute a traditional Thai plant medicine that has a long history of treating male sexual dysfunction. In a three-month, randomised, double-blind clinical trial on volunteers with erectile dysfunction, the results revealed that 82 per cent improved significantly and, in addition, did not experience side-effects.

SAW PALMETTO is a treatment for benign prostatic hypertrophy and can probably play a part in treating erectile dysfunction that is the result of enlargement of the prostate (*see p.370*).

CAUTION

• See p.69 before taking a herbal remedy and, if you are already taking prescribed medication, consult a herbalist first.

• Consult a herbalist before taking one of the traditional herbal remedies for erectile dysfunction as many are potentially toxic.

• Do not take ginseng for more than six weeks without a break.

---

and sperm motility. Kidney *Jing* and *Yin* are largely responsible for the health of the sperm and fertility. Male sexual function also depends on a sound psychological state. Severe shock or fright can directly disorder kidney function.

KIDNEY YANG DEFICIENCY can lead to loss of libido (sex drive) and erectile dysfunction. The man is cold, listless and pale. He may have to get up several times at night to pass water. Typically, his back and knees are weak and sore. For this condition, a Chinese herbalist may prescribe a combination of Restore the Right Kidney Pill (*You Gui Wan*) and Special Pill to Aid Fertility (*Zan Yu Dan*).

KIDNEY YIN DEFICIENCY generates "false heat" that can excite the kidneys and briefly fire up the libido, but sexual activity cannot be sustained. A man with kidney *Yin* deficiency may be treated with a modified and combined version of the Six-Flavour Rehmannia Formula (*Liu Wei Di Huang Wan*) and Restore the Left Decoction (*Zuo Gui Yin*).

LIVER QI STAGNATION As the liver meridian passes through the external genitals, liver *Qi* stagnation can also be a cause of erectile dysfunction. The flow of liver *Qi* can be obstructed by mental stress, resentment or anger. Liver *Qi* stagnation is typically found in men who are stressed by work or home circumstances, leading to a loss of libido and erectile dysfunction. The main prescription is Rambling Powder (*Xiao Yao San*).

QI AND BLOOD DEFICIENCY In TCM, anxiety, shock and emotional highs and lows are thought to affect the function of the heart, which governs blood flow. Overwork, poor diet, irregular eating patterns, worry and anxiety can damage the spleen so that it fails to make sufficient *Qi* and blood, thereby undermining sexual performance. Prolonged or severe illness can also cause *Qi* and blood deficiency.

Heart-blood and spleen-*Qi* deficiency can be a cause of erectile dysfunction, since lack of *Qi* and blood cannot sustain an erection. This type of erectile dysfunction is made worse by fatigue. The man may be treated with a modified Return the Spleen Decoction (*Gui Pi Tang*).

At least 20 per cent of men in their 70s have persistent erectile dysfunction

---

feeling more relaxed and energetic is likely to increase libido.

Research indicates that red Korean ginseng has constituents that can specifically improve sexual function in men with erectile dysfunction.

Siberian ginseng (*Eleutherococcus senticosus*) also contains steroidal saponins and has demonstrated a range of effects – antifatigue, antistress, antidepressant and an ability to enhance the immune system – that may also help men to overcome erectile dysfunction.

Chinese Herbal Medicine

Practitioners of Traditional Chinese Medicine (TCM) consider that a man's ability to achieve and maintain an erection is primarily dependent on his kidneys and liver functioning properly. A review summarising the TCM approach to treating male infertility and erectile dysfunction was published in 2001.

Kidney *Yang* and the fire of the kidneys (*Ming Men* – "the Fire of Life Gate") govern the functional aspects of an erection

"DAMP HEAT" that can settle in the genital area and disrupt sexual function can be brought on by an over-rich diet, too much hot and spicy food and/or drinking alcohol or smoking. Overwork or excessive lifting, standing or sexual activity can damage kidney *Qi*, *Yin* and *Yang*. The main treatment is a modified version of Two Marvel Powder (*Er Miao San*), with the addition of other damp-removing herbs and a tonic herb to boost the liver and kidneys.

> **CAUTION**
>
> See p.69 before taking a herbal remedy and, if you are already taking prescribed medication, consult a herbalist first.

Bodywork Therapies

OSTEOPATHY AND CHIROPRACTIC If a man is experiencing pelvic pain as well as erectile dysfunction, the nerve supply to the pelvic organs from the low back may be irritated. Specialised prostatic massage by an osteopath or chiropractor may resolve both problems.

Breathing Retraining

Learning to breathe properly (*see p.62*) may help to relieve the anxiety that accompanies erectile dysfunction, and which may often be part of the cause. This is particularly true if fatigue is an associated symptom, since men who hyperventilate are often too tired to have sex. (*See Anxiety, p.414, for suitable breathing methods.*)

Acupuncture

Acupuncture is one of many traditional Chinese remedies for erectile dysfunction, which is thought of as "withered *Yang*". Although there are few controlled trials in this somewhat controversial area, acupuncture is worth a try – it is safe and relatively free of side-effects, but there is certainly no guarantee of cure.

A preliminary trial of men with erectile dysfunction gave them two electro-acupuncture treatments a week for one month. The results showed that 15 per cent of the participants had better erections, and sexual activity improved in 31 per cent of the men.

Another preliminary trial achieved good results in more than half the men treated. However, in the only controlled trial of electroacupuncture for erectile dysfunction, a placebo produced as good an improvement in sexual function as acupuncture. So, in everyday terms, there is a one in two chance that electroacupuncture would be a useful treatment for erectile dysfunction.

Acupuncture should generally be given weekly for six to eight sessions; if there is no response it should be discontinued. If it is beneficial then consider maintenance treatments on a monthly basis until no further treatment is required.

Anxiety is the most common cause of temporary erectile dysfunction

Psychological Therapies

PRIMARY TREATMENT **COUNSELLING AND SEX THERAPY** Sexual dysfunction in men occurs in several categories. At the sexual arousal stage, men sometimes find themselves unable to achieve an erection (erectile failure). At the orgasm stage, ejaculation may be too quick (premature ejaculation) or may be delayed or absent (male orgasmic disorder). Some men experience pain during intercourse (dyspareunia). Erectile dysfunction may be treated by sex therapy.

ERECTILE DYSFUNCTION is treated by a form of graded exposure. A sex therapist will ask the couple to caress each other, but to avoid the penis (non-genital sensate focus) until they become relaxed with each other. The man's partner stimulates the penis gently until an erection is achieved and then stops until the erection subsides. The couple repeat this process until (as usually happens) the man is not only able to experience an erection – indeed, he comes to expect one.

PREMATURE EJACULATION is readily treatable and high success rates have been reported. The therapist helps the man to relax and become less anxious through cognitive therapy and relaxation training.

The man's partner then employs the "squeeze technique" which was developed by the sex researchers W.H. Masters and V.E. Johnson.

In this technique, the partner stimulates the man until he almost reaches orgasm, and then squeezes the tip of the penis until the urge for orgasm dissipates. This procedure is repeated several times until the man starts to gain more control.

Some research suggests that it is important for the couple to maintain this technique and use it on a continuing basis, as longer-term follow-up studies have shown that some men relapse and experience erectile dysfunction again.

Mind–Body Therapies

Although there is virtually no research into the use of mind–body therapies in the treatment of erectile dysfunction, stress and anxiety have a major impact on the condition, so mind–body therapies may help to relieve it. Try practising a stress-management technique, such as guided imagery, relaxation and breathing on a regular basis. Concentrate on communicating and enjoying sensual and affectionate experiences with your partner.

HYPNOTHERAPY In one trial, in which men underwent three hypnosis sessions a week (reducing to one per month over a six-month period), 75 per cent of men showed improvement.

> **PREVENTION PLAN**
>
> The following may help to prevent erectile dysfunction:
>
> - Practise relaxation.
> - Communicate well with your partner.
> - If you are a smoker, stop.
> - If you drink heavily, reduce your intake.
> - If you are a diabetic, keep it well controlled.

Children's Health

A child's immune system is constantly being exposed to new, potentially harmful organisms. In most cases, a healthy diet and plenty of exercise gives enough resilience to combat most common ailments. When children are ill, their self-healing systems can be supported with rest and attention, coupled with the occasional supplement, antibiotic or homeopathic remedy.

NAPPY RASH

Nappy rash, in which the area of skin covered by the nappy becomes sore and inflamed, is a common problem in babies. It affects nearly all babies at some point and can make them irritable. If possible, the best way to deal with nappy rash is to prevent it in the first place by cleaning and drying the area thoroughly, changing nappies frequently and applying a barrier cream at the first sign of redness. Nappy rash may be treated with antifungal creams if *Candida* is involved. Self-help includes barrier creams, probiotics and homeopathic medicines.

WHAT ARE THE SYMPTOMS?

- Redness in the nappy area (but not in the skin folds and creases)
- Sometimes, a scaly rash similar to cradle cap in the nappy area

WHY MIGHT MY BABY HAVE THIS?

PREDISPOSING FACTOR

- Insufficient nappy changing

TRIGGERS

- Irritation of sensitive skin by ammonia in urine
- Food sensitivity
- Candida overgrowth causes redness in the creases of the skin where urine does not reach

TREATMENT PLAN

PRIMARY TREATMENTS

- Self-help measures, including barrier creams (*see Helping your child*)
- Antifungal creams (for *Candida*)

BACK-UP TREATMENTS

- Eliminate food sensitivities
- Probiotic supplements
- Homeopathic medicines
- Calendula or chamomile ointments

For an explanation of how treatments are rated, see p.111.

WHY DOES IT OCCUR?

Nappy rash usually begins when ammonia in the urine or faeces irritates the delicate skin of the nappy area. It becomes worse if the baby's nappy is not changed frequently, or if the nappy area is not cleaned thoroughly at each nappy change. Sometimes, perfumed baby-care products or certain laundry detergents can irritate a baby's skin and cause or worsen nappy rash. If the rash is present in areas not directly in contact with a soiled nappy, such as the creases between the legs and groin, it may be due to an infection, such as candidiasis.

HELPING YOUR CHILD

PRIMARY TREATMENT The following measures can prevent and treat the rash:

- Change your baby's nappies at least 8 times a day. Thoroughly clean the nappy area with water (not perfumed baby wipes) and ensure it is completely dry.
- Use a barrier cream, such as zinc and castor oil or chamomile or calendula ointment at the first sign of redness.
- Let your child be nappy-free as much as possible. Exposing the affected skin to sunlight for a short while may also help.

TREATMENTS IN DETAIL

Conventional Medicine

PRIMARY TREATMENT If your baby's rash does not clear up in a few days, take him or her to your doctor. If there is an associated *Candida* infection, the doctor might prescribe an antifungal cream. Occasionally, a mild corticosteroid cream is prescribed for a few days to reduce inflammation.

Nappy rash makes the skin red, sore, spotty and uncomfortable. Left untreated, the skin may become blistery.

Nutritional Therapy

FOOD SENSITIVITY may sometimes give rise to nappy rash, perhaps during the weaning period when you introduce your child to new foods. Some babies may have a cows' milk intolerance. (*For more details about food sensitivity, see p.39.*)

CANDIDA ALBICANS If a breastfeeding mother takes probiotics, or gives them to her baby, a nappy rash caused by *Candida* may be alleviated.

Homeopathy

The same medicines recommended for other types of dermatitis (*see Eczema, p.167*) are often effective for nappy rash. These include *Rhus toxicodendron*, *Sulphur* and *Calcarea carbonica*. They should be given in the 6C strength. Crush one tablet or two pills between two teaspoons and give a small amount, dry on the tongue, 3 times a day at least 10 minutes before or after a feed. These medicines are not available as creams.

ORAL THRUSH

Oral thrush is a fungal infection caused by an overgrowth of *Candida albicans* in the mouth. White patches are visible on the tongue and on the lining of the baby's mouth. Common in babies under a year old, oral thrush can cause the baby's mouth to feel sore and make it reluctant to feed. The condition is sometimes associated with nappy rash caused by the same fungus. Treatments include antifungal creams, a *Candida*-elimination diet (for the mother if she is breast-feeding), probiotics and the homeopathic medicine *Borax*.

WHAT ARE THE SYMPTOMS?

- Creamy-yellow or white spots in the mouth that are difficult to rub off
- Sore mouth, which may lead to reluctance to feed

WHY MIGHT MY BABY HAVE THIS?

PREDISPOSING FACTORS

- Impaired immunity
- Use of some antibiotics

TREATMENT PLAN

PRIMARY TREATMENTS

- Antifungal drops and gels
- Anti-*Candida* diet (for the mother)

WORTH CONSIDERING

- Probiotics
- Homeopathic remedy *Borax*

For an explanation of how treatments are rated, see p.111.

WHY DOES IT OCCUR?

Candida albicans is a yeast organism that is naturally present in the mouth and the gut. An overgrowth of the yeast in the mouth results in oral thrush if the oral bacteria that keep it in check are disturbed by certain antibiotics.

Some complementary practitioners say that a dietary imbalance may also disturb the bacteria. As well as young children, oral thrush can affect the elderly and people with impaired immunity.

SELF-HELP

If you bottlefeed your baby, take care to thoroughly sterilise all equipment.

TREATMENTS IN DETAIL

Conventional Medicine

PRIMARY TREATMENT **ANTIFUNGAL DROPS AND GELS** The doctor will examine your baby's mouth and may take a mouth swab to check for the presence of *Candida albicans*. If oral thrush is confirmed, the doctor may prescribe an antifungal treatment, such as nystatin, to be applied to the baby's mouth.

Oral thrush usually improves shortly after starting the treatment, and should clear up within a week, but it may recur.

PREVENTION To prevent *Candida* from overgrowing in the future, breastfeeding mothers may be prescribed an antifungal cream for their nipples. If you bottlefeed your baby, make sure all the equipment you use is thoroughly sterilised by immersing it in boiling water.

The white or creamy-yellow spots of oral thrush affect a baby's mouth, gums, soft palate and tongue. They form a distinctive coating that is hard to wipe away.

Nutritional Therapy

PRIMARY TREATMENT **CANDIDA ALBICANS**, the yeast responsible for oral thrush, thrives on sugar. Eliminating or reducing sugar and refined carbohydrates, such as white flour products, can help to starve yeast out of the system. To help clear oral thrush in a breast-fed baby, the mother can cut back on her intake of sugar and refined carbohydrates, and take probiotics.

PROBIOTICS (healthy gut bacteria supplements) may be very useful in treating oral thrush. You can give probiotics to your baby by adding the contents of a capsule or a powder to water or another drink.

Homeopathy

Borax is a specially prepared homeopathic medicine for oral thrush. Babies who respond to *Borax* may be nervous and jumpy. Crush one tablet or two pills of the 6C strength between two teaspoons and give a small amount, dry on the tongue, 3 times a day at least 10 minutes before or after a feed.

TEETHING

Teething is the eruption of primary (milk) teeth in babies and small children. The eruption of a new tooth through the gum can be uncomfortable; babies may cry and be difficult to settle as a result. A teething baby may also be less willing to feed and may not sleep well at night. Treatments include rubbing a teething gel on to the baby's gums, giving liquid paracetamol or homeopathic *Chamomilla*. Letting a baby gnaw on a chilled teething ring or other suitably hard object can also help to bring relief.

WHAT ARE THE SYMPTOMS?

In babies and small children:

- Dribbling
- Crying
- Flushed cheeks
- Red, swollen gums where the tooth is emerging
- Reluctance to feed

IMPORTANT

Fever, vomiting and diarrhoea are not symptoms of teething, although they may occur during teething. See your doctor if your baby develops any of these symptoms as they may indicate an infection.

TREATMENT PLAN

PRIMARY TREATMENTS

- Pain relief (*see Helping your child*)
- Homeopathic medicine *Chamomilla*

For an explanation of how treatments are rated, see p.111.

WHY DOES IT OCCUR?

A child's first tooth usually emerges at about six months of age and the remaining primary (milk) teeth by the age of three. The process of teething continues until the mid-teens, as the secondary teeth replace the primary teeth. As the root of a tooth grows, the tooth breaks through the skin of the gums, causing pain – more so from the canines and molars than from the incisors.

HELPING YOUR CHILD

PRIMARY TREATMENT Help to relieve the pain and discomfort of teething with the following measures:

- Let your baby gnaw on a cold, hard object, such as a teething ring. Do not put the ring in the freezer. You could also try vegetables such as celery sticks or marshmallow root.
- Rub an over-the-counter teething gel containing anaesthestic on to the baby's gums. Rubbing the gum without the gel may help, too.
- Consider giving liquid paracetamol to babies over three months (do not give aspirin to children as there is a risk of Reye's syndrome).
- Keep the baby's face dry, as dribbling can cause a face rash. Give the baby plenty of water to replace the fluids.
- Give the baby diluted chamomile tea.
- Bathe the baby in a bath with lavender.

Homeopathy

CHAMOMILLA is the standard homeopathic treatment for teething. It is sometimes prepared in the form of fine granules known as homeopathic teething granule (marketed as Teetha by Nelson's in the UK), which are convenient to give to babies. *Chamomilla* pills in the 6C strength contain exactly the same homeopathic medicine. Both the pills and granules are made of lactose (milk sugar) which tastes slightly sweet, so getting the baby to take them is not a problem.

Chamomilla is likely to help when the baby gets very cross and can only be soothed by vigorous movement: the baby quietens when rocked, picked up or walked around, only to start crying again as soon as the movement stops.

Give *Chamomilla* in the 6C strength. Crush one tablet or two pills between two teaspoons and give a small amount, dry on the tongue, 3 times a day at least 10 minutes before or after a feed.

ORDER OF PRIMARY TEETH

A baby's primary, or "milk", teeth are already developing at the time of birth. The first teeth to come through, either the top or bottom jaw, are usually the incisors, which often cause no pain. The rest of the primary teeth come through in no particular order. The canines and molars are often the most painful.

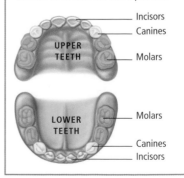

UPPER TEETH — Incisors, Canines, Molars

LOWER TEETH — Molars, Canines, Incisors

HEAD LICE

Head lice are tiny, almost transparent, wingless insects that infest the scalp, where they suck blood and cause irritation and itching. Their eggs, known as nits, are laid close to the scalp and can be seen as tiny white specks attached to the hair shafts. Infestations of head lice are common in school-age children, especially in girls, who tend to have long hair. Treatments include the use of products containing insecticides, wet combing with conditioner and applying neem, turmeric and other herbal remedies to the scalp.

WHAT ARE THE SYMPTOMS?

- Itchiness of the scalp, which may be intense
- Small, white specks (nits) at the base of the hair shafts near the scalp
- The presence of lice themselves (tiny, almost transparent, wingless insects)

WHY MIGHT MY CHILD HAVE THESE?

TRIGGERS

- Close contact with someone with headlice
- Sharing a hat or comb that is infested with lice

TREATMENT PLAN

PRIMARY TREATMENTS

- Insecticidal shampoos
- Wet combing
- Herbal shampoos, such as neem, turmeric and quassia

For an explanation of how treatments are rated, see p.111.

WHY DOES IT OCCUR?

Head lice (*Pediculus capitis*) are adapted to live on the scalp and neck hairs of humans. Children are more commonly infested than adults and the lice are usually transmitted by close head-to-head contact and by sharing items, such as hair accessories, hats and combs. Their presence on your child's scalp is not an indication of poor hygiene or sanitation.

Adult head lice live by sucking blood from the scalp and cannot live for more than a day without a feed. The females can lay about six eggs a day and are able to lay about 100 eggs in total. The female has to be inseminated by a male for the eggs to hatch. In general, an infested scalp may have ten or so adults, but hundreds of eggs that are either dead, hatched or viable.

After applying conditioner to your child's head, use a fine-toothed comb to carefully remove the lice and eggs from the hair shafts.

TREATMENTS IN DETAIL

Conventional Medicine

Once you have confirmed that your child has head lice, check the hair of the rest of the family and inform a teacher or nurse at your child's school.

PRIMARY TREATMENT **INSECTICIDAL SHAMPOOS** A number of over-the-counter shampoos containing insecticides, such as malathion and permethrin, are effective treatments though there may be some skin irritation. Head lice can become resistant to chemicals that are used too much in certain areas. As a result, the treatments recommended may vary in different areas, depending on the resistance patterns. You usually need to apply the products twice, with a week between treatments (*see right*). A third shampoo a week later should make sure. Always follow the directions carefully.

PRIMARY TREATMENT **WET COMBING** If you want to avoid using chemicals, thoroughly wet your child's scalp and hair, then use a fine-toothed comb to remove the head lice and nits. Perhaps the best way is to apply plenty of conditioner to the wet hair before painstakingly combing for up to half an hour. Wipe the comb on a piece of tissue after every stroke. Rinse the hair thoroughly and make sure that you dispose of the tissue. Repeat the combing every 2–4 days for two weeks or more.

CAUTION

Consult your doctor before treating a child under the age of two or a child with allergies, eczema or asthma.

THE LIFE CYCLE OF HEAD LICE

The eggs of a head louse hatch after 7–10 days. The nymphs mature after 10–14 days when they, too, can lay eggs. In order to synchronise the shampooing of your child's hair with the life cycle of the lice, you need to do three weekly insecticidal shampoo treatments from the time you discover the lice. The first kills any live lice. A week later, the second would kill those that had hatched between days one and seven. The third kills those that had hatched on day 10 – the last day that an egg could hatch.

A nymph spends about 8 days developing inside an egg case, which becomes almost transparent at the time of hatching.

Evolution has endowed the six legs of the adult head louse with the ability to grasp the shaft of a human hair.

When to shampoo your child's hair

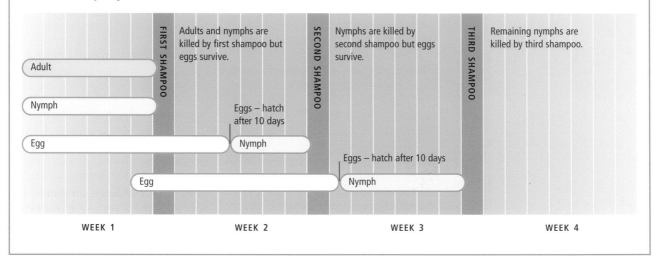

FIRST SHAMPOO — Adults and nymphs are killed by first shampoo but eggs survive.

SECOND SHAMPOO — Nymphs are killed by second shampoo but eggs survive.

THIRD SHAMPOO — Remaining nymphs are killed by third shampoo.

Adult

Nymph

Egg

Eggs – hatch after 10 days

Nymph

Egg

Eggs – hatch after 10 days

Nymph

WEEK 1   WEEK 2   WEEK 3   WEEK 4

Western Herbal Medicine

There are many traditional approaches to treating head lice; some are effective. Apply one of the following remedies to a child's wet hair, then comb it through. A water-based remedy can be left in, but an oil-based remedy needs to be washed out. The eggs (nits) are not destroyed by the treatment so the application needs to be repeated regularly for 2–3 weeks, by which time all the eggs will have hatched and the newly emerged head lice can be killed.

PRIMARY TREATMENT **NEEM** (*Azadirichta indica*), an oriental tree found in much of tropical Asia, is a safe and generally effective insecticide, anti-malarial and insect repellant herb. It is strongly bitter and its main active constituents (liminoids) are toxic to many parasites, including lice. An infusion made from the leaf or the seed oil are the most common preparations used.

PRIMARY TREATMENT **TURMERIC** (*Curcuma longa*) powder or decoction is commonly mixed with neem to treat head lice in India. An Indian study involving 814 people with lice found the combination 98 per cent effective – though treatment also included boiling clothing and bedding, thereby minimising chances of reinfection.

PRIMARY TREATMENT **QUASSIA** (*Picrasma spp.*) is a specific herbal treatment for head lice in many parts of the world. An infusion of the powdered wood, or a tincture, is applied to the hair and scalp. Clinical studies have found it effective for head lice and other infestations.

ESSENTIAL OILS may help to clear infestations. Use various combinations (ideally, with neem seed oil as a base), allow them to soak into the scalp after being thoroughly combed in, then rinse. Good essential oils include aniseed (*Pimpinella*

anisum), eucalyptus (*Eucalyptus globulus*), geranium (*Pelargonium spp.*), clove (*Syzygium aromaticum*), rosemary (*Rosmarinus officinalis*), tea tree (*Melaleuca alternifolia*), lemon (*Citrus limonum*) and lavender (*Lavandula angustifolia*). The appropriate dosage levels are important, particularly when treating children, so purchase a prepared product or see a medical herbalist.

PREVENTION PLAN

The following may help to prevent your child from having head lice:

- Encourage your child not to share hats or combs with other children who may have head lice.

- Check your child's hair regularly so that any problem that develops can be treated early.

CROUP

Croup is a common complaint that is characterised by noisy breathing and a barking cough. It particularly affects children between the ages of six months and three years, and occurs mainly in the autumn and winter. Boys seem to be more susceptible to croup than girls, but the reason for this is not known. Treatment for croup involves putting the child in a steamy atmosphere but giving doses of vitamin C, gentle massage and homeopathy may help. Severe cases need corticosteroids.

WHAT ARE THE SYMPTOMS?

- Barking cough, which may be worse at night
- Noisy breathing, especially on inhaling
- Hoarseness, often noticed when the child is crying
- Symptoms of croup are usually mild, but occasionally breathing may be severely affected

WHY MIGHT MY CHILD HAVE THIS?

PREDISPOSING FACTORS

- Upper respiratory tract infections

TREATMENT PLAN

PRIMARY TREATMENTS

- Increase the humidity (*see Helping your child*)
- Corticosteroids (for severe cases)

BACK-UP TREATMENTS

- Vitamin C supplements
- Massage
- *Aconite* and other homeopathic medicines

For an explanation of how treatments are rated, see p.111.

WHY DOES IT OCCUR?

Croup often follows the symptoms of a common cold, such as a runny nose, by one or two days. In an attack, the trachea narrows, restricting the flow of air to the lungs and causing noisy breathing and a characteristic barking cough.

Most children recover from croup completely within a week, but the condition may recur until they reach about the age of five. At this age, the airways are wider and less likely to become significantly narrowed in response to a viral infection.

HELPING YOUR CHILD

PRIMARY TREATMENT The following measures may help to relieve the symptoms:
- Give your child plenty of fluids to drink.
- Increase the humidity of your child's room with a humidifier, a boiling kettle or a bowl of steaming water (take care not to let the child touch it), or sit together in a steamy bathroom. The moist air may help to ease congestion and discomfort, reducing the intensity and frequency of coughing bouts.
- Give your child a chest rub that includes oil of eucalyptus and lavender.
- Sometimes, breathing the cool air outside for a few minutes is helpful.

IMPORTANT

In a severe case of croup, breathing may become difficult and rapid or laboured. A child's lips and tongue may take on a bluish colour due to lack of oxygen (cyanosis). If your child is having difficulty breathing or if cyanosis develops, call an ambulance.

TREATMENTS IN DETAIL

Conventional Medicine

PRIMARY TREATMENT **CORTICOSTEROIDS** Oral or inhaled corticosteroids may be prescribed to help relieve inflammation. Children with severe symptoms will need to be treated in hospital.

Nutritional Therapy

VITAMIN C SUPPLEMENTS The research evidence is mixed but vitamin C may reduce the symptoms and duration of viral infections. For children aged two and over, give 1g of vitamin C a day, divided into three or four doses and administered as a powder dissolved in a drink. If the vitamin C loosens the bowels, reduce the dose until the bowel habit returns to normal.

Bodywork Therapy

MASSAGE Gently massaging a sick, coughing and wheezing child can relax the tense muscles of the upper chest and throat and so ease the breathing.

Homeopathy

ACONITE, SPONGIA AND HEPAR SULPHURIS For over 150 years, homeopaths have treated croup with a sequence of these three medicines. Preferably, each should be given in the 30C potency. Place two pills on the child's tongue (crush them between two teaspoons if necessary for very young children). As with all homeopathic medicines, the pills should be chewed or sucked, not swallowed whole. Give half-hourly for the *Aconite* and hourly for the *Spongia* and *Hepar sulph*.

GLUE EAR

In glue ear, or chronic secretory otitis media, the middle ear becomes filled with a thick, sticky fluid, which can cause partial hearing loss. Since glue ear often develops in the years when a child is acquiring language, it may cause a delay in speech and language development. Glue ear is more common in boys for reasons that are not known and sometimes runs in families. It is treated by eliminating food sensitivities, manipulation and homeopathy. In some cases, there is a need for grommet insertion or autoinflation.

WHAT ARE THE SYMPTOMS?

Symptoms develop gradually and may not be noticed at first. They may seem less severe at times but are usually worse in winter. They may include:

- Partial deafness
- Speech or pronunciation that is immature for a child's age
- Behavioural problems due to frustration at not being able to hear and therefore understand properly
- Slow progress at school

WHY MIGHT MY CHILD HAVE THIS?

PREDISPOSING FACTORS

- Middle ear infection
- Parents who smoke
- Having Down's syndrome or a cleft palate
- Hay fever and other allergic conditions
- A family trait
- Food sensitivity

TREATMENT PLAN

PRIMARY TREATMENT

- Food elimination diet

BACK-UP TREATMENTS

- Grommet insertion
- Autoinflation
- Homeopathy

WORTH CONSIDERING

- Reducing sugar intake
- Nutritional supplements
- Bodywork therapies

For an explanation of how treatments are rated, see p.111.

WHY DOES IT OCCUR?

The middle ear must be full of air so that the normal vibrations of the eardrum can be transmitted via the ossicles (the tiny bones of the middle ear) to the inner ear. The air comes from the throat to the middle ear via the Eustachian tube.

If one or both of the Eustachian tubes become blocked, as sometimes happens following middle ear infections, air cannot reach the middle ear and fluid is secreted from the lining of the tube. This fluid thickens and prevents the normal vibrations of both the eardrum and the ossicles. In some cases, the reason for the blockage of the tube is unknown.

One way of noticing glue ear is if your child shows signs of impaired hearing. This becomes evident if he or she turns the volume of the television up high or sits very close to it.

Glue ear is more common in children whose parents smoke and in children with allergic conditions, such as hay fever. Children who have Down's syndrome or who are born with a cleft palate are also at greater risk of developing glue ear.

In most cases, glue ear will settle with time, but sometimes it persists and may result in permanent impairment of hearing. Glue ear is rare in children over the age of eight because, as a child grows, the Eustachian tubes widen and are less likely to become blocked.

IMPORTANT

If you think your child has a hearing problem, consult your doctor as soon as possible.

TREATMENTS IN DETAIL

Conventional Medicine

If you suspect your child has glue ear, consult your doctor, who will examine your child's ear with a viewing instrument called an otoscope. Often, the doctor will recommend waiting for a time to see whether the condition resolves.

If the child continues to have difficulties, or if there are hearing problems, the doctor will refer the child to an ear, nose and throat (ENT) specialist. The specialist will re-examine the child's ears and may refer the child for hearing tests and tympanometry, in which the movements of the eardrum are assessed.

GROMMET INSERTION In some cases, the specialist may recommend the insertion of a grommet for persistent glue ear associated with hearing loss. This procedure, which is carried out under a general anaesthetic, involves making a small hole in the eardrum to allow the fluid to drain away. A tiny tube (a grommet) is then inserted to allow air to enter and circulate in the middle ear. These tubes often fall out within a year and the eardrum heals. In some cases, the procedure is repeated. Occasionally, during the same operation, the child's adenoids are removed, which may reduce the risk of further episodes of glue ear.

AUTOINFLATION may be recommended as a means of relieving symptoms of glue ear. This manoeuvre aims to open up the Eustachian tube by raising the pressure in the nose – for example, the child tries to blow up a balloon through a small plastic tube inserted into the nostril.

GLUE EAR

The three ossicles of the middle ear conduct sound vibrations from the eardrum to the oval window of the inner ear. When a thick, sticky fluid fills the middle ear and prevents the normal vibrations of the ossicles and the eardrum, a child's hearing is impaired.

Ossicles

Ear canal

"Glue" in middle ear

Middle ear

Eustachian tube

Nutritional Therapy

| PRIMARY TREATMENT | **FOOD ELIMINATION DIET** Good evidence suggests that food sensitivity is a common factor in recurrent glue ear and ear infections. A 2001 study found that milk, eggs, beans, citrus fruit and tomatoes were the most likely culprits. Eliminating the suspect food led to a significant reduction of symptoms in most patients. Reintroducing suspect foods into the diet tended to provoke a recurrence of glue ear. (*For more details about food sensitivity, see p.39.*)

REDUCE SUGAR INTAKE Try restricting the child's sugar intake if ear infections or glue ear are recurrent. Although sugar intake has not been studied in direct relation to ear problems, it is known that sugar consumption can impair immune function.

SUPPLEMENTS A 2002 study of children showed that a daily multivitamin and mineral tablet, along with some cod liver oil, may help to prevent ear infections and reduce the need for antibiotics. Give half a teaspoon of cod liver oil each day.

PROBIOTICS Antibiotics given to a child with recurrent ear infections can disturb the normal balance of beneficial bacteria in the gut. In the long term, this can lead to problems with irritable bowel syndrome (*see p.222*), yeast overgrowth (*see p.40*) and food sensitivity (*see p.39*). To avoid this, try giving the child probiotic supplements in capsule form for one to two months. If necessary, you can open the capsule and add the contents to a drink or dessert.

N-ACETYLCYSTEINE Evidence suggests that taking 200mg of the amino acid supplement N-acetylcysteine (NAC) twice a day may help to treat glue ear. It is anti-inflammatory and may help to break down mucus. In a 2000 study, NAC significantly reduced the recurrence of glue ear, the need for re-inserting grommets, the number of episodes of ear problems and the frequency of visits to an ear, nose and throat clinic.

XYLITOL Studies suggest that xylitol, a naturally occurring sugar found in some fruits, can interfere and prevent the growth of some bacteria, thereby possibly protecting against recurrent ear infections.

Bodywork Therapies

Studies reveal that most glue ear problems get better on their own, whatever treatment is used. This makes it difficult to verify the claims of parents and practitioners, many of whom testify that massage, cranial osteopathy and chiropractic can improve a child's glue ear problem by draining the middle ear.

Homeopathy

Glue ear is one of the paediatric conditions most frequently treated by homeopathy. The many reports of success stories are backed up by a clinical trial in 1999, which suggested that homeopathy might be more effective than routine GP care. However, more research is needed.

Glue ear is commonly triggered by acute middle ear infection and it appears that glue ear is more likely to follow if this infection is treated with antibiotics. Clinical trials and studies of the outcome of treatment suggest that homeopathy is an effective treatment for acute middle ear infection. The following should be given as two 6C pills or tablets, 3 times a day.

KALIUM SULPHURICUM is the most commonly used medicine for glue ear. Children who respond to *Kali. sulph.* experience deafness with clicking in the ears when they swallow. They have a tendency to catarrh with thick, lumpy discharge – for instance, down the back of the nose.

PULSATILLA Children who respond to *Pulsatilla* have rather similar symptoms to those who respond to *Kali. sulph.*, but the child also tends to be weepy, whingey and clingy, but quickly cheers up after a cuddle.

OTHER REMEDIES If these medicines do not work or seem inappropriate, consult a skilled homeopath for other remedies.

PREVENTION PLAN

The following may help to prevent your child developing glue ear:

- Give your child gum sweetened with xylitol to chew.
- If you are a smoker, then stop.
- Don't give a dummy (pacifier).
- Breast-feed for the first few months if possible and include fresh fruit and vegetables in the child's diet.
- Avoid antibiotics.

WHAT ARE THE SYMPTOMS?

- Prolonged crying that takes place at approximately the same time each day, usually in the evening
- Lack of response to comforting measures, such as holding or feeding
- Sometimes, drawing the legs up to the chest as if in pain
- The crying may be made worse if the baby is tired or is in an unfamiliar environment

WHY MIGHT MY CHILD HAVE THIS?

PREDISPOSING FACTOR

- Living with smokers

TRIGGERS

- Food sensitivity
- Drinking cows' milk

TREATMENT PLAN

PRIMARY TREATMENTS

- Soothing the baby (see *Helping your child*)
- Avoiding cows' milk

WORTH CONSIDERING

- Food elimination diet
- Stabilising blood-sugar levels
- Manipulation
- Homeopathic medicine *Chamomilla*
- A weak, sweetened infusion of chamomile or mint

For an explanation of how treatments are rated, see p.111.

COLIC

Colic is a condition in which an otherwise healthy baby regularly has episodes of prolonged, vigorous crying, often for up to three hours. Colic and the screaming is of course distressing for parents. Colic clears up on its own and does no harm, but may be helped if cows' milk is avoided and if the baby is allowed to feed on demand. Some babies have been helped with homeopathy or cranial osteopathy.

WHY DOES IT OCCUR?

No one knows why colic occurs. It is not thought to be due to an illness, abdominal pain or wind. In some instances, the baby may be sensitive to formula cows' milk. Breast milk is less rich, plentiful and satisfying in the evening. Colic often begins when a baby is a few weeks old and usually stops at about four to five months. Colicky babies typically eat and gain weight well and do not have more health problems than babies without colic.

HELPING YOUR CHILD

PRIMARY TREATMENT Try these simple measures to cope with colic:

- Rock your baby, walk around with him or her, or go for a drive in your car.
- If you breast-feed, rest in the afternoon so your early evening milk is replenished.
- Burp your baby frequently.
- Give a little chamomile or mint tea.
- Gently massage your baby's abdomen.

TREATMENTS IN DETAIL

Conventional Medicine

The doctor will check there is no underlying cause for the symptoms and that the baby is otherwise well. Over-the-counter remedies, such as gripe water, may provide relief, but they are not backed up by medical evidence.

IMPORTANT

Consult your doctor or health visitor for advice and support if you cannot cope with a colicky baby's prolonged crying. Consult your doctor if your baby develops symptoms that are not part of colic, such as a fever or vomiting.

Nutritional Therapy

PRIMARY TREATMENT **AVOID COWS' MILK** Babies may react to infant formulas based on cows' milk. Switching to a formula based on soya, goats' or cows' milk specially treated to break down the large protein molecules (hydrolysates) within it can be very effective. Breastfed infants with colic often improve when cows' milk is also eliminated from their mother's diet. Milk from rice, oats and calcium-enriched soya make good alternatives for the mother.

FOOD ELIMINATION DIET Evidence suggests that eliminating cabbage, broccoli, cauliflower, onion and chocolate from a breastfeeding mother's diet may help.

STABILISE BLOOD-SUGAR LEVELS Feeding on demand may dramatically reduce the incidence of colic, possibly because it avoids a fall in the child's blood-sugar levels.

Bodywork Therapy

MANIPULATION Colic almost always improves on its own after a few months. so the value of treatment is often hard to establish. Chiropractic, cranial osteopathy or craniosacral therapy may also help, but as yet they are unsupported by research.

Homeopathy

CHAMOMILLA is the classical medicine for colic. Crush a pill of 6C strength between two teaspoons and give a few granules on the tip of a spoon when the baby has colic. If the baby needs them more than four times a day, you probably need to increase the strength or use another medicine, such as *Colocynthis* or *Magnesia phosphorica*. If in doubt, or you think the medicine may be inappropriate, consult a homeopath.

For an explanation of how treatments are rated, see p.111.

CHILDREN'S FEVERS

A fever, in which the body's temperature rises above 38° C (100° F), is not an illness in itself but is a symptom of one. Fever is one of the body's responses to infection and enhances its defence mechanisms. The body generates extra heat as the immune responses fight off viruses or bacteria. More uncommonly, a children's fever may be a response to an inflammatory disease or other non-infectious diseases. The aim of treating a fever is to keep the child hydrated and to improve the immune response.

WHAT ARE THE SYMPTOMS?

- Body temperature rises above 38° C (100° F)
- Shivering
- Chills may result when the body temperature falls

WHY MIGHT MY CHILD HAVE THIS?

TRIGGERS

- Infection
- Inflammation
- Allergy

TREATMENT PLAN

PRIMARY TREATMENTS

- Fluids and other self-help measures (*see Helping your child*)

BACK-UP TREATMENTS

- Vitamin C supplements
- Homeopathic medicines

WHY DO THEY OCCUR?

The body's temperature is controlled by the hypothalamus, which is located in the brain and acts like a thermostat. In a fever, the body raises its temperature to the higher level set by the hypothalamus by moving blood from the skin to the interior, reducing the amount of heat radiating from the body. Shivering, which involves the muscles contracting, may also help to increase heat production. When the hypothalamus resets the temperature at a lower level, the body throws off the extra heat by moving blood outwards to the skin and sweating.

HELPING YOUR CHILD

PRIMARY TREATMENT If your child is uncomfortable, try the following measures:

- Keep your child cool and comfortable – give plenty of cool drinks (such as water with fresh lemon juice), loosen clothes and moisten the skin with a flannel soaked in tepid water.
- Give liquid paracetamol (not aspirin) to children over three months.

IMPORTANT

- Call an ambulance or go straight to hospital if you detect meningitis (a fever plus severe headache, dislike of bright lights, neck pain on moving the head forwards, confusion or drowsiness, a rash of flat spots that do not fade when pressed with a drinking glass).

- If a baby under six months has a fever, consult a doctor without delay.

- An unexplained persistent or recurring high temperature needs full medical investigation.

TREATMENTS IN DETAIL

Conventional Medicine

Children who develop a fever in response to an upper respiratory tract infection, such as a cold (*see p.200*), usually recover after two to three days without requiring any medical attention or treatment.

However, if your child runs a high temperature (over 39°C/102°F), consult your doctor. Also, if the temperature stays high for 48 hours, even if everything else seems normal, consult your doctor, because a persistent fever may mean a bacterial infection, which could be serious.

Nutritional Therapy

VITAMIN C SUPPLEMENTS Give a child 500–1,000mg of vitamin C a day, divided into three or four doses, to help resolve a fever associated with a minor infection.

Homeopathy

ACONITE AND BELLADONNA For the early stages of acute fevers, the two most commonly used medicines are *Aconite* and *Belladonna*. In both cases, the fever comes on quickly and the child's temperature may be quite high. These medicines should ideally be given in the 30C strength, in two pills or tablets every 1–2 hours until the fever settles. You can give 6C pills if the 30C strength is not available.

OTHER MEDICINES may be required after the initial stage of the fever and should be given in the 6C strength every 2 hours. These medicines include *Ferrum phosphoricum*, *Gelsemium* and *Mercurius solubilis*.

TONSILLITIS AND ENLARGED ADENOIDS

The tonsils, which are at the back of the throat, and the adenoids, which are at the back of the nasal cavity, form part of the body's defences against infection. In tonsillitis, the tonsils are infected with bacteria or a virus, causing inflammation and a sore throat. The adenoids may become enlarged, often as a result of recurrent infections or an allergy. Mild cases may be helped with herbal and homeopathic remedies, antibiotics or a food elimination diet. Severe, recurrent cases may need surgery.

WHAT ARE THE SYMPTOMS?

Tonsillitis symptoms usually develop over 24–36 hours and may include:

- Sore throat and difficulty swallowing
- Fever
- Headache
- Enlarged lymph nodes in the neck

Symptoms of enlarged adenoids tend to appear gradually over time and may include:

- Breathing through the mouth and snoring during sleep
- Persistently blocked or runny nose

WHY MIGHT MY CHILD HAVE THIS?

TRIGGERS
- Recurring viral infection
- Food sensitivity (possibly)

TREATMENT PLAN

PRIMARY TREATMENTS
- Fluids and liquid paracetamol (*see Helping your child*)
- Food elimination diet (prevention)
- Herbal gargles

BACK-UP TREATMENTS
- Antibiotics (in some cases)
- Vitamin and mineral supplements
- Homeopathy
- Herbal tinctures and teas

WORTH CONSIDERING
- Chinese herbal medicine
- Lymphatic pump techniques
- Massage and chiropractic
- Surgery (for recurring tonsillitis or adenoids that are blocking airways)

For an explanation of how treatments are rated, see p.111.

WHY DOES IT OCCUR?

Tonsillitis is common in children because their tonsils are exposed to many infections for the first time. The tonsils become smaller with age and tonsillitis occurs less frequently in adults. Symptoms tend to become milder as a child grows older and have usually disappeared completely by the time adolescence is reached.

Tonsillitis may be recurrent and eventually result in the enlargement of the tonsils. Enlargement of the tonsils and adenoids may block the upper airway. In some cases, it causes obstructive sleep apnoea, in which breathing is interrupted for brief periods during sleep.

Enlarged adenoids may also predispose a child to recurrent infections of the middle ear and, in some cases, to glue ear (*see p.388*). Permanently enlarged tonsils and adenoids may be due to an allergy – commonly to house-dust mite or to moulds.

HELPING YOUR CHILD

PRIMARY TREATMENT You can relieve some of the symptoms of your child's tonsillitis with the following measures:

- Bring down your child's temperature by sponging with tepid water and giving liquid paracetamol. (Avoid giving your child aspirin because of the risk of Reye's syndrome.)
- Give your child frequent drinks, such as water or diluted fruit juice, but in small quantities.
- Older children can eat ice cream or ice lollies, or suck throat lozenges.

- Relieve a sore throat in young children by giving them cold, non-acidic drinks such as milk.
- Older children can gargle with warm, salty water, or with manuka honey, which is antibacterial and soothing to the throat.

TREATMENTS IN DETAIL

Conventional Medicine

Your doctor will diagnose tonsillitis from the symptoms and an examination. However, a throat swab may be sent to the laboratory to look for a bacterial cause. Paracetamol and similar drugs may help to calm the fever and discomfort. In some cases, antibiotics are prescribed.

SURGERY Surgical removal of the tonsils (tonsillectomy) is not commonly performed today. A doctor might recommend it if a child is repeatedly unwell and missing school, but children tend to "grow out" of recurrent tonsillitis.

Tonsillectomy may be advised for severe, recurrent tonsillitis. Tonsillectomy and adenoidectomy may be recommended in cases of persistent obstruction and when obstructive sleep apnoea is present.

Nutritional Therapy

PRIMARY TREATMENT **FOOD ELIMINATION DIET** Clinical experience suggests that recurrent tonsillitis is often related to food sensitivity, commonly to dairy products, such as milk, cheese, yoghurt and ice cream. In practice, when these suspect foods are eliminated from the affected child's diet, the tonsillitis attacks generally become far less common or disappear altogether. (*For more details about food sensitivity, see p.39.*)

VITAMIN AND MINERAL SUPPLEMENTS
Children with recurrent tonsillitis infections may be helped if they take a multivitamin and mineral supplement each day by ensuring good nutrient levels. Studies indicate that the balance of many vitamins and minerals may be disturbed in individuals who have regular bouts of tonsillitis. A 2001 study found that patients who suffered with chronic tonsillitis had decreased levels of vitamins B1, B2 and C.

There is some evidence to suggest that zinc levels can be especially low in individuals who have recurring tonsillitis. A 1998 study found that taking a vitamin E supplement was effective in the treatment of recurring tonsillitis.

> **CAUTION**
>
> Consult your doctor before giving zinc or vitamin C with antibiotics (*see p.46*).

TONSILS AND ADENOIDS

The tonsils and adenoids are composed of lymphatic tissue that is rich in white blood cells and forms an important part of the body's first line of defence against invading organisms, such as bacteria and viruses. Infected tonsils swell up and become inflamed, making it painful to swallow. Enlarged adenoids can block both the nasal passage, making it difficult to breathe through the nose, and the Eustachian tubes that allow air to reach the middle ears.

The location of the tonsils and adenoids

Tongue

Adenoids

Tonsils

Larynx

The tonsils are two almond-shaped glands of lymphatic tissue located at the back of the throat. The pair of adenoids are located above the throat at the back of the nasal cavity.

Homeopathy

In a 1994 clinical trial, homeopathic medicines, such as *Sulphur, Calcarea carbonica, Belladonna, Pulsatilla* and *Silica*, were used to treat children (aged between 18 months and 10 years) who had repeated upper respiratory tract infections, such as tonsillitis, and ear infections. Not all the children had enlarged tonsils, but among those who did fewer tonsillectomies and adenoidectomies were required, and fewer courses of antibiotics if they received homeopathy, rather than placebo tablets.

The following medicines can safely be used on a self- (or family) treatment basis (*see p.77 for details of doses*). If you are in doubt or the response to treatment is poor, consult a qualified homeopath.

CALCAREA CARBONICA is one of the main medicines for children with chronically enlarged tonsils and adenoids. Children who respond to *Calc. carb.* are often big and chubby, and they sweat on their heads at night. They are often stubborn, and may have various fears, waking at night crying and frightened. They often love eggs.

SILICA Children who respond to *Silica*, in contrast to those who respond to *Calc. carb.*, tend to be small and slim, with fine hair and delicate skin. Appearances may be deceptive because they can be quite determined and stubborn. But they often feel the cold and seem to "pick up every cold that is going around". They often have cold, clammy hands and feet, and may have weak or deformed nails.

BARYTA CARBONICA Those children who respond to *Baryta carb.* may have really big tonsils and sometimes large, firm glands in the neck. They often have delayed development: they are slow to talk or read for no obvious reason, and they may be very shy. They may also have sweaty, smelly feet.

SULPHUR A number of other medicines may be required, including *Sulphur*. Those children who respond to *Sulphur* are hot-blooded, throwing off their bedclothes at night. They are generally strong-willed, determined and messy. They often have skin trouble, particularly eczema.

PULSATILLA Children who respond to *Pulsatilla* tend to cry easily and become whingey, clinging to their mothers when ill. Their noses become blocked with excessive amounts of yellow or green mucus, which can trickle down into their throats, making them cough, particularly at night.

Western Herbal Medicine

Sore throats are much better treated in the first instance by herbal medicines than by antibiotics. This is a condition that is suitable for self-treatment, but consult a health professional if symptoms persist and do not respond to treatment.

PRIMARY TREATMENT **HERBAL GARGLES** are an effective way to alleviate sore throats. There are three main categories of herbs for gargles. One or two herbs from each category should be combined together.

TANNIN HERBS In the first category are astringent herbs that contain tannin, which has the ability to coagulate the protein of infecting bacteria. These herbs include tormentil (*Potentilla erecta*), bayberry (*Myrica cerifera*) bark, agrimony (*Agrimonia eupatoria*), plantain (*Plantago major*), oak (*Quercus robur*) bark and raspberry (*Rubus idaeus*) leaves.

HERBS WITH ESSENTIAL OILS In the second category are herbs with antibacterial essential oils. These herbs include sage (*Salvia officinalis*) leaf, hyssop (*Hyssopus officinalis*), thyme (*Thymus serpyllum*), chamomile (*Matricaria recutita*), marigold (*Calendula officinalis*) flowers and myrrh (*Commiphora myrrha*).

MUCILAGE HERBS In the third category are herbs containing mucilage, a gum-like substance that can soothe an inflamed throat. These herbs include marshmallow (*Althea officinalis*) root or leaf, mullein (*Verbascum thapsus*), aloe vera (*Aloe vera*) juice, liquorice (*Glycyrrhiza glabra*), slippery elm (*Ulmus rubra*) and Iceland moss (*Cetraria islandica*).

MAKING THE GARGLES Use two parts of the mucilage herbs, two parts of tannin herbs to one part of the herbs with essential oil. (If using myrrh, add 15 drops of tincture to a gargle.)

To make the gargles, boil the roots or barks first, then add the volatile oil-bearing and mucilage herbs in the last five minutes of the simmering period. Strain off the fluid and allow to cool. Gargle every 2–4 hours daily during the acute phase.

USEFUL RECIPES:
Sage sore throat soother
Take a handful of fresh garden sage or half a handful of dried sage and simmer it for 20 minutes in 500ml of water with the lid on the pan. Strain and add a tablespoon of cider vinegar and a teaspoon of honey. Allow to cool, then gargle 3–4 times daily during the acute phase of the infection. Keep left-over fluid in the fridge.

Cider vinegar and honey gargle
Use one tablespoon of cider vinegar to a glass of warm water and add one to two teaspoons of honey. Gargle the mixture 2–4 times daily during the acute phase.

INTERNAL HERBAL TREATMENTS A herbal practitioner would prescribe internal treatments for a child with recurring tonsillitis, using perhaps tinctures of the following herbs, either individually or in a combination: echinacea (*Echinacea angustifolia*), wild indigo (*Baptisia tinctoria*), golden seal (*Hydrastis canadensis*), myrrh, the root of burdock (*Arctium lappa*), the herb or root of figwort (*Scrophularia nodosa*), thyme, sage, hyssop, marshmallow (*Althea officinalis*), agrimony and andrographis (*Andrographis paniculata*).

The tinctures made with these herbs all combat the bacteria that cause a sore throat as well as easing the soreness. You can drink teas made of thyme, sage and hyssop to support your immune system's resistance and aid the mucous membranes of the throat.

> **CAUTION**
>
> See p.69 before giving a herbal remedy and, if your child is already taking prescribed medication, consult a medical herbalist first.

Chinese Herbal Medicine

Chinese herbs for treating sore throat include burdock seed, figwort (*Scrophularia ningpoensis*) root, puff ball (*Lasiosphaera fenzlii*), dyer's woad (*Isatis tinctoria*) root, pigeon pea (*Sophora subprostata*), honeysuckle (*Lonicera japonica*), forsythia (*Forsythia suspensa*), field mint (*Mentha arvensis*), liquorice (*Glycyrrhiza glabra*), blackberry lily rhizome (*Belamcanda chinensis*) and balloonflower (*Platycodon grandiflorus*) root.

Sore throats are treated according to the pattern of symptoms they present to the practitioner. A "wind–heat" presentation is marked by an aversion to cold, as well as fever, headache, generalised aching, red tonsils, sore throat, difficulty in swallowing and a red tip to a tongue tip that has a thin yellow coat. It is treated with Honey-

suckle and Forsythia Powder (*Yin Qiao San*), which can be taken in pill form or as a decoction.

A more serious presentation is the development of "throat–fire toxin". The patient may have a high fever, thirst, restlessness and swelling of the tonsils with an abscess or pus formation on the surface.

> ## Tonsillitis in pre-school children is usually caused by a virus

The TCM doctor may use a variation of Coptis Decoction to Clear the Throat (*Huang Lian Qing Hou Yin*).

> **CAUTION**
>
> Do not treat a child with Chinese herbs without first consulting a Chinese herbalist for a correct diagnosis.

Bodywork Therapies

LYMPHATIC PUMP TECHNIQUES can be used, but only if a child happily tolerates bodywork. Experience suggests that specific osteopathic methods, known collectively as "lymphatic pump techniques", can increase the immune system's response to infection. They markedly increase the levels of defensive white blood cells for up to 24 hours.

MASSAGE AND CHIROPRACTIC Bodywork therapists would aim to boost the immune system of a child through a general, nonspecific massage. Consult a licensed chiropractor or osteopath if you want advice about this approach to prevention.

> **PREVENTION PLAN**
>
> **The following may help prevent your child developing tonsillitis:**
>
> - Give your child plenty of fresh fruit and vegetables.
> - Give your child a daily multivitamin and mineral supplement.

MUMPS

Mumps is a relatively mild viral illness that was common in children before the MMR (measles, mumps and rubella) vaccine was introduced. In most cases, the virus causes characteristic swelling and inflammation of the parotid salivary glands, located below and just in front of the ears. Swelling may be on both sides of the face or on one side only. Treatment depends on the severity of the symptoms and involves giving fluids and paracetamol Homeopathic medicines may also help.

WHAT ARE THE SYMPTOMS?

Symptoms usually begin two to three weeks following infection with the virus and may include:

- Pain and swelling on one or both sides of the face, below and in front of the ear, lasting for about three days
- Pain on swallowing
- Sore throat
- Fever

WHY DOES IT OCCUR?

Mumps is caused by a paramyxovirus and is spread via coughs and sneezes or by direct contact with the saliva of an infected person. Symptoms are mild in most people and absent in a few. An individual with mumps is infectious from three days before swelling to seven days afterwards.

HELPING YOUR CHILD

PRIMARY TREATMENT The following can make your child more comfortable:

- Give plenty of cool fluids to drink to help prevent dehydration.
- If your child is over three months old and has a fever, try liquid paracetamol.
- Give a nutritious diet.

TREATMENTS IN DETAIL

Conventional Medicine

Always consult your doctor if a child is very young or very ill and you suspect they have mumps. Your doctor will usually diagnose mumps from the characteristic swelling below and in front of the ears. There is no specific treatment except for dealing with the symptoms (*see above*). It is best to keep the child at home.

Adolescent boys may develop a severe inflammation of one or both testes for which a strong painkiller is needed. If other sites of the body are affected, the relevant symptoms will be treated accordingly.

Nutritional Therapy

VITAMIN C AND ZINC SUPPLEMENTS Though no trials have been done, for children aged two and over it is safe to give

The characteristic swollen cheeks in mumps are the result of swelling of the parotid salivary glands, which are below and in front of the ears.

500–1,000mg of vitamin C divided into three or four doses during the day and 10–15mg of zinc once or twice a day for the period of the illness.

Homeopathy

The medicines *Mercurius solubilis*, *Pulsatilla* and *Belladonna* may safely help a child with mumps and should be given as two pills in the 6C strength, 3 or 4 times a day. If in doubt, or the response to the treatment is poor, consult a qualified homeopath.

There is no evidence that homeopathic vaccination works. Your homeopath should not recommend them, as the vaccinations will lull you into a false sense of security.

IMPORTANT

A boy or man who thinks he may have contracted the disease, or been exposed to someone with it, and has swollen testes should see his doctor without delay.

TREATMENT PLAN

PRIMARY TREATMENT

- Fluids and liquid paracetamol (*see Helping your child*)

BACK-UP TREATMENTS

- Vitamin C and zinc supplements
- *Mercurius solubilis* and other homeopathic medicines

For an explanation of how treatments are rated, see p.111.

MEASLES

Measles is a viral illness that causes fever and a rash. It is a highly infectious disease that mainly affects young children. It is relatively uncommon in the developed world due to immunisation, usually as part of the combined MMR (measles, mumps and rubella) vaccine. However, in the developing world, where immunisation is rare, measles and its complications killed an estimated 600,000 children in 2002. Treatment involves relieving the symptoms, boosting vitamin A levels and increasing the immune system's response to infection.

WHAT ARE THE SYMPTOMS?

Symptoms usually begin around ten days following infection with the virus and may include:

- High fever, runny nose and cough
- Reddened, painful, watery eyes
- White spots on a red base on the inside of the cheeks (Koplik's spots)
- After three to four days, a red rash that starts on the face and behind the ears, before spreading down the body. The rash does not itch and lasts about a week

WHY DOES IT OCCUR?

The measles virus is transmitted through minute airborne droplets of saliva that are scattered when an infected person coughs and sneezes. Measles is contagious from the onset of the cold-type symptoms until five days after the distinctive rash appears. Symptoms usually disappear about a week or more after the rash appears, unless complications develop. One measles infection should confer lifelong immunity.

In otherwise healthy, well-nourished children measles is usually not serious, although the child may feel very ill. However, complications, such as conjunctivitis, middle ear infections and bacterial pneumonia, can occur, especially if the child is malnourished or if his or her immune system is depleted. In rare cases (about 1 in 1,000), the brain may be affected and inflamed (viral encephalitis), sometimes with permanent damage.

At first, the spots in a measles rash appear on the face and behind the ears, before spreading over the whole body. They are initially separate and then gradually merge together to form a blotchy large-scale rash.

HELPING YOUR CHILD

PRIMARY TREATMENT Try the following measures to allow your child to recover from the illness, to bring down the fever and to relieve discomfort:

- Let your child sleep as much as possible. Allow your child to rest in bed or be up and about around the home, according to how he or she feels, but prevent him or her from becoming tired.
- Keep your child cool – loosen the clothes and moisten the skin with a flannel soaked in tepid water.
- Encourage your child to drink plenty of cool fluids to prevent dehydration. Thirst is often absent and dehydration is a real danger, especially for babies. Offering lots of small sips is usually best, especially when nausea is a problem. A plastic medicine dropper that holds a few fluid ounces is useful.
- A child with a fever can go from cold to hot very quickly; follow his cues and let him throw off the covers if he wants.
- Don't force food on a child with a fever. Let him decide when and what to have,

IMPORTANT

If your child vomits, develops earache, has a severe headache, becomes drowsy, starts breathing abnormally or experiences a febrile convulsion, call your doctor at once.

TREATMENT PLAN

PRIMARY TREATMENT

- Fluids and liquid paracetamol (*see Helping your child*)

BACK-UP TREATMENTS

- Vitamin A supplements
- Vitamin C and zinc supplements (may protect or reduce the severity)
- Homeopathic medicines

For an explanation of how treatments are rated, see p.111.

but avoid too much sugar which may slow immune responses down.

- Give liquid paracetamol to children over three months (aspirin should not be given to children under 12 years because of the risk of Reye's syndrome).
- Rarely, if your child's temperature rises quickly, he or she may have a febrile convulsion. Don't worry – remove nearby objects and surround the child with pillows and cushions. The convulsion will soon subside. Consult a doctor straightaway and prevent your child from becoming cold afterwards. (*See also Children's fevers, p. 391.*)

TREATMENTS IN DETAIL

Conventional Medicine

Doctors usually make the diagnosis from just the symptoms and an examination. However, blood tests may also be used for confirmation. No treatment is usually needed, other than measures to relieve the symptoms (*see Helping your child, left*). Keep your child at home. Complications will need treatment, such as antibiotics for bacterial pneumonia.

IMMUNISATION Most babies in the UK are immunised against measles with the MMR (measles, mumps, rubella) vaccine. An injection into the thigh or upper arm is given at 12–15 months, with a booster dose before going to school. Fears that the MMR vaccine may contribute to the development of autism were shown to be unfounded by research published in 2004. Many parents, however, remain unconvinced. A few doctors offer the choice of a "single measles" immunisation.

> **CAUTION**
>
> If you are concerned about letting your child be immunised with the MMR vaccine, consult your doctor.

Nutritional Therapy

Encourage your child to drink plenty of cool fluids, especially if there is a fever. This will help to prevent dehydration and is likely to help speed the healing and recovery process. Restricting a child's intake of

refined sugar may help, as it is known that sugar consumption can impair certain immune functions.

VITAMIN A SUPPLEMENTS appear to have an important role in the treatment of measles. Evidence from research suggests that vitamin A deficiency has the effect of

making both measles, and its complications, more likely. A study undertaken in California in 1992 found that about 50 per cent of supposedly well-nourished children who were infected with measles were relatively deficient in vitamin A.

In a 2002 review, vitamin A supplementation in young children with measles was described as one of the best-proven, safest and most cost-effective interventions in international public health.

The World Health Organisation recommends giving 200,000 IU per day for two days to children over two years of age with measles when vitamin A deficiency may be present. (For infants, this recommended dose can be reduced to about 100,000 IU.) At this dose there is evidence of a reduced risk of complications and mortality.

During a measles epidemic, half these recommended doses can safely be given to children, even if they are not vitamin A deficient. The vitamin A can be given until symptoms disappear.

VITAMIN C SUPPLEMENTS have immune-stimulating and antiviral properties that might help in the treatment of measles. For children aged two years and over, it is safe to give a daily dose of 500–1,000mg of vitamin C supplements, divided into three or four doses throughout the day. If this loosens your child's bowels, reduce the dose until a normal bowel pattern returns. Stop giving the supplements once the child feels better.

> **CAUTION**
>
> Consult your doctor before giving vitamin C with antibiotics (*see p.46*).

Homeopathy

The following medicines (*Pulsatilla, Euphrasia, Bryonia* and *Sulphur*) should be given in a dose of two pills or tablets of the 6C strength every 6 hours. Increase the dose to every four hours if it seems to help, but the effect does not last.

Febrile convulsions only occur in about 1 in 200 cases of measles in the UK

PULSATILLA is the homeopathic medicine most commonly required for measles. As is often the case with homeopathy, *Pulsatilla* is prescribed on a "whole person" basis (*see Constitutional prescribing, p.73*).

The child who is likely to benefit from *Pulsatilla* becomes whingey and weepy when he or she has measles, and becomes better from attention and affectionate cuddles. There is a thick, yellowish discharge from the nose and sometimes from the eyes, gumming them up.

There are some rather unusual paradoxical features that strongly suggest *Pulsatilla* would be helpful. For instance, the child has a dry, sticky mouth, but is not thirsty; and although the child is chilly, easily feeling the cold, he or she wants fresh air, his or her nose is less blocked and he or she feels generally better from having the window open or a fan playing on him or her.

OTHER MEDICINES that may help include *Euphrasia* if conjunctivitis is a problem or *Bryonia* for a dry, painful, hacking cough. If the measles drags on, *Sulphur* may help – the child feels hot and is lethargic, the rash turns purple and may become itchy.

> **PREVENTION PLAN**
>
> **The following measures may help to prevent measles:**
>
> - Arrange for your child to have the MMR vaccine.
> - Give plenty of fruit and vegetables to ensure a plentiful supply of protective antioxidants.

RUBELLA

Rubella, or German measles, is a viral illness that usually causes no more than a mild rash and a fever. However, it is a serious problem for unborn babies. It is less common than it used to be due to routine immunisation, with the MMR (measles, mumps and rubella) vaccine. It usually settles by itself after a few weeks, and is treated by taking fluids, paracetamol and sometimes supplements. Homeopathy may also help.

WHAT ARE THE SYMPTOMS?

Symptoms usually begin around two to three weeks following infection with the virus and may include:

- Fever, which is usually mild in children but may be high in adolescents and adults
- Swollen lymph nodes, particularly those at the back of the neck and behind the ears
- After two to three days, a pink rash, which appears first on the face and then spreads down the body. The rash does not itch and usually clears within three days

WHY DOES IT OCCUR?

The rubella virus is spread via coughs and sneezes. An individual with rubella is very contagious from roughly a week before the pink rash appears until a week after it goes. One infection confers lifelong immunity.

HELPING YOUR CHILD

PRIMARY TREATMENT The following measures may enable you to help your child feel more comfortable:

- Let your child sleep as much as possible.
- Allow him or her to rest or to get up and play as she or he feels inclined.
- Give plenty of cool fluids, such as water with a little lemon juice added, to help prevent dehydration.
- If the child is over three months of age and has a fever, give liquid paracetamol (but do not give aspirin as there is a risk of Reye's syndrome).
- Provide little tempting meals with foods your child likes and preferably some nutritious fruits and vegetables.

TREATMENTS IN DETAIL

Conventional Medicine

Children should have the MMR vaccine, which is particularly important for girls. If a woman may have rubella, a doctor will arrange blood tests to confirm diagnosis. There is no specific treatment except for dealing with the symptoms (*see Helping your child*). Keep infectious children at home, away from other people.

Nutritional Therapy

VITAMIN C SUPPLEMENTS There is some evidence that orange juice may lessen the symptoms of German measles and acceler-

The pink rash of German measles first appears on the face. It gradually develops on the body and then on the arms and legs.

ate the production of antibodies in the blood. Giving sips of freshly squeezed orange juice, which should be diluted with the same amount of water, throughout the day may help your child to recover from a rubella infection.

However, supplemental vitamin C is likely to provide some additional benefit. Give 500–1,000mg vitamin C supplements each day, divided into three or four doses. If this regime loosens the bowels, reduce the dose and stop the treatment when your child recovers.

Homeopathy

Rubella in children is often mild and does not require treatment. If symptoms are troublesome, consult a homeopath, or you can safely use medicines such as *Belladonna*, *Ferrum phosphoricum*, *Gelsemium*, *Pulsatilla* and *Euphrasia* (*for dosages, see p.77*).

IMPORTANT

If you are pregnant, are not immune to rubella and think you may have contracted the disease or been exposed to someone with it, see your doctor for blood tests without delay.

TREATMENT PLAN

PRIMARY TREATMENTS

- Rest, fluids and liquid paracetamol (*see Helping your child*)

WORTH CONSIDERING

- Vitamin C supplements
- *Belladonna* and other homeopathic medicines

For an explanation of how treatments are rated, see p.111.

WHOOPING COUGH

Whooping cough, or pertussis, is a highly infectious bacterial illness that was common in children before immunisation against it became routine. The infection causes characteristic fits of severe coughing that end with a "whoop" as an affected child inhales. Whooping cough is most serious in babies under a year, for whom it can be life-threatening, and it remains serious for children under the age of two. Integrated treatments include antibiotics and nutritional and other strategies to support the immune system.

WHY DOES IT OCCUR?

Whooping cough is caused by the bacterium *Bordetella pertussis*, which infects and inflames the windpipe and airways in the lungs. The bacteria are spread by coughs and sneezes. The initial stage of whooping cough may last one to two weeks. During this time, the child is highly infectious. Symptoms become worse before subsiding, usually within four to ten weeks if there are no complications. However, a dry cough may persist for some time.

An attack of whooping cough does not give complete immunity, but a second attack is usually milder and may not be recognised as whooping cough. There are potential complications, including convulsions, pneumonia and bronchiectasis (permanent widening of the airways). Babies may briefly stop breathing after the coughing fits.

TREATMENTS IN DETAIL

Conventional Medicine

Your doctor will probably be able to diagnose the illness from the distinctive sound of your child's cough. This diagnosis can then be confirmed by testing swabs taken from the nose.

IMPORTANT

If your child is under a year old and seems to have whooping cough, contact your doctor immediately. Most children have the DTP immunisation at two, three and four months, as well as before they start school.

PRIMARY TREATMENT **ERYTHROMYCIN** If whooping cough is diagnosed in the initial phase, then giving the antibiotic erythromycin may stop the disease from progressing or decrease its severity. If an unimmunised child is exposed to the infection, erythromycin should be given as a preventive measure.

HOSPITAL TREATMENT Seriously ill children will be admitted to hospital for monitoring and other measures, including intravenous fluids and oxygen if necessary.

Nutritional Therapy

MULTIVITAMIN/MINERAL SUPPLEMENTS may boost the child's immune system. During an infection, restrict sugar intake and give a children's multivitamin and mineral supplement. Some nutrients, especially vitamin C and zinc, may help to maintain and stimulate the function of the immune system. If an ear infection accompanies whooping cough, treat it in the same way as glue ear (*see p.388*).

Homeopathy

The main homeopathic medicines for whooping cough are *Belladonna*, *Drosera* and *Cuprum metallicum*.

PREVENTION It has sometimes been claimed that "homeopathic immunisation", using a nosode (a homeopathic medicine made from a disease product) of whooping cough called *Pertussin* or *Coquelchin* is an effective alternative to DTP immunisation. However, there is no scientific evidence to support this and homeopaths do not recommend it.

WHAT ARE THE SYMPTOMS?

Symptoms usually begin 1–3 weeks following infection and may include:

- A mild fever, headache or flu-like symptoms
- Rash that appears as crops of small red spots. The spots become itchy and fluid-filled, then dry out and form scabs
- Discomfort in the mouth if spots develop there
- Possible complications include bacterial infections of the rash

WHY MIGHT MY CHILD HAVE THIS?

PREDISPOSING FACTOR

- Weakened immune system

TREATMENT PLAN

PRIMARY TREATMENTS

- Fluids, paracetamol, etc. (*see Helping your child*)
- Antiviral drugs (in some cases, e.g. when immunity is compromised by other illnesses or drugs)

BACK-UP TREATMENTS

- Antibiotics (if a secondary infection occurs)
- Nutritional therapy
- *Rhus toxicodendron* and other homeopathic medicines

For an explanation of how treatments are rated, see p.111.

CHICKENPOX

Chickenpox, also known as varicella, is a contagious viral illness that is common in children. It is caused by the varicella zoster virus and results in a characteristic rash of fluid-filled spots which are usually widespread over the body. Chickenpox is usually mild in children, but symptoms tend to be more severe in young babies, adolescents and adults. The main aim of treatment is to fight the virus and to enhance the function of the immune system.

WHY DOES IT OCCUR?

The varicella zoster virus, which causes chickenpox, is transmitted through airborne droplets contained in the coughs and sneezes of infected people. It can also be transmitted by direct contact with the rash of spots and blisters.

Once the rash appears, the tiny red spots quickly turn into itchy, fluid-filled blisters These dry out within 24 hours and form scabs. Several crops of spots can appear.

Someone with chickenpox is infectious from about two days before the rash appears until the last spots have formed scabs, usually 10–14 days after the onset of the rash.

COMPLICATIONS Bacterial infection of the blisters caused by scratching the sometimes unbearably itchy rash is the most common complication of chickenpox. Newborn babies and people with weakened immune systems (such as those who are undergoing chemotherapy) are more likely to have a more serious chickenpox infection and may also develop other complications, such as pneumonia.

THE RELATIONSHIP OF CHICKENPOX WITH SHINGLES People who have had chickenpox are then immune to the disease and cannot catch it again. However, the virus remains dormant in nerve cells and may be reactivated later in life, causing shingles (*see p.165*). People who have not had chickenpox can catch it from someone with shingles, but only via direct contact with the shingles rash and not via coughs and sneezes. However, it is not possible to develop shingles without having first had chickenpox, even if it was only a very mild episode a long time ago.

The chickenpox rash first affects the skin on the body, then spreads to the face and limbs. The spots become itchy, fluid-filled blisters that dry out and then form scabs.

HELPING YOUR CHILD

PRIMARY TREATMENT For a child with a mild infection who does not need to see a doctor, try the following measures:

- Let him rest.
- Help to reduce the fever by stroking his skin with a cool flannel.
- Encourage him to drink plenty of cool fluids to prevent dehydration. Thirst is

IMPORTANT

Pregnant women who develop chickenpox, or who are exposed to the infection and think they may never have had the infection, should see their doctor.

often absent and dehydration is a real danger, especially for babies. Offering lots of small sips is usually best, especially when nausea is a problem. A plastic medicine dropper that holds a few fluid ounces is useful.

- Follow your child's cues about whether to bundle up or throw off the covers: fevers can go up and down.
- Don't force food on a child with a fever. Offer tasty, favourite foods, but avoid giving too much sugar, which may slow immune responses.
- To relieve the discomfort of chickenpox, give liquid paracetamol to children over three months (but do not use aspirin as there is a risk of Reye's syndrome).
- A bath with plenty of warm water that contains either a handful of bicarbonate of soda or two cups of powdered oatmeal can be soothing.
- Use cotton wool to gently dab calamine lotion on to the spots to relieve the itching. Alternatively, you can apply a gel of chickweed (*Stellaria media*) and/or a paste made from slippery elm (*Ulmus rubra*) powder, baking soda and water to the spots.
- Keep your child's fingernails short and try to prevent him from scratching the spots and blisters, which could lead to skin infections. Babies may need to wear mittens to stop the scratching.

TREATMENTS IN DETAIL

Conventional Medicine

If your child is otherwise healthy, the infection is likely to be mild and will not need treatment. The child will normally recover fully between 10 and 14 days after the onset of the first crop of the chickenpox rash. Simply focus on relieving the itching and preventing your child from scratching the blisters (*see Helping your child*). Permanent scars may result from blisters that have been scratched and become infected.

PRIMARY TREATMENT Babies or individuals with reduced immunity, such as those who are undergoing chemotherapy or who are HIV positive, should see a doctor at once regarding possible treatment with antiviral drugs.

Chickenpox does not usually require any treatment, although antiviral drugs, such

as aciclovir, may be considered for adults. Antiviral drugs may limit the effects of the varicella infection but they need to be administered in the early stages of the disease if they are to be of help.

Antibiotics are needed if a secondary bacterial infection of the rash occurs.

IMMUNISATION A vaccination against varicella has been developed. However, it is not recommended for immunising healthy children in the UK. The health services in some other countries, such as the US and Australia, have introduced a programme of varicella immunisation as a routine measure for children who are aged between 12 and 18 months.

> **CAUTION**
>
> Antiviral drugs have potential side-effects: ask your doctor to explain these to you.

> **CAUTION**
>
> Consult your doctor before giving vitamin C with antibiotics (*see p.46*).

Homeopathy

Chickenpox is usually a mild disease in young children, settling without complications. However, it can be a severe illness in people with a suppressed immune system (which occurs, for example, as a side-effect of certain drugs).

RHUS TOXICODENDRON The classical homeopathic treatment for chickenpox is *Rhus tox.* This medicine is frequently helpful, particularly if the rash is very itchy and is accompanied by small blisters. Give your child two pills of the 6C strength, 4 times a day until the rash heals (*see p.77*).

Chickenpox during pregnancy, especially the second half, can endanger the baby

---

Nutritional Therapy

PRIMARY TREATMENT **VITAMIN C SUPPLEMENTS** Although no conclusive clinical trials have been performed, vitamin C supplements may be able to boost the immune system of children with chickenpox. They may help to fight the infection, encourage healing and speed recovery. The recommended dose is 500–1,000mg of vitamin C supplements per day, divided into three or four doses.

VITAMIN A SUPPLEMENTS Studies show that the chickenpox infection causes a lowering of vitamin A levels in children. Consequently, giving 3,000–5,000 IU of vitamin A every day for 10 days from the start of infection seems to help children with chickenpox.

If they are given at the very start of the chickenpox infection, vitamin A supplements may be effective in shortening the duration of the illness. Moreover, the supplements may also help to protect against complications, such as pneumonia, conjunctivitis and gasteroenteritis.

OTHER MEDICINES *Belladonna* or *Aconite* are two homeopathic medicines that may help in the early stages of the infection, where there is fever and the child is generally unwell. *Aconite* is likely to help if the child feels both chilly and frightened. *Belladonna* is appropriate if the child feels hot and flushed.

Pulsatilla may help with children who are miserable, clingy and tearful with the illness. They may have a fever, but strangely are not thirsty. *Antimonium tartaricum* has a reputation for helping when the skin rash is slow to settle.

> **PREVENTION PLAN**
>
> **The following may help to prevent your child from catching chickenpox:**
>
> - Avoid people infected with either chickenpox or shingles.
> - Give a daily multivitamin and mineral supplement, as well as a diet rich in fruit and vegetables.
> - An immunisation against varicella.

ADHD

Attention deficit hyperactivity disorder (ADHD) is characterised by high levels of activity, impulsiveness and inattention. In some cases, hyperactivity and impulsiveness predominate; in others, the main problem is difficulty in concentrating on a given activity. ADHD is more common in boys than girls, and seems to run in families. Treatment may involve reducing and/or managing the symptoms through counselling, drugs, nutrition, manipulation, herbs, homeopathy and psychological therapies.

WHAT ARE THE SYMPTOMS?

Symptoms of ADHD usually become apparent between the ages of 3 and 7 years, and are often noticed after a child starts school. They may include:

- Almost constant physical activity
- Impulsiveness
- Short attention span and difficulty paying attention in a classroom situation
- Difficulty following simple instructions
- Inability to complete simple tasks
- Tendency to talk constantly and interrupt others
- Difficulty waiting and taking turns
- Learning difficulties
- Startle response, in which a child is excessively jumpy from quite mild stimuli, such as sudden noises

WHY MIGHT MY CHILD HAVE THIS?

PREDISPOSING FACTORS

- Genetic factors
- Fetal hypoxia (inadequate oxygen reaching the brain) in the womb or during birth
- Family stress

TRIGGERS

- Food sensitivity
- Low blood-sugar levels
- Exposure to metals, such as lead, mercury and manganese, in the environment

WHY DOES IT OCCUR?

ADHD belongs to a group of behaviours that also includes attention deficit disorder (ADD) and hyperkinetic disorder (HKD). The causes of ADHD are not fully understood. It is not a result of poor parenting, as is sometimes believed. Nor should it be confused with the normally boisterous activity of healthy children. Genetics, conditions in the uterus during pregnancy and environmental factors, such as family stress and toxic metals, may play a part.

TREATMENT PLAN

PRIMARY TREATMENTS

- Behaviour management
- Talking therapies
- Emotional support
- Drugs (e.g. Ritalin)

BACK-UP TREATMENT

- Nutritional therapy

WORTH CONSIDERING

- Massage
- Chiropractic
- Osteopathy
- T'ai chi and yoga
- Individualised homeopathy
- Avoiding lead and other environmental hazards

For an explanation of how treatments are rated, see p.111.

Children can outgrow ADHD, although some of them may carry aspects of the disorder, such as problems with attention, into adulthood.

HELPING YOUR CHILD

The following techniques can help you to manage your child's ADHD:
- Establish a routine that your child can clearly understand and easily follow.
- Create simple rules and boundaries, and make sure that you stick to them.
- Reinforce acceptable behaviour with rewards and discourage unacceptable behaviour with sanctions.
- Organise activities that help to increase your child's concentration.
- Keep distractions to a minimum.
- Arrange plenty of physical activities so that your child can let off steam.

TREATMENTS IN DETAIL

Conventional Medicine

The advice of various specialist professionals and consultants, such as a paediatrician and a child psychologist, may be needed to diagnose ADHD. This is because there are many factors to consider and no one definitive test. ADHD may be diagnosed if a child consistently shows the distinctive symptoms of hyperactivity, impulsiveness and attention difficulties over a period of six months or more and in more than one environment (for example, at home, school or in hospital).

PRIMARY TREATMENT **COMBINED APPROACH** Treatment of ADHD requires a combined approach, which may include drugs in some cases. Therapy that aims to modify behaviour may be recommended (*see Psychological Therapies, p.405*), while the parents may be given support and advice on managing the child, often through counselling and self-help groups.

PRIMARY TREATMENT **DRUGS** The drugs doctors most commonly prescribe are stimulants, such as methylphenidate (Ritalin) and dexamphetamine, which may help to reduce the symptoms of ADHD. These drugs are prescribed by specialists who will monitor the children carefully. Every year or so the drugs may be stopped for short periods of time to see whether they are still needed.

Tricyclic antidepressants, such as amitriptyline, may improve behaviour in some children with ADHD.

> **CAUTION**
>
> Drugs for ADHD have a range of side-effects: ask your doctor to explain these to you.

Nutritional Therapy

ELIMINATE FOOD SENSITIVITIES ADHD is sometimes amenable to a nutritional approach, when certain foods seem to be associated with an increased risk of mood and behaviour disturbance. Eliminating caffeine, sugar and food additives (artificial flavourings, colourings, preservatives) from the child's diet may help to control the symptoms of ADHD.

Children suffering from food intolerance are likely to have dark circles or bags under their eyes. During bouts of uncontrollable behaviour, their cheeks and/or

STABLE BLOOD-SUGAR LEVELS Episodes of low levels of blood sugar (hypoglycaemia) appear to be a common feature in children with ADHD. Starving the brain tissue of its prime fuel (sugar) can provoke significant problems with mood. Low blood-sugar levels also tend to cause the body to secrete more of the hormone adrenaline, which can make children anxious and/or aggressive.

Blood-sugar problems are likely if a child either craves sweet foods or becomes very irritable if he or she does not eat regularly and on time. These children will often respond to a diet designed to stabilise blood-sugar levels (*see p.42*).

ESSENTIAL FATTY ACIDS Children with ADHD may have nutrient deficiencies. They are especially likely to lack healthy fats known as essential fatty acids (EFAs). Common symptoms of EFA deficiency include dry, flaky skin, frequent urination and excessive thirst.

EFAs (*see p.34*) play an important role in the function of the brain. Possibly the most important in this respect are two omega-3 fatty acids, known as eicosapentaenoic acid (EPA) and docosahexaenoic acid (DHA), which are found in oily fish, such as salmon, mackerel and sardines, or in fish oil supplements. In practice, it is worth trying about 1g of concentrated fish oils two or three times every day. It is harmless and could be beneficial.

NUTRITIONAL SUPPLEMENTS There is good evidence that many children do not receive adequate amounts of key nutrients in their diets. Many vitamins and minerals, such as B vitamins, selenium and magnesium, are important for brain function and

and does seem to improve mood and behaviour in some children.

Other evidence points to magnesium and zinc as being particularly helpful. Giving a child a total of 100–200mg of magnesium supplements and 15mg of zinc supplements per day is recommended.

Homeopathy

Certain homeopathic medicines, including *Stramonium*, *Hyoscyamus*, *Belladonna*, *Cina*, *Lycopodium*, *Calcarea carbonica*, *Sulphur* and *Causticum*, may help children with ADHD. Homeopathic treatment of ADHD is complex. Although these medicines can safely be used on a self-help basis at home, it is always best to consult a qualified practitioner.

STRAMONIUM is an important medicine when there has been a background of trauma, including abuse and fostering. Symptoms indicating *Stramonium* may be appropriate include fears of the dark, water or other things related to the original trauma. Children may also exhibit fits of destructive rage.

Other symptoms indicating *Stramonium* include "startle responses", night terrors and intrusive thoughts or flashbacks to traumatic events.

HYOSCYAMUS Children who respond to *Hyoscyamus* are described as wild, manic and difficult or impossible to control. They may talk very rapidly and display sexualised behaviour.

BELLADONNA Children who respond to *Belladonna* are oversensitive to noise, light and jarring, which make them "jump". They become very hot and flushed, and may be confused and delirious when really worked up.

CINA is a useful medicine for physically aggressive children who are constantly arguing and fighting with others, and who throw tantrums when they are disciplined or told what to do.

CALCAREA CARBONICA Children who respond to treatment with *Calc. carb.* tend to be big and plump, with especially big heads. Characteristically, they sweat a lot on the head at night.

About 1.7 per cent of the population in the UK has the symptoms of ADHD or ADD

ears may turn very red. While any food may give rise to these types of unwanted reaction, the most common culprits are wheat, dairy products, chocolate, citrus fruits and eggs. Children may often crave the foods that they are sensitive to (*see The elimination diet, p.39*).

are known to affect mood. Studies show that some children with ADHD have low levels of certain nutrients such as magnesium, zinc and B vitamins.

Giving a child a daily multivitamin and mineral supplement may help to ensure that they have an adequate nutrient intake

Typically, they are not hyperactive, but find it hard to concentrate, and they are often very stubborn. Their development may be delayed – for example, they may start talking late. They also have many fears, including fear of animals and death, even a fear that their parents will die or desert them. As a result, they often experience nightmares.

LYCOPODIUM is one of the most useful homeopathic medicines for school phobia: the child screams and cries or complains of stomachache when it is time to go to school. In fact, they often have "tummy ache", particularly wind and bloating, and may have "bilious attacks", in which they vomit. They have difficulty concentrating, particularly in the afternoon. These children lack self-confidence and fear being alone. They are shy and awkward with strangers, but can be bossy and bad-tempered with family and friends.

ticularly of the dark. They may also exhibit compulsive and perfectionistic behaviour. When they become teenagers *Causticum* children can become both rebellious and highly idealistic.

Environmental Health

Hyperactivity is a disease in which various aspects of the modern environment appear to play a major role. For example, it may be triggered by exposure to organic toxins and many people with attention and hyperactivity disorders are exquisitely susceptible to distraction from electronic devices, such as television.

A first step in dealing with hyperactivity in children should be to avoid or minimise their exposure to heavy metals, such as lead, mercury or manganese. This is especially important for pregnant women and for developing children whose bodies readily incorporate the toxic compounds.

amount of lead incorporated into the child's bones.

A technique called chelation (binding a metal and filtering it from the bloodstream by chemical means) is one way of dealing with lead in the body, but there is no guarantee this will work, even in acute high-dose lead poisoning.

Supplementing with calcium (*see p.37*) may work, since calcium takes preference over lead when the metals are absorbed and incorporated in the body.

MERCURY, like lead, is notorious for interfering with the normal development of nerves. The organic form is particularly dangerous. You can decrease your child's exposure to mercury by limiting the amount of fish, especially oily fish, that he or she eats.

Although many fish oil supplements contain DHA (*see Essential fatty acids, p.403*), which has been shown to help with several behavioural issues, make sure the brand of fish oil you use has been conclusively determined not to contain heavy metals. If in doubt, look for a product that has been distilled.

> ## If one identical twin has ADHD, the other nearly always has it, too

SULPHUR Children who respond to *Sulphur* are typically highly active, hot and scruffy. They are "into everything" and seem to make a mess everywhere they go. No matter how carefully they are dressed in the morning, they soon get dirty and scruffy. They like to be the centre of attention and make trouble if they are not. They are often irritable and self-centred; seeming to have no regard for the feelings of others, they may be bullies.

Children who respond to *Sulphur* are typically "hot-blooded", throwing off the bedclothes at night and thirsty for cold drinks, and often have skin problems, especially eczema.

CAUSTICUM Children who respond to *Causticum* are both sensitive and excitable. Unlike *Sulphur* children, they are very aware of, and intensely sympathetic to, the suffering of others.

A *Causticum* child may burst into tears for the slightest reason, especially when they witness cruelty to animals, even in a story. They may also have many fears, par-

LEAD can have a devastating effect on the development and function of nerves, especially those in the central nervous system. Evidence suggests that it is increasingly probable that a child who has been exposed to lead will have problems with hyperactivity. Where possible, take the following measures to minimise your child's exposure to lead:

- Limit their exposure to lead-containing paints in older homes.
- Before using, run water for at least a minute through household pipes that may contain lead-based solder.
- Make sure your child drinks cold, not hot, tap water (or filter your water with an approved portable filter or a reverse osmosis system).
- Do not let your child eat or drink from leaded crystal or improperly glazed ceramic dishes or containers.
- Check that remedies, including calcium supplements, are lead-free.

Significant lead exposure can be detected by testing a child's blood or, in cases of long-term exposure, by measuring the

MANGANESE has been associated with hyperactivity problems, according to a few studies. Since manganese is a recent addition to petrol in the US and Canada, more evidence may emerge in the future about its role in ADHD.

ELECTRONIC STIMULATION There is ample research that demonstrates what common sense tells us: over-stimulation by television, video games or loud noises can exacerbate a child's problems with attention and hyperactivity.

The rapid-firing bombardment of the senses and the neural circuitry by electronic entertainment devices could make anybody inattentive and "wired". If a child is prone to hyperactivity, this kind of stimulation can make the problem worse and should be discouraged.

PHYSICAL EXERCISE Another kind of stimulation, however, can ease the symptoms of hyperactivity: physical exercise can be highly therapeutic for people who are prone to ADHD. Encourage your child to play sport, take regular exercise or engage in a physical activity.

Bodywork Therapies

MASSAGE can be a very useful technique for managing children with ADHD. One study in 1998 suggests that children who receive 15 minutes of massage after school each day for 10 days experience an improvement in their concentration and behaviour, and a reduction in their hyperactivity. The massage consists of five minutes on the neck, five minutes across the base of neck and shoulders, and five minutes on the spinal region.

The researchers strongly urge considering the use of massage in helping children with ADHD, either in conjunction with a standard treatment or as a substitute, especially when medication is having undesirable side-effects.

CHIROPRACTIC Some case reports suggest that hyperactivity and associated behavioural conditions respond well to chiropractic care.

CRANIAL OSTEOPATHY and craniosacral methods of manipulation have also been used in the treatment of children with ADHD. The benefits may be greatest when the problems being treated are related to obstetrically complicated deliveries.

T'ai Chi and Yoga

Movement and bodywork may be able to help to calm children and adolescents with ADHD. For example, research at the Touch Research Institute at the University of Miami Medical School in the USA has shown that t'ai chi, as well as massage, can markedly reduce ADHD symptoms.

T'AI CHI In a 2000 study, adolescents with developmental problems who had been diagnosed with ADHD did t'ai chi exercise classes twice weekly for five weeks, in the early afternoon. During the 30-minute classes the adolescents improved their conduct and exhibited less anxiety, "day dreaming", displays of inappropriate emotions and hyperactivity.

YOGA Research at the University of Sydney in Australia in 2003 suggested that yoga can help boys with ADHD manage their behaviour while they are not taking any medication. Following 20 weeks of practis-ing yoga in weekly one-hour classes, the boys' restless and/or impulsive behaviour was reduced – although their ADHD was still present.

Psychological Therapies

PRIMARY TREATMENT **BEHAVIOUR MANAGEMENT** The main focus of the various talking therapies is to help the parents manage a child's or young person's behaviour. Parents often feel overwhelmed and powerless to help their children. This sometimes ends up in a spiral of "coercive parenting" in which parents try to force their children to do things or behave in certain ways – but the real result is that they bring out the worst in each other. Most of the psychological research has been carried out using systems therapies (*see p.107*) because the focus of these is on family interactions.

Training both parents and children to manage their behaviour simultaneously has been shown to reduce conflicts and non-compliance in children with ADHD. This form of training has also been evaluated for children with conduct and behaviour problems, and has been shown to reduce their problematic and oppositional behaviour.

PRIMARY TREATMENT **TALKING THERAPIES** aim to help a child or young person regulate their behaviour and become more reflective. Despite considerable interest in developing cognitive behavioural therapy (CBT) for these children, the results have so far been disappointing, even when the children are also given medication.

Skills training has brought some success in improving children's social skills and behavioural therapy, in which rewards are given for "acceptable" behaviour, shows short-term improvement.

Anger-control training, in which children engage in role play to find ways of coping with situations, has shown initial promise in the treatment of ADHD.

The practice of some of the above skills in a school environment has also been attempted with some success. While some of the behavioural methods have only shown short-term improvement, their use in the classroom on a more regular basis has shown promise. This process involves teaching behavioural techniques to teachers so that they can help to make a child with ADHD become a more integral part of the classroom culture.

MULTIMODAL TREATMENT A combination of medication and talking therapies becomes more effective than the sum of the treatments when they are used separately and individually. One advantage of this multimodal approach appears to be that a lower dosage of medication can be given, thus reducing the occurrence of side-effects.

Mind–body Therapy

Biofeedback may benefit children with ADHD. A small controlled study of EEG (brainwave) biofeedback found that it was more effective than placebo treatment.

> As many as a third of children with ADHD in the UK may be clinically depressed

PREVENTION PLAN

The following may help to prevent your child developing ADHD:

- Don't drink alcohol in pregnancy.
- Make sure your child's diet contains a only a minimum amount of caffeine, sugar and additives.
- Avoid family stress caused by arguments, conflicts, etc.
- Avoid exposing your child to toxic levels of metals, such as lead, mercury and manganese.
- Limit the amount of time your child spends watching television or playing computer or video games.
- Encourage your child to exercise.

Mind & Emotions

Mental and emotional problems can disturb the roots of a person's existence, affecting their self-esteem and ability to cope with the pressures of the modern world. Advances in our understanding of the way the mind and body are interrelated have led to new ways of coping with these disorders, which range from touch and movement therapies to drugs, nutritional supplements, psychological therapies and stress-management techniques.

COPING WITH STRESS

A physical or mental challenge such as a car speeding towards us or a work deadline looming provokes the "fight or flight" stress response, which involves physical reactions, such as an increase in heart rate and sweating, and psychological reactions, such as intense concentration. Everyone faces a certain amount of stress and it only becomes a problem when it is too much for the individual to handle. There is a wide range of therapeutic measures that aim to reduce the symptoms and to help the person better manage stressful situations.

WHAT ARE THE SYMPTOMS?

Physical symptoms of stress include:

- Tiredness
- Frequent headaches, caused by tension
- Muscle pains
- Worsening symptoms of any other diseases present
- Inability to cope physically

Psychological symptoms of stress include:

- Anxiety
- Tearfulness
- Irritability
- Lack of concentration
- Difficulty with decision-making
- Problems with sleeping
- Loss of appetite
- Low energy levels and lack of motivation
- Inability to cope psychologically

WHY MIGHT I HAVE THIS?

PREDISPOSING FACTORS

- Anxious personality
- Poor general health
- Lack of social support

TRIGGER

- Accumulation of many "daily hassles" or major life events

WHY DOES IT OCCUR?

In the "flight-or-fight" response, stress hormones, such as adrenaline, noradrenaline and cortisol, pour into the body's systems. As digestion slows, the muscles tense up; the liver releases sugar and fats as energy for sudden action and the heart rate rises. If this energy and tension are not discharged, the effects can accumulate and affect every major organ and body system, causing or worsening existing diseases and conditions, including gastrointestinal disorders, arthritis, diabetes, chronic back pain, angina, hypertension, sleep disorders and cancer.

TREATMENT PLAN

PRIMARY TREATMENTS

- Self-help measures
- Counselling
- Psychotherapy
- Stress-management programmes

BACK-UP TREATMENTS

- Nutritional therapy
- Breathing retraining
- Western herbal medicine
- Touch therapies
- Homeopathy
- Acupuncture
- Mind–body therapies

For an explanation of how treatments are rated, see p.111.

Coping with life events, such as bereavement, divorce, giving a public presentation or moving house, can be emotionally and physically demanding. In a different way, so is boredom or an accumulation of minor irritations, such as being stuck in a traffic jam and losing the house keys. The degree to which people become stressed under these circumstances depends on their personality traits and how well they have learned to cope with pressure. Stress only becomes a problem when it is too much for the individual and when it interferes with the ability to relax and cope with life.

People vary in their capability to cope with stress on a physical and on an emotional level. Enhancing this capability in one area will improve the other, so taking more exercise to improve physical functioning will also increase the ability to cope with emotional stress.

SELF-HELP

PRIMARY TREATMENT The following measures may help you deal with stress:

- Aim for optimum health by eating a balanced diet and taking regular exercise (exercise is an excellent stress-reliever).
- Reduce your intake of caffeine and other stimulants, as well as addictive substances, such as tobacco and alcohol.
- Make time to enjoy aspects of your life that give your mind a break from sources of stress.
- Keep in touch with friends and family – this will make you feel supported and may help increase your self-confidence.
- Learn relaxation techniques (*see p.99*).
- Anticipate times of stress and prepare yourself to deal with them.
- List what you have to do and prioritise.

TREATMENTS IN DETAIL

Conventional Medicine

PRIMARY TREATMENT **COUNSELLING AND PSYCHO-THERAPY** If you are feeling stressed and are having difficulty coping, or believe that stress is affecting your physical or emotional health, you may wish to speak to your doctor, who will talk to you about possible underlying causes and check your general health. Your doctor may recommend the preventive measures described (*see Self-Help, left*) and may advise you to have counselling or another form of psychotherapy.

Nutritional Therapy

STRENGTHEN ADRENAL FUNCTION Stress can lead to weakened adrenal glands and taking steps to strengthen adrenal function does seem to help individuals cope better with the stress in their lives (*see p.44*).

MAGNESIUM may help to alleviate stress by improving the function of the adrenal glands and by counteracting the magnesium depletion in the body that stress can induce. One study with fighter pilots found that taking 400mg of magnesium supplements a day reduced the stress-induced rises in noradrenaline. You may find taking 300–500mg of magnesium per day is useful during times of stress.

PROBIOTICS Studies suggest that excessive stress can cause the depletion of beneficial bacteria, such as species of *Lactobacillus* and *Bifidobacteria*, in the intestinal tract. Try taking a probiotic in times of stress.

> **CAUTION**
>
> Consult your doctor before taking magnesium with ciproflaxin, warfarin or spironolactone (*see p.46*).

Homeopathy

It is difficult to generalise about particular treatments for stress, not only because of the individualised nature of prescribing medicines, but also because of the variety of stresses and different ways that people cope, or fail to cope, with stress.

HOW THE BODY RESPONDS TO STRESS

The brain and adrenal glands work together to control the stress responses. There are two types: the fast "fight or flight" stress response occurs when your brain detects a threat such as a car hurtling towards you. Adrenaline is released into the bloodstream to prepare your body for immediate action. If stress is prolonged, for example as the result of a heavy workload, the hormone ACTH is released, which makes the adrenal glands secrete corticosteroid hormones. These have a damaging effect on the body.

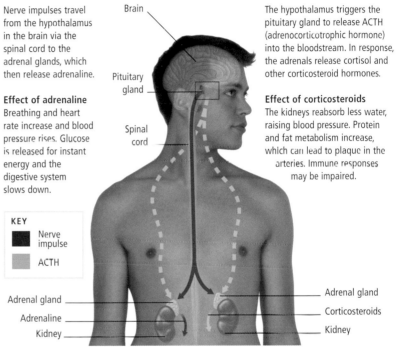

IMMEDIATE RESPONSE

Nerve impulses travel from the hypothalamus in the brain via the spinal cord to the adrenal glands, which then release adrenaline.

Effect of adrenaline
Breathing and heart rate increase and blood pressure rises. Glucose is released for instant energy and the digestive system slows down.

KEY
- ■ Nerve impulse
- ▨ ACTH

Brain

Pituitary gland

Spinal cord

Adrenal gland
Adrenaline
Kidney

LONG-TERM RESPONSE

The hypothalamus triggers the pituitary gland to release ACTH (adrenocorticotrophic hormone) into the bloodstream. In response, the adrenals release cortisol and other corticosteroid hormones.

Effect of corticosteroids
The kidneys reabsorb less water, raising blood pressure. Protein and fat metabolism increase, which can lead to plaque in the arteries. Immune responses may be impaired.

Adrenal gland
Corticosteroids
Kidney

NUX VOMICA is the classical homeopathic medicine for stress. The typical "picture" of *Nux vomica* is of the efficient, hard-driving businessman who finds himself waking early in the morning, fretting about the problems of the day that lie ahead and is unable to get back to sleep. He feels exhausted in the morning and it takes several cups of coffee to get him going.

Very impatient and irritable, he is annoyed by what he perceives as inefficiency or stupidity. As the day wears on, he feels better, gradually relaxing, perhaps with the help of rich or spicy food, alcohol, nicotine or other drugs. Yet the cycle starts again early next morning.

There may be physical symptoms, such as a stuffy head cold, sore throat, indigestion and bowel problems – in particular, a constant urge to pass stools, with or without success.

KALIUM PHOSPHORICUM In contrast to *Nux vomica*, this homeopathic medicine is useful for people who have a very different reaction to stress. Their main feature is fatigue, particularly mental exhaustion, combined with weak memory and trouble with concentration, headaches, disturbed sleep with bad dreams and a tendency to pick up infections.

CALCAREA CARBONICA can help with stress at work, especially for the solid, reliable worker who gets jaded with work, waking at night in a sweat worrying that he or she will be unable to cope.

LYCOPODIUM may be the appropriate medicine for serious, conscientious people in responsible and intellectually demanding posts who get depressed and lose self-confidence.

PHOSPHORIC ACID can help when intellectual and emotional stress combine – for instance, exam stress and difficulties with relationships that teenagers experience.

NATRUM MURIATICUM is important for the consequences of bottled-up, long-term emotional stress, which the sufferer does not like to talk about.

Western Herbal Medicine

Adaptogenic herbs can help with stress and its associated fatigue, debility, anxiety and depression. They improve vitality, staying power, memory and concentration, and include ginseng (*Panax ginseng*), Siberian ginseng (*Eleutherococcus senticosus*) and astragalus (*Astragalus membranaceus*).

Repeating the rosary prayer or a yoga mantra can slow down your breathing rate

The so-called nervine herbs help to support an overtaxed nervous system. They include skullcap (*Scutellaria laterifolia*), wild oat (*Avena sativa*), vervain (*Verbena officinalis*) and damiana (*Turnera diffusa*).

Stress with anxiety and depression can be helped by valerian (*Valeriana officinalis*), lemon balm (*Melissa officinalis*) and St John's wort (*Hypericum perforatum*).

Passionflower (*Passiflora incarnata*), hops (*Humulus lupulus*), valerian, chamomile (*Matricaria recutita*) and lemon balm can all help to improve the quality and duration of sleep and to ease stress and relieve nervous tension.

Cramp bark (*Viburnum opulus*) relaxes tense muscles often associated with stress. Soaking in a lavender oil bath (add 10–15 drops of the essential oil to a hot bath) can help ease away the stresses of a busy day.

> **CAUTION**
> • See page 69 before taking a herbal remedy and, if you are already taking prescribed medication, consult a medical herbalist first.
> • Do not take St John's wort with warfarin antidepressants or antibiotics, and do not take Siberian ginseng for if you have high blood pressure.

Breathing Retraining

If you are affected by stressful feelings and events, learn breathing techniques (*see p.62*) because certain breathing patterns can have an "anti-arousal" effect that reduces the sympathetic (alarm) response triggered when we are faced with potentially demanding events or stimuli. Yoga breathing patterns can reduce physiological and psychological arousal during threatening and non-threatening situations.

Touch Therapies

EFFECTS OF TOUCH Research into the calming, anti-stress effects of touch therapies, such as massage and reflexology, have consistently shown that they commonly lead to a reduction in production of cortisol and other stress hormones. Touch therapy has helped people with asthma, anorexia, breast cancer, burns, depression, chronic fatigue, diabetes and HIV. It is also useful for preterm infants and during labour, as well as in people suffering post-traumatic stress disorder.

GIVING MASSAGE When highly stressed individuals learn to give massage – for example, parents massaging their hyperactive children or grandparents massaging their grandchildren – both givers and receivers of the massage show reduced stress levels. In a study, grandparents reported less anxiety and fewer depressive symptoms. They also reported improved mood and self-esteem, as well as reduced pulse rates and decreased cortisol levels.

REFLEXOLOGY calms people with stressful problems, including hospitalised patients, parents of babies in intensive care and people with a range of health conditions, such as migraine and bowel and sleep disturbances. General foot massage may also help: in many studies when reflexology is compared with general foot massage, the benefits seem very similar.

Acupuncture

Acupuncture can help balance an individual's energy and possibly avoid stress. In situations of acute anxiety and concern, acupuncture may be given daily or every other day, but in general weekly treatments are the preferred option, and benefit should be apparent in six to eight sessions.

Mind–Body Therapies

While some patients visit doctors complaining of stress, more often they complain of gastrointestinal disturbances, pain, insomnia, fatigue or other symptoms. The mainstay of treatment is appropriate counselling, lifestyle advice, reassurance, addressing specific issues and other non-pharmaceutical treatments.

PRIMARY TREATMENT **STRESS-MANAGEMENT PROGRAMMES** using behavioural and mind–body approaches are widely employed to reduce stress. Among the mind–body skills and therapies that have been found to be effective are regular physical exercise, clinical biofeedback, muscle relaxation and psychotherapy.

Guided imagery (*see p.99*), which combines the techniques of deep relaxation and positive suggestion, is a powerful way of managing stress. Eight studies found that, relative to control groups, guided imagery sessions were effective at reducing the physical and emotional signs of stress in groups of smokers, surgical patients, cardiac and cancer patients, and in otherwise well people who reported high stress levels. Moreover, the effects were stronger when patients practised the skills on their own.

Relaxation, practised with or without guided imagery, is highly recommended, as it can improve the ability to cope with the inevitable stresses of everyday life.

> **PREVENTION PLAN**
>
> The following may help to prevent the development of excess stress:
> • Eat a nutritious diet.
> • Take regular exercise.
> • Practise relaxation regularly.

PHOBIAS

A phobia is a persistent, irrational fear of an object, situation or activity that compels a person to avoid it obsessively. A fear of something, such as dogs or high places, that causes occasional unease but does not disrupt everyday life is not a phobia. People with genuine phobias can be severely restricted, with their lives affected in many different ways. Their phobias usually develop in late childhood or during adolescence and early adulthood. Phobias are principally treated with exposure therapy but breathing retraining can also be helpful.

WHAT ARE THE SYMPTOMS?

Exposure to the object of the phobia, or sometimes even thinking about it or imagining it, may cause the following symptoms:

- Dizziness and feeling faint
- Palpitations (awareness of an abnormally rapid heartbeat)
- Sweating, trembling and nausea
- Shortness of breath

WHY MIGHT I HAVE THESE?

PREDISPOSING FACTORS

- Traumatic childhood experience
- Lack of self-esteem
- Anxious personality

TREATMENT PLAN

PRIMARY TREATMENTS

- Exposure therapy, sometimes in combination with certain antidepressants
- Breathing retraining

WORTH CONSIDERING

- Nutritional therapies
- Homeopathy
- Other psychological therapies

For an explanation of how treatments are rated, see p.111.

WHY DO THEY OCCUR?

SIMPLE OR COMPLEX PHOBIAS Phobias are often classed as being either simple or complex. Simple phobias are specific to a single object, situation or activity, such as a fear of flying, fear of spiders or fear of enclosed spaces. Complex phobias involve several component fears.

A fear of open or public spaces (agoraphobia) is a complex phobia that may involve, for example, fear of being alone in a public place and of being trapped in a public place with no exit. Social phobias, in which people are afraid of embarrassing themselves or being humiliated, are also considered complex phobias.

CAUSES Phobias often have no identifiable cause. Sometimes, however, a simple phobia can be traced back to a traumatic experience in childhood. Simple phobias appear to run in families, but this is thought to be because children learn the fear from a family member. The causes of complex phobias are less clear, but they seem to develop from a general tendency to anxiety. People who lack self-esteem are more likely to develop social phobias or agoraphobia.

AVOIDANCE A phobic person is aware that his or her fear is irrational but is still compelled to avoid the object or situation that he or she fears. Exposure to the object of the phobia causes a physical reaction ("fight or flight"), often with sweating and a rapid heartbeat. A factor that is common to all phobias is avoidance of the object of the phobia and this may severely limit a person's activities. Anxiety and panic attacks (*see p.414*) sometimes develop in relation to the phobia.

TREATMENTS IN DETAIL

Conventional Medicine

PRIMARY TREATMENT — Your doctor will suggest psychological therapies, which are the mainstay of conventional treatment for all kinds of phobias (*see Psychological Therapies, p.412*). When there are symptoms of depression (*see p.436*), certain antidepressants may be helpful when prescribed in combination with psychological therapy. Most commonly, these drugs are tricyclics, such as clomipramine; but selective serotonin re-uptake inhibitors (SSRIs) are sometimes used.

Nutritional Therapy

The nutritional measures described for anxiety (*see p.414*) are also relevant for people with phobias. These include balancing blood-sugar levels, avoiding caffeine and taking supplements, such as magnesium, selenium or a multivitamin and mineral combination.

Homeopathy

Homeopathy is helpful for treating the phobic "terrain", i.e. the background of anxiety and phobias. Some homeopathic medicines may help with specific fears, among them *Argentum nitricum, Phosphorus, Stramonium, Lycopodium, Calcarea carbonica* and *Silicea.*

ARGENTUM NITRICUM Probably the most useful medicine is *Arg. nit.* It is suitable particularly for claustrophobia and fear of heights, especially if associated with a distressing impulse to jump. People who respond to this medicine are hot, twitchy and impulsive. They seem to have a problem with managing their time, always seeming to be in a hurry and getting into a terrible state before any important event. The anxiety associated with the phobia may express itself in physical manifestations, including diarrhoea, burping, vertigo and tremor.

PHOSPHORUS may be appropriate for people who have a fear of the dark. People who respond to *Phosphorus* are excessively sensitive, both to their physical and their human environment. They may be hypersensitive and sense that they can "feel vibes", though not always accurately. They are greatly affected by thunderstorms: they may fear them or develop a headache before a storm breaks.

STRAMONIUM may also be appropriate for people who fear the dark. *Stramonium* may help when someone is praying and trembling and really beside themselves with fear. Apart from the dark, they may also fear animals, ghosts or water.

LYCOPODIUM Various fears make up parts of the "picture" of other homeopathic medicines. For instance, *Lycopodium* is frequently a valuable medicine for children with a phobia about school and for adults whose stagefright makes them anxious before appearing in public.

CALCAREA CARBONICA People whose constitution fits the *Calc. carb.* "picture" tend to have many fears, especially of disease and death.

SILICEA People who respond to *Silicea* (aslo called *Silica*) fear needles and pins, and may feel faint at the suggestion of a blood test. But in all cases, the person's overall "picture" must fit the remedy if the treatment is to be of help. It is therefore essential to consult an experienced homeopath (*see p.73*).

Breathing Retraining

PRIMARY TREATMENT Evidence confirms that combining breathing retraining with manual therapy (to assist in freeing the muscles of the chest and other respiratory structures) can reduce the anxiety and help people cope with phobic reactions. This will often completely eliminate phobic behaviour. Where a phobia has deep-rooted emotional or psychological causes, breathing retraining might have to be used alongside psychotherapy or cognitive behavioural therapy.

In one major study, more than 1,000 phobic patients (mainly people suffering from agoraphobia – the fear of open/public places) were treated using techniques such as breathing retraining, physical therapy and relaxation. On the whole, their symptoms took one to six months to disappear, with some younger patients requiring only a few weeks. A year after the treatment, 75 per cent of former patients were free of all their symptoms; a further 20 per cent had only mild symptoms. Only about 1 patient in 20 failed to respond to the treatment.

HYPERVENTILATION It has been estimated that approximately 60 per cent of people who experience phobias or exhibit phobic behaviour have hyperventilation as part of their symptom picture.

The main characteristic of hyperventilation is an habitual tendency to breathe in a shallow way with just the upper chest, rather than the deeper breathing that uses the diaphragm. This leads to excessive exhalation of carbon dioxide, so that the person gets used (habituated) to having low levels of this important regulatory gas in their bloodstream.

TESTING CARBON DIOXIDE TOLERANCE A low tolerance to carbon dioxide can help to identify people who hyperventilate. A simple test can be used in which a person is asked to exhale and wait until there is a an urgent "need to breathe". During the holding time, carbon dioxide levels will be rising, and the "need to breathe" represents that moment when the level of carbon dioxide triggers a message to the respiratory centre in the brain, requesting that breathing start again.

This test is a reasonably accurate way of assessing a person's current tolerance to carbon dioxide. "Normal" is thought to be between 25 to 30 seconds. Under 15 seconds is thought to represent a low tolerance of carbon dioxide.

Another test for carbon dioxide tolerance is to ask a person to breathe air that contains increased levels of carbon dioxide and then assess their reaction by finding out when feelings of panic and phobia start. Using this approach, researchers have reported that childhood anxiety disorders are all associated with carbon dioxide hypersensitivity.

YOGA AND THE BUTEYKO METHOD A major part of breathing retraining involves using techniques, such as slow exhalation as in yoga-type exercises and periodic holding of the breath, that help the person slowly, over a period of months, to be become accustomed to increasingly higher levels of carbon dioxide in the blood. The breath-holding method forms a part of the Russian Buteyko breathing retraining method (*see also Asthma, p.205*).

When breathing retraining is applied regularly, the benefits include reduced feelings of anxiety, far fewer panic attacks and, most importantly, a lessening or vanishing of phobic feelings. (*For details of a breathing sequence, see p.62.*)

Psychological Therapies

Phobias can be severely restricting, creating a powerfully negative impact on a person's life in many different ways. In general, they are divided into two main categories: simple or specific phobias and complex or social phobias.

Therapies from the cognitive behavioural model (*see p.106*) have been shown to be particularly effective for both categories. Exposure therapy is probably the most commonly used for simple or specific phobias, which include animal phobias and the fear of flying. Eye movement desensitisation and reprocessing (EMDR) may also be effective.

The more complex social phobias, such as the fear of open spaces (agoraphobia), are more difficult to disentangle and need more psychological reprogramming of a person's thinking and perception.

You can try to tackle your own phobia if you think it is mild enough by following the three steps of the phobia desensitisation sequence (*see p.413*).

PRIMARY TREATMENT **EXPOSURE THERAPY** is most commonly used as a treatment for simple phobias. As the name suggests, exposure therapy (or graded

PHOBIA DESENSITISATION

The aim of this phobia desensitisation sequence is to reduce your fear response and replace it with a relaxation response. Take it slowly: do not attempt all the steps in a single day. Spread them over several days or more if you prefer. You need to feel completely comfortable with each step before moving on to the next. As you feel ready, you can use photos or video clips of the object or situation that triggers your phobia before attempting to encounter it in real life. This self-desensitisation sequence is only suitable if you have a mild phobia. Do not hesitate to seek professional help if you need it.

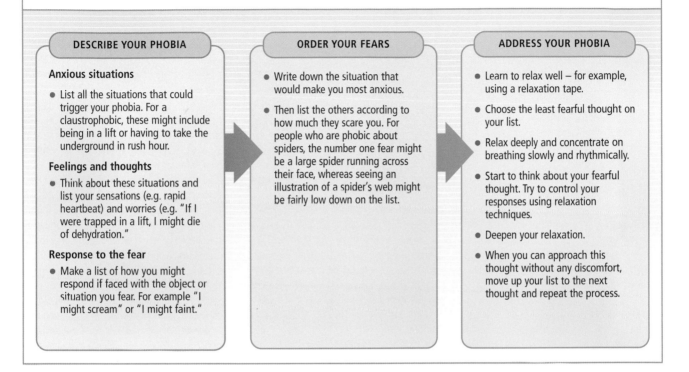

DESCRIBE YOUR PHOBIA

Anxious situations

- List all the situations that could trigger your phobia. For a claustrophobic, these might include being in a lift or having to take the underground in rush hour.

Feelings and thoughts

- Think about these situations and list your sensations (e.g. rapid heartbeat) and worries (e.g. "If I were trapped in a lift, I might die of dehydration."

Response to the fear

- Make a list of how you might respond if faced with the object or situation you fear. For example "I might scream" or "I might faint."

ORDER YOUR FEARS

- Write down the situation that would make you most anxious.
- Then list the others according to how much they scare you. For people who are phobic about spiders, the number one fear might be a large spider running across their face, whereas seeing an illustration of a spider's web might be fairly low down on the list.

ADDRESS YOUR PHOBIA

- Learn to relax well – for example, using a relaxation tape.
- Choose the least fearful thought on your list.
- Relax deeply and concentrate on breathing slowly and rhythmically.
- Start to think about your fearful thought. Try to control your responses using relaxation techniques.
- Deepen your relaxation.
- When you can approach this thought without any discomfort, move up your list to the next thought and repeat the process.

exposure) consists of gently introducing patients to the very thing, situation or event that makes them anxious. For example, someone with a spider phobia will initially be asked to imagine a spider, then to view a drawing of a small spider, until they stop being anxious. Next, the patient is asked to look at a more detailed drawing while their anxiety reduces to a manageable level and they become desensitised.

The patient progresses at his or her own pace and eventually may be presented with a real spider. The therapist may hold the spider until the patient's anxiety subsides sufficiently (a technique known as modelling) and may consequently invite the patient to touch or hold it (a technique known as *in vivo*).

Video and virtual reality technology have been used to expose patients to their fears, and a review found that 70–80 per cent of patients showed significant clinical improvement. The *in vivo* method seems to be particularly effective.

One advantage of gradual exposure therapy is that it can be brief. For instance, people with a fear of going to the dentist can be treated using between two or four sessions. People with animal phobias have been treated in a single two-hour session and in one study using exposure and modelling, 90 per cent of subjects remained free of their phobias one year later.

The mode in which the exposure therapy is delivered – whether it is carried out in an individual, couple, family or group setting – has also been examined and the use of group treatment has been shown to be effective.

EYE MOVEMENT DESENSITISATION AND REPROCESSING (EMDR) is based on exposure therapy and has shown promising results. (*For a description of EMDR, see Post-Traumatic Stress Disorder, p.422.*)

COGNITIVE THERAPY While the use of cognitive therapy (this is cognitive behav-ioural therapy without a behavioural component, such as exposure therapy or EMDR) has not been shown to make a significant difference with simple phobias, it seems to help people with the more complex social phobias.

Cognitive therapy focuses on how the patient perceives and thinks about the event or situation that disturbs them. Facilitating the patient to review their thoughts and change them has been shown to help as an adjunct to exposure therapy in social phobias.

According to one review, cognitive behavioural therapy is an effective method of treating social phobias. It would appear that a combination of cognitive and exposure methods rather than one or other alone is the most effective form of treatment. Social skills training, which is designed to promote a more productive and positive interaction with other people, may also have a positive effect on resolving social phobias.

ANXIETY AND PANIC DISORDER

Feeling worried or anxious occasionally and with reason is appropriate and normal. When anxiety becomes the usual response to ordinary situations and interferes with everyday life, it is considered a disorder. Panic disorder is a common, recurrent and unpredictable type of anxiety. Anxiety disorders may be present without panic attacks. Treatment involves psychological therapies, the occasional use of drugs, control of blood-sugar levels, supplements, massage, breathing exercises, homeopathy, herbs and mind–body therapies.

WHAT ARE THE SYMPTOMS?

Symptoms of anxiety disorder include:

- Headaches
- Abdominal cramps, sometimes with diarrhoea and vomiting
- Frequent urination
- Sweating, flushing and tremor
- Constricted feeling in the throat
- Being on edge, with a sense of foreboding
- Inability to concentrate
- Repetitive worrying thoughts
- Disturbed sleep patterns, sometimes with nightmares

Symptoms of a panic attack include:

- Intense anxiety
- Shortness of breath
- Sweating, trembling and nausea
- Rapid heartbeat
- Dizziness and fainting
- Constricted feeling in the throat
- Feeling of unreality and fears about loss of sanity

WHY MIGHT I HAVE THIS?

PREDISPOSING FACTORS

- Genetic factors
- Stress overload
- Trait anxiety

TRIGGERS

- Caffeine
- Blood-sugar imbalance
- Stressful event, such as a death in the family

WHY DOES IT OCCUR?

The term "anxiety disorders" covers a group of psychological conditions that are related to excessive worries and fears. They include generalised anxiety disorder, panic disorder, acute stress disorder, post-traumatic stress disorder (*see p.422*), phobias (*see p.411*) and obsessive-compulsive disorder (*see p.419*).

TREATMENT PLAN

PRIMARY TREATMENTS

- Self-help measures (*see Self-help*)
- Cognitive behavioural therapy
- Drugs, such as benzodiazepines
- Breathing retraining

BACK-UP TREATMENTS

- Drugs, such as beta-blockers and antidepressants (short term only)
- Nutritional therapy
- Exercise and massage
- Acupuncture
- Western herbal medicine

WORTH CONSIDERING

- Homeopathy
- Environmental health measures

For an explanation of how treatments are rated, see p.111.

All of these conditions are marked by feelings of apprehension, uneasiness or tension, which range from being mild to incapacitating. Physical symptoms can include muscle tension, shaking or trembling, shortness of breath, palpitations (*see p.258*) and sweating.

Anxiety disorders usually start in middle age and are more common in women than in men. Sometimes, an anxiety disorder develops after a stressful event, such as a death in the family. However, often the anxiety has no identifiable cause. In some cases, it forms part of a depressive illness.

Poor bonding between parents and children or an abrupt separation of a child from a parent may also play a part in some anxiety disorders.

TRAIT ANXIETY Anxiety disorders appear to be caused by a complex interaction of psychological, physical and genetic influences. Some people are more prone to anxiety than others. For example, the likelihood of developing an anxiety disorder is increased if you have close relatives with anxiety disorders or phobias (*see p.411*) or if you experienced a traumatic event in your childhood.

Those with high "trait anxiety" (a long-standing tendency rather than simply being temporarily anxious) are more likely than most to perceive a stressful situation or sensation as dangerous or threatening. Their response is to feel apprehensive, upset or distressed. Also called neuroticism, this trait often runs in families and involves a rapid and excessive "flight-and–fight" arousal response.

GENERALISED ANXIETY DISORDER (GAD)

Some anxiety is normal. Persistent, exaggerated worry is not. Everyone feels some anxiety, even on a daily basis. But people with generalised anxiety disorder (GAD) have a constant anxiety, often without any obvious cause, yet enough to interfere with normal life. Typical symptoms of GAD are:

- Persistent worry and anxiousness about events that are unlikely to occur.
- Inability to shut off these constant anxious thoughts.
- Muscular tension, aches and soreness.
- Restlessness, an inability to relax and a lack of energy.
- Feelings of dread.
- Sweating, hot flashes or a dry mouth.
- Dizziness and lightheadedness.
- Insomnia (having trouble falling or staying asleep).
- Shakiness or trembling.
- Concentration problems.
- Irritability or can be startled easily.
- Stomach problems (nausea, diarrhoea).

SELF-HELP

| PRIMARY TREATMENT | The following measures may help if you have panic attacks:

- Practise relaxation exercises (*see p.99*).
- Try "rebreathing" into a paper bag.
- Slow your breathing to 10 breaths or less per minute.
- Try one of the homeopathic medicines discussed below.

TREATMENTS IN DETAIL

Conventional Medicine

A doctor may recommend relaxation exercises together with counselling to help with stress management or other psychological therapies, such as cognitive behavioural therapy (*see Mind–body therapies, below*), to help control anxiety and panic attacks.

| PRIMARY TREATMENT | **BENZODIAZEPINES** In rare cases, when an individual is undergoing an extremely stressful period,

benzodiazepines, such as diazepam, may be prescribed, but only on a short-term basis as they are associated with high risks of dependence. If dependence occurs, increasing doses are needed to achieve the same effect and withdrawal symptoms such as restlessness and severe anxiety may occur.

BUSPIRONE Studies have shown that the drug buspirone helps to relieve anxiety; it takes about two weeks to have an effect and is used for short periods only.

BETA-BLOCKERS are prescribed in some cases to help control the physical symptoms of anxiety, but they have no effect on the psychological features of the condition.

ANTIDEPRESSANTS When anxiety is part of a depressive illness, antidepressants may be prescribed. Some, such as paroxetine, venlafaxine and other selective serotonin uptake inhibitors (SSRIs), have been found to help relieve the symptoms of anxiety and panic disorders.

Some antidepressants, for example the tricyclic antidepressants group, have been shown to help improve the symptoms of panic disorders in some people.

CAUTION

Drugs to relieve anxiety and panic attacks may have side-effects: ask your doctor to explain these to you.

Nutritional Therapy

BALANCE BLOOD-SUGAR LEVELS An imbalance in the levels of blood sugar is a common factor associated with anxiety. The body generally attempts to correct a fall in blood sugar by secreting adrenaline, which stimulates the release of sugar from the liver. Adrenaline is certainly one hormone in the body that is well known to provoke feelings of anxiety and even panic.

Several studies show that one of the symptoms of hypoglycaemia (low levels of

COPING WITH ANXIETY

Anxiety is a normal response to a worrying event or threatening situation. However, it is not the situation or event itself but the accompanying thoughts that generate anxiety. Here are four steps to help you reduce a panic attack.

- Is the problem actually yours? Sometimes, people get needlessly upset over distressing events that do not actually threaten their well-being.
- Write down the essence of the problem and the worst-case scenario.
- Then list ways to solve the problem. For example, if you are worried about intruders, could you install window locks or a burglar alarm? Choose the solution that seems most practical and break it down into steps.
- To gain a sense of perspective, talk through your anxieties with a sensible friend.
- Stress-management measures, such as taking plenty of exercise and relaxing regularly, can also help to restore your calm and well-being.

sugar in the blood) in diabetes is anxiety, and clinical experience suggests that even non-diabetics can be prone to anxiety at times when blood-sugar levels are lower than ideal. (*For a diet to steady blood-sugar levels, see p.42.*)

In practice, individuals prone to anxiety will tend to put more strain on their adrenal glands. This seems to be especially true for individuals who feel weak or anxious if a meal is skipped. (*For more on adrenal function, see p.44.*)

AVOID CAFFEINE A very important dietary factor that often features in anxiety is caffeine. It is a stimulant and can provoke symptoms of anxiety and nervousness. A 2002 study found that it may exaggerate responses to the stressful events of normal daily life. In the study, caffeine (equivalent to that found in four small cups of coffee) raised blood pressure and elevated the production of adrenaline.

Anxiety disorders and related illnesses affect 5 per cent of the population

Individuals suffering from anxiety and panic attacks seem to be sensitive to the amount of caffeine found in just one cup of coffee. If you are prone to anxiety and panic attacks, it is probably advisable to avoid caffeine altogether.

MAGNESIUM SUPPLEMENTS Studies show that magnesium deficiency can enhance stress reactions and that emotional stress, such as anxiety, can increase the need for magnesium. Supplementing the diet with magnesium may be valuable for sufferers of anxiety. Taking about 200mg of magnesium supplements twice daily may help to reduce symptoms.

MULTIVITAMIN/MINERAL SUPPLEMENT A good nutritional status may be helpful to those who suffer from anxiety and panic attacks. A 2000 study showed that a multivitamin and mineral supplement taken for 28 days was associated with a consistent and significant reduction in anxiety and perceived stress.

SELENIUM SUPPLEMENTS The trace mineral selenium seems to have a particular role to play in regulating mood. A 1991 study found that taking 100mcg a day of selenium lead to a general improvement in mood and a reduction in feelings of anxiety, especially in those individuals with low levels of selenium in the diet.

Selenium supplementation may be particularly beneficial in the UK where daily intakes of this nutrient tend to be low.

CAUTION

Consult your doctor before taking magnesium with ciproflaxin and warfarin, or with iron and warfarin, or with spironolactone (*see p.46*).

Homeopathy

COMPLEX HOMEOPATHY In a clinical trial, a complex homeopathic medicine called Anti-Anxiety, which contains *Ignatia*, *Asa foetida* and *Valeriana officinialis*, was found to be effective in treating anxiety.

IGNATIA Many homeopathic medicines may be helpful in anxiety, depending on the type of anxiety and the person who has it. Perhaps the most frequently appropriate

medicine for acute anxiety triggered by an emotional shock is *Ignatia* (for dosages, see p.73). Typically, the anxiety this medicine relieves is characterised by hypersensitivity of all the senses: noises seem too loud, lights too bright, and so on. There is also great emotional hypersensitivity and changeability, as well as various kinds of spasms, including nervous coughs and tics. The "keynote" is said to be paradoxicality – for instance, there is a sensation of a lump in the throat, but liquids are more difficult to swallow than solids.

ACONITE is another homeopathic medicine that is useful in acute situations, often triggered by a physical shock or acute physical illness. Typically, the patient is very anxious, feels very chilly and thinks she or he is about to die.

CONSTITUTIONAL TREATMENT If anxiety is long-term, you may need to visit a homeopath for constitutional treatment (*see p.72*). Perhaps the most common medicines are *Argentum nitricum*, *Calcarea carbonica* and *Arsenicum album*.

ARGENTUM NITRICUM patients often have many fears, particularly claustrophobia and fear of heights, associated with a distressing impulse to jump from high places. They typically suffer from severe anticipa-

CALCAREA CARBONICA presents a very different picture. The anxiety may be less obvious on the surface, but is deep seated. These people are often solid, conscientious types, but have many fears, particularly about being seriously or incurably ill. They tend to "niggle" – they turn small things over and over in their minds. On the physical side they tend to be chilly, but sweat easily, especially on the head and neck.

ARSENICUM ALBUM patients are different again. They tend to be perfectionists who get very upset if everything is not tidy and organised. They get very anxious even if they have minor illnesses; where there is nothing to worry about, they will find something. On the physical side, they are usually very chilly and may have skin problems, including eczema, psoriasis or just dry, flakey skin.

CAUTION

Some homeopathic medicines, including *Ignatia*, are antidoted by coffee. This means that the medicine is rendered ineffective.

Western Herbal Medicine

RELIEVING SYMPTOMS It is unrealistic to expect a herbal medicine to "cure" an anxiety that is disrupting someone's life. Herbal medicines can help to relieve the symptoms of anxiety, such as muscle tension, headaches, palpitations and sleep disturbance, and to reduce the intensity with which anxiety can grip the person's mind.

SHORT-TERM RELIEF to enable the person to implement changes that will lower anxiety levels is an aim of the herbal approach. For example, better quality and duration

---

> People with panic disorder may become so afraid of an attack that they develop a phobia

---

tion, getting into a terrible state in advance of important events, with physical symptoms often relating to the intestines, including bloating, belching and diarrhoea. They also tend to feel too hot.

of sleep usually lead to improved self-confidence and vitality, increasing the person's chances of taking more exercise, improving their diet, getting through a relationship breakdown and so forth.

In the longer term, the aim would be to prescribe herbs that will strengthen the function of the neuro-endocrine system (nerves and hormones), while helping the person to develop life patterns so they became less dependent on an "adrenaline economy" – in other words, overactivity of the sympathetic nervous system.

Typically, herbal remedies are selected to match the specific anxiety exhibited by the individual patient. Limeflowers (*Tilia euro-*

ANTI-ANXIETY BREATHING

One of the effects of experiencing anxiety and panic disorders is to change your pattern of breathing, forcing you to breathe more quickly and more shallowly from the upper chest. This has an effect on your body chemistry, leading to a cycle of tension and stress. If you feel that you are about to become anxious, or are on the verge of a panic attack, try to practise the two steps of the anti-anxiety breathing technique shown here. You can either stand, sit or lie down on your back – whatever is appropriate and comfortable for you at the time.

Place your hands, with the fingers spread out, below your ribcage and either side of your torso. Concentrate on your diaphragm and breathe deeply for several breaths.

Then, with your eyes closed, place your hands on your upper chest and concentrate on sending several breaths down through your lungs to the diaphragm.

pea) or lemon balm (*Melissa officinalis*) relieve anxiety (anxiolytic). Both can also treat nervous palpitations, strengthening parasympathetic nervous activity on the heart, that in turn dampens the nervous irritability producing heart irregularity.

OVER-THE-COUNTER REMEDIES You can take a range of herbal medicines to relieve anxiety. Most are suitable for self-medication as well as for practitioner use. You can buy many over-the-counter formulations (including the herbs listed below) as tablets or capsules, though the quality of such products can be very variable. For the best results, consult a qualified herbalist.

VALERIAN (*Valeriana officinalis*) is a relaxant and mild sedative, taken for nervous overactivity, insomnia and muscle tension. Clinical trials have shown valerian extracts improve sleep quality and duration, with few side-effects. A 1995 clinical study found valerian, combined with St John's wort (*Hypericum perforatum*), was as effective as amitryptyline in treating depressive anxiety, yet with far fewer side-effects.

PASSION FLOWER (*Passiflora incarnata*) is a sedative herb that is used principally for combating sleep disturbance, but it is equally useful in relieving anxiety.

WITHANIA (*Withania somnifera*) is a relaxant and restorative herb. It is particularly useful in treating the exhaustion and enervation that accompany long-term anxiety.

> **CAUTION**
>
> Before taking a herbal remedy, see page 69 and, if you are already taking prescribed medication, consult a medical herbalist first.

Environmental Health

TOXIC EXPOSURES Anxiety, weakness, fatigue and difficulty in concentrating are common symptoms in people after they have been exposed to toxic compounds. The symptoms result either from toxic injury to the nervous system, or to emotional or psychological responses to the exposure, or to both.

According to some research, an acute exposure that requires medical care is more likely to result in psychological symptoms, such as anxiety, than chronic low levels of toxic exposure. In fact, there is still doubt about whether or not chronic exposures could lead to an anxiety disorder. Anxiety responses to toxic exposures show some similarity to post-traumatic stress disorder (*see p.422*).

Anxiety problems may develop in people with a history of past serious exposures to environmental toxicants, or who live in close proximity to known environmentally dangerous sites.

There are many factors that affect whether or not someone will develop anxiety or other psychological problems from living or working close to a hazardous site. For example, symptoms may be more likely if the exposure was accidental or involuntary, or if there was a feeling of a lack of community control over the safety regulations in place. In addition, anxiety and worry that develop near such sites may depend on whether or not the person has a history of acute exposure to the relevant compounds or if the compounds from the site have a perceptible odour. Some people may continue to have psychological symptoms, such as anxiety, after toxic exposures; these symptoms are more likely if the person was stressed before the event happened, or if he or she had a severe enough exposure to warrant a visit to an accident and emergency department.

CHEMICALS Panic attacks may be brought on by certain chemicals, such as the cyanoacrylate and organic solvents in Superglue. Research into other compounds, such as ammonia from a diazo printer, ozone from a photocopier or chlorine from a pulp mill factory, support this finding. The panic reactions were often unpredictable and the particular compounds irritated skin and mucous membranes.

If you have panic attacks, it is not necessary to avoid all possible chemical triggers because people react to them in an unpredictable fashion. There is no evidence that avoidance helps to prevent panic attacks from developing or improves the symptoms of panic attacks.

However, some people have a learned or conditioned response to a particular chemical so that when they smell, inhale or contact the chemical again at a later date, they experience a panic attack.

Just as a particular chemical can elicit a panic attack, classical (Pavlovian) conditioning can be used to allay anxiety. For example, if a distinct essential oil is used during a series of relaxing massages, then

women with a background of depression and anxiety were much better after a four-month programme of aerobic exercise combined with appropriate medication.

Breathing Retraining

PRIMARY TREATMENT Breathing retraining is a valuable tool for easing anxiety states. If your breathing is too shallow, it disrupts your body's biochemistry, which can contribute to feelings of anxiety (*for breathing exercises, see pp.57 and 62*).

In 1999, a Dutch study involved a combination of breathing retraining (learning to slow down the rate, and to improve abdominal breathing) together with phys-

very acute, in which case treatment can be given two or three times a week. In general, you would usually expect some benefit to emerge over six to eight treatment sessions, with the possibility that long-term maintenance may be required.

Mind–body Therapies

PRIMARY TREATMENT **COGNITIVE BEHAVIOURAL THERAPY** The most effective non-drug approaches involve cognitive-behavioural therapy (CBT). Many research studies confirm the effectiveness of CBT for treating anxiety disorders. In some circumstances, it may even replace medication in treating the symptoms of anxiety related ailments such as obsessive-compulsive disorder and post-traumatic stress disorder.

OTHER APPROACHES Studies confirm the efficacy of mind–body treatments, such as guided imagery, relaxation, hypnosis, meditation and clinical biofeedback, in all types of anxiety and across all age ranges. They work well combined with CBT and medication – the latter is sometimes required if the anxiety is disabling. Patients report feeling more in control of their symptoms; positive benefits have been sustained in follow-ups as long as six years. Self-help audiotapes and/or multimedia self-help programmes have also been effective.

Meditation can relieve and prevent anxiety and panic attacks. Some forms may be more effective than others, but it is important to adopt a technique that you feel comfortable doing on a regular basis.

Anxiety and panic disorders can be greatly eased with professional help

---

the scent of the oil will come to be associated with relaxation. A small bottle of the oil can then be carried around and smelled at the first sign of anxiety to help induce a state of relaxation.

Exercise and Massage

People who are anxious or prone to panic attacks are recommended to take regular aerobic exercise and to receive a regular massage. Both practices have been shown to be effective ways of reducing feelings of anxiety and apprehension, on their own and in combination with each other, or with medication.

For example, research at the Touch Research Institute in Miami, USA, has shown in numerous studies that massage reduces feelings of anxiety, as well as the presence of elevated levels of "stress" hormones, such as cortisol. In a 2003 study, the effects of massage and movement therapy (50-minute sessions, twice weekly, for three weeks) were compared with the effects of relaxation on anxiety experienced by people with chronic pain. The results showed that the greatest reduction in anxiety (and pain) levels was achieved by those receiving massage and movement therapy.

A 2002 study showed that over 50 per cent of a group of middle-aged men and

iotherapy designed to release tense muscles that were hampering the breathing process. The researchers found that there was a clear link between the rate of breathing and the development of symptoms of anxiety, and that slowing this rate was the key to the successful treatment.

In 1993, research looked at the effects of breathing retraining on anxiety experienced by people with chronic fatigue, compared with non-fatigued anxious individuals. The results were varied and the researchers concluded that "Breathing retraining is of benefit, not only in restoring more normal patterns of breathing but also in reducing anxiety, particularly in patients without the complication of chronic fatigue".

Acupuncture

Clinical experience suggests that acupuncture is often useful to help people cope with anxiety and panic attacks. In addition, there are good scientific theories explaining how acupuncture could alter the balance of chemical messengers in the brain in a way that would be likely to benefit people with these conditions.

Often, several acupuncture treatments are required, given on a weekly basis – unless the particular anxiety disorder is

---

PREVENTION PLAN

The following may help you to prevent an anxiety or panic disorder:

- Take plenty of regular exercise to relax muscle tension.

- If you feel a panic attack is imminent, practise slow, diaphragmatic breathing.

- Reassure yourself that the feelings you are having in your body are not dangerous and will soon pass off.

- Avoid caffeine and other stimulants.

- Eat a nutritious diet to help you maintain steady blood-sugar levels.

OBSESSIVE–COMPULSIVE DISORDER

In obsessive–compulsive disorder (OCD), unwanted thoughts enter the mind repeatedly. These often involve anxieties about safety, hygiene or security of possessions. The unwanted thoughts are often accompanied by anxiety and irresistible urges to carry out compulsive actions over and over again. Treatment may involve psychotherapy techniques and adopting ways of relieving anxiety, including breathing retraining and controlling blood-sugar levels.

WHAT ARE THE SYMPTOMS?

The most common symptoms of obsessive–compulsive disorder include:

- Intrusive and irrational mental images
- Repeated attempts to resist irrational or unwanted thoughts
- Repetitive behaviour that cannot be resisted

WHY MIGHT I HAVE THIS?

PREDISPOSING FACTORS

- Genetic influence
- Tendency to perfectionism and inflexibility
- Difficulty dealing with stressful events

TREATMENT PLAN

PRIMARY TREATMENTS

- Exposure, ritual prevention and other cognitive behavioural techniques

BACK-UP TREATMENTS

- Antidepressants (in some cases)
- Exercise
- Breathing retraining
- Diary-keeping

WORTH CONSIDERING

- Homeopathy
- Nutritional therapy

For an explanation of how treatments are rated, see p.111.

WHY DOES IT OCCUR?

People with OCD are obsessed with something in their lives, as if a particular thought, urge or fear has them in its grasp. Again and again, the obsession returns like repetitive bouts of mental hiccups. The compulsions are ritual actions that are attempts to banish an obsession.

A tendency to develop obsessive–compulsive disorder sometimes runs in families. The disorder is often associated with depressive illness. It is possible to have an obsessive–compulsive personality, which is characterised by inflexibility and continually striving for perfection. People with this type of personality are at an increased risk of developing the disorder.

Examples of common compulsive actions are handwashing, checking that windows and doors are locked, making sure that keys are safely in their place and arranging items on a desk in a precise manner. The same action is performed over and over again – sometimes hundreds of times a day – because each time it brings only a temporary sense of relief from anxiety. The disorder can interfere with normal life and so may cause a great deal of distress.

IMPORTANT

OCD is not a condition that is suitable for self-diagnosis and self-treatment. Consult your doctor if you think you have the symptoms of OCD. As in all personality and mental health problems, expert advice and supervision is essential in treating OCD.

TREATMENTS IN DETAIL

Conventional Medicine

Your doctor should be able to diagnose obsessive–compulsive disorder from a description of your symptoms. He or she will recommend psychological treatments, such as "ritual prevention", in which the individual must learn to resist performing a compulsive action (*see Psychological Therapies, p.421*).

ANTIDEPRESSANTS Certain types of antidepressant drugs may help some people, although psychological therapy is the main treatment. Drugs include clomipramine and selective serotonin re-uptake inhibitors (SSRIs), including fluoxetine.

CAUTION

Antidepressant drugs may cause side-effects: ask your doctor to explain these to you.

Nutritional Therapy

Nutritional strategies have not been shown to help OCD, but since the condition usually involves an underlying anxiety, they are worth considering as part of an overall self-help programme (*see Anxiety, p.414*).

RELIEVING ANXIETY Anxiety is a prominent feature in some individuals with OCD and one nutritional factor that is commonly seen in conjunction with anxiety is blood-sugar imbalance. When blood-sugar levels fall, the body generally attempts to correct this by secreting the hormone adrenaline, which stimulates the release of sugar from the liver. Adrenaline is certainly one hormone in the body that is well known to provoke feelings of anxiety and even panic. Clinical experience suggests that even non-diabetics can be prone to anxiety at times when blood-sugar levels are lower than ideal. (*For more on blood-sugar balance, see p.42.*)

IMPAIRED ADRENAL FUNCTION In practice, individuals who are prone to OCD or anxiety can have weakness in the adrenal glands. This seems to be especially true for individuals who feel weak or anxious if a meal is skipped. (*For more on impaired adrenal function, see p.44.*)

AVOID CAFFEINE Caffeine is a stimulant, and can provoke symptoms of anxiety and nervousness. Individuals suffering from anxiety seem to be sensitive to the amount of caffeine found in just one cup of coffee. For individuals prone to OCD or anxiety, it is probably advisable to avoid caffeine.

MAGNESIUM SUPPLEMENTS Studies show that magnesium deficiency can enhance the way some people react to stress and that emotional stress, such as anxiety, can increase the need for magnesium. Magnesium supplementation may be valuable for people who are prone to anxiety. Taking 200mg of magnesium supplements twice daily may help people with OCD to reduce their anxiety.

CAUTION

Consult your doctor before taking magnesium with ciproflaxin, warfarin or spironolactone (*see p.46*).

Homeopathy

Although there is no research on the homeopathic treatment of OCD, some practitioners report that they have been able to help patients. Treatment of this condition requires skilled homeopathic prescribing from an experienced practitioner (*see Constitutional prescribing, p.73*). Among the medicines that may help are *Thuja occidentalis, Aurum metallicum, Silicea* and *Anacardium*.

OBSESSIONS AND COMPULSIONS

People with OCD become obsessed with something that takes over their lives. They attempt to deal with these obsessions by endlessly repeating a ritual action known as a compulsion. The table below lists some of the more common obsessions as well as some of the particular compulsive actions that may be expressed in OCD.

OBSESSION	COMPULSION
Germs and cleanliness	• Repeatedly hand-washing and scrubbing, sometimes until the skin is raw and bleeding
Security and safety	• Repeatedly checking that both doors and windows are locked • Repeatedly checking that keys are put in the "safe place" • Repeatedly checking that the oven/iron has been turned off
Preoccupation with exactness, or perfect order	• Rearranging objects, e.g. lining shoes up, straightening pictures • Counting or sorting objects
Religious anxieties	• Overly time-consuming mental rituals and prayers • Repeating "good" thoughts in order to counteract "bad" thoughts
Worries about harm to self or others	• Repeatedly checking that self or others are alright
Running out of things	• Buying more than necessary, shopping in a ritualistic pattern
Worries about diseases, e.g. cancer	• Repeated self-checking, e.g. blood pressure

---

THUJA OCCIDENTALIS is perhaps the most commonly indicated homeopathic medicine for both obsessional and intrusive thoughts. Those who respond to *Thuja occidentalis* may be preoccupied by a disease, such as cancer, and feel the need to follow rituals to avoid it. They may have strange feelings about their body – for instance, that there is an animal moving around inside their abdomen, or that they are very fragile.

Their facial skin may be greasy and they may have multiple warts and other skin blemishes. The problems sometimes seem to have been triggered by immunisations or other long-term medical treatment.

AURUM METALLICUM is often the medicine of choice when the patient is very depressed and obsessed with thoughts of death or suicide. Frequently, the problem is worse in winter and at night. The patient may become very angry over minor things. The compulsive behaviour may be associated with sinusitis or palpitations.

SILICEA People who respond to *Silicea* (also called *Silica*) may be obsessed with counting or sorting small objects. These patients tend to be shy and show signs of fatigue. They may also feel the cold, but have cold, clammy hands and feet, and weak nails and hair.

ANACARDIUM Patients who respond to *Anacardium* have a curious sensation that their mind and body are separated, or that they are being controlled by an external force. They may also suffer from bouts of violent anger, gaps in their memory and sometimes skin problems, especially hives.

Exercise

Both physical exercise and breathing (*see Breathing Retraining, right*) can be very useful in managing the symptoms of OCD, but they should be incorporated into a general programme of treatment that might include medication as well as cognitive behaviour modification (*see Psychological Therapies, right*).

Canadian researchers report that regular exercise may help many people who suffer from psychiatric disorders, including phobias (*see p.411*) and OCD. A review of all the major studies of anxiety disorders and exercise, dating back to 1981, reported that strength training, running, walking and

Breathing Retraining

The anxiety-relieving effect of breathing retraining may help people with OCD. Practising yoga-type breathing (*see p62*) can be a useful part of the treatment programme for anyone who has an anxiety-related disorder.

Psychological Therapies

FAMILY HELP One of the most important steps in helping people to overcome their OCD is to get them to recognise that there are, in fact, effective ways to treat their condition. This is where family members (and friends) can be most useful – they need to learn as much as possible about the causes and treatment of OCD and to keep abreast of developments.

When people with OCD continue to deny they have a problem or persistently refuse treatment, then there is little that can be done for them. However, once the person accepts that he or she has OCD,

ritual prevention, with cognitive therapy. Exposure often helps the patient cope with the anxiety and the obsession, while ritual prevention works on reducing the compulsive behaviours.

Exposure and ritual (or response) prevention consists of gradually exposing the patient to the thing or the event that they find distressing, and asking the patient not to respond with the ritual that they normally use to alleviate the anxiety.

For example, some people with OCD may respond to thoughts about having germs on their skin by obsessively washing their hands. In this case, the patient would be asked to think deliberately about the germs and then to refrain from handwashing. While this is likely to be distressing to start with, the distress usually subsides until eventually the patient can have the distressing thought and not feel a compulsive need to wash their hands.

DIARY-KEEPING is another important aspect of treating OCD, especially if combined with CBT. Patients may be asked to keep a diary between therapy sessions, recording their thoughts and how they were triggered. They would also be asked to note how they responded to the thoughts as a way of alleviating the anxiety. This diary would then be used in the following therapy session to plan the next stage of the treatment.

A typical diary entry may have the following headings: time; thought; trigger (what initiated the thought?); response (what were your actions?); duration (how long did your response last?); and feelings.

For example, someone who is obsessed with cleanliness might have the following diary entry:

- Time: 8.30am.
- Thought: The table is dirty.
- Trigger: Crumbs on the breakfast table.
- Response: Repeatedly scrubbed the table.
- Duration: How long did your response last? 20 minutes.
- Feelings: Initially relief, then anxiety and anger because I was late for work.

Regular diary-keeping may help you to recognise patterns of behaviour and to identify the ways in which you can make changes. For example, if each bout of compulsive behaviour lasts on average for 30 minutes, you could aim to gradually reduce this time.

Up to a half of adults with OCD say that their disorder began during childhood

other forms of aerobic exercise can help to alleviate mild to moderate depression (*see p.436*), and may also help to relieve other mental disorders, including anxiety, OCD and substance abuse.

Some experts are concerned that a devotion to regular exercise may itself represent a form of obsessive–compulsive behaviour. However, several research studies refute this idea. One evaluated the personalities of more than 200 men and women recruited from gymnasiums and concluded that "Contrary to prediction, excessive exercisers were not found to have lower self-esteem, more external locus of control or to be more obsessive–compulsive than moderate exercisers.... These findings suggest that exercise is not an expression of a dysfunctional personality."

To support this, a different Canadian study that involved 55 aerobic-class regulars concluded that people who regularly attend aerobic classes are not more likely to have OCD.

then there is a good chance that the disorder can be brought under control and managed effectively.

Family members can also join in with the therapy to help them understand the rituals and to introduce them to step-by-step ways of gradually (not abruptly) disentangling normal family life from the OCD rituals.

It is important to avoid making negative comments, as only calm support and encouragement can help to bring about a positive outcome to treatment. Joining a support group provides an opportunity for family members to share experiences and worries, to learn new ways of coping and to help them lead their own lives.

PRIMARY TREATMENT **COGNITIVE BEHAVIOURAL THERAPY (CBT)** By far the most common form of treatment for OCD comes from cognitive behaviour therapy (CBT) techniques, which combine behavioural therapy, such as exposure and

WHAT ARE THE SYMPTOMS?

Symptoms may occur straight after the event or weeks, months or even years later and include:

- Involuntary thoughts about the traumatic experience and repeated reliving of the event
- Panic attacks
- Avoiding reminders of the event and refusing to discuss it
- Disturbed sleep and nightmares
- Disrupted concentration
- Irritability

WHY MIGHT I HAVE THIS?

PREDISPOSING FACTORS

- Previous traumatic experience
- High trait anxiety
- Being under 16 or over 60

TRIGGER

- Witnessing or being involved in a traumatic event

TREATMENT PLAN

PRIMARY TREATMENTS

- Different types of psychological therapy, sometimes in combination with antidepressants
- Eye movement desensitisation and reprocessing (EMDR)

BACK-UP TREATMENT

- Breathing retraining

WORTH CONSIDERING

- Nutritional therapy
- Homeopathy
- Massage therapy

For an explanation of how treatments are rated, see p.111.

POST-TRAUMATIC STRESS DISORDER

Post-traumatic stress disorder (PTSD) is a persistent disturbing reaction following a traumatic and highly stressful experience. Sometimes, the reaction is delayed. The kinds of event that cause PTSD include natural disasters, serious accidents and being attacked. Treatment may involve counselling, psychological therapy, homeopathy and measures such as breathing retraining and massage which help to relieve anxiety.

WHY DOES IT OCCUR?

Witnessing or being involved in a stressful event, such as a traffic accident, mugging or an earthquake, can trigger intense emotions. Sometimes, symptoms last for years. Children and elderly people are at higher risk of developing PTSD, as are people with anxiety disorders (*see p.414*) and those who lack support.

People with PTSD may feel emotionally numb, detached from life and distanced from family and friends. However, they may also experience great anxiety in response to reminders of the traumatic experience. They may also become depressed. Sometimes, the disorder can lead to drug or alcohol abuse. People who have already had PTSD once are more likely to experience it again if they are faced with another traumatic event.

TREATMENTS IN DETAIL

Conventional Medicine

PRIMARY TREATMENT Through discussion, a doctor can diagnose PTSD and determine the severity of symptoms. The main part of treatment is likely to be psychological (*see Psychological Therapies, p.423*).

IMPORTANT

PTSD is not a condition that is suitable for self-diagnosis and self-treatment. Consult your doctor as soon as you suspect you have the symptoms of PTSD. If the symptoms are disabling, don't hesitate to seek urgent medical advice.

Certain antidepressants, such as selective serotonin re-uptake inhibitors (SSRIs), may be recommended in some cases.

CAUTION

Drugs for PTSD have side-effects: ask your doctor to explain these to you.

Nutritional Therapy

Nutritional treatment of PTSD overlaps with treatment for other ailments in which anxiety is a significant factor. See also anxiety (*see p.414*), depression (*see p.436*), phobias (*see p.411*) and coping with stress (*see p.408*). (*For more on adrenal imbalance, see p.44.*) PTSD may also be associated with reductions in immune function and can be treated accordingly.

AVOID CAFFEINE Caffeine is a stimulant that can provoke symptoms of anxiety and nervousness and so should be avoided by people with PTSD.

SUPPLEMENTS Studies show that magnesium deficiency can enhance stress reactions and that emotional stress can increase the need for magnesium. In practice, magnesium supplementation does seem to be valuable for individuals who are persistently anxious. Taking 200mg of magnesium twice daily can help.

A good nutritional status is important for those who suffer from anxiety and stress. If you have PTSD, take a multivitamin and mineral supplement each day; in one study doing this for 28 days was associated with a consistent and significant reduction in anxiety and perceived stress.

Homeopathy

There are a number of reports that homeopathic medicines help people with PTSD, particularly children in foster care who have suffered physical and sexual abuse and adult survivors of childhood sexual abuse. Medicines used include *Stramonium*, *Platina*, *Ignatia*, *Staphysagria*, *Causticum* and *Opium*. Consult an experienced homeopath who can make a constitutional diagnosis (*see p.73*).

STRAMONIUM is an important medicine for some of the most distressing symptoms of PTSD, such as night terrors, startle responses and intrusive thoughts or flashbacks to traumatic events. The person may have fears of the dark, water or other things related to the original trauma, as well as fits of destructive rage.

IGNATIA People who respond to *Ignatia* may appear hysterical. They are hypersensitive, both emotionally and physically. It is said to be a medicine of paradoxes – for instance, there is often a sensation of a lump in the throat, making swallowing difficult, yet liquids are more difficult to swallow than solids.

STAPHYSAGRIA The "keynote" feature of *Staphysagria* is said to be "suppressed indignation". It is suitable for people who may have suffered a sexual assault or abusive relationship as an adult, and are tremendously angry about what has been done to them. But this may be bottled up and expressed through physical symptoms, particularly recurrent sterile cystitis or urethral syndrome. Sometimes, the anger is expressed, making these people prickly and difficult to deal with.

CAUSTICUM complements *Staphysagria* because it is often appropriate for use after *Staphysagria*. A typical feature of people who respond to *Causticum* is their strong sense of justice and feelings of empathy with those who have been unjustly treated.

OPIUM When physical injury played an important part – for instance, in PTSD that follows a traffic accident, war experience or another violent episode – homeopathic *Opium* may be indicated as a potential medicine. A typical feature of a person who responds to *Opium* is that they may feel "spaced out" or withdrawn, becoming either very timid or else reckless by losing their sense of danger or abusing alcohol or other drugs.

Breathing Retraining

PTSD involves a great deal of anxiety, which responds to strategies for breathing retraining (*see p.62*).

Many experts believe that the quality of an individual's sleep is extremely important in the PTSD process, and that sleep disruption, whatever its cause, has important influences on the trauma recovery process for many people.

Disturbed sleep is often associated with sleep-disordered breathing (SDB), which may involve sleep apnoea (brief periods when breathing stops), snoring and a tendency to nightmares. Feeling sleepy during the day is a consequence and exaggerates the PTSD symptoms.

Treating the breathing component of SDB might help sleep quality and thereby the PTSD symptoms. To find out if this is true, one research study evaluated the benefits of using a CPAP (continuous positive airway pressure) breathing mask that delivers oxygen and helps to maintain normal airflow during sleep. The results were remarkable, not just in terms of better sleep, daytime well-being and reduced nightmares, but also in relation to all the PTSD symptoms.

Other research has found similar benefits – when a person's breathing improves, their sleep improves and so, usually, do their PTSD symptoms.

Massage Therapy

Researchers evaluated the benefits of massage therapy for children affected by a major hurricane disaster who had severe symptoms of PTSD, such as anxiety, depression and behavioural outbursts. A group of 60 children were divided into two sets, one of which received massage (30 minutes of back massage administered twice weekly for a month). The other set spent the same amount of time watching non-stimulating video cartoons – the children sat quietly with psychology graduate students, who maintained physical contact either with the child sitting on the graduate's lap or with an arm around the child.

After one month, the children who had received massage showed significant differences compared to the other set. Their anxiety and depression had improved, their stress hormone (cortisol) levels were

Survivors of a trauma who blame themselves may be more at risk of severe or long-term PTSD

lower and they were better able to relax. The researchers in the study noted that "Unlike several other forms of treatment, such as psychotherapy or pharmacological treatment, massage therapy could be continued in a cost-effective way if it were taught to parents."

Psychological Therapies

PRIMARY TREATMENT The talking therapies used to treat PTSD include cognitive behavioural therapy (CBT) techniques, such as systematic desensitisation, exposure therapy, anxiety management and stress inoculation. Eye movement desensitisation and reprocessing (EMDR) and psychodynamic approaches are also used.

EXPOSURE TECHNIQUES In a review of treatments for PTSD, three studies of exposure therapy showed some positive

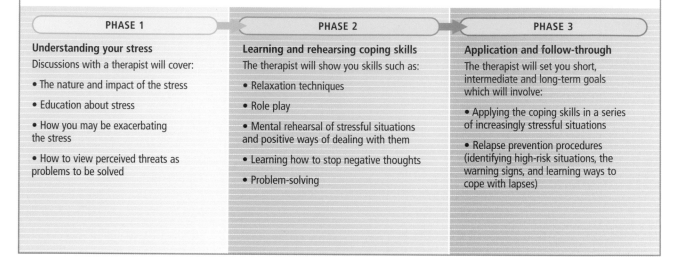

STRESS INOCULATION TRAINING

People with PTSD can benefit from stress inoculation training because it not only helps them to cope with the aftermath of their particular trauma, but also inoculates them against future stressors. The technique follows three stages: understanding the stress that is affecting them; learning and practising the skills needed to cope with the particular stressful event; and applying the coping skills to future situations. SIT can take up to 12 months to be effective and may need booster and follow-up sessions.

PHASE 1

Understanding your stress

Discussions with a therapist will cover:

• The nature and impact of the stress

• Education about stress

• How you may be exacerbating the stress

• How to view perceived threats as problems to be solved

PHASE 2

Learning and rehearsing coping skills

The therapist will show you skills such as:

• Relaxation techniques

• Role play

• Mental rehearsal of stressful situations and positive ways of dealing with them

• Learning how to stop negative thoughts

• Problem-solving

PHASE 3

Application and follow-through

The therapist will set you short, intermediate and long-term goals which will involve:

• Applying the coping skills in a series of increasingly stressful situations

• Relapse prevention procedures (identifying high-risk situations, the warning signs, and learning ways to cope with lapses)

---

and some less positive results. Another study found that, after having exposure therapy, patients reported a significant reduction in the number of PTSD symptoms. (*For a description of the techniques, see Phobias, p.411.*)

STRESS INOCULATION TRAINING (SIT) consists of helping patients to respond in different ways to traumatic and stressful situations (*see box, above*). SIT combines role play, relaxation techniques, modelling (where the therapist literally shows the patient different ways of responding) and some techniques used in changing thought patterns. SIT therapy has been effective in reducing PTSD symptoms, such as anxiety and intrusive thoughts, in rape victims. Compared to exposure therapy, SIT appears to be the most promising technique.

ANXIETY MANAGEMENT uses techniques, such as relaxation training (*see p.99*), biofeedback and stress management, which provide significant benefit for people with PTSD.

SYSTEMATIC DESENSITISATION (SD) is a cognitive technique that uses relaxation to help a patient gradually and systematically desensitise their trauma under controlled conditions. SD has been studied in a num-

ber of research studies and there is some evidence that it is effective.

Other studies showed support for SD in the treatment of victims of rape. Although the research is promising, there are a number of difficulties in the design of the studies which mean that the evidence so far is inconclusive.

PRIMARY TREATMENT **EYE MOVEMENT DESENSITISATION AND REPROCESSING (EMDR)** is a relatively new therapy that was designed specifically for the treatment of PTSD. It is beginning to accrue an evidence base that suggests it may be an astonishingly and rapidly effective treatment for people with PTSD.

According to the theory, rapid eye movements (which are known to occur when dreaming) take place when the brain moves information in short-term memory to long-term memory. The former type of memory tends to be emotional, whereas the latter is not.

In EMDR, the person treated thinks about the most important features of the trauma while the therapist moves his or her fingers in front of the person's eyes producing rapid eye movements. This reawakens the memory and it may cause a minor reaction, which the experienced practitioner must carefully control.

According to the theory, however, EDMR helps to move the traumatic memories into long-term storage, defusing their emotional charge. In many cases, so the emerging research suggests, patients within a few sessions recall the trauma without the previous terrifying feelings.

PSYCHODYNAMIC METHODS are widely used in the treatment of PTSD. One of the problems with working with traumatised people is that it is sometimes not clear how much the traumatic incident itself has created the problems and how much symptoms are due to earlier difficulties that the traumatic incident has exacerbated. It seems likely that those people most likely to develop PTSD are those who have been previously traumatised and/or who have an anxious personality.

Psychodynamic methods help people to distinguish between the two. They involve the therapist listening to the person's account of their experiences and exploring the connections between what the person is thinking, doing and feeling in their present life and past experiences.

Evidence is promising but limited and the research has had some criticisms. However, psychodynamic methods have been found to be just as effective as hypnotherapy and systematic desensitisation.

WHAT ARE THE SYMPTOMS?

- Hallucinations
- Hearing voices that do not exist
- Having lots of irrational thoughts and fixed, strange beliefs, especially of being controlled by other people or persecuted
- Believing that trivial events are of great significance
- Lack of emotions or quite inappropriate emotions, such as laughing at bad news
- Rambling speech
- Difficulty concentrating
- Periods of agitation and restlessness, alternating with periods of stupor

WHY MIGHT I HAVE THIS?

PREDISPOSING FACTORS

- Genetic factors
- Substance abuse
- Omega-3 fatty acid deficiency
- Folic acid deficiency
- Abnormal levels of histamine

TRIGGER

- Stressful life event

IMPORTANT

Because of their irrational thoughts and delusions, schizophrenics may behave in ways that are dangerous to themselves or others. If this is the case, they should be seen urgently by a psychiatrist or other appropriately trained professional.

SCHIZOPHRENIA

Schizophrenia is a severe mental illness that impairs the person's sense of reality, leading to irrational behaviour and disturbed emotional reactions. Contrary to popular belief, it does not mean that people have split personalities. People with schizophrenia may hear voices, which contributes to their bizarre behaviour. They often have problems maintaining relationships with other people and holding down jobs. Treatment with antipsychotic drugs aims to control symptoms. Supplements, exercise and massage may also have a role.

WHY DOES IT OCCUR?

Schizophrenia is a brain disorder often mistakenly described as a split personality. It can develop at any age, but most commonly in the late teens and early 20s. However, the onset in women may be later than in men. At first, there may be signs of confused, shocking or irrational behaviour, involving a loss of a sense of reality and an inability to function socially, either at work or in relationships with family and friends. Together with this sense of social isolation, there may be a number of other symptoms (*see left*), involving disturbed emotional reactions, hallucinations, illusions, delusions and unusual speech patterns.

TREATMENT PLAN

PRIMARY TREATMENTS

- Emotional and practical support from various services and groups
- Antipsychotic and other drugs, including chlorpromazine
- Cognitive behavioural therapy in some cases, and psychosocial treatment

WORTH CONSIDERING

- Omega-3 fatty acids and folic acid
- Homeopathy
- Exercise
- Massage
- Mind–body therapies

For an explanation of how treatments are rated, see p.111.

No single cause of schizophrenia has been identified, but genetic factors are implicated (*see chart, p.426*) and possibly abnormalities in the levels of certain neurotransmitters in the brain, such as dopamine and serotonin. A stressful life event, such as a bereavement or serious illness, can trigger the disorder in a person who is susceptible. Substance abuse may also be a factor.

The condition affects approximately one per cent of people worldwide and may begin gradually or come on suddenly. Some people have episodes of illness with periods of complete recovery in between, while in others the disorder is continuous.

Left to themselves without treatment, people with schizophrenia are prone to self-neglect or even self-harm, and about 10 per cent commit suicide. Rarely, there may be violence towards others.

BRAIN ABNORMALITIES Advances in brain-imaging techniques have revealed that some people with schizophrenia, but not all, have enlarged ventricles (the fluid-filled cavities in the brain). Research also suggests that inappropriate nerve connections in the brain, generated while the foetus was developing in the womb, could subsequently cause abnormalities during puberty and adolescence.

In 2004, researchers reported that there were distinct abnormalities in the auditory cortex (the area of the brain that decodes nervous impulses conducted from the inner ears and thereby governs hearing) in those with schizophrenia.

However, as yet it is far from clear whether schizophrenia has a single cause, or even that it is predominantly due to an abnormality in brain biochemistry.

RISKS OF DEVELOPING SCHIZOPHRENIA

Schizophrenia is a disease with a strong family link as the chart below shows. If you have an identical twin with schizophrenia, you stand an almost 50 per cent chance of developing the disease yourself. This risk drops as the degree of relationship decreases. A person's susceptibility to schizophrenia is closely linked with a range of genes, so susceptibility can be passed through family lines. However, family dynamics can also strongly influence the development of psychological problems.

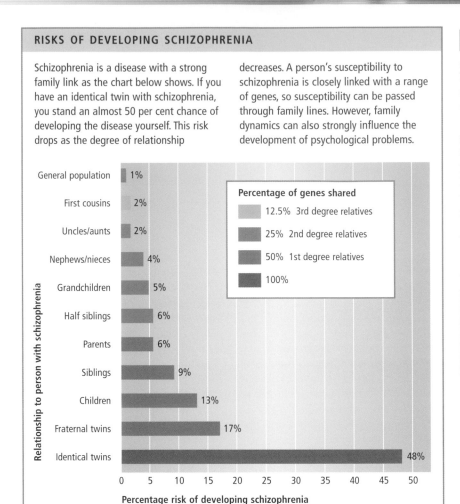

Percentage of genes shared
- 12.5% 3rd degree relatives
- 25% 2nd degree relatives
- 50% 1st degree relatives
- 100%

Relationship to person with schizophrenia:
- General population — 1%
- First cousins — 2%
- Uncles/aunts — 2%
- Nephews/nieces — 4%
- Grandchildren — 5%
- Half siblings — 6%
- Parents — 6%
- Siblings — 9%
- Children — 13%
- Fraternal twins — 17%
- Identical twins — 48%

Percentage risk of developing schizophrenia

ANTIPSYCHOTICS are the main drugs that are used to treat schizophrenia. They exert their effect by blocking the action of the neurotransmitter dopamine. Control of symptoms may take up to three months.

Antipsychotics include the following groups: phenothiazines, such as chlorpromazine; butyrophenones, such as haloperidol; thioxanthines, such as flupentixol. If individuals have problems remembering to take their medication, they can receive it in the form of injections into muscle every 1–5 weeks. In some cases, drugs are combined with cognitive behavioural therapy (*see Psychological Therapies, p.427*), which may help with delusions.

CAUTION

Antipsychotic drugs for treating schizophrenia have a range of side-effects: ask your doctor to explain these to you.

Nutritional Therapy

OMEGA-3 FATTY ACIDS, such as eicosapentaenoic acid (EPA) and docosahexaenoic acid (DHA), have been shown to be deficient in schizophrenic patients. These omega 3-fatty acids (*see p.34*) can be found in foods such as oily fish, such as mackerel, salmon and sardines.

One study showed that the lower the levels of these fatty acids are in the body, the more severe the symptoms of schizophrenia tend to be. Studies suggest that people with schizophrenia who take EPA supplements alone or in combination with normal medication show improvement in their symptoms. Taking 1 or 2g of EPA supplements per day may be useful (in combination with normal medication) in the treatment of schizophrenia.

FOLIC ACID (FOLATE) Studies suggest that folic acid deficiency is also common in those with the disease. Good sources are leafy green vegetables, organ meats, whole grains, fortified bread and nuts. One study showed that giving supplements to folate-deficient schizophrenics (in addition to standard treatment) brought significant improvements in their condition and their ability to function normally. Moreover, the folic acid supplement appeared to increase

SELF-HELP

If you or a loved one have schizophrenia, the following may prove useful (once an effective treatment has been established):

- Discuss your condition with your family, friends, employer and colleagues. Try to establish a good balance of support – you don't want to feel smothered by their attention, but if people are too remote, you may feel isolated.
- Don't put yourself under too much pressure or stress by trying to do too many things. On the other hand, avoid boring and meaningless activities – try to do things that suit you and your temperament.
- Identify situations that make you feel stressed and ask your friends and family to help you to establish ways of dealing with them.
- Join a self-help group that can provide you and your family with support.

TREATMENTS IN DETAIL

Conventional Medicine

The doctor will be able to make a full assessment by talking to the patient as well as to a close relative or friend, if possible. Admission to hospital is usually necessary to begin with where various drug treatments are prescribed.

EMOTIONAL AND PRACTICAL SUPPORT play an important role in helping to care for a person who has schizophrenia in the long term. There is a range of services available, from helplines, self-help groups and residential care, as well as charities who can offer practical help with both employment issues and financial benefits. Such services also assist the families of people with the disease, who often find they require a great deal of support and help, too.

the effectiveness of standard pharmaceutical drugs given for schizophrenia. Taking 400–800mcg of folic acid supplements per day is recommended.

VITAMIN C Studies have shown that many people with schizophrenia excrete vitamin C more quickly than others. As a result, those with the disease may benefit from taking 1g of vitamin C per day.

HISTAMINE There is some possibility of a relationship between levels of histamine in the blood and schizophrenia. Some nutritionists employ a blood test to assess "histamine type" and then give appropriate supplementation. About half of all patients with schizophrenia have low levels of

histamine. They may be helped by taking various nutrients, such as vitamin B3, folic acid, vitamin B12, zinc and manganese, that can help to increase the levels of histamine in the body.

About 20 per cent of people with schizophrenia have high levels of histamine in their bodies. Nutrients that may help these people include vitamin C, calcium and the amino acid methionine.

CAUTION

Consult your doctor before taking vitamin C with antibiotics or warfarin, or omega-3 fatty acids/fish oils with warfarin, or folic acid with anticonvulsants or methotrexate (*see p.46*).

Homeopathy

Schizophrenia is a serious condition, so support from trained professionals, such as psychiatrists, nurses and psychiatric social workers, is required. There is no published research on the homeopathic treatment of schizophrenia, and certainly homeopathic medicines should not be used alone. But some homeopaths report being able to help people with long-term problems related to schizophrenia.

Exercise

Studies have demonstrated that people with schizophrenia have increased rates of gastrointestinal, respiratory and cardiovascular disease. This is likely to be due to high rates of smoking and obesity, accompanied by a poor diet, lack of exercise and the side-effects of medication.

If it is possible to achieve higher levels of physical activity, along with a better diet and improved lifestyle habits, general health should improve, too. Since increased exercising alone has been shown to be helpful in a variety of mental illnesses, such as depression (*see p.436*), it is possible that people with schizophrenia may also benefit.

> ## Treatment allows about 1 in 5 people with schizophrenia to make a full recovery

Massage

One small and uncontrolled German study found that massage was useful for treating chronic schizophrenia. Ten people who had chronic schizophrenia were given massage to the feet, back and neck, to increase their awareness of their body limits. (Some people with schizophrenia lose the awareness of where their body begins and ends.) Being massaged by a highly experienced and competent practitioner may help them to reconnect with their body.

Massage therapy is clearly relaxing, as recorded by physiological measurements of skin conductance (the skin's capacity to conduct an electric current) and slowing of the heart rate. Patients reported that they felt more relaxed, too. Although the number of patients who participated in the study was too small to draw any firm conclusions, the results do suggest that massage and other forms of body therapy might be worth considering for schizophrenic patients.

This study supports ideas that have been put forward for a more holistic approach to treating schizophrenia by incorporating different forms of bodywork and movement therapies, as part of the overall care of the individual.

Mind–Body Therapies

Mind–body therapies, such as yoga, relaxation and guided imagery (*see p.99*) may have a role in reducing the stress associated with schizophrenia. Expressive therapies, such as art, music, dance and drama, have been widely used in psychiatric settings. They can help to integrate the emotions and elevate mood.

Psychological Therapies

PRIMARY TREATMENT **COGNITIVE BEHAVIOURAL THERAPY (CBT)** Although talking therapies are not recommended as the main treatment for complex mental health problems such as schizophrenia, cognitive behavioural therapy, which helps people to change their patterns of belief and behaviour, may be useful in reducing delusions in some patients.

PRIMARY TREATMENT **PSYCHOSOCIAL TREATMENTS** Once the antipsychotic drugs (*see Conventional Medicine, left*) have reduced or relieved their psychotic symptoms, people with schizophrenia need help with fitting in with the world at large. They need to develop their communication skills, build their self-confidence, discover their motivation and establish relationships with other people. In addition, because their illness has probably developed during the crucial years of their education and training, they have been, more often than not, prevented from following a particular career path.

Various forms of psychosocial therapy can help to improve social functioning. Such treatments may take place at home, in the workplace, in the community or at the hospital. They include rehabilitation (which helps with everyday skills, such as money management, as well as vocational training) and psychotherapy, which involves regular appointments with a mental health professional to help people to learn about themselves and deal with their particular problems.

OTHER PSYCHOLOGICAL THERAPIES are available both for people with schizophrenia and for their carers. These include counselling, family intervention and group therapy, and doctors can advise on the suitability of each.

WHAT ARE THE SYMPTOMS?

Alcohol dependency

- A compulsion to drink; lack of control over amount consumed; drinking in the mornings
- Increased tolerance to the effects of alcohol; larger amounts needed to achieve desired effects

As dependency increases:

- Night sweats; vomiting in morning
- Withdrawal symptoms, including tremor, nausea and sweating, sometimes only a few hours after the last drink
- A severe withdrawal state, delirium tremens, can develop up to three days after the last drink. Addict has severe tremor, agitation, sweating and hallucinations. Requires urgent hospital treatment.

Drug dependency

- Mood changes
- Changes in energy levels
- Changes in ability to concentrate
- Faster or slower speech
- Increased or decreased appetite
- Withdrawal symptoms depend on addictive drug involved, but may include: anxiety and restlessness; sweating that alternates with chills and shivering; confusion; muscle aches and abdominal cramps; vomiting; diarrhoea; seizures

Nicotine dependency

- Cravings for tobacco
- Irritability, mood swings, anxiety

WHY MIGHT I HAVE THESE?

PREDISPOSING FACTORS

- Genetic predisposition
- Culture of drinking or drug taking
- Poor stress management

TRIGGERS

- Blood-sugar imbalance
- Nutrient deficiencies
- Prostaglandin (PGE1) deficiency

SUBSTANCE DEPENDENCY

Substance dependency is the excessive and compulsive use of a substance, such as alcohol or heroin, which may take priority over all other things in a person's life. Dependency is distinguished from abuse by a craving for the substance and withdrawal symptoms when the substance is unavailable. Dependency on alcohol and drugs is more common in men. Treatment varies according to the substance involved, but in each case the addict needs support, counselling and, commonly, the short-term use of medication to help with withdrawal.

WHY DO THEY OCCUR?

The causes of substance dependency are complex and vary with the substance used. For example, alcohol dependency may run in families, as a result of genetic factors and/or cultural influences. It can also develop as the result of drinking to overcome anxiety (*see p.414*), low self-esteem or depression (*see p.436*). Social drinking and stress (*see p.408*) may increase the risk of dependency. Similar reasons may apply to dependency on a drug, whether it is taken for recreational or medical reasons, such as insomnia (*see p.448*) or depression.

TREATMENT PLAN

PRIMARY TREATMENTS

- Advice and emotional support
- Drugs where appropriate
- Psychological therapies

BACK-UP TREATMENTS

- Nutritional supplements

WORTH CONSIDERING

- Diet to balance blood sugar
- Homeopathy
- Acupuncture
- Breathing retraining and yoga
- Mind–body therapies
- Massage

For an explanation of how treatments are rated, see p.111.

ALCOHOL DEPENDENCY Alcohol has a direct effect on the organs and tissues of the body and may cause a number of diseases when used to excess. The compulsion to drink gradually worsens (*see Symptoms, left*). Long-term dependency on alcohol is the most common cause of severe liver disease and may also damage the pancreas and stomach.

People who drink heavily tend to neglect their nutrition and eat poor diets. Consequently, they may be deficient in vitamins, in particular vitamin B1. Deficiency of this vitamin can cause neuropathy (*see p.127*) and dementia (*see p.133*).

Several psychiatric disorders are also related to alcohol addiction, including anxiety (*see p.414*), depression (*see p.436*) and suicidal behaviour. Alcohol dependency is likely to lead to social problems, including difficulties with personal relationships and achievement at work.

NICOTINE DEPENDENCY Smoking can be highly addictive because it releases nicotine into the bloodstream. Once in the body, nicotine affects the transmission of nervous impulses and sets up a pattern of dependency that is hard to break.

The toxic substances in the smoke damage the mucous membranes that line the lungs, preventing the tiny hairs (cilia) from clearing the mucus from the alveoli, bronchioles and bronchi. Smokers commonly develop a distinctive cough and a shortness of breath. Carcinogens in the smoke increase the risk of developing lung cancer in heavy smokers, while pipe and cigar smokers are prone to developing mouth cancer and cancer of the larynx.

Smoking can cause permanent damage to the heart and blood vessels, probably through the actions of nicotine and carbon monoxide. Smokers are at risk of developing atherosclerosis (narrowing of the arteries), coronary artery disease (*see p.252*) and stroke (*see p.148*).

Smoking is implicated in a number of other problems, such as peptic ulcers and reduced fertility in both men and women, while pregnant women who smoke put their unborn babies at risk.

DRUG DEPENDENCY Some drugs available on prescription are as likely to cause dependency as illegal and recreational drugs, such as heroin and marijuana. For example, benzodiazepines (anti-anxiety and sleeping drugs) have strong addictive qualities; opiate analgesics (painkillers) can also cause substance dependency.

The risk of dependency varies with the drug being used. For example, heroin may cause dependency after only a few doses. Once in the brain, it binds to the opioid receptors on certain nerves. At first, this process may cause a pleasurable sensation. However, increasingly large quantities of an addictive drug are often needed to produce the desired effect, and physical withdrawal symptoms may develop if the drug is stopped.

The use of certain drugs, such as cocaine, amphetamines and LSD, can induce a state of psychosis in which the person who takes them can experience hallucinations, feelings of persecution and extreme excitement or lack of emotion.

As well as mental problems, misuse of certain drugs may cause physical damage; for example, repeated snorting of cocaine can result in destruction of the nasal septum which separates the nostrils, and the use of ecstasy may cause kidney and liver failure. The sharing of needles by intravenous drug abusers carries a risk of hepatitis B and HIV infection (*see p.470*).

IMMEDIATE RELIEF

When you have cravings, try:
- Massaging your ear or hands to stop the craving if you are a smoker.
- The homeopathic medicine *Nux vomica* to help reduce withdrawal symptoms, such as nausea and retching.
- Distracting yourself with exercise, chewing gum, reading, watching TV, etc.
- Calling a friend or a helpline.

TREATMENTS IN DETAIL

Conventional Medicine

PRIMARY TREATMENT **ALCOHOL DEPENDENCY** The problem of alcohol dependency requires a great deal of support and understanding, as well as advice on how to keep up the motivation to follow the programme through. In addition to psychotherapy on an individual basis, support groups, such as Alcoholics Anonymous (AA), play an important role in treatment for many people. At AA, recovered alcoholics help uncontrolled drinkers follow a 12-step programme in a bid to give up alcohol.

Some doctors prescribe benzodiazepine drugs, such as diazepam, over a period of days on a reducing schedule to help you cope with the symptoms of alcohol withdrawal. However, these drugs must only be used for a short period as they rapidly cause dependency.

Certain drugs aim to prevent a return to drinking. These include acamprosate, which, when used in combination with counselling, may help to maintain abstinence. The drug disulfiram can also be prescribed. It causes unpleasant symptoms, including vomiting, flushing of the face, palpitations and severe headaches, when combined with even a small amount of alcohol. The effects of drinking larger amounts of alcohol with the drug are serious and may include abnormal heart rhythms and collapse, so it is important not to drink for some time before and after taking disulfiram.

PRIMARY TREATMENT **DRUG DEPENDENCY** The treatment varies to an extent on the drug involved, but in all cases emotional support and advice on withdrawal will be beneficial. Specific treatment may be required for some individuals; for example, the drug methadone may be prescribed in a schedule of reducing doses to help those withdrawing from heroin.

PRIMARY TREATMENT **NICOTINE DEPENDENCY** It may be very hard to give up smoking, but you are never too old to benefit. If you need help, consult your doctor who may recommend one of the various aids that will help to prevent the cravings for nicotine. These include special nicotine-containing chewing gum or patches. You may also benefit from joining a support group or contacting a telephone helpline that is staffed by ex-smokers (*see p.486 for contact details*).

CAUTION

Drugs aimed at preventing dependency may have side-effects: ask your doctor to explain these to you.

Nutritional Therapy

BALANCING BLOOD SUGAR Alcohol craving can be associated with fluctuations in the level of sugar in the bloodstream. When blood-sugar levels drop, the body tends to crave foods that replenish sugar quickly, such as sweet foods or alcohol. Clinical experience, as well as some scientific research, suggests that many individuals can successfully reduce their alcohol consumption by eating a wholesome diet, which balances their blood sugar (*see p.42*).

INCREASING THE INTAKE OF NUTRIENTS Research demonstrates that alcoholics very often lack key nutrients, especially the B vitamins, zinc and magnesium. Studies on alcoholics have shown that when they supplement their diet with nutrients they can reduce alcohol consumption.

Increasing the intake of nutrients through eating a balanced diet is also associated with both reduced alcohol craving and increased abstinence from alcohol. Individuals who want to stop drinking alcohol or reduce their alcohol consumption might do well to take a good-quality

> Government figures suggest that nearly 10 per cent of the population are alcohol dependent

multivitamin and mineral, combined with a B-complex supplement which provides 25–50mg of vitamins B1, B2, B3, B5 and B6 each day.

ESSENTIAL FATTY ACIDS People who are dependent on alcohol may also be deficient in essential fatty acids (EFAs). One of the final breakdown products of these EFAs when they are metabolised in the body is a hormone-like molecule, known as prostaglandin E1 (PGE1). This is thought to have mood-enhancing and antidepressant actions in the brain. Alcoholics are often deficient in both PGE1 and gamma-linolenic acid (GLA), the molecule from which it is made.

Studies suggest that supplementing the diet with EFAs can help to reduce alcohol intake and prevent symptoms of withdrawal. Taking 1g of evening primrose oil, which is rich in GLA, three times a day might help to control drinking alcohol in the long term.

GLUTAMINE The amino acid glutamine appears to help reduce alcohol cravings. In a 1957 study, 9 out of 10 alcoholics thought that glutamine, taken at a dose of 1g per day, reduced their desire for alcohol.

> **CAUTION**
>
> Consult your doctor before taking omega-3 fatty acids/fish oils with warfarin (*see p.46*).

Homeopathy

Case series reports show that individualised homeopathic treatment may be helpful for alcoholism, reducing craving and the frequency of relapses. The most commonly used medicines are *Nux vomica, Sulphur* and *Staphysagria*. If you are trying to give up smoking, alcohol or drugs, visiting a homeopath for a constitutional assessment may help (*see p.73*).

NUX VOMICA In the treatment of hangover and alcohol withdrawal symptoms, the most commonly used medicine is *Nux vomica*. It is helpful for symptoms including nausea, retching, headaches, muscular twitching and cramps. Symptoms are usually associated with irritability, poor sleep and early waking.

ACUPRESSURE FOR SMOKING CESSATION

Researchers from the Touch Research Institute at the University of Miami in the US have demonstrated that massaging particular areas of the hand can help to relieve stress and anxiety in smokers who crave the nicotine in tobacco. Benefits include reductions in both the intensity and frequency of the nicotine craving. Regular practice of the acupressure sequence shown here is soothing and may help smokers who are trying to give up. Try the sequence at the first sign of a craving.

1. Place one thumb and forefinger at the junction of the other thumb and forefinger. Squeeze thumb and forefinger together for 30 seconds. Change hands and repeat.

2. Hold one hand in the other hand, with the thumb on top. Press down with the thumb and rotate it around the palm for 30 seconds. Change hands and repeat.

3. Use the thumb and fingers of one hand to massage, from base to tip, each of the fingers of the other hand (above). Massage each joint thoroughly. Change hands and repeat.

4. With the palm of one hand massage the fingers of the other hand by pushing them up and stretching them back. Do this five times. Change hands and repeat.

SULPHUR is usually prescribed on a constitutional basis (*see p.73*). It is said that *Sulphur* may help the tendency to substance dependency. Individuals who respond to *Sulphur* are typically warm and do not feel the cold. They are untidy sometimes to the point of being scruffy or smelly, argumentative or garrulous, and thirsty. They often have skin problems that may be very itchy.

STAPHYSAGRIA is another useful medicine. The main feature of patients who respond to this medicine is that they are angry and indignant about what they see as injustices done to them in the past.

PREVENTION Constitutional treatment, particularly with *Sulphur*, may help those people who are inclined towards substance dependency resist the temptation.

Massage

Massage induces calm, eases anxiety and generally reduces feelings of stress. There is a great deal of reporting of how massage and other "anti-arousal" methods help people to break their dependency on a substance. However, the research evidence to support this is limited.

People who stop smoking can experience marked withdrawal symptoms, including intense cravings, anxiety and depressed mood. Anecdotally, massage has been shown to reduce this anxiety and to improve mood.

A simple self-massage of the hand (*see illustration, left*) during the period of cravings may reduce anxiety and withdrawal symptoms and may result in smoking far fewer cigarettes per day.

Breathing Retraining and Yoga

Learning to breathe slowly (taking 10 breaths per minute) and rhythmically can ease the feelings of anxiety that relate to dependency on substances, such as alcohol. Anti-anxiety exercises involving yoga-type breathing induce calm and reduce feelings of apprehension, anxiety and panic (*see p.62*). A 2002 survey by The Yoga Biomedical Trust in the UK showed that yoga therapy can benefit people who are addicted to tobacco and alcohol.

Acupuncture

Acupuncture can help people who seek to break their dependency on a drug, alcohol or nicotine. The Gateway Clinic in the UK, for example, has developed a successful detoxification programme for substance dependency that includes acupuncture treatment. Many studies also suggest that ear acupuncture can prove useful, although a review of the scientific research concluded that it is too early to make definitive recommendations.

Curiously, it does not seem to matter whether the acupuncturist uses specifically selected acupoints or randomly chosen points (the so-called "sham acupuncture") – the benefits appear to be the same.

Acupuncture, whether real or sham, has often been shown, particularly in smoking trials, to help roughly the same percentage of people as other approaches, such as hypnosis and chewing nicotine-containing gum. At least one study indicates that a traditional Chinese acupuncture approach appears to work very well in controlling alcoholics who have relapses.

Acupuncture treatment for substance dependency may need to be provided very frequently – for instance, in one study on alcohol abuse treatment was provided every other day for two months. However, this can be expensive and time-consuming so people should consider carefully before they make a commitment.

Mind–Body Therapies

STRESS Substance dependencies cover a wide array of disorders, ranging from tobacco and smoking to cocaine abuse and alcoholism. It appears that people who have difficulty dealing with stress are more prone to drug and alcohol dependency and more likely to relapse (*see also Excess stress, p.408*).

Most major theories of substance dependency postulate that stress has an important role in increasing drug use and relapse. Many animal studies and some human laboratory studies (where people come into a structured setting) have shown that exposure to stress increases the likelihood of continuing dependency.

Human research into the relationship between stress and substance dependency is largely correlational (not causal), often anecdotal and, at times, contradictory. However, evidence is growing that stress, in addition to the drug itself, plays a key role in perpetuating drug abuse and relapse. The psychological and/or biochemical mechanisms underlying this association remain unclear.

TREATMENTS Mind–body therapies that can reduce stress are evidently useful in treating substance dependencies. A few but important research studies indicate that mind–body techniques and self-care practices, such as transcendental meditation (TM) and clinical biofeedback, are useful complementary additions to the Alcoholics Anonymous (AA) treatment.

It is well worth trying meditation (*see p.98 for a sequence*) or taking up yoga, as they may be able to help with detoxification, treatment and relapse prevention.

Psychological Therapies

PRIMARY TREATMENT Talking therapies account for much of the treatment for substance misuse. The model adopted depends on which of the two main ways in which the practitioner understands the substance misuse: the disease model and the learned behaviour model.

DISEASE MODEL This is probably the most commonly held model. Substance misuse is viewed as a disease that, once developed, cannot be "cured" (i.e. "once an alcoholic or addict always an alcoholic or addict"). The focus is on how to cope with the disease and how to manage life while "in recovery". The goal is total abstinence. The main proponent of this view is known as the 12-step, or Minnesota, model and is practised by the collective "anonymous" groups, such as Alcoholics Anonymous.

Much of the research on treatments using the Minnesota model has been criticised for poor methods. However, some more robust studies support it, with about a third of clients maintaining abstinence after one year. More research is needed.

LEARNED BEHAVIOUR MODEL The other main model views substance misuse as a learned behaviour that can be unlearned. While it recognises that the substance can have addictive properties, the main focus is on practising different ways of behaving and thinking, i.e. cognitive behavioural therapy (CBT) and a return to "controlled use" is considered a relevant goal alongside abstinence. The main theory – the Cycle of Change – focuses on the cyclical nature of dependence (be it on a substance, such as alcohol, or a behaviour, such as eating, gambling or sex). At first, the person is unaware of the potential problems of their behaviour (Pre-contemplative), followed by a period of thinking about their dependency (Contemplation); then they may decide to act to change (Action). They may maintain this change, but more often they return to their original pattern (Relapse) and start the cycle again.

The cycle may be repeated several times before the person moves into a dependency-free life. At each stage of the cycle, different interventions may be used, including motivational interviewing, CBT and relapse prevention.

WHAT ARE THE SYMPTOMS?

- Feelings of sadness and apathy
- Fatigue and lethargy
- Sleep problems, often oversleeping but also disturbed sleep and early waking
- Overeating, with a craving for sweet foods and carbohydrates, leading to weight gain
- Loss of self-esteem
- Tension and irritability
- Decreased sex drive

WHY MIGHT I HAVE THIS?

TRIGGER

- Lack of sunlight

TREATMENT PLAN

PRIMARY TREATMENTS

- Bright light therapy
- Antidepressants

BACK-UP TREATMENTS

- Vitamin D and other nutritional measures

WORTH CONSIDERING

- Homeopathy
- Exercise
- Psychological therapies

For an explanation of how treatments are rated, see p.111.

SEASONAL AFFECTIVE DISORDER

In seasonal affective disorder (SAD), episodes of depression occur in the autumn and winter months. This is thought to be because of reduced daylight. While many people experience SAD as a mild "blue" feeling, others have disabling symptoms. Treatment aims to lift the mood and to relieve the depression. Light therapy is the main treatment for SAD and has good results, but exercise, vitamin D, homeopathy and psychological therapies may also help.

WHY DOES IT OCCUR?

Many functions of the body, such as body temperature and the secretion of hormones into the bloodstream, follow an approximately 24-hour cycle, known as a circadian rhythm. The organs, tissues and cells of the body seem to respond to the slow environmental cycle of day and night. This response is co-ordinated by a biological clock in part of the brain called the hypothalamus, which links the nervous system and the endocrine system of hormones. Like the conductor of an orchestra, the hypothalamus, together with the pituitary gland to which it is connected, synchronises the physiology and biochemistry of the body.

There are two general categories of SAD: one that starts in the winter and the other that starts in the summer. The second is much rarer than the first, but both have similar symptoms.

MELATONIN is thought to be a key hormone in the development of SAD because of its importance in the regulation of sleep (*see p.448*). The pineal gland in the brain produces melatonin mostly at night when there is no daylight and the body is asleep. The blood level of melatonin reaches its peak in the middle of the night but melatonin is almost undetectable in the day.

When the melatonin cycle and the sleep cycle are out of synchrony, an imbalance in the hypothalamus may result and the depression associated with SAD may develop. This asynchrony and imbalance is thought to be due to fewer hours of daylight and a lack of sunlight in the autumn and winter months. When longer days return in spring, some people with SAD experience a short-lived period of high levels of activity. For others, the symptoms of SAD disappear gradually with the spring.

SELF-HELP

The following may help you to cope with the symptoms of SAD:

- Buy a light box for use at home. Make sure you follow the manufacturer's instructions and work with your doctor to derive the most benefit.
- Try to establish whether you are more of a "lark" (more active in the morning) or an "owl" (more active in the evening). Owl types begin to produce melatonin later than lark types. Synchronising the time when you use the light box with the timing of your melatonin cycle can be beneficial.
- Take regular exercise, preferably outside in natural daylight.

TREATMENTS IN DETAIL

Conventional Medicine

Your doctor will ask you carefully about the history of your symptoms to exclude any other psychological causes or an underlying physical cause. Investigations may also be arranged to help the doctor with the diagnosis.

PRIMARY TREATMENT **BRIGHT LIGHT THERAPY** There is fairly good evidence to support treating SAD with a course of bright light therapy (phototherapy) given

People with seasonal affective disorder can be treated by exposure to a bright light. Each day, they sit in front of a bright screen for a period of time to compensate for lack of sunlight in winter months.

on a daily basis, usually early in the morning. The individual is exposed to fluorescent light from a light box with a similar spectrum to daylight. It is thought that the light needs to be at least 2,500 lux (a measurement of light intensity). Each treatment usually lasts for between 30 and 60 minutes. Light therapy may be helpful in treating both mild and severe SAD.

PRIMARY TREATMENT **ANTIDEPRESSANTS** Selective serotonin re-uptake inhibitors (SSRIs), such as fluoxetine, may also help to relieve the depressive symptoms.

> **CAUTION**
>
> SSRIs may have side-effects: ask your doctor to explain these to you.

Nutritional Therapy

Depression is the primary symptom of SAD, and may be helped by various approaches (*see Depression, p.436*). There is evidence that some people with SAD have low thyroid function, so taking steps to maintain thyroid health may prove useful (*for more information, see p.310*).

Overeating, craving sweet foods and weight gain are also characteristic of SAD and regulating blood-sugar levels may help to control these (*see p.42*).

VITAMIN D supplements may be useful to improve mood in people with SAD. It has been suggested that the seasonal symptoms of SAD may be due to changing levels of vitamin D3, a nutrient made by the action of sunlight on the skin, and that this can improve mood through the brain chemical serotonin. In one study, subjects were given 400IU, 800IU or no vitamin D3 for five days during late winter. Results showed that the vitamin significantly enhanced positive mood. In another study, 30 days of treatment with vitamin D completely resolved depression in a group of people with SAD, whereas light treatment did not. If you have SAD, taking 400–800IU vitamin D3 daily may help.

> **CAUTION**
>
> Consult your doctor before taking vitamin D with verapamil (*see p.46*).

Homeopathy

AURUM METALLICUM Although there is no published research, some homeopaths report good results in the treatment of SAD. The medicine most often recommended is *Aur. met.* People who respond to this medicine may be seriously depressed, even to the extent of brooding about death or suicide. Although

depressed, they may fly into a rage because of a minor annoyance or from being contradicted. As well as SAD, they may also have palpitations and sinusitis.

Exercise

It is well known that exercise can usually improve mild to moderate depressive symptoms, so a study was performed to evaluate the relative benefits of combining exercise and bright light on the mood of people affected by seasonal changes in light availability. Ninety-eight people completed an eight-week study in which it was found that both exercise and bright light effectively relieved depressive symptoms. However, bright light seemed to be more effective, suggesting that SAD is not quite the same as mild clinical depression.

Psychological Therapies

While the main method of treating SAD is by using light, or phototherapy, and medication, promising research suggests that including talking therapies in the treatment plan can be beneficial. For example, interpersonal therapy has helped patients cope with the associated relationship difficulties, such as feelings of isolation or alienation, of SAD. Cognitive therapy has also been used with promising results.

There are also potentially promising results for a combination of talking therapies and medication for people who do not respond to light therapy.

A family member who is depressed can have a profound effect on the rest of the family and systemic therapy as a means of support is recommended. In this form of psychological therapy, a practitioner helps the group to cope better with the depressed person.

> **PREVENTION PLAN**
>
> **The following may help you to avoid succumbing to SAD:**
>
> - Use a light box at home, with advice from your doctor.
> - Take plenty of exercise, preferably outside in natural daylight and when the sun is shining.

COPING WITH BEREAVEMENT

Adjusting to the death of a loved one, close relative or friend takes time. The grieving process usually has several stages, the length of which varies between individuals. However, at any one time an individual may experience a mix of emotions. Throughout the grieving process, people may vacillate between focusing on their loss and distracting themselves with work or making plans for the future. Help is available in the form of support, counselling, breathing retraining and homeopathy.

WHAT ARE THE SYMPTOMS?

- Shock
- Feeling numb and detached
- Anxiety symptoms, such as inability to sleep and loss of appetite
- Sadness, and possibly anger, guilt or fear

TREATMENT PLAN

PRIMARY TREATMENTS

- Self-help measures (see right)
- Support and counselling

WORTH CONSIDERING

- Breathing retraining
- Homeopathy

For an explanation of how treatments are rated, see p.111.

WHY DOES IT OCCUR?

The initial reaction to bereavement is usually one of shock and of feeling numb and detached. This reaction is normal and shields the bereaved person from the immediate impact of the loss. The effects of grief (see p.435) are common at this stage, and they may include the inability to sleep and loss of appetite.

INTENSE EMOTIONS Following the initial shock, a person may be overcome by intense emotions, including sadness but also anger, guilt and fear. Thinking constantly about the loss is normal. As the mind adjusts to the idea of loss and accepts the reality of it, a bereaved person may feel bleak, apathetic and confused and have no hope for the future. In extreme cases a bereaved person may feel suicidal.

ACCEPTANCE As time passes, the bereaved person comes to accept the loss and achieves a new normality. The bereavement process eventually results in being able to remember happy times and hope to be happy again without forgetting the person they loved. These feelings are part of the normal grieving process. However, if very intense emotions last for a long time; if a person does not stop grieving, even after several years; or if a person cannot grieve at all, this process has been interrupted and special advice is needed.

IMPACT ON HEALTH The sense of loss that a person experiences in bereavement can provoke strong physical and emotional reactions, which may have serious effects

on health. Bereaved spouses, especially men, are at increased risk of dying from either disease or suicide in the year following their bereavement. In addition, bereavement increases a person's risk of developing depression (see p.436).

SELF-HELP

PRIMARY TREATMENT Everyone grieves differently – there is no "normal" way – but the following may help:

- Talk to family and friends – even if it is painful – don't bottle up feelings.
- Keep up regular routines and avoid making sudden changes in your life.
- Try to get plenty of sleep and take regular exercise.
- Accept that uncomfortable emotions, such as anger and bitterness, are normal and will pass in time.
- However tempting, don't drown your feelings in alcohol or drugs.
- Keep a diary or write poetry – some find pouring out their grief on paper is helpful, while others find comfort in putting together a photo album of the person.
- Give yourself plenty of time: it can take months or years to fully accept the death of someone close.

IMPORTANT

You should consult your doctor if you feel you need help or advice coming to terms with a bereavement, and particularly if you develop overwhelming feelings of helplessness or depression or if you feel suicidal.

- For some, homeopathic *Ignatia* may relieve symptoms (*see below*).
- Join a self-help group for support.
- Read about other people's experience of grief and bereavement, and join in discussions on the Internet if you like.

Conventional Medicine

People often go to see their doctor after the death of a loved one. Doctors may have long-standing relationships with the family and can provide important emotional support and spend time talking to family members. The doctor may also recommend bereavement counselling to help individuals come to terms with their loss. Emotional support and understanding are also available through organisations for those who have been bereaved. It is possible to attend a group session or have counselling on a one-to-one basis.

Breathing Retraining

Research has shown that approximately one-third of people who experience acute episodes of hyperventilation can trigger a repeat episode by recalling a bereavement. The emotion caused by bereavement or loss, when unexpressed because of the inability to grieve openly, may be a major trigger for hyperventilation.

If you find that your grief is causing your breathing to be disturbed, breathing retraining (*see p.62*) can help. However, underlying psychological issues also need to be dealt with. Learning to breathe correctly only deals with the hyperventilation, not with the feeling of grief itself.

Homeopathy

IGNATIA is the most frequently indicated medicine for immediate reactions to bereavement. People who respond to *Ignatia* may feel numb and unreal, emotionally hypersensitive, with occasional paradoxical reactions, such as inappropriate or hysterical laughter. They may experience a lump in the throat and muscular twitching.

NATRUM MURIATICUM is the classical medicine for long-standing, unresolved reactions to grief. Typically, those helped

---

STAGES OF GRIEF

Not everyone will pass through each grief stage, and not necessarily in the order below. A grieving person may cycle between stages, appearing to progress, then move back to an earlier stage. Some psychologists see grieving as a series of tasks that have to be accomplished before the bereaved can reach acceptance and recovery.

STAGE	BEHAVIOUR	POSSIBLE DURATION
Shock	Usually the first response. May include numbness, pain or apathy.	Usually lasts no more than 2 weeks.
Denial	Refusal to acknowledge the death ("It can't be true").	Usually an early feature. Duration varies.
Disorganisation	Inability to do the simplest thing. May feel restless, aimless, helpless and lonely.	
Anger/Guilt	Includes self-blame, irritability or anger towards God, fate, doctors or the deceased.	Begins almost at once. Peaks 2–4 weeks.
Bargaining	Acknowledges the loss, but tries to bargain ("If only I could…" or "If only I had…").	
Mourning/ Depression	As denial breaks down, grief, mourning and depression set in. A painful and lonely stage.	Can recur at any time, but becomes less frequent and intense.
Anxiety	Worry about control of feelings or of going mad. Apprehension about the future.	
Restitution	Attending rituals, such as the funeral, and accepting the reality of the loss.	
Resolution	Gradual acceptance of the death and that life goes on.	
Re-integration	Forging new relationships and goals. The deceased has a special place in the memory.	Can take many months or years.

---

by *Nat. mur.* could not express grief at the time – for instance, they may not have cried at the funeral. They may be cast in the role of coper, the person who "keeps their head, when all around are losing theirs". They may put on a brave face, coping and caring for others, but privately feel desperately depressed.

CAUSTICUM is often appropriate for carers who have looked after a relative or friend with great dedication for a long period. Anger, particularly about injustice, may be a strong feature.

CAUTION

Some homeopathic medicines, including *Ignatia*, are made ineffective by coffee.

Psychological Therapy

PRIMARY TREATMENT **COUNSELLING** Talking to someone outside the immediate family can help the bereaved person to express their feelings, cope with the reaction of others and adjust to life without the person who has died.

DEPRESSION

Depression is a state of mind in which persistent feelings of sadness are accompanied by a loss of interest in life and a lack of energy. Repetitive, worrying thoughts and a constant sense of foreboding may also be present. It affects about 1 in 10 people in the UK and is one of the most common mental health disorders. Women are twice as likely as men to be diagnosed with depression. A range of treatments may be called upon – from counselling, medication and supplements to aerobic exercise, homeopathy, herbs and psychological therapies.

WHAT ARE THE SYMPTOMS?

In depression, feelings of sadness are often worse in the morning and persist to some degree for the rest of the day. Other symptoms include:

- Loss of interest and enjoyment in work or leisure activities
- Difficulty concentrating
- Low self-esteem
- Feeling guilty
- Tearfulness
- Difficulty with decision-making
- Early waking, or excessive sleeping
- Reduced sex drive
- Physical symptoms, such as a low energy levels, decreased appetite and constipation
- Symptoms of anxiety and panic attacks are common

WHY MIGHT I HAVE THIS?

PREDISPOSING FACTORS

- Genetic factors
- Stress or violence at home or work
- Isolation

TRIGGERS

- Stressful life events
- Loss of a family member or friend
- Following childbirth
- Seasonal affective disorder
- Food sensitivity
- Blood-sugar imbalance

IMPORTANT

You should consult your doctor if you develop overwhelming feelings of helplessness or depression or if you feel suicidal.

WHY DOES IT OCCUR?

Depression may occur in response to a particular stressful event or situation. The trigger for depression is often a loss of some kind, whether through break-up of an important relationship or a bereavement (*see p.434*). Other factors include family traits, stress, chronic pain, disease or having a disability. However, often there is no apparent cause.

Some factors may cause an increased susceptibility to depression. These include a traumatic experience in childhood, such as the death of a parent, and having a close relative with a history of depression. Hormonal changes in women that occur after childbirth (*see p.362*) may also be associated with depression.

How depression develops is not yet fully understood, but low levels of neurotransmitters (chemicals released from nerve endings that transmit impulses to another nerve) in the brain, such as serotonin and noradrenaline, and hormones are thought to play a role.

TREATMENT PLAN

PRIMARY TREATMENTS

- Lifestyle measures (*see Self-Help*)
- Support
- Antidepressant drugs
- St John's wort

BACK-UP TREATMENTS

- Nutritional therapy
- Exercise
- Acupuncture
- Homeopathy
- Western herbal medicine
- Mind–body therapies
- Psychological therapies

WORTH CONSIDERING

- Environmental health measures
- Massage

For an explanation of how treatments are rated, see p.111.

SELF-HELP

PRIMARY TREATMENT If you are recovering from depression, the following measures may help you:

- List the tasks you have to do each day, with the most important at the top.
- Complete these tasks one at a time and think about what you have achieved.
- Practise relaxation every day (*see p.99*).
- Take regular exercise to relieve stress.
- Eat a nutritious diet (*see p.44*).
- Get involved in an activity (sport, pastime, hobby, etc.) to stop yourself from thinking too much about your worries.
- Join a support group so you can share your thoughts and experiences with like-minded people.

TREATMENTS IN DETAIL

Conventional Medicine

Your doctor may arrange for blood tests to rule out physical illnesses that could be affecting your mood and energy. Your doc-

SELECTIVE SEROTONIN RE-UPTAKE INHIBITION

Depression is thought to be associated with a low level of the chemical serotonin in parts of the brain. Serotonin is normally produced by the brain and helps to control mood. When serotonin is reabsorbed, in a process known as re-uptake, by the nerve endings that produce it, the level of stimulation falls. Specific drugs that selectively inhibit this re-uptake can help to reduce the likelihood of depression.

How SSRIs work

BEFORE THE DRUG

When a nerve impulse reaches the nerve ending, serotonin is released. It crosses the synaptic space, stimulates the next nerve cell and is then reabsorbed.

AFTER THE DRUG

An SSRI drug can block the re-uptake of serotonin by occupying the exact places on the nerve ending where the molecules of serotonin would be reabsorbed.

electrical current briefly between two electrodes applied to either side of the head. Another technique, transcranial magnetic stimulation, is an alternative to ECT.

> **CAUTION**
>
> ECT and drugs used to treat depression can cause side-effects: ask your doctor to explain these to you. Conventional antidepressants should not be taken at the same time as herbal ones, such as St John's wort.

Nutritional Therapy

While depression is predominantly a psychological problem, it can also have biochemical triggers. Problems include low thyroid function (*see p.319*), anaemia and/or iron deficiency, SAD (*see p.432*), food sensitivity (*see p.39*) and blood-sugar imbalance (*see p.42*).

FOOD ELIMINATION DIET This can be worth trying if you have reasons to suspect that foods are triggering your depression (*see p.39*). Certain foodstuffs, such as sugar, caffeine, alcohol and artificial sweeteners, may upset brain chemistry. Removing these from the diet may lead to a significant improvement in mood.

OMEGA-3 FATTY ACIDS Evidence is starting to accumulate that links depression with abnormalities in fatty acid metabolism and deficiencies in dietary fatty acid intake. The omega-3 essential fatty acids, such as EPA and DHA (*see p.34*), found in oily fish, such as salmon and mackerel, seem to be most important in this respect.

Countries where people eat plenty of oily fish, such as Japan and China, have substantially lower rates of depression, and, in general, people who eat fish regularly are less likely to report feeling depressed. In addition, low levels of omega-3 fatty acids are often found in the blood of depressed individuals.

Supplementing the diet with omega-3 fatty acids, especially EPA, is often useful in treating depression. A dose of 1g of EPA (found in about 3g of concentrated fish oil) each day may be helpful.

THIAMINE (VITAMIN B1) deficiency can cause depression. Thiamine supplements

tor may suggest one or a combination of treatments. A reduction in alcohol intake should be advised, as alcohol can aggravate depression. Exercise may be recommended as it can improve general well-being.

PRIMARY TREATMENT **SUPPORT** Psychotherapy may be suggested; for example, cognitive therapy (*see Mind–body Therapies, p.440*) has been shown to be beneficial. Emotional support from family and friends is very important; support groups may also be beneficial. In addition, help may be needed to cope practically with specific problems, such as unemployment and financial difficulties.

PRIMARY TREATMENT **ORAL DRUGS** Your doctor may prescribe drugs; the exact drug selected depends on the symptoms and the possible side-effects. Symptoms may start to improve after about two weeks. In some cases, the drug may need to be changed if it is not effective (sometimes, more than one drug needs to be tried) or if it causes unacceptable side-effects.

Your doctor may prescribe one or more drugs from these antidepressant groups:

- Selective serotonin re-uptake inhibitors (SSRIs), such as fluoxetine and paroxetine, affect serotonin (*see box, above*).
- Tricyclic antidepressants, such as amitriptyline and dothiepin, are commonly prescribed. They interfere with the reabsorption of serotonin and noradrenaline so that high levels of these neurotransmitters remain in the body.
- Monoamine oxidase (MAO) inhibitors, such as phenelzine, may be used when other drugs fail to work. They block the action of an enzyme that makes serotonin and noradrenaline inactive.

There are various newer drugs, including reboxetine, which may help when energy levels are low, and mirtazapine, which can be used to help sleep.

ELECTROCONVULSIVE TREATMENT (ECT) is occasionally recommended for very severe depression when other treatments fail. A course of ECT is carried out under a general anaesthetic and involves passing an

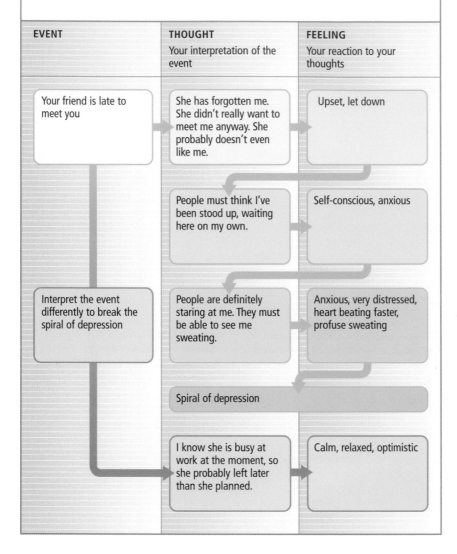

SPIRAL OF DEPRESSION

One of the features of depression is the spiral of negative thoughts and feelings that is triggered by a seemingly innocuous event. Thoughts and feelings feed off each other until the spiral goes out of control. A way of preventing this is to interpret the event differently as soon as possible and to think positively about it.

EVENT	THOUGHT Your interpretation of the event	FEELING Your reaction to your thoughts
Your friend is late to meet you	She has forgotten me. She didn't really want to meet me anyway. She probably doesn't even like me.	Upset, let down
	People must think I've been stood up, waiting here on my own.	Self-conscious, anxious
Interpret the event differently to break the spiral of depression	People are definitely staring at me. They must be able to see me sweating.	Anxious, very distressed, heart beating faster, profuse sweating
	Spiral of depression	
	I know she is busy at work at the moment, so she probably left later than she planned.	Calm, relaxed, optimistic

CAUTION

Consult your doctor before taking omega-3 fatty acids or fish oils with warfarin, or folate (folic acid) with anticonvulsant drugs or methotrexate (*see p.46*).

Homeopathy

Depression is a common problem and much can be done to help. Talking through feelings is beneficial: a problem shared is a problem halved. Do not suffer alone, as the nature of the disease is to make you feel worthless and stops you making the effort to seek help.

Case series suggest that depression responds to homeopathic treatment, but it is a very variable condition, and many different homeopathic medicines are potentially appropriate. Unless you have a good knowledge of homeopathy, you will probably need to consult a practitioner.

Among the more commonly suggested homeopathic medicines are *Natrum muriaticum*, *Sepia*, *Lachesis*, *Pulsatilla* and *Aurum metallicum*.

NATRUM MURIATICUM is often the medicine for "copers" – people who seem in control, kind and caring to others, yet hiding the black mood they feel inside. Their problems are often triggered by relationship problems. Sometimes, they have the unfortunate habit of falling in love with unsuitable people for the wrong reasons, such as misplaced pity. They are good listeners but have difficulty expressing their own feelings and may get annoyed if others pry or try to help.

SEPIA People who respond to *Sepia* are similar in this respect – they resent fuss and sympathy. But in other respects, *Sepia* is different. For instance, *Nat. mur.* people empathise (perhaps too much) with others, but *Sepia* people are emotionally flat – they cannot be bothered with others, even their close family.

A very important feature of *Sepia* is the temporary improvement brought on by vigorous activity: working out or dancing lifts the mood. In women, there is a loss of sex drive; in men, there may be sexual promiscuity. In women, the depression may be triggered by having a baby.

may be helpful even when deficiency does not exist. A double-blind trial in female college students who were not deficient in thiamine found their mood benefited from taking 50mg a day for two months. Taking a dose of 25mg of thiamine a day would be safe in the long term.

FOLATE (FOLIC ACID) is another vitamin that seems to be involved in depression. Studies reveal that up to a third of people with depression have low folate levels. Supplementing the diet with 500mcg per day of folate may help to relieve depression.

SELENIUM A deficiency of selenium is associated with a significantly greater incidence of depression and other negative mood states. Selenium supplementation seems to have a beneficial impact on mood, especially in people who are only slightly deficient in the mineral (as is the case in the UK, where many people are borderline deficient). Eating plenty of foods rich in selenium, such as shellfish, eggs and mushrooms, or taking selenium supplements appears to improve mood. If you have depression, try taking 100mcg of selenium per day.

LACHESIS If depression is associated with the menopause, a woman may respond to *Lachesis*. There is often severe hot flushing and the depression may be accompanied by jealousy or excessive suspiciousness. People who respond to this medicine are often talkative, and for some reason hate tight clothes, especially collars.

PULSATILLA Depression that responds to *Pulsatilla* is often characterised by great weepiness, dithering and indecision. The people who are helped by the medicine may feel temporarily much better for company and talking about their problems (unlike *Nat. mur.* and *Sepia* patients).

AURUM METALLICUM may be useful for people with really serious depression who have suicidal thoughts. In people whom it helps, depression is often seasonal, worse in winter and at night. It may be accompanied by painful sinusitis.

Western Herbal Medicine

PRIMARY
TREATMENT **ST JOHN'S WORT** (*Hypericum perforatum*) Though a range of herbal remedies exists for the treatment of mild to moderate depression, attention inevitably focuses on St John's wort, which over the last 10 years or so has become the key herbal remedy for what is an increasingly common condition.

Since 1996, when the *British Medical Journal* published a ground-breaking analysis, endorsing the herb's use in depression, St John's wort has become first choice treatment for non-severe depression. With about 30 clinical trials showing positive results in lifting depression, and a remarkably low incidence of side-effects, St John's wort is a safe and effective treatment for depressive illness.

Unusually, St John's wort is safe for self-treatment, though depression is frequently a condition that requires professional help. St John's wort can be taken as an infusion or extract and generally needs to be taken for at least 10 days before its antidepressant activity takes effect.

It has been used for depressive states since the time of the ancient Greeks, but herbal practitioners also see St John's wort as a herb of choice in conditions in which the nervous system is under stress, such as shingles (*see p.165*), sciatica (*see p.272*) and

nervous exhaustion. It combines well with valerian (*Valeriana officinalis*) in depression to promote sleep and relaxation; and with black cohosh (*Cimicifuga racemosa*) in depression linked to the menopause.

OTHER HERBAL MEDICINES that can prove valuable in depression include: lemon balm (*Melissa officinalis*), which is a gentle sedative with a positive, uplifting effect; liquorice (*Glycyrrhiza glabra*), which is a tonic and restorative that supports liver and adrenal gland function; ginkgo (*Ginkgo biloba*), which stimulates the circulation, protects the nerves and has some antidepressant activity; and schisandra (*Schisandra chinensis*), which is a nerve tonic that improves memory and mental performance.

Herbal practitioners will combine these with other herbs that strengthen liver function and elimination, support circulation, particularly to the central nervous system, and stimulate adrenal gland activity.

> CAUTION
>
> See page 69 before taking a herbal remedy and, if you are already taking prescribed medication, consult a medical herbalist first. Do not take St John's wort with antidepressants, warfarin or antibiotics.

Environmental Health

STRESS The majority of research demonstrates higher rates of depression in individuals unable to cope with stressful situations or who lack strong inner belief about themselves. Factors that can trigger a recurrence of depressive symptoms are many and varied. Environmental factors such as poor housing and pollution can cause stress. For example, research suggests individuals who lived near the Chernobyl power plant in Ukraine, a site of a major nuclear disaster in 1986, experienced depression from chronic stress.

SEASONAL PATTERNS, such as changes in weather, temperature and light, affect the body and mind in numerous ways and may lead to symptoms of depression. They may result in physiological changes that sometimes lead to reduced mental stability and increases in symptoms of depression. Case studies indicate that lack of natural light potentially causes increased anxiety and depression (*see also SAD, p.432*). Evidence also suggests that experiencing sunlight and the beauty of nature can help relieve symptoms in some depressed people.

Depression and suicide are increasing faster among young people than any other age group

WAR Non-military personnel may experience symptoms of depression during times of war. Some researchers claim that the many symptoms, including depression and memory loss, that have been linked with "Gulf War syndrome" may represent injury to the nervous system. Among the possible causes for this injury are exposure to chemical warfare agents, pesticides, extremes of heat and cold, blowing dust, and smoke from oil well fires. This supports other studies that show a possible connection between exposures to certain solvents in the workplace and symptoms of depression.

HOME ENVIRONMENT People who have a low income and/or live in poor housing have demonstrated a higher prevalence of depressive symptoms. Higher rates of depression can also be found in areas of high crime or other community violence. Relocating to another home will not necessarily resolve depressive symptoms, but re-evaluating your surroundings is an important step to improving the symptoms you are experiencing.

Another aspect of the home environment that might be relevant to depression is the amount of television that families watch. For example, as children spend more time watching television, they are less likely to participate in enriching activities with their parents, eroding the parental–child bond; this could lead to depression in the parents.

Massage and Exercise

MASSAGE has been shown in numerous research studies to be a useful treatment in depression. It helps relieve depression in child and adolescent patients, adolescent mothers, people with chronic fatigue and immune deficiency, cancer patients, people with chronic pain and those who are depressed as a result of work-related stress.

AEROBIC EXERCISE has been shown to help alleviate even major depression. It increases self-esteem, improves mood, reduces anxiety, enhances the ability to handle stress, and encourages better sleep, in both adults and children. If you suffer from depression, take up walking, running, or other aerobic exercise, for 20 minutes three times a week.

Research has also shown that other forms of exercise, including martial arts, have the potential to offer similar benefits.

Acupuncture

There is good evidence that acupuncture can have fundamental effects upon the brain's chemical messages. It would therefore be reasonable to suggest that acupuncture may be useful for treating depression. In fact, there are at least three clinical trials indicating that acupuncture is as effective for depression as some conventionally used antidepressants.

Usually, prolonged treatment is needed. Acupuncture treatment should be given on a weekly basis for eight to ten weeks. If it proves to be valuable, then maintenance treatments may be required, depending on how the symptoms respond.

Mind–Body Therapies

PSYCHOTHERAPEUTIC APPROACHES These include cognitive behaviour therapy (*see right*), behavioural therapy (especially mind–body stress-management programmes), psychodynamic approaches (*see right*) and solution-oriented brief therapy.

Many experts believe that combining psychotherapy or behavioural therapy with SSRIs is more effective for depression than either treatment alone – at least in women.

RELAXATION AND GUIDED IMAGERY (*see p.100*) have been shown to improve mood and to decrease depressive symptoms in women who have recently had a baby, those with cancer or who have just had an operation, people with multiple sclerosis, healthy adults and college students. The antidepressant effects of guided imagery and relaxation may result from reduced anxiety and an increased sense of control over life stresses.

A very low-cost programme, based upon mind–body skills, such as relaxation and/or guided imagery, can provide people with powerful self-help tools for overcoming their depression. Those who are able to practise these techniques at home are likely to need fewer medical resources and have increased quality of life, greater longevity and better overall health.

Psychological Therapies

AVOIDING ISOLATION Social isolation can cause or worsen the symptoms of depression. If you are prone to depression, it is vital to spend time with your friends and to participate in some form of community event where the group dynamics can provide excitement and release tension.

TALKING THERAPIES Four of the five talking therapy approaches (*see p.106*) can be of value in treating depression: these are psychodynamic, cognitive behavioural therapy (CBT), humanistic therapy and interpersonal therapy (IPT). A great deal of research has been published on the employment of these approaches. Overall, reviews suggest that therapies from the CBT group tend to be most effective.

THE PSYCHODYNAMIC APPROACH recognises that depressed people have developed a very negative self-image, which usually begins in childhood. They are often highly critical of themselves, engaging in a self-punishment that is expressed as a kind of internal battle. They may "invite" other people to join in with and so confirm their negative self-image.

This process is largely unconscious so that the goal of the therapy is to make the process more conscious: the therapist "declines the invitation" and gains an understanding of the internal conflict via the therapeutic relationship. As a result, new opportunities for emotional assimilation and insight open up for the client. Evidence suggests that this form of therapy is effective in both an individual and a group setting.

THE COGNITIVE BEHAVIOURAL THERAPY APPROACH is not dissimilar to the psychodynamic approach and is based around negative thinking. The therapist's goal is to help the client identify their negative thoughts, often by using a "thought diary" and thinking about alternatives. Other people's behaviour patterns, which often confirm the negative thoughts, are also identified – alternative behaviour is generated and tried out by the client in "homework tasks".

Problem-solving techniques can help clients to manage their lives so that they feel less overwhelmed by the world. A wealth of evidence supports the use of CBT in the treatment of depression, both with individuals and in groups.

THE HUMANISTIC APPROACH aims to provide a supportive and non-judgemental environment in which clients can explore their difficulties and provide a solution for themselves. Research suggests that a humanistic therapy, such as client-centred therapy, helps people who are depressed and that no significant advantage is gained by combining it with medication.

INTERPERSONAL THERAPY tends to focus more on the client's present personal relationships and how they are contributing to the feeling of depression. The goal of the therapy is to review these relationships and explore new potential ways of relating to other people. Interpersonal therapy has been shown to be particularly effective with adolescents.

> People who are depressed dream up to three times more than people who are not depressed

EATING DISORDERS

People with eating disorders use overeating, purging or rigidly restricting their food intake to help them cope with their problems. Those with anorexia deliberately lose weight until they are unhealthily thin, while people with bulimia repeatedly binge on food, after which they may force themselves to vomit or take laxatives. Some people have anorexia and bulimia at the same time. The multidisciplinary approach to treatment, which involves support, psychotherapy, medication and supplements, aims to help them cope better with underlying feelings.

WHAT ARE THE SYMPTOMS?

Anorexia nervosa:
- Refusal to maintain a reasonable body weight
- Obsession with food and food-related activities, such as cooking
- Preoccupation with body weight and shape
- Weight loss – which may be concealed with baggy clothing
- Distorted view of body shape
- Use of appetite suppressants and laxatives
- Rigid routine of excessive exercise
- Dry skin and sparse hair

If anorexia continues for some time, physical symptoms may include:
- Extreme weight loss
- Wasting of the muscles
- Swollen ankles
- Fine body hair on limbs and trunk
- Irregular or absent periods

Bulimia:
- Major fluctuations in body weight
- Eating alone and in secret
- Preoccupation with weight control
- Guilt/self-disgust after binge eating
- Vomiting
- Use of laxatives and other drugs to affect weight loss

If binge eating and purging become established, features may include:
- Abdominal pain and swelling following a binge
- Physical weakness
- Eroded teeth
- Bleeding from oesophagus lining
- Disturbed heart rhythm and impaired kidney function

WHY MIGHT I HAVE THESE?

PREDISPOSING FACTORS
- Low self-esteem
- Perfectionist, high-achieving personality

WHY DO THEY OCCUR?

ANOREXIA NERVOSA usually develops in adolescence and is more common in girls and women than in boys and men. The condition can cause changes in levels of hormones that may affect growth and development during adolescence and may interfere with normal menstruation in girls and women. In severe cases, the weight loss caused by anorexia is extreme and can be life-threatening.

Anorexia is a condition that occurs almost entirely in developed countries and is much more prevalent in the middle and upper classes. The importance placed on having a perfect, slim body in many countries can lead people of normal size to diet without reason, especially if they have low self-esteem. Anorexia often occurs in young people, especially girls, who are under pressure to succeed in a family in which success is overemphasised. The condition is also common in professions in which being slim is highly valued, such as dance, gymnastics and modelling.

OVEREATING Anorexia may alternate with bouts of overeating. People who starve themselves or overeat as a means of coping with the stress of their feelings can end up in a cycle of starvation, secret binge eating, induced vomiting and depression (*see p.436*). The overeating eases the stress, but a short time later feelings of guilt and shame take over, culminating in depression. The cycle is further complicated by worries about weight.

BULIMIA usually develops in early adulthood and is more common in women. Bouts of bulimia are sometimes triggered by stress. The pattern of binge eating followed by purging may become habitual and the cycle may be difficult to break. Unlike anorexia, bulimia does not usually lead to severe weight loss. However, repeated vomiting can have a number of effects, including dehydration and chemical imbalances in the blood, and can also cause the teeth to become eroded.

TREATMENT PLAN

PRIMARY TREATMENTS
- Emotional support
- Psychotherapy and counselling
- Antidepressants (in some cases)
- Hospital therapy (for severe anorexia)

BACK-UP TREATMENTS
- Blood-sugar stabilising diet (bulimia) and other nutritional therapies

WORTH CONSIDERING
- Massage and exercise
- Homeopathy

For an explanation of how treatments are rated, see p.111.

IMPORTANT
As soon as you suspect you have an eating disorder, consult your doctor. If you don't feel able to do this, talk to a sympathetic friend or relative first.

Conventional Medicine

PRIMARY TREATMENT **ANOREXIA NERVOSA** is difficult to treat. Studies suggest that around 40 per cent of anorexics who are treated make a full recovery. However, it can be fatal.

Psychotherapy (*see Psychological Therapies, p.443*) may be recommended to address the disorder itself – for example, in terms of the distorted body image and underlying reasons for its development. As well as dealing with the emotional problems behind the disorder, treatment aims to encourage the person to eat a balanced diet and so return to an acceptable weight.

Hospital admission may be needed if the weight loss is very severe and there are physical symptoms, such as dizziness and extreme weakness. There may also be chemical imbalances and vitamin deficiencies that need treating.

Antidepressant drugs may be prescribed if there are symptoms of depression.

PRIMARY TREATMENT **BULIMIA** Cognitive behavioural therapy and other forms of psychotherapy are likely to be recommended (*see Psychological Therapies, p.443*). Certain antidepressants, such as monoamine oxidase (MAO) inhibitors and fluoxetine, may also be helpful. The prognosis for bulimia tends to be better than for anorexia.

Nutritional Therapy

ANOREXIA NERVOSA Individuals with anorexia often have multiple nutrient deficiencies, a factor that might have a major impact on both psychological and physical health. Taking a high-potency multivitamin and mineral supplement each day may help to prevent or reverse these.

One nutrient that appears to be particularly beneficial for anorexics is zinc, which has many important functions in the body, such as the normalisation of brain function and perception. In a 1990 study, a daily dose of 45–90mg of zinc led to weight gain in 17 out of 20 anorexics after periods ranging between 8 and 56 months. In a 1994 double-blind study, 14mg of zinc per day doubled the speed of weight increase in a group of anorexic women.

A 2002 review of the scientific literature concluded that zinc therapy should be included in the treatment of anorexia because it enhances the rate of recovery by increasing weight gain and reducing levels of anxiety and depression.

Anorexic individuals may benefit from taking 45–90mg of zinc per day. Because zinc can induce copper deficiency, about 3–6mg of copper should be taken with this dose of zinc. Once improvement is seen, the dose of zinc may be reduced, and the anorexic individual should try to eat a nutritious, varied diet.

BULIMIA Blood-sugar imbalance seems to play an important role in bulimia. In a 1984 study, a group of bulimic women were put on a diet designed to maintain stable blood-sugar levels. It excluded all alcohol, caffeine, refined sugar, white flour products, monosodium glutamate and flavour enhancers. All the women in the study stopped bingeing while they were on this regime, and were still binge-free two and a half years later. (*For more information on blood-sugar instability, see p.42.*)

Another factor that may play a part in bulimia is depression, which may be associated with low levels of serotonin. Serotonin, which generally induces feel-good emotions, is made in the brain from an amino acid called tryptophan, which is found in foods, such as meat, tofu, almonds, peanuts, pumpkin seeds, sesame seeds and tahini (sesame seed paste). Tryptophan is absorbed into the brain more efficiently when carbohydrate is present, which might explain why people often gravitate towards sweet or starchy foods when they are upset or stressed.

In a 1989 study, bulimic women were given either 3g of tryptophan or a placebo each day for about a month. Those taking tryptophan were also given 45mg of vitamin B6 per day, as this nutrient is thought to help the conversion of tryptophan into serotonin. Those who took the tryptophan and vitamin B6 found their mood, eating behaviour and feelings about eating improved compared to the bulimic women taking the placebo.

Tryptophan is not available over the counter in many countries, including the UK and the US. However, 5-hydroxytryptophan (5-HTP), which is the substance tryptophan is converted into before it is made into serotonin, is a good alternative. The recommended dose is 50mg of 5-HTP, taken 2 or 3 times a day.

> **CAUTION**
>
> Consult your doctor before taking 5-HTP with zolpidem, venlafaxine, fluvoxamine, fluoxetine, sumatriptan or paroxetine, and before taking zinc with antibiotics (*see p.46*).

ANOREXIA CYCLE

In anorexia, the person becomes trapped in a cycle in which their distorted body image (a mistaken view that they are overweight) is reinforced by changes in their physique due to malnutrition and, possibly, the diet drugs and laxatives that they have been taking. Once established, this anorexia cycle is very difficult to break.

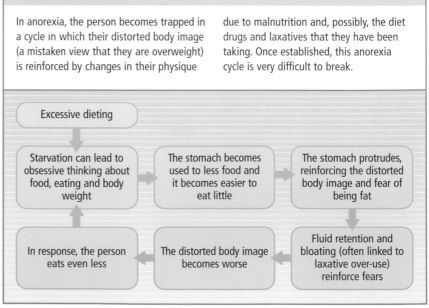

Excessive dieting

Starvation can lead to obsessive thinking about food, eating and body weight

The stomach becomes used to less food and it becomes easier to eat little

The stomach protrudes, reinforcing the distorted body image and fear of being fat

Fluid retention and bloating (often linked to laxative over-use) reinforce fears

The distorted body image becomes worse

In response, the person eats even less

Homeopathy

Individualised homeopathy may be helpful in conjunction with other methods. Generally, eating disorders require skilled treatment from a qualified homeopath. Among the most frequently indicated medicines are *Ignatia*, *Arsenicum album*, *Tarentula*, *Pulsatilla* and *Phosphorus*. These are prescribed according to the individual's constitution and characteristics (*see p.73*).

IGNATIA Conditions that respond to *Ignatia* are often triggered by some kind of emotional shock, such as a bereavement (*see p.434*) or a relationship break-up. The person is emotionally and physically oversensitive. *Ignatia* is said to be a medicine of paradoxes: for instance, there is often a sensation of a lump in the throat, making swallowing difficult, but liquids are more difficult to swallow than solids.

ARSENICUM ALBUM People who respond to *Arsen. alb.* are often excessively perfectionist, making impossible demands on themselves. They tend to be very tidy and organised – great planners who get upset if their plans go awry. They feel the cold excessively and often have dry, flaky skin.

TARENTULA is made from the poison of the spider of the same name. People who respond to it are restless even to the point of being twitchy and making involuntary movements. They love music and dancing, and feel better for them.

PULSATILLA is appropriate for people who are very changeable in their mood and in their symptoms. People who respond to *Pulsatilla* may be extremely faddy eaters and particularly dislike fatty and rich food. Despite having a dry mouth, they are not thirsty. They are weepy, but quickly cheer up after a sympathetic chat.

Women who respond to this medicine often have disturbances of the menstrual cycle, particularly very irregular or variable periods. They often feel worse in the premenstrual period.

PHOSPHORUS may be helpful for bulimics, particularly those whose favourite binge food is ice cream. People who respond to this medicine tend to feel better in the morning and from a short nap. They often

have irrational fears and phobias (*see p.411*), particularly of being alone in the dark and of storms. They may be oversensitive and find they are able to "pick up vibes" from around them.

> **CAUTION**
>
> Some homeopathic medicines, including *Ignatia*, are antidoted by coffee. This means that the medicine is rendered ineffective.

Massage and Exercise

Regular massage is recommended for people who have eating disorders. In various studies, massage has been shown to reduce dissatisfaction with body image in people with either anorexia and bulimia. Massage also reduces associated levels of anxiety and depression.

Research also shows that exercise therapy significantly improves anxiety feelings associated with bulimic behaviour, although it did not produce any change in the bulimic

behaviour itself. People with eating disorders are recommended to take up walking, running, or other forms of aerobic exercise, for 20 minutes three times a week.

Psychological Therapies

PRIMARY TREATMENT **ANOREXIA NERVOSA** People with anorexia often have a distorted view of their body shape – what to most people would be considered thin, they may view as excessively fat. They may respond to various approaches, particularly to the systemic and psychodynamic therapies. Approaches vary: someone with anorexia can have therapy with his or her family, on a one-to-one basis, or in a group with other people who have the disease.

Anorexia is a very serious condition and can be life-threatening, so sufferers may need to be treated in hospital to bring their weight under control. Once weight loss is no longer a danger, treatment outside hos-

pital may begin. Initially, the treatments often consist of medical care and programmes designed to increase weight in the short term, with talking therapies aiming to address the longer-term problems.

A 1991 review examined a variety of treatments for patients with severe anorexia. These consisted of inpatient treatment with an outpatient follow-up and an outpatient group who had psychodynamic individual, family or group therapy. All these forms of treatment were effective, although the members of the solely outpatients group (who were probably less severely anorexic) remained well for a longer time.

A 2000 review of treatments for younger patients (aged 12 to 30) with anorexia concluded that the most effective method of treatment was a family therapy that used a mixture of systemic interventions and education about the risks of anorexia. There has been remarkably little research on the effectiveness of cognitive behavioural therapy (CBT) research for anorexia, although this is being addressed.

About half of all those with anorexia are able to recover and maintain a healthy weight

PRIMARY TREATMENT **BULIMIA** For people with bulimia, the fear of gaining weight is alleviated by self-induced purging, which may be vomiting and/or taking laxatives. The purging normally follows a period of binge eating.

Many studies support the use of CBT in bulimia, either given to individuals or to people in groups. It is effective when combined with psycho-education, which is usually carried out in a group setting and attempts to explain psychological theory in a user-friendly, often experiential, way. For example, participants are invited to have an anxiety-provoking thought and to notice what happens in their body.

Interpersonal therapy also looks promising for eating disorders and has compared favourably with CBT when researched. Psychodynamic therapy has also been shown to be useful. People with binge-eating disorder have also been effectively treated with CBT.

OBESITY

Obesity is the accumulation of excess body fat that raises a person's body mass index (BMI) to over 30 (*see p.445*). Carrying excess weight puts a strain on the body's organs and joints, and increases the risk of potentially fatal disorders. A surfeit of appetising and widely available fatty and sugary foods combined with sedentary lifestyles are making obesity increasingly common in the developed world. Treatment largely involves changing to a healthy diet and taking regular exercise. Drugs, acupuncture, stress-reduction techniques and surgery may also be used.

WHAT ARE THE FEATURES?

- A BMI of over 30 (*see p.445*)
- Accumulation of excess body fat

WHY MIGHT I HAVE THIS?

PREDISPOSING FACTORS

- Overeating
- Sedentary lifestyle
- Diet rich in fats
- Diet rich in sugary foods (high-glycaemic index carbohydrates)
- Genetic factors
- Stress and other psychological factors
- Dietary imbalances
- Rarely, low thyroid function

TREATMENT PLAN

PRIMARY TREATMENTS

- Lifestyle measures (*see Self-Help*)
- Weight-reducing diet (on rare occasions in combination with drugs or surgery)
- Exercise and increased lifestyle activity

BACK-UP TREATMENTS

- Nutritional therapy
- Mind–body therapies

WORTH CONSIDERING

- Acupuncture
- Homeopathy

For an explanation of how treatments are rated, see p.111.

WHY DOES IT OCCUR?

Obesity is defined as having a BMI of 30 or more, but a BMI of between 25 and 30 can also have detrimental effects on health. The risks are greater if fat collects around the abdomen (apple-shaped), as tends to occur in men and post-menopausal women, rather than the hips (pear-shaped).

Obesity occurs when food intake (measured in calories) provides more energy than the body needs. It is usually brought about by overeating and lack of exercise. Lifestyle and psychological factors, such as stress, depression and anxiety, which often lead to "emotional eating" may play a role.

Obesity is only relatively rarely the result of a medical disorder, such as an underactive thyroid gland (*see p.319*). Some drugs, such as oral corticosteroids, can cause an increase in weight. Obesity appears to run in families. Genetic factors and learning bad eating habits are both likely to play a role.

FAT CELLS in white adipose tissue, which normally protects joints and organs, stores the excess energy. At birth, we are born with approximately 5 billion fat cells, or adipocytes, which contain triglycerides, but throughout childhood and adolescence the number increases so that an average adult has 25–30 billion.

Normally, the body establishes an energy equilibrium and a steady body mass index (*see right*). However, when the calorie intake persistently exceeds energy needs, the adipose tissue multiplies, either in the number or size of the fat cells, or both. Fat cells, once formed, are not lost but stay in the body for life. As a result, someone who becomes overweight and then obese may have as many as 200 billion fat cells.

FOETAL PROGRAMMING It seems that babies who do not receive enough nutrients in the first six months in their mother's womb are more likely to become obese later in life. The theory goes that the shortage of nutrients means that the body's organs (brain, heart, kidneys, liver and pancreas) are programmed differently, as if their development and function were primed for a life of scarcity. If they then face a life in which food is plentiful, their appetite malfunctions and they find it hard not to overeat. As a result, mothers who are obese, diabetic or malnourished may be passing on obesity to future generations.

OBESITY EPIDEMIC According to the World Health Organization, obesity is rapidly becoming more common in developed and developing countries. It predicts there will be approximately 300 million cases by 2005. In the UK in 2003, more than half the population were overweight and 1 in 5 English adults were obese – a rise of almost 70 per cent for men and almost 25 per cent for women since 1993. Childhood obesity is also on the increase. In 1998, almost 1 in 10 children between 2 and 4 years old, and in 2001, 16 per cent of 6–15 year olds, were classified as obese. Experts predict that if these trends continue, 1 in 3 adults, 1 in 5 boys and 1 in 3 girls could be obese by 2020.

DETRIMENTAL EFFECTS ON HEALTH Governments' policies need to encourage healthy choices about eating and diet. Obesity is the major public health problem of our age. Obesity contributes to conditions such as osteoarthritis (*see p.289*), because it increases the strain on the knees and hips. It can also increase the risk of developing serious health problems, such as coronary artery disease, stroke and high blood pressure.

Obesity is also a risk factor for type 2 diabetes (*see p.314*) and cancer of the colon. Of particular concern is the increasing incidence of type 2 diabetes, which used to be mainly confined to overweight adults, among children.

SELF-HELP

PRIMARY TREATMENT For sustained and permanent weight loss, focus on making long-term changes to your eating habits.

- Don't try a crash/fad/starvation/liquid diet. They don't work and could damage your health in the long term.
- Aim to lose about 2–3 kg a month.
- Eat a nutritious diet based on whole grains, low-fat dairy products, lean meat and plenty of fruit and vegetables. Concentrate on quality rather than quantity.
- Cut out foods (soft drinks, crisps, sweets and alcohol) that only deliver calories and have no other nutritional value.
- Keep to hand a stock of nuts, fruit, oat cakes and other healthy snacks.
- Eat some protein with every meal and limit your intake of high-glycaemic index foods such as bagels and pasta.
- Hide the frying pan and grill, bake or steam food instead.
- Increase the amount of regular exercise you take. Try using a pedometer to give you feedback on the amount of physical activity you have performed each day. You can set targets, such as 10,000 steps a day, and use them to motivate yourself.
- Diet with a friend or join a slimming club for morale-boosting support.

TREATMENTS IN DETAIL

Conventional Medicine

Your doctor will measure your weight and height to calculate your BMI (*see above*) and will discuss with you your diet and the amount of exercise you take. Your blood may be tested to measure the level of sugar, cholesterol and, rarely, hormones.

PRIMARY TREATMENT **DIET** The mainstay of treatment is a reduction in calorie intake, while ensuring a balanced intake of nutrients, and then a permanent change in

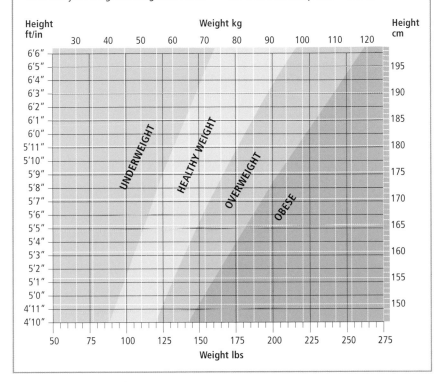

BODY MASS INDEX (BMI)

A BMI of 20 to 25 is healthy, 25 to 30 is overweight and over 30 indicates obesity. To work out yours, multiply your height in metres by itself (e.g. 1.6m x 1.6m = 2.56). Then find your weight in kilograms. Divide your weight by your height squared to give your BMI. For example, a woman who is 1.6m (5 feet 3 inches) tall and weighs 65kg (10 stone) has a BMI of 25 (1.6 x 1.6 = 2.56. 65 divided by 2.56 = 25.39).

eating habits to maintain the weight loss. Your doctor can advise you about healthy eating habits and how to lose weight slowly and steadily. He or she may give you a diet sheet or refer you to a dietician. The balanced diet should be combined with an exercise programme. Psychotherapy may play a role in modifying attitudes to food and eating patterns. Losing a great deal of weight is a long-term venture, and a great deal of support is needed from doctors, dieticians, relatives or slimming clubs.

DRUGS are occasionally considered for obesity, but everyone who takes them must also follow a strict diet. Some have been banned in the UK due to their potential effects on the heart and circulatory system. The two that are available in the UK are sibutramine, which acts on the brain to suppress appetite, and orlistat, which reduces the absorption of fat in the gut. However, weight tends to be regained after the drugs are stopped.

SURGERY should be used only for very severe obesity. There are various options. In gastroplasty, the stomach is stapled to limit the amount of food that can be eaten at one time, although eating small but very frequent meals may put the weight back on. Intestinal bypass surgery effectively short-circuits the digestion but causes chronic diarrhoea. Liposuction is not useful.

CAUTION

Drugs and surgical procedures for obesity have potential side-effects and risks: ask your doctor to explain these to you.

Nutritional Therapy

Obesity is created by consuming more calories than are burned in the body. As a result, the main conventional approaches to it are centred around restricting calorie intake and/or increasing exercise. However, experience suggests that specific imbalances can be very common in cases of overweight and obesity, and identifying and correcting them can be key to successful long-term weight loss. They may include low thyroid function, blood-sugar imbalance, food sensitivity and gut flora imbalance.

FAT, CARBOHYDRATE AND OBESITY Many weight-loss diets restrict the intake of fat because it contains 9 kilocalories per gram, whereas carbohydrate contains 4. However, in 2002, a comprehensive review concluded that dietary fat was not a major factor in weight gain, and that restricting fat alone is unlikely to bring long-term benefits in terms of weight reduction.

HEALTHY FATS The fats to use in a healthy diet designed for weight loss are the essential fatty acids found in extra-virgin olive oil, nuts, seeds, avocados and in oily fish, such as salmon, trout, mackerel, herring and sardines. Although not as harmful as once thought, saturated fats, such as those in red meat and dairy products, are still best eaten sparingly.

UNHEALTHY FATS Probably the most harmful fats in the diet (and therefore the ones most important to avoid) are the trans-fatty acids of partially hydrogenated fats. These can be found in most margarines and in fast and processed foods. (*For more on different types of fat and their effects on health , see p.34.*)

EXCESS CARBOHYDRATE Growing evidence suggests that the burgeoning rates of overweight and obesity in industrialised nations are fuelled by excessive consumption of carbohydrates (starches and sugars). High-glycaemic index foods (*see chart, p.43*), which release sugar quickly into the blood, seem to be the most problematic. They tend to cause the body to secrete large amounts of the hormone insulin, which encourages the conversion of sugar into fat. Studies show that high insulin secretion is associated with weight gain.

High blood-sugar levels also tend to mean the body is using carbohydrate, not fat, as its energy source. Long-term studies in animals have shown that diets based on high-glycaemic index starches are more likely to promote weight gain. In general, diets based on low-glycaemic index foods

BURNING THE CALORIES			
Choosing simple everyday activities rather than the labour-saving alternatives can make a big difference to your calorie balance (the difference between the number of calories you take in and burn		off). The table below provides some everyday examples that compare the sedentary option with the more active, calorie-burning alternative. (NB: figures use a basal metabolic rate of 60 kcal per hour.)	
SEDENTARY	**KCAL**	**ACTIVE**	**KCAL**
Driving to work (20 mins)	50	Cycling to work (30 mins)	140
Taking lift up one floor	0.1	Walking up a flight of stairs	5
Using a car-wash	10	Washing and waxing car by hand	300
Employing a gardener	0	Gardening and mowing the lawn (30 minutes)	150
Employing a cleaner	0	Heavy housework, e.g. scrubbing floors (1 hour)	225
Sitting and waiting 30 minutes for pizza delivery	30	Cooking for 30 minutes	100
Letting the dog run round the garden (30 mins)	30	Taking dog for brisk 30-minute walk	125
Shopping on-line (1 hour)	90	Shopping in supermarket (1 hour)	200
Taking the bus (20 mins)	30	Walking, carrying shopping (30 mins)	120
Using remote control to change TV channel	0.1	Walking across room to change channel	3
Total calories expended:	**240.2**	**Total calories expended:**	**1368**

may help weight loss because they moderate levels of sugar and insulin in the body. Low-glycaemic index starches have more fibre and help to control the appetite, so that fewer calories are consumed. (*For more about blood-sugar balance, see p.42.*)

SNACKING AND WEIGHT GAIN Most weight-loss regimes advise against eating between meals on the basis that this puts additional calories into the body. However, healthy snacking may help to control the appetite and prevent overeating at meals, and may also help to stabilise the body's levels of sugar and insulin. A 1964 study found that people eating six little meals rather than three normal-sized ones lost weight and had more stable levels of blood sugar.

Snacking may also reduce the appetite and the overall quantity of food eaten in a day. In a 1999 study, overweight men ate a large breakfast and then nothing for five hours. Another group ate the same food but it was divided into five hourly meals. At an "all you can eat" lunch, the men who had had regular hourly snacks ate a quarter less than the men who just had one large breakfast. The "snackers" also had more favourable insulin and blood-sugar levels. A 1996 review on this subject concluded that snacking has distinct benefits for weight loss. Healthy snacks for most people include fresh fruit and nuts.

OVERWEIGHT CHILDREN are facing major health problems. Research has shown that by addressing the problems of obesity and low fitness levels early in the child's life, a significant step can be taken towards reversing the negative trends of this potentially dangerous condition. It is not easy to help children change their eating habits. But the extra calories in a fizzy, sugary drink and a packet of crisps can be enough to tip the balance from having just enough calories to having too many. Try to restrict these kind of snacks. The extra few grams of fat deposited every day become the kilograms that cause disability in the long term.

Homeopathy

Little scientific evidence indicates that homeopathy helps in obesity, and it is certainly no substitute for diet and lifestyle changes. But some practitioners feel they can help with constitutional homeopathic prescribing. The medicines they usually recommend are *Calcarea carbonica* and *Graphites* (*see p.73*).

Exercise

PRIMARY TREATMENT There is some disagreement regarding the precise role of exercise. Some studies suggest that it helps to reduce weight, while others say its chief benefit is to maintain (rather than to assist) weight loss. However, there is no doubt that regular exercise, such as walking, cycling and swimming, is important, whether you are overweight or not. If you are obese, exercise should not be extreme or prolonged, but brisk walking for half an hour a day will make a substantial difference to your well-being and should assist weight loss and maintenance. In a 2003 study, a combination of increased general exercise and an appropriate diet were shown to offer major health benefits. Weight loss, improved cardio-respiratory fitness and reduced cholesterol levels were all maintained after the programme for a period of six months.

PRIMARY TREATMENT **LIFESTYLE ACTIVITY** Studies indicate that incorporating more activity into your daily life could be even more beneficial than formal exercise sessions. A 1999 study examined the short- and long-term benefits produced by a low-fat diet of about 1,200 calories per day when it was combined with either structured aerobic exercising or moderate-intensity lifestyle activity (for example, walking to the shops rather than driving, performing more work outdoors and using stairs rather than the lift when possible). Changes in body weight, body composition, cardiovascular risk profiles and physical fitness were assessed at 16 weeks and again at one year. Overall, those doing more lifestyle activity lost significantly more weight and managed to keep it off for longer compared to those doing aerobic exercise. Cholesterol levels reduced significantly in both groups.

It is crucial to encourage overweight children to exercise regularly. Try to incorporate enjoyable activities and exercise, such as playing games or going swimming together, into the family routine.

Acupuncture

Acupuncture over the stomach meridian point in the ear may help to suppress appetite. The treatment involves wearing a tiny "ear stud". Pressing it whenever you feel hungry can help to control appetite. However, the four clinical trials that evaluated this approach indicated only marginal benefit. It is worthwhile persisting with acupuncture, probably for four to six weeks, but if there is no obvious effect then discontinue treatment.

Mind–Body Therapies

BEHAVIOUR MODIFICATION has traditionally been used for weight management, along with diet, exercise, nutritional education and other techniques. Individual and/or group psychological treatment is often recommended, especially for people who are significantly obese.

Diet, exercise and other strategies will often achieve some short-term weight loss, but long-term weight management is not usually possible without tackling the factors that cause overeating in the first place. Most people struggle through the "yo-yo process" of losing and gaining weight repeatedly, becoming more and more frustrated and disappointed each time. Weight-management treatments are often unsuccessful in the long run because they focus on reducing excessive and unhealthy eating rather than on understanding the forces that produce such behaviour.

STRESS can negatively influence weight. Stress and unsuccessful efforts to manage it can have a "double-whammy" effect. First, stress affects the body directly through hormonal changes that can have profound and negative effects on the body's metabolic systems, even influencing how and where fat is stored. Second, psychological stress and distress can affect weight indirectly by encouraging people to comfort eat and to avoid taking exercise.

Mind–body practices, such as autogenic training and visualisation, can engage the full power of the mind to help you manage your weight. Yoga, relaxation breathing or guided imagery (*see p.100*) can be a part in an overall weight-loss plan. This is not to suggest that effective weight management is simply a case of "mind over matter", or that you can magically lose weight through thinking or visualising your fat cells melting away. However, when it comes to managing weight, the mind does matter and there is a growing body of scientific research to back up this statement.

STRESS EATING Studies have shown that being stressed all the time may contribute to the tendency to accumulate fat, particularly in the abdomen. Stress hormones, such as cortisol, are released, which alter the metabolic processes responsible for the proper utilisation of fat. Research in 2000 also suggests that leptin, a neurotransmitter produced in fat cells and involved in regulating appetite, is also released. With plenty of cortisol and leptin circulating in the body, food intake is increased, a phenomenon scientists term "stress eating". Often, when individuals are under stress, they will eat to excess or consume high-calorie foods, triggering weight gain. Mind–body practices, used both at home and as part of a supervised weight-loss programme, can reduce stress and enhance the ability to both lose weight and maintain a lifelong desirable weight.

PREVENTION PLAN

The following may help to prevent you from becoming obese:

- Eat a nutritious diet.
- Take plenty of exercise.

SLEEP DISORDERS

Adequate sleep is important for maintaining good health. If you sleep well, you wake up feeling refreshed and ready to deal with the day ahead; if you sleep badly on a regular basis, your ability to cope with life can suffer. Common sleep problems include trouble falling asleep, waking up in the night or too early in the morning, and feeling sleepy during the day. Sometimes sleep disorders can be treated with simple lifestyle measures such as exercise and dietary changes, but in addition there is a range of therapies that may help.

WHAT ARE THE SYMPTOMS?

Symptoms of insomnia include:
- Regular inability to fall asleep or to stay asleep
- Excessive tiredness

Symptoms of sleep apnoea include:
- Breathing during sleep is interrupted for 10 seconds or more at least five times an hour
- Sleep is restless and not refreshing
- Loud snoring
- Sleepiness during the day
- Morning headaches

WHY MIGHT I HAVE THESE?

PREDISPOSING FACTORS

Insomnia:
- Stress
- Illness, such as asthma, that causes problems at night
- High intake of caffeine or alcohol
- Food sensitivity
- Blood-sugar instability

Sleep apnoea:
- Being male, especially between 40 and 60 years of age
- Being overweight
- Drinking alcohol
- Smoking

TRIGGERS
- Depression and anxiety
- Emotional upset

IMPORTANT

If you think your sleeping problems may be part of depression, see your doctor.

WHY DOES IT OCCUR?

Most people experience changes in their sleep patterns at some point in their lives. These may be due to, or made worse by, behaviour associated with stress, such as drinking too much alcohol or working late into the night. Sleep disorders are caused by, and contribute to, other problems, such as depression (*see p.436*), anxiety (*see p.414*), SAD (*see p.432*) and fibromyalgia (*see p.298*). In some cases, a sleeping disorder is caused by an underlying medical disorder, such as an overactive thyroid gland (*see p.319*).

Sleepiness during the day may simply be a reflection of a difficulty getting to sleep or of staying asleep at night. In a few cases, it is caused by sleep apnoea, a condition mainly affecting middle-aged men in which breathing is repeatedly interrupted during sleep. This is often due to the soft tissues of the throat relaxing and blocking the flow of air.

THE RIGHT AMOUNT OF SLEEP In general, adults should sleep for about seven or eight hours each night. Teenagers need an hour or so more, whereas babies need as much as 16 hours a day. Pregnant women in their first trimester usually sleep for a few more hours a day than normal. Older people usually sleep less than younger adults. If you feel sleepy during the day, or fall asleep the moment your head hits the pillow, it is likely that you need more sleep.

TREATMENT PLAN

PRIMARY TREATMENTS
- Simple lifestyle measures (*see Self-Help*)
- Treatment of underlying disorders
- Caffeine withdrawal
- Blood-sugar stabilising diet
- Valerian
- Behavioural therapy (for chronic insomnia)

BACK-UP TREATMENTS
- Sleeping tablets
- Massage and exercise
- Bodywork and movement therapies
- Homeopathy
- Western herbal medicine
- Acupuncture
- Mind–body therapies

For an explanation of how treatments are rated, see p.111.

SELF-HELP

PRIMARY TREATMENT If sleep eludes you, the following measures might help:
- Avoid drinking large amounts of tea, coffee and cola in either the afternoon or the evening.
- Give up smoking, because nicotine is a stimulant that can keep you awake.
- Avoid drinking alcohol.
- Do not eat large meals late in the evening – you won't have time to digest the food.
- Take plenty of regular exercise, but not in the evening as this can overstimulate.
- Go to bed at the same time each night and wind down first by listening to

music or soaking in a warm bath.

- Add five drops of lavender oil to an evening bath or burn them in an aromatherapy vaporiser to scent the room.
- Keep your bedroom for sleeping rather than eating, watching TV, reading, etc.
- If you are unable to fall asleep, get up and do something rather than lie in bed awake and frustrated.
- Invest in heavy curtains, blackout blinds or an eyemask if early morning light bothers you.
- Practise yoga eye exercises (see p.451).

(see p.451)

TREATMENTS IN DETAIL

Conventional Medicine

Tackling problems that are worrying you may help you sleep better, as may following preventive advice (see Self-Help, p.448). Counselling may be appropriate to help resolve issues that are troubling you.

PRIMARY TREATMENT **TREATING AN UNDERLYING DISORDER** If sleeping problems are persistent, it may be worth seeing your doctor, who will discuss your symptoms with you to look for evidence of an underlying physical or psychological cause. Investigations may be arranged if necessary. For example, if sleep apnoea is suspected, sleep studies may be performed, in which breathing, heart rate and blood oxygen levels are monitored during sleep. Underlying conditions are then treated where possible.

SLEEPING TABLETS do not treat the cause of the sleep disorder but may be prescribed occasionally to help restore a normal sleep pattern. Benzodiazepines may be prescribed, but only on a short-term basis as they are addictive. If dependency does occur, increasing doses are needed to achieve the same effect and withdrawal symptoms such as restlessness and severe anxiety may result.

Your doctor may prescribe other sleeping tablets, such as zopiclone and zolpidem, which do not last as long in the body. However, they may also be associated with dependency.

In elderly patients, sleep medications can cause falls or respiratory depression. They can interact with other medications or alcohol, and can disrupt natural circadian rhythms. The next-day after-effects of sleep medications can be similar to the effects of sleep deprivation itself.

OTHER DRUGS Over-the-counter drugs containing antihistamines are available. When poor sleep is associated with depression (see p.436), antidepressants may help.

> **CAUTION**
>
> Sleeping tablets (including ones bought over the counter) can affect the ability to drive and operate machinery. These effects can last until the next day and are made worse by drinking alcohol. Sleeping pills may cause other side-effects: ask your doctor to explain these to you.

Nutritional Therapy

PRIMARY TREATMENT **AVOID CAFFEINE** Dietary factors can play an important part in determining the ability to get to sleep. A common cause of sleeplessness is caffeine, which has stimulant effects in the body. Studies have shown that coffee and tea drinkers are more likely to suffer from sleep disruption, an effect that appears to be related to caffeine's ability to enhance arousal. The effects of caffeine can linger for up to 20 hours, so cutting it out or at least avoiding it after breakfast may be necessary to regularise sleep patterns. Caffeine sensitivity tends to get worse with age.

FOOD SENSITIVITY/ALLERGY may also be an underlying problem in sleep disorders. Foods causing allergic reactions are known to increase the heart rate, among other reactions, hence they can cause or aggravate insomnia. Children and infants suffering from persistent sleeplessness may well be intolerant to cows' milk. Studies show that exclusion of cows' milk from the diet may normalise sleep in some children. (For more on food sensitivity, see p.39.)

PRIMARY TREATMENT **STABILISE BLOOD SUGAR** Some people find that while getting to sleep is not a problem, they tend to wake in the middle of the night. Often, they can feel alert at this time and have difficulty getting back to sleep. In practice, this problem is often related to a drop in the level of sugar in the bloodstream during the night. Normally, the body tries to keep an adequate and stable blood-sugar level while we sleep. If the level falls, the body secretes certain hormones, notably adrenaline (which increases arousal), to correct this.

The secret to ensuring a good night's sleep for some people is to maintain a stable level of blood sugar throughout the night. An evening meal based on protein (meat, fish, eggs), vegetables and a limited amount of starch should help. A snack of some fruit and/or nuts taken an hour before bedtime may help to maintain blood-sugar levels through the night, and therefore may help sleep. (For more information about blood-sugar levels, see p.42.)

TRYPTOPHAN SUPPLEMENTS Sleep is induced by the production of certain brain chemicals, including a substance called serotonin. In the body, serotonin is made from the amino acid tryptophan. Low levels of tryptophan in the body can lead to insomnia. Supplementing with 5 hydroxytryptophan (5-HT), an intermediary in the production of serotonin from tryptophan, may help to induce and maintain sleep. The normal recommended dose is 50mg of 5-HT supplements, taken an hour before bedtime. Malted-milk products are high in tryptophan and may have a sleep-promoting effect.

> **CAUTION**
>
> Consult your doctor before taking 5-HTP with zolpidem, fluoxetine, paroxetine, venlafaxine, fluvoxamine or sumatriptan (see p.46).

Homeopathy

There are a number of homeopathic remedies available for sleeping disorders. For the medicines described below, take two 6C pills twice a day. In addition, there are proprietary remedies available in the UK, including Noctura, made by Nelson's. Avena sativa compound, made by Weleda, has a similar composition, but comes in a liquid form. The usual dose is 5–10 drops in a little warm water, about one hour before bed.

NUX VOMICA For insomnia, one of the mostly commonly suitable remedies is *Nux* *vomica.* The type of person this medicine helps typically wakes at 5 or 6am, feeling grouchy and "out of sorts", perhaps with a headache or indigestion.

COFFEA helps when the problem is going off to sleep – often, there has been too much mental stimulation during the day and the person lies awake, too excited to sleep and with many thoughts spinning around their head.

KALIUM PHOSPHORICUM may help when the person is exhausted, "too tired to sleep" and is woken by bad dreams.

CALCAREA CARBONICA Medicines for bad dreams include *Calc. carb.* Typically, the person it helps wakes up in a cold sweat from vivid, anxious dreams. There are often other constitutional features suggesting this medicine (*see Constitutions and constitutional prescribing, p.73*).

KALIUM BROMATUM is another useful medicine for vivid, disturbing dreams that are often of a sexual nature. As well as having sleep problems, the people *Kali. brom.* helps often also have acne and difficulty in concentrating.

RHUS TOXICODENDRON AND LACHESIS Medicines for unrefreshing sleep include *Rhus tox.* and *Lachesis.* The former is suitable when the problem is restlessness – the person feels they have "tossed and turned all night". *Lachesis* patients may complain of "waking feeling more tired than they went to bed", waking feeling wretched, often with a left-sided headache. These patients sometimes wake with a jerk, just as they are dropping off to sleep. There may be constitutional features (*see p.73*).

NUX MOSCHATA is a useful medicine for attacks of overpowering drowsiness during the day. An unusual feature of the people who respond to this medicine is an extreme dryness of the mouth.

Western Herbal Medicine

Herbal medicines are used worldwide for sleep disorders and can be a safe, effective and non-addictive solution to the problem. A herbal approach is likely to work well in relieving or at least ameliorating temporary sleep disorders – the occasional disturbed night's sleep or short-term insomnia resulting from an emotional upset. However, herbs are less likely to help in entrenched sleep disorders, though there is still scope for them.

Most sleep disorders involve difficulty in getting off to sleep, waking for variable lengths of time during the night or early waking and an inability to return to sleep. Preparing for sleep by relaxing and unwinding beforehand is important.

Most commonly available herbal remedies that aid sleep (*see below*) can be safely used at home. If self-medication proves ineffective, seek professional advice. The herbal practitioner will consider factors not directly linked to sleep, such as the state of the circulation, digestion, liver and the nervous system, and prescribe appropriate remedies.

PRIMARY TREATMENT **VALERIAN** (*Valeriana officinalis*) has a long history of use for sleep disorders, proving especially useful when nervous overactivity and anxiety are factors. It has been fairly well researched and is extremely safe. Clinical studies indicate that extracts improve sleep quality and increase the time spent in deeper sleep. Drowsiness on waking is not common but can occur, as people have different levels of sensitivity to the herb.

In one double-blind clinical trial, 44 per cent of those taking valerian reported having perfect sleep, while 89 per cent reported improved sleep. Valerian combines well with St John's wort (*Hypericum perforatum*) for sleep disturbance that is linked with depression (*see p.436*), which typically results in poor-quality sleep and early morning waking.

OTHER HERBAL REMEDIES that are commonly used to improve sleep include passionflower (*Passiflora incarnata*), Californian poppy (*Eschscholzia californica*), scullcap (*Scutellaria laterifolia*) and hops (*Humulus lupulus*). These and other sedative remedies are often combined together in proprietary blends and are available in tablet and capsule form. For the best results, make sure you purchase quality herbs from reputable manufacturers.

Alternatively, make an infusion of one of the following and drink a cup before retiring. Chamomile (*Matricaria recutita*) is a gentle, relaxing and antispasmodic herb, which is helpful when tension is a factor. It is also valuable for children with disturbed sleep – it is a traditional remedy for nightmares. Lemon verbena (*Lippia citriodora*) is pleasant-tasting and mildly sedative. Limeflower (*Tilia cordata*) is a mild sedative that helps when anxiety is a factor. If required, these herbs may also be taken during the night, as they are mild-acting and the exact dosage is not critical.

> **CAUTION**
>
> See page 69 before taking a herbal remedy and, if you are already taking prescribed medication, consult a medical herbalist first. Do not take St John's wort with antidepressants, warfarin or antibiotics.

Bodywork and Movement Therapies

MASSAGE may help to restore normal sleep patterns. Studies have shown a benefit of massage therapy in improving disturbed sleep patterns in those who have chronic migraines (*see p.119*) and in those with the chronic muscle pain and fatigue symptoms of fibromyalgia (*see p.298*).

When sleep is disturbed as the result of a serious illness, acupressure in combination with massage was shown to be helpful – in one study it helped people with kidney disease who were receiving regular dialysis.

MODERATE EXERCISE or other physical activity, if taken regularly, may be useful for those with sleep disorders and there are studies to support this. Avoid exercising late in the day, as this can make getting to sleep difficult.

People who have sleep apnoea may briefly wake hundreds of times every night

EYE EXERCISES

These yoga eye exercises will keep your eye muscles strong and active, and will also help you to sleep. In each case, do not move your head, only your eyes. Close and relax your eyes for about 30 seconds before moving on to the next exercise.

Exercising your eye muscles

1. Keep your head still and look ahead. Look up and then down 10–15 times.

2. Look left and right as far as possible. Repeat 10–15 times.

3. Move the eyes diagonally 10–15 times one way, then the other.

4. Move the eyes in a 180-degree arc, looking upwards 10–15 times.

5. Finally, move the eyes in a 180-degree arc looking downwards 10–15 times.

YOGA EYE EXERCISES Traditional Hatha yoga eye movement exercises can effectively induce a sense of relaxation to help you get to sleep. The eye exercises consist of "drawing" a vertical line by moving the eyes up and down as far as they will go for between 10 and 15 repetitions (*see illustration, above*).

The procedure is repeated making a repetitive horizontal line (side to side), and then two diagonal lines, relaxing the eyes in their normal posture in between exercises. After the linear exercises, use your eyes to make two 180-degree arcs, upper and lower, making a clockwise and then a counter-clockwise circle. In studies, 90 per cent of individuals report sleep to be rapidly approaching by the time the latter part of the exercise is performed.

YOGA MEDITATION Practising yoga meditation may help insomnia. A study in 2000 showed that practising yoga meditation effectively increases the levels in the body of melatonin, a hormone that assists in normalising sleep patterns.

CHIROPRACTIC AND OSTEOPATHY Some reports suggest that chiropractic and osteopathy may treat sleep disorders, but only if the cause lies in disturbed mechanics of the spine having an adverse effect on the nervous system. For example, a case report discussed the effectiveness of spinal adjustment in the relief of poor sleeping patterns (and disturbed behaviour) of a 12-month-old toddler.

Acupuncture

Acupuncture has been widely used in the treatment of insomnia and other sleep disorders, although there are only a small number of clinical trials for these specific conditions. A traditional Chinese doctor would make a specific diagnosis, and then therapy and treatment may be needed over a prolonged period. In practice, acupuncture can sometimes give immediate relief from sleep disorders and may have a long-term beneficial effect, making it a useful means of prevention.

Treatment should initially be given on a weekly basis, and some improvement should be observed after six to eight sessions. If this proves to be effective, then long-term maintenance treatments may be required to prevent the insomnia returning.

Mind–Body Therapies

There are three types of sleep disturbance. In the first, there is a "sleep latency period" of greater than 30 minutes, i.e. it takes more than 30 minutes to get to sleep. The second involves a "waking after sleep onset" of greater than 30 minutes, i.e. you wake after about 30 minutes of sleep. The third involves waking early, with feelings of fatigue and drowsiness during the day, and this regularly recurs.

Although certain medical conditions need to be ruled out, long-term insomnia is most commonly due to a behavioural or psycho-physiological problem. Temporary sleeplessness during stressful life events is usually the result of anxiety (*see p.414*).

Insomniacs tend to have higher than normal levels of anxiety and depression, low self-efficacy (when a person feels unable to influence or control their behaviour or the course of daily events) and high performance anxiety – all of which can be either a cause or an effect of sleeplessness. Hormonal changes and drug use, including prescription drugs, cigarettes and alcohol, can also cause insomnia.

PRIMARY TREATMENT **BEHAVIOURAL THERAPY** has been repeatedly demonstrated to be the most effective long-term approach to chronic insomnia, in both general and specific groups. The main categories of behaviour therapy for insomnia are stimulus control (using a bed only for sleeping), a sleep hygiene programme (advice to help you sleep), keeping a sleep log, cognitive control (turning off the "racing mind") and progressive relaxation. These methods are often combined.

RELAXATION reduces sleep-onset insomnia (not being able to get to sleep), with or without stimulus control measures. However, effects are better when the two are combined. Guided imagery programmes combine progressive relaxation with pleasant suggestions for cognitive control, turning off the "racing mind" that characterises much chronic insomnia.

Practising relaxation skills can help individuals of all ages cope with chronic insomnia, although effects will be stronger if lifestyle change recommendations are also followed (*for a relaxation and guided imagery sequence, see p.100*).

WHAT ARE THE SYMPTOMS?

- Stumbling over and repeating certain words or sounds

WHY MIGHT I HAVE THIS?

PREDISPOSING FACTORS

- Genetic factors
- Emotional stress in childhood

TRIGGERS

- Fatigue
- Stressful situations such as talking on the telephone or in public

STAMMERING

Stammering, also known as stuttering, is a disorder that interferes with the continuous flow of speech. It is a common problem – about 1 per cent of the adult population are affected. Stammering varies between individuals, but is usually characterised by repetition of certain sounds, pauses and lengthening of words that are different from normal fluent speech. Speech and language therapy aims to build self-confidence, nurture social skills, improve communication and develop fluency control.

WHY DOES IT OCCUR?

There is no single reason why a person stammers, but given that speech is a complex process involving 37 muscles and thousands of nerves, it is not surprising that sometimes there can be a problem.

Each stammerer is different and the disorder seems to be caused by a combination of many factors. Having a close relative with a speech disorder increases the risk of a person developing a stammer, and the condition is much more prevalent in men and boys. Emotional stress in childhood may be a factor in some people. Stammering is often made worse by stress, fatigue or particular situations.

DEVELOPING A STAMMER The disorder usually starts in early childhood (between 2 and 6 years of age), when it may not cause much concern to the child. In fact, it can be difficult to spot because as they learn to speak, all young children naturally pause and repeat sounds or words.

Between 8 and 12 years, stammering may start to cause concern. In adolescence and adulthood, the speech disorder and lack of fluency can cause considerable frustration and embarrassment, and usually affects self-confidence.

THE PROCESS OF SPEAKING seems to involve a "planning" and an "articulation" stage, which need to be synchronised to be effective. If a significant gap develops between these two stages, or the timing of the synchrony is disrupted, stammering may result. One theory suggests that too much self-monitoring is a factor. Stammerers may find themselves caught in a vicious circle – they feel self-conscious and worried about making mistakes, which in turn causes stammering.

IMAGING THE BRAIN Research with techniques such as transcranial magnetic stimulation (TMS) reveal there may be a "neurological switch" in the brain that affects how we monitor speech. The fact that the presence of people activates some mechanism that makes stammerers stumble over words seems to support this.

PET (positron emission tomography) scans reveal that people who stammer may use the wrong side of their brains when they try to speak. It seems as though the right hemisphere is interfering with the left, which is usually more active in the production of speech. During times when stammerers are more fluent, their PET scans appear to show more similarities with those of people who do not stammer.

TREATMENT PLAN

PRIMARY TREATMENT

- Self-help measures (*see Helping your child*)
- Speech and language therapy

BACK-UP TREATMENTS

- Psychological therapies

WORTH CONSIDERING

- Homeopathy
- Relaxation and breathing

For an explanation of how treatments are rated, see p.111.

PRIMARY TREATMENT Speech and language therapists recommend the following:

- Encourage everyone in the family to take turns at talking. If a young child is constantly interrupted by older siblings, he or she may not be getting enough practice at speaking.
- Give your child your full attention: make eye contact and speak slowly.
- Play with your child and make plenty of time to talk together.
- Listen carefully and respond positively to what your child says rather than criticising how he or she says it.
- Give your child the opportunity to speak voluntarily rather than repeatedly asking him or her questions.
- Develop a daily routine and make family life at home as calm as possible, to avoid children feeling rushed for time and under pressure.
- Praise your child for things he or she does well in order to build up his or her self-confidence.

TREATMENTS IN DETAIL

Conventional Medicine

If a child is stammering and it is causing distress or concern to the child or to the parents, a doctor can refer them to a speech and language therapist. Older children and adults who stammer should also consult speech and language therapists who specialise in stammering.

PRIMARY TREATMENT **SPEECH AND LANGUAGE THERAPY** Therapists talk and play with a child in order to assess his or her speech. They also watch to see how the parents and other carers interact with the child. They will offer advice and support to parents on the kind of measures that help to prevent the stammer.

When treating an older child or an adult, therapists take a more holistic approach, looking not only at the speech itself, but also at how the stammering is affecting the individual's life. The subsequent treatment focuses on building up self-confidence and developing social skills as well as finding ways of coping with the stammer. Treatment may be given on an individual basis or in groups, and there are various techniques that are taught to the stammerer, such as slowing down the rate of speech and paying particular attention to breathing patterns.

Speech and language therapy has a high success rate in young children. In teenagers and adults, the problem becomes more complex to treat as the stammering is now

> ## Two-thirds of children who spontaneously stammer are fluent by the time they are adults

likely to be inextricably linked with the feelings it has caused, such as a lack of self-confidence. However, benefit can still be gained in many cases.

Homeopathy

Some homeopathic medicines, such as *Stramonium, Hyoscyamus, Agaricus muscarius* and *Zincum metallicum*, are used for the treatment of stammering.

STRAMONIUM is suitable for excitable children who flail their limbs when they try to get words out, and may have night terrors.

HYOSCYAMUS may be used for excitable children who try to talk too fast and "trip over their words".

AGARICUS MUSCARIUS AND ZINCUM METALLICUM are both suitable for people whose stammering is associated with twitchiness. People who respond to *Agaricus muscarius* may have tics of the face and elsewhere, and suffer from itchy chilblains. People who respond to *Zinc. met.* have fidgety, restless legs.

CAUSTICUM, LYCOPODIUM AND SULPHUR may help adults and children when prescribed on a constitutional basis (*see p.73*).

Relaxation and Breathing

Breathing patterns are inextricably linked with speech. Speech and language therapists teach deep breathing techniques as part of their treatment, but in addition for long-term speech fluency individuals who stammer may benefit from learning relax-ation and yoga-type diaphragmatic breathing, which helps to reduce anxiety.

Psychological Therapies

Voice problems can have significant social and psychosocial consequences. As a result, talking therapies need to treat the effect of stammering on self-image and self-esteem as well as the process of stammering itself. Therapists may use one or a combination of the following therapies.

HUMANISTIC THERAPIES emphasise the importance of the therapeutic relationship rather than the technical expertise of the therapist (*see p.107*). The client-centred approach focuses on giving the patient who stammers the space to provide their own solutions to their difficulties.

Gestalt therapy (*see p.99*) may be combined with a 12-step approach which is similar to that used in the recovery from substance use (*see p.428*). Here, the emphasis is on achieving three essential stages of recovery – awareness of the process of stammering, acceptance of the problem and change.

HYPNOSIS has had some positive results and is used for helping the person who stammers relax and increase their self-esteem, as well as attempting to address the stammering directly. Hypnosis has also been used in conjunction with other therapies, such as rational emotive behavioural therapy (*see p.103*).

COGNITIVE BEHAVIOURAL THERAPY is probably the most widely used and most researched form of psychological therapy for stammering. CBT focuses on the stammerers' beliefs about themselves, their ability to speak fluently and other people's reaction to their stammering. It also aims to help patients reassess their perception of themselves as potentially fluent speakers, and to overcome critical and judgemental notions that can inhibit change.

Allergies & Systemic Disorders

The holistic nature of integrated medicine is particularly appropriate for conditions that affect the whole body. Allergies can often be controlled through diet, and for chronic illnesses, the complementary therapies such as acupuncture, homeopathy, herbs and talking therapies can ease symptoms and offer enhanced emotional stability, support and a sense of control.

FOOD ALLERGIES AND INTOLERANCES

True food allergy is not common but can be very dangerous. The immune system reacts instantly to the food, forming immunoglobulin E (IgE) antibodies that may cause the skin and the mucous membranes to swell. In a severe reaction, blood pressure may drop suddenly, causing anaphylactic shock. By contrast, food intolerances are more common and do not involve an immune response. Symptoms occur after eating certain foods, but these are never acute or severe. In both cases, identifying and avoiding problem foods is essential.

WHAT ARE THE SYMPTOMS OF FOOD ALLERGIES?

Symptoms occur almost immediately:

- Itching and swelling of the lips, mouth and throat
- Itchy red rash (*see* Hives, *p.176*)
- Shortness of breath and wheezing

WHAT ARE THE SYMPTOMS OF FOOD INTOLERANCES?

Symptoms usually occur a few hours after eating the food:

Lactose intolerance

- Bloating and wind
- Diarrhoea

Fructose intolerance

- Stomach cramps
- Vomiting
- Weakness and dizziness
- Hunger and sweating

Amine intolerance

- Irritation of the skin, mouth, stomach and intestinal tract
- Hives
- Mouth ulcers
- Nausea and stomach cramps
- Diarrhoea
- Headaches

WHY MIGHT I HAVE THIS?

PREDISPOSING FACTORS

- For food allergies, having other atopic conditions, such as asthma (*see p.205*)
- In babies, temporary lactose intolerance may follow gastroenteritis
- Genetic predisposition
- Prolonged stress, in some cases
- Gastroenteritis and drugs that affect the permeability of the intestinal lining

WHY DOES IT OCCUR?

FOOD ALLERGIES The symptoms of food allergies are caused by an abnormal or exaggerated immunological response to one or more proteins in a particular food. Various theories have been put forward to explain why food allergy develops in infancy rather than later in life. It has been suggested that babies have an immature immune system and that their stomachs produce less acidic juices, allowing more proteins to reach the small intestine and trigger allergic responses. The majority of food allergies tend to resolve in early childhood. However, some, such as peanut allergy, may be life-long.

Food allergy seems to be more common in children with other atopic conditions, such as asthma (*see p.205*) and eczema (*see p.167*). Relatively few foods are responsible for the majority of allergic reactions. Common allergenic foods include cow's milk, eggs, peanuts, tree nuts, fish and shellfish.

FOOD INTOLERANCES may have a variety of causes, including a lack of certain chemicals in the body. One example of this is lactose intolerance. It is caused by insufficient amounts of the enzyme lactase, which is needed to break down the sugar lactose found in milk. Lactose intolerance is common in people of Afro-Caribbean, Asian and Mediterranean descent and it also seems that as people grow older they produce less lactase and therefore may be more likely to develop lactose intolerance.

Another substance that people are commonly intolerant of is the sugar fructose, which is found naturally in fruit and is added to fizzy soft drinks, juices and sports drinks. Amines (found in bananas, tomatoes, oranges, avocados, mushrooms, wine and Parmesan cheese) can also cause intolerances, and so too can the chemical MSG,

TREATMENT PLAN

PRIMARY TREATMENTS

- Elimination diet
- Antihistamines and other drugs

BACK-UP TREATMENTS

- Nutritional therapy

WORTH CONSIDERING

- Homeopathy
- Acupuncture
- Bodywork therapies

For an explanation of how treatments are rated, see p.111.

IMPORTANT

If someone with a known food allergy develops a rash, swelling in the lips or face or difficulty breathing, administer adrenaline using an Epipen in the thigh and call for an ambulance. If no Epipen is available, call for an ambulance immediately.

FOOD SENSITIVITY AND THE "LEAKY GUT" THEORY

One theory concerning the development of food sensitivity concentrates on the permeability of the intestinal lining. Some researchers believe that if the intestinal lining is more permeable than normal, it allows incompletely digested food proteins to be absorbed into the bloodstream, where the immune system reacts to them and becomes sensitised to them. According to the "leaky gut" theory, this then gives rise to an allergic reaction whenever the food concerned is eaten. The theory has yet to be widely accepted.

Absorption of food in the intestine

Food particles, represented here by coloured shapes, are broken down as digestion progresses (*arrow*). When they are small enough, they pass through the intestinal wall and into the bloodstream.

The "leaky gut" theory states that if the intestinal wall becomes more permeable than normal, it allows incompletely digested food proteins to enter the bloodstream, provoking an immune reaction.

an additive in tinned soups, ready meals and Chinese food. Intolerance of gluten, which is found in wheat products, is known as coeliac disease and is another form of severe food intolerance.

TREATMENTS IN DETAIL

Conventional Medicine

DIAGNOSING FOOD ALLERGY The doctor will first take a careful history to determine what the offending food might be and whether the time between eating the food and the onset of symptoms suggests an allergic response. Possible investigations include skin prick tests, in which dilute solutions are made from foodstuffs. A drop of each solution is put on the skin, which is pricked with a needle; the skin is then monitored for a reaction. These tests are not always reliable because a significant number of people who test positive to a certain food will not have allergic symptoms when they eat it. However, negative results are more reliable and virtually rule out the possibility of allergy to the food tested.

In some cases of suspected food allergy, blood samples are taken and antibody levels to certain food proteins measured. Known as RAST tests, these investigations are less reliable than skin tests.

If a skin test or a RAST test for a particular food is positive and the diagnosis is backed up by the symptoms described, the food should be tested using a double-blind food challenge. In this test, responses are monitored to the food and to a placebo. These are presented in such a way that neither the patient nor the investigator knows which is which.

DIAGNOSING FOOD INTOLERANCE There is no specific group of tests to investigate food intolerance apart from testing for gluten and lactose intolerance. Often, the diagnosis is made from a description of the symptoms. However, in certain cases, such as lactose intolerance, specific tests may be appropriate.

PRIMARY TREATMENT **TREATMENT FOR FOOD ALLERGY** The treatment aim for food allergies is to avoid the offending food. Antihistamines may be taken if the

food is mistakenly ingested and severe swelling and shock (anaphylaxis) require medical urgent treatment with intravenous drugs. For this reason, people with known food allergies are given easy-to-use injectable doses of adrenaline (known as Epipens) to keep with them and use if the signs of an allergic reaction develop (*See also Hives, p.176*).

Nutritional Therapy

It has been suggested that food intolerances are more likely to occur when the mucous membrane lining the intestines becomes excessively permeable, allowing large food-derived molecules and breakdown products to pass from the intestines into the bloodstream and triggering intolerance responses. This is known as the "leaky gut" hypothesis (*see above*).

Many food intolerance reactions of this nature are not mediated by the immune system through the production of IgE antibodies (as occurs in true allergic reactions). It is possible that some non-immune mechanisms may also be involved in food intolerance.

PRIMARY TREATMENT **ELIMINATION DIET** Although many tests claim to identify sensitive foods (*see p.39*), their reliability has yet to be conclusively proved. The elimination diet is regarded by many practitioners of nutritional medicine as the most accurate way of testing for food intolerance. In this approach, all likely problem foods are removed from the diet for several weeks. Initially symptoms may actually worsen, but if, as usually happens, an improvement in symptoms is seen, foods are added back into the diet, one at a time, and a note is made of which foods cause a recurrence of the symptoms. (*See p.39 for further details of elimination diets.*)

Improving digestive function may help reduce a tendency to food intolerance, because more complete digestion of food ensures that it is not absorbed in a partially digested form. (*See p.39 for ways to improve the digestion.*)

Homeopathy

Homeopathy is reputed to be helpful for children who are intolerant of cow's milk protein (this is not the same as lactose intolerance, in which the body cannot digest the milk sugar lactose). The most commonly appropriate medicines are *Silicea*, *Calcarea carbonica*, *Magnesia carbonica* and *Natrum carbonicum* and in order to get a correct diagnosis it is best to take your child to a homeopath. If sensitive children continue to have milk, other problems may develop, including runny nose, asthma and skin rashes.

Homeopathic pills usually include lactose, which theoretically might cause problems if you are lactose intolerant. However, the amount of lactose is very small and is unlikely to cause trouble. If it does, homeopathic medicines can be made from sucrose pills or as liquid.

SILICEA AND CALCAREA CARBONICA In children who respond to *Silicea* and *Calcarea carbonica*, milk often causes vomiting. Children who respond to *Silicea* tend to be small and wiry, with fine hair and delicate skin. However, appearances may well be deceptive because these children can actually be quite determined, set in their ways and stubborn.

By contrast, children who respond to *Calcarea carbonica* are often big and chubby, and they may sweat on their heads at night. They are often stubborn, and may have various fears that cause them to wake at night crying and frightened. Another key feature of these children is that they often love eggs.

NATRUM CARBONICUM AND MAGNESIA CARBONICA In children who respond to *Natrum carbonicum* and *Magnesia carbonica*, the problem is more likely to be diarrhoea. Features that suggest *Natrum carbonicum* include a lot of nasal catarrh and symptoms such as headaches brought on by the sun. Symptoms that suggest *Magnesia carbonica* include abdominal swelling and diarrhoea that resembles frog spawn. An affected baby may also have a sour smell, even after bathing.

Bodywork Therapies

MASSAGE AND REFLEXOLOGY If stress may play a part in your food intolerance, massages or reflexology sessions may help.

Sustained destructive emotions, such as anxiety, anger and fear, influence the intestinal tract and may lead to an increased likelihood of intestinal permeability. Massage and reflexology can help to reduce stress levels and so might improve the function of the digestive tract in the long term.

OSTEOPATHY AND CHIROPRACTIC Food intolerances may at times be related to incomplete breakdown of food, which can arise if there is inadequate production of digestive enzymes and acids. Osteopaths and chiropractors believe that digestive dysfunction can be caused or aggravated by a number of structural factors, including spinal restrictions, which cause the nerves supplying the digestive organs to become "irritable".

Clinical experience suggests that another structural factor that can contribute to digestive dysfunction is the presence of trigger points (particularly sensitive areas) in the muscles of the abdominal wall. Bodywork practitioners believe that these can influence the underlying digestive organs, such as the stomach and pancreas, and reduce their secretion of digestive juices. This in turn has an impact on how well the body is able to digest food.

Osteopathic, chiropractic and soft-tissue manipulation methods may help to treat both spinal restrictions and trigger points. If you have food intolerances, visiting a practitioner may be worthwhile, but so far no hard evidence is available.

Acupuncture

Acupuncture does not cure food intolerance, but it can help to relieve many of the symptoms caused by it.

Food intolerance is usually associated with a specific traditional Chinese diagnosis called "damp heat" that involves the lung, large intestine, spleen and stomach, and the liver and gallbladder meridians. Treating these with repeated acupuncture, based on a traditional Chinese diagnosis, can certainly help relieve many symptoms caused by food intolerance.

Traditional acupuncture can be used to strengthen an individual's constitution, and as such would be given on a weekly basis for eight or ten weeks.

> Food intolerance may cause discomfort but it is never life-threatening, unlike food allergy

PREVENTION PLAN

The following measures may help to prevent your child from developing food sensitivities:

- Breast-feed your baby exclusively for the first six months. If possible, avoid giving formula or introducing solid food before six months.

- When introducing solids, begin with only rice-based foods. Do not give milk (as a drink) until after the first year, or nut products until three years.

ALLERGIC RHINITIS

In allergic rhinitis, the membrane lining the nose becomes irritated and inflamed due to an allergic reaction when certain airborne substances are inhaled. Some people are only affected at a particular time of year (this is called seasonal allergic rhinitis, or hay fever), while others have it throughout the year (perennial allergic rhinitis). The first line of defence against allergic rhinitis is to identify and avoid allergens. Once this has been done, other measures including drugs, herbs, dietary changes and homeopathy may help to relieve symptoms.

WHAT ARE THE SYMPTOMS?

- Itching sensation in the nose
- Frequent sneezing
- Blocked, runny nose
- Itchy, red, watery eyes
- Headaches
- Nosebleeds, if nasal lining becomes very inflamed

WHY MIGHT I HAVE THIS?

PREDISPOSING FACTORS

- Genetic tendency
- Food sensitivities (*see p.456*)

TRIGGERS

- Exposure to allergens, such as house-dust mites or pollen

TREATMENT PLAN

PRIMARY TREATMENTS

- Lifestyle changes
- Drugs
- Elimination diet

BACK-UP TREATMENTS

- Nutritional supplements
- Western herbal medicine
- Environmental health measures
- Homeopathy

WORTH CONSIDERING

- Hydrotherapy
- Massage
- Breathing retraining
- Acupuncture

For an explanation of how treatments are rated, see p.111.

WHY DOES IT OCCUR?

In response to inhaling a trigger substance, specialised immune cells, called mast cells, release histamine, a chemical that triggers inflammation and the other symptoms of allergic rhinitis.

Seasonal allergic rhinitis, commonly called hay fever, is usually due to pollen from grass, trees, flowers or weeds. By contrast, perennial allergic rhinitis may be caused by house-dust mites, animal dander, feathers and mould spores.

It is important to confirm with your doctor that your symptoms are truly due to an allergy. Often, people with non-allergic rhinitis are misdiagnosed, since they experience the same runny nose, nasal congestion, sneezing and watery eyes that someone with allergic rhinitis experiences. In some cases rhinitis may be due to a viral infection instead of an allergy. Once you have identified the triggers for your allergic rhinitis, you can take appropriate steps to avoid them.

Several factors may influence allergic rhinitis. For instance, food sensitivity seems to be a common component of allergy in people who also have hay fever.

Some practitioners believe that shallow breathing using just the upper chest may also be a factor, because it causes the blood to become too alkaline and makes histamine levels in the body rise. This makes allergic responses such as rhinitis more likely. Other practitioners believe that trigger-point activity in the muscles of the face may make rhinitis symptoms worse by altering mucus secretion from the mucous membranes in the nose and sinuses.

Both seasonal and perennial allergic rhinitis are more common in people who have other conditions with an allergic component, such as asthma. Both types of allergic rhinitis sometimes run in families, suggesting that genetic factors may play a part in their onset.

SELF-HELP

PRIMARY TREATMENT For perennial allergic rhinitis try the following:

- Avoid furry animals.
- Only use pillows containing synthetic stuffing and cover pillows and mattresses with plastic.
- Have bare wood floors instead of carpet, particularly in the bedroom, and wash the floor often.

For seasonal allergic rhinitis:

- In summer avoid going outside before 10am (when the pollen count is at its highest).
- Keep doors and windows closed at night when possible.
- Wear dark glasses outside to help prevent eye irritation.

(*See also Environmental Health, p.462*)

TREATMENTS IN DETAIL

Conventional Medicine

PRIMARY TREATMENT Your doctor will take a careful history to identify possible allergens. Skin-prick tests may be arranged to help identify the allergens that are involved. In these tests, small amounts of allergens are applied to the skin to see if there is a reaction.

Specific allergens should be avoided as far as this is practical, but clearly it is not always possible to avoid certain allergens, such as pollen, for example.

HOW ALLERGIC REACTIONS OCCUR

In an allergic reaction, the immune system responds inappropriately to a substance that normally would cause no reaction at all. After the first exposure to the substance, the immune system becomes sensitised to it and produces antibodies against it. Further exposures to the substance then cause an allergic reaction, in which the antibodies bind to specialised immune cells known as mast cells. The allergens link the antibodies and destroy the mast cells, which release a substance called histamine. Histamine causes an inflammatory response in the body and is responsible for the symptoms associated with allergy, such as sneezing, a runny nose and itchy, watery eyes. Antihistamine drugs work by blocking histamine receptor sites on tissue cells, preventing histamine from attaching to them.

Mast cell destruction and histamine release

Allergen
Antibody
Released histamine
Antibodies linked by allergen
Histamine within cell

Repeated exposure to an allergen causes antibodies previously produced in response to it to bind to the surface of mast cells, which contain histamine.

The allergens bind to and link the antibodies, which causes the cell to burst and release the histamine that it contains. Histamine causes inflammation in the body.

PRIMARY TREATMENT | **DRUGS** Various treatments help to relieve the symptoms of allergic rhinitis. Oral and topical (locally applied) antihistamines can be bought over the counter. You should bear in mind that topical treatments may irritate the lining of the nose. Anti-inflammatory drugs, such as sodium chromoglycate, may provide some relief. Decongestants, such as xylometazoline, are available as drops to relieve nasal blockage. Their effects can gradually wear off after a week or so and symptoms may worsen when they are stopped. Low-dose corticosteroids can be used as nasal spray or drops. Small amounts may be absorbed into the bloodstream, but are unlikely to cause side-effects unless use is excessive or prolonged. If the symptoms persist, a short course of oral corticosteroids may be prescribed.

CAUTION

Drugs for allergic rhinitis can cause a range of possible side-effects: ask your doctor to explain these to you.

Nutritional Therapy

PRIMARY TREATMENT | **FOOD ELIMINATION DIET** A diet that excludes common problem foods has been shown to help some people with allergic rhinitis. While the effect of such a diet on allergic rhinitis symptoms has not been studied specifically, in practice identification and elimination of problem foods often seems to help control symptoms. Dairy products are renowned for their ability to stimulate mucus formation and experience shows that eliminating dairy products from the diet is often beneficial. *(For more information about food sensitivities, see p.456.)*

VITAMIN C The chemical histamine triggers the allergic response. Vitamin C has a natural antihistamine effect in the body and there is some evidence it can help control hay fever symptoms and symptoms of perennial allergic rhinitis.

If you have allergic rhinitis, take 1g of vitamin C two to three times a day while symptoms persist.

QUERCETIN Another useful natural agent for the treatment of hay fever and allergic rhinitis is quercetin. Quercetin appears to have the ability to reduce the release of histamine from mast cells. Some evidence suggests that quercetin may be a useful supplement for alleviating symptoms of both seasonal allergic rhinitis and perennial allergic rhinitis. If you have allergic rhinitis, try taking 400mg of quercitin two or three times a day.

Homeopathy

There is strong evidence that several homeopathic approaches to hay fever are successful. These include isopathy, in which hay fever is treated with homeopathic dilutions of pollen and the homeopathic medicine *Galphimia glauca*. There are also studies indicating that homeopathic complexes are effective.

ISOPATHY In clinical trials conducted by Dr David Reilly of the Glasgow Homoeopathic Hospital, *Mixed Grass Pollen* 30C had a beneficial effect on the symptoms of allergic rhinitis.

COMPLEX HOMEOPATHY involves taking a combination of homeopathic medicines likely to be beneficial. It is often the most practical form of homeopathy for simple self-treatment. You can buy the homeopathic complex *Allium, Euphrasia and Sabadilla*, often known simply as "AES". It is marketed by Nelsons in the UK under the brand name *Pollenna*. AES can bring fast relief when nasal congestion is due to allergy. However, homeopaths believe that visiting a homeopathic practitioner for individualised treatment with medicines such as *Arsenicum album, Arsenicum iodatum* or *Sulphur* is required to obtain the full benefit of homeopathic treatment.

Western Herbal Medicine

Allergic rhinitis often responds well to herbal treatment. Appropriate herbs can reduce the severity of symptoms even in those who have had allergic rhinitis for a long time, helping to reduce irritation and improve nasal breathing. A herbal practitioner will assess the state of the mucous membranes, digestive system and immune function. You may be advised to avoid sugar and dairy products, which can exacerbate symptoms. The practitioner will also take into account emotional factors. He or she will then combine a mix of herbs according to your specific needs.

EYEBRIGHT AND PLANTAIN are often prescribed to strengthen mucous membranes and relieve irritability and inflammation. Eyebright (*Euphrasia officinalis*) is an astringent, tonic herb that helps to dry up excessive watery secretions. Plantain (*Plantago major*), which is rich in a soothing substance called mucilage, can soothe sore, dry mucous membranes. Both can help to relieve sneezing. Research suggests that they have anti-inflammatory, antioxidant and immune-modulating actions.

ELDERFLOWER AND ECHINACEA are both thought to have a direct antiviral action. Elderflower (*Sambucus nigra*) is given to treat chronic upper respiratory infection and echinacea (*Echinacea spp.*) to restore normal immune function.

NETTLE, GINKGO AND GERMAN CHAMOMILE help to reduce the underlying allergic tendency. These herbs have anti-allergenic, antihistamine and anti-inflammatory actions. A 1990 placebo-controlled clinical trial involving 69 patients investigated nettle (*Urtica dioeca*) as a treatment for allergic rhinitis. It was found to be "moderately effective" by 58 per cent of those taking it, compared to 37 per cent in the placebo group. Ginkgo (*Ginkgo biloba*) and chamomile (*Matricaria recutita*) also have an anti-inflammatory action.

MILK THISTLE AND DANDELION Both milk thistle (*Silybum marinum*) and the common dandelion (*Taxacum officinale*) aid detoxification in the body by stimulating the function of the liver and the digestive system. This detoxification is thought indirectly to improve the health of mucous membranes.

> **CAUTION**
>
> See p.69 before taking a herbal remedy and, if you are already taking prescribed medication, consult a herbalist first.

Bodywork Therapies

TRIGGER-POINT DEACTIVATION AND MASSAGE Trigger points (sensitive areas) in certain muscles of the face and neck can increase secretions from the mucous membranes lining the nose and sinuses. Trigger points can be deactivated by acupuncture, as well as by manual pressure and stretching techniques such as those used by osteopaths, massage therapists (particularly those with a neuromuscular therapy training) and some physiotherapists and chiropractors. Therapeutic massage can also assist the drainage of lymphatic fluid and may help to decongest the area.

Breathing Retraining

Shallow breathing, using just the upper chest, can cause respiratory alkalosis, in which the blood becomes too alkaline. This causes histamine levels in the body to rise, heightening allergic responses such as allergic rhinitis. Learning yoga-type diaphragmatic breathing exercises can help; they reduce respiratory alkalosis by improving the mechanics and efficiency of breathing. To do them, breathe in through the nose after fully exhaling through pursed lips ("kiss" position). Take as long as is comfortable to exhale fully, and when you sense that it is time to breathe in, close the mouth and pause for a count of one, then inhale through the nose.

TRIGGER POINTS IN ALLERGY

The symptoms of allergic rhinitis may be made worse by trigger points, sensitive areas in muscles that can affect nearby tissues and cause pain. Trigger points in facial and neck muscles may be responsible for causing pain in various areas of the head. They may also cause an increase in secretions from the mucous membranes in the nose, making catarrh worse. Osteopaths, acupuncturists and other practitioners can deactivate trigger points using a variety of different methods.

Areas affected by trigger points

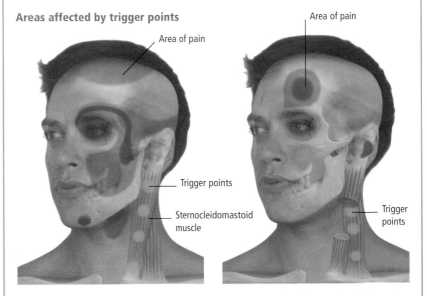

Area of pain

Area of pain

Trigger points

Sternocleidomastoid muscle

Trigger points

Trigger points in the sternocleidomastoid muscle in the neck may be responsible for pain that is felt in the area of the sinuses and on the back and top of the head.

Trigger points in other muscles in the neck may be responsible for pain that is felt in the forehead above the left eye, behind the ear and at the back of the head.

Hydrotherapy

A traditional yoga technique involving nasal saline inhalation, in which a warm salt-water solution is poured through the nose, usually offers rapid relief from allergic rhinitis (*see p.199*). A special ceramic pot, known as a "neti lota" pot, makes this procedure easy to perform. Fill the pot with warm water and add enough salt so the solution tastes like tears. Stand over a sink, tilt your head far to one side so your ear is parallel to the floor, and pour the solution into the upper nostril, allowing it to drain through the lower nostril. Repeat on the other side. This procedure may be performed two or three times a day.

> CAUTION
>
> Nasal saline inhalation should not be done by children under the age of 12.

Acupuncture

Acupuncture has been used for both chronic sinusitis and perennial and seasonal allergic rhinitis. The clinical trials in this area are limited and not particularly rigorous, but in practice acupuncture seems to be of real value in treating this acute and often distressing condition.

acupuncture can have quite a long-term effect and it may encourage the hay fever to disappear altogether.

Environmental Health

The severity of allergic rhinitis is greatly affected by the environment. Consequently, avoidance of triggers is the most effective strategy whenever possible.

POLLEN If your allergic rhinitis is seasonal (hay fever), avoid being outside when pollen counts are highest. Concentrations of airborne pollen usually peak between 5am and 10am. Throughout the allergy season it is best to be in an air-conditioned environment and keep the windows shut. A high-efficiency particle air (HEPA) filter may be useful.

You should get someone else to mow the lawn if you have outdoor seasonal allergies. If you must do outdoor work when the pollen count is high, a respirator-type mask may be useful, but remember that allergens can enter the body and trigger symptoms via the eyes as well as the nose and mouth. Allergic conjunctivitis, causing teary and itchy eyes, often accompanies allergic rhinitis. The use of sealing goggles may look strange but can help you to avoid an attack of allergic rhinitis and conjunctivitis.

DUST MITES In the home, dust mites (microscopic organisms that live in bedding, upholstered furniture and carpeting) and pets are leading causes of perennial allergic rhinitis. If you are sensitive to dust mites, consider removing the carpet and having wooden floors. If this is not possible, have someone else vacuum regularly while you are out of the house. Do not return for two or three hours to allow any airborne particles to settle (or use a HEPA filter). If you need to vacuum yourself, wear a mask while doing so, then leave the house for a few hours afterwards. Use double-thickness vacuum bags or special allergy vacuum bags to limit the spread of airborne allergens.

It helps to keep the humidity in your home below 40 or 50 per cent, as this limits dust-mite reproduction. You can control humidity levels with a dehumidifier and by using air conditioning in summer. Wash your bedding weekly in a wash that is hot, and remove any cuddly toys from the bed. The use of mite-impermeable mattress covers and pillowcases alone will not make much difference, but is probably beneficial when used along with other measures.

PETS If you have tested positive for allergy to pets (usually cats), it would be best not to have a pet. If this is not possible, the bedroom at least should become a pet-free haven. Special pet shampoos may or may not be effective, but a weekly bath for your pet seems important.

INDOOR MOULDS are another indoor allergen worth noting, although they typically are responsible for more asthma than rhinitis symptoms.

There are numerous species of fungi that can be found in the home, either from spore entry through windows or through growth indoors. Mould can often be seen around leaky pipes, on basement carpets and in bathrooms lacking adequate ventilation. Wipe away any obvious mould using a solution of dilute bleach (make sure the room is adequately ventilated), and eliminate damp conditions that favour its growth by using a dehumidifier. Maintain heating, ventilation and air-conditioning systems with regular inspections. When cleaning mould, be sure to wear a particle mask to limit exposure.

Glue ear and nasal polyps frequently co-exist with perennial allergic rhinitis

A traditional Chinese diagnosis is usually required, and treatment will need to be repeated on several occasions.

If you have seasonal allergic rhinitis and want to use acupuncture as a preventive treatment, you should have two or three sessions before the hay-fever season in preparation, and two or three sessions during the season itself. If acupuncture works for you during a particular hay-fever season, then you should try a similar regime each summer, just prior to when you are expecting the hay fever to occur. If treatment works for three or four years, it might be worthwhile to try a hay-fever season without acupuncture. Sometimes

Keep in mind that many people introduce outdoor allergens into their houses without thinking. For example, people who have allergies to tree pollen may attribute their increase in symptoms at Christmas time to dust mites or other indoor allergens, when actually the Christmas tree is the culprit. Fresh flowers brought into the house may have the same effect.

OUTDOOR MOULDS, such as *Alternaria*, can also cause problems. If exposure to mould triggers your allergy symptoms, stay clear of outdoor places where it may be found, such as old sheds, garages, barns and storage areas.

GLANDULAR FEVER

Glandular fever, also known as infectious mononucleosis, is caused by infection with the Epstein-Barr virus (EBV). It is characterised by a sore throat, swollen lymph glands and fatigue, which in some cases can persist for weeks afterwards. It is most common in adolescents and young adults; one attack provides lifelong protection against getting the infection again. The integrated approach involves treating the symptoms, eating a nutritious diet to help the immune system fight the virus, having massages and taking homeopathic remedies.

WHAT ARE THE SYMPTOMS?

Symptoms usually begin 4–6 weeks following infection with the virus. They may come on gradually or abruptly, and include:

- Fever and sweating
- Sore throat that may cause difficulty swallowing
- Enlarged and tender lymph glands in the neck
- Headache
- Tiredness
- Poor appetite
- Complications are uncommon, but include bacterial throat infections. The spleen is often enlarged

WHY MIGHT I HAVE THIS?

TRIGGER

- Contact with someone who has the Epstein-Barr virus

TREATMENT PLAN

PRIMARY TREATMENTS

- Painkillers
- Fluids
- Rest
- Antibiotics (for a throat infection)

BACK-UP TREATMENTS

- Dietary changes
- Multivitamin and mineral supplements

WORTH CONSIDERING

- Lymphatic pump techniques
- Homeopathy

For an explanation of how treatments are rated, see p.111.

WHY DOES IT OCCUR?

Infection with EBV is very common – about 90 per cent of the population are infected by the age of 50. However, many people with EBV infection do not develop symptoms and therefore do not know that they have the infection. Glandular fever, which may result from infection with EBV, has been associated with chronic fatigue syndrome (*see p.474*).

The virus is transmitted in the saliva, which is why it is called the "kissing disease". It enters the body through the nose or throat, and causes B lymphocytes to multiply rapidly and produce IgM antibodies to fight the virus. As a result of the huge numbers of lymphocytes in the body, the lymph nodes in the neck, throat and nose swell and the throat feels sore. The spleen is also enlarged. In some people, the symptoms clear up within about two weeks; in others, there is persistent lethargy lasting for weeks or months afterwards.

TREATMENTS IN DETAIL

Conventional Medicine

A diagnosis may be made from the symptoms. Your doctor may also arrange for blood tests to confirm the diagnosis.

PRIMARY TREATMENT **SYMPTOM RELIEF** Measures to relieve symptoms include painkillers for headaches, drinking plenty of fluids and rest if there is a fever. Vigorous exercise should be avoided while the spleen is enlarged and for a few weeks afterwards. Any complications will be treated; for example, antibiotics may be given for a bacterial throat infection.

Nutritional Therapy

DIETARY CHANGES Support the immune system by eating a nutritious diet, based on whole, unrefined foods, and restrict sugar, which can impair immune function.

Support for the immune system can be supplied by taking a high-potency multivitamin and mineral preparation each day. Alternatively, take a daily dose of 500–1,000mg of vitamin C and 10–25mg of zinc (balanced with 1mg of copper for every 15mg of zinc) while symptoms last.

Homeopathy

MERCURIUS SOLUBILIS Of the several medicines that may be helpful, *Mercurius solubilis* is probably the most frequently used. People who respond to it have a sore throat with swollen glands and excessive saliva that is painful to swallow. *Merc. sol.* is best taken as the 30C dilution, two pills four times a day. If the 30C dilution is not available, use the 6C dilution instead.

OTHER REMEDIES People who respond to *Ailanthus* may have a blotchy red rash, headache and muscular pain, with throat ulcers that make swallowing difficult. *Baryta carbonicum* is useful for persistent glandular fever.

Bodywork Therapies

Evidence suggests that osteopathic methods known as lymphatic pump techniques can increase immune response. They markedly increase blood levels of B and T lymphocytes for up to 24 hours. General, non-specific massage by a trained practitioner may have a similar effect.

CANCER SUPPORT

In cancer, cells grow uncontrollably because their normal regulatory mechanism has been damaged. Most types of cancer form solid tumours in a specific area of the body. The options for treating cancer are increasing and research continues into new types of treatment. Some people with cancer can now be cured and in others, the disease and its symptoms can largely be controlled. Dietary changes, acupuncture, bodywork therapies and talking therapies can play important roles in supporting conventional cancer treatment.

WHAT ARE THE SYMPTOMS?

The symptoms of cancer depend mainly on where it arises and what type of cancer it is. However, the following symptoms may be associated with cancer:

- A lump, which is often firm and painless, e.g. in the breast
- Changes in the appearance of a mole, as well as itchiness or bleeding
- A wound that does not heal
- Blood in the urine
- Blood in sputum
- Unexplained changes in bowel habits
- Blood-stained discharge or bleeding from the vagina or anus
- Persistent hoarseness or changes in the voice
- Difficulty swallowing
- Unaccustomed or very severe headaches

There may also be more general symptoms, including:

- Weight loss
- Fatigue
- Nausea and loss of appetite

WHY MIGHT I HAVE THIS?

PREDISPOSING FACTORS

These depend on the type of cancer.

- Genetic predisposition for some types of cancer
- Smoking for lung cancer
- Being over 65 for prostate and many other cancers
- Exposure to strong sunlight for skin cancer
- Various poorly understood dietary and environmental factors

WHY DOES IT OCCUR?

There are many factors that contribute to the development of cancer. In some cases, a susceptibility to developing cancer is genetic. For example, genes have been identified that play a role in the development of breast cancer, ovarian cancer, bowel cancer and prostate cancer. Sometimes an environmental cause can be identified. For example, smoking has been shown to be the main cause of lung cancer in as many as 70 per cent of cases, and exposure to the ultraviolet rays in strong sunlight causes most cases of malignant melanoma (the most serious type of skin cancer). In many instances, avoiding the cancer-causing agents can significantly reduce the chances of developing a specific type of cancer.

Cancer develops more often in older people because their cells have had more time to accumulate genetic damage and because the immune system, which acts to repair damage to cells, becomes less efficient with age. As life expectancy has increased in the developed world, the incidence of cancer has also increased.

Common sites for cancer include the skin, breast, lung, bowel and prostate gland. It may also affect the lymph nodes (leukaemia) or blood-forming cells in the bone marrow (lymphoma). Once established, cancer may spread through the blood and lymphatic systems, causing secondary cancers, which are known as metastases. These often occur in the liver, lungs, bone and brain.

TREATMENT PLAN

PRIMARY TREATMENTS

- Surgery
- Chemotherapy
- Radiotherapy
- Hormonal and biological therapies
- Drugs for pain relief and other symptoms
- Talking therapies

BACK-UP TREATMENTS

- Nutritional therapy
- Exercise

WORTH CONSIDERING

- Western and Chinese herbal medicine
- Homeopathy
- Lymphatic drainage and massage
- Acupuncture and acupressure

For an explanation of how treatments are rated, see p.111.

TREATMENTS IN DETAIL

Conventional Medicine

Cancer may be identified during routine screening, for example during a mammogram. Screening aims to identify cancer or

IMPORTANT

See your doctor promptly if you develop any of the symptoms listed (*see left*).

pre-cancerous changes that may later lead to cancer (in the case of cervical smears) before symptoms develop. However, in many cases, the disease is diagnosed when symptoms are investigated.

There are a number of options available for cancer treatment. The one that is recommended will depend on several factors, including the type of tumour and whether there is any spread (metastasis). Treatment may aim to cure the cancer, slow its growth or to relieve symptoms.

The support of medical and nursing staff, friends and family, support workers and self-help groups is often key to helping a person come to terms with a diagnosis of cancer and to cope with treatment. Friends and family may also need support. (*For details of support organisations, see p.486.*)

INVESTIGATIONS for cancer vary depending on the symptoms. Blood tests are commonly performed to check for anaemia and assess the function of various organs, including the liver and kidneys. Imaging tests, such as X-rays, ultrasound or CT scanning, may be used to look at an area of the body in more detail.

In some cases, viewing instruments are passed into a part of the body (such as the airways of the lungs, the bladder, the digestive tract or the abdomen) and samples of tissue (biopsies) are taken to look for cancer cells. If cancer is found, the type of cancer cell will be identified, which will help when recommending the most appropriate treatment option.

If cancer is diagnosed, further tests may be needed to look for evidence of cancer spread to nearby lymph nodes or to other parts of the body.

| PRIMARY TREATMENT | **SURGICAL TREATMENT** Solid tumours diagnosed at an early

stage are often removed surgically. The surgeon may also take some of the surrounding tissue to improve the chances of removing all the cancer cells. Nearby lymph nodes may also be removed, sometimes in order to look for evidence of cancer spread.

In some cases, palliative surgery may be performed to relieve symptoms. Other treatments, such as chemotherapy and radiotherapy (*see below*), may be given in addition to surgery; these additional therapies are known as adjuvant therapies.

| PRIMARY TREATMENT | **CHEMOTHERAPY** aims to destroy cancer cells by damag-

ing the genetic material they contain. A combination of cytotoxic (cell-destroying) drugs is often given through a drip into the bloodstream. In addition to destroying cancer cells, these drugs can damage other rapidly dividing cells in the body, such as those in the hair follicles and those that line the mouth. The specific side-effects caused by chemotherapy depend on the drug or drugs that are used.

Cytotoxic drugs may affect the production of blood cells by the bone marrow, causing anaemia and predisposing to infections. Nausea is often a side-effect of these drugs, but this can usually be relieved successfully by the antinausea drugs now available. Hair loss may occur too, but this is temporary.

| PRIMARY TREATMENT | **RADIOTHERAPY** Like chemotherapy, radiotherapy also

aims to destroy cancer cells by damaging their genetic material. In radiotherapy, high-intensity radiation is delivered to the site of the cancer by a machine as a series of treatments. Alternatively, some cancers are treated with sources of radiation placed inside the body in or very near the affected area. The specialist carefully calculates the necessary dose to keep the radiation delivered to nearby healthy tissues to the minimum possible.

| PRIMARY TREATMENT | **HORMONE THERAPY** can be used to treat certain cancers,

such as breast cancer. In some cases of breast cancer, growth of the tumour is influenced by the female hormone oestrogen. Drugs, such as tamoxifen, can be given to suppress the action of oestrogen. Hormone therapy may also be used to treat prostate cancer.

| PRIMARY TREATMENT | **BIOLOGICAL THERAPY** is a term that covers a variety of

treatments. Some of these can help the body's immune system react against and destroy cancer cells. The use of these drugs is limited to specific cancers.

The protein erythropoietin may be given as a biological therapy. Erythropoietin occurs naturally in the body and causes the bone marrow to produce red blood cells. It can therefore be helpful when anaemia develops as a side-effect of cytotoxic drugs.

HOW CANCER DEVELOPS

Our cells divide to produce new cells. Cancer arises when cells divide faster than is necessary to replace lost cells. In the example of skin cancer shown below, the cells that form skin are dividing uncontrollably. As the number of rapidly dividing cells increases, a tumour forms.

Skin cancer

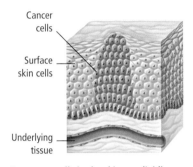

Cancer cells
Surface skin cells
Underlying tissue

Cancerous cells in the skin are dividing too fast.

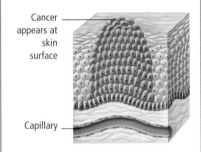

Cancer appears at skin surface
Capillary

The cancerous cells accumulate and eventually form a mass, which is known as a tumour.

Cells enter blood-stream

Cancerous cells grow into nearby tissues. If they reach the bloodstream and lymph system, they may spread.

COMPLEMENTARY THERAPIES FOR SIDE-EFFECTS

Chemotherapy and radiotherapy are powerful anti-cancer treatments but they have a range of side-effects. Try the following therapies and self-help measures to relieve these.

SIDE-EFFECTS	HELPFUL TREATMENTS
Chemotherapy	
Nausea and vomiting	• Acupuncture • THC (the active ingredient in marijuana) • Ginger • Fennel • Slippery elm • *Ipecac* 6x • Acupressure to wrist (*see p.154*)
Loss of appetite	• THC (the active ingredient in marijuana)
Diarrhoea	• Slippery elm • Acidophilus capsules to balance gut flora
Decreased immune function	• Echinacea • Astragalus • Pau d'arco • Andrographis • Cat's claw
Sore mouth	• Tincture of myrrh and golden seal as mouthwash
Sensitivity to sun	• High-factor sun block
Hair loss	• Scalp cooling during chemotherapy treatment
Fatigue	• Relaxation and gentle exercise • Nourishing diet with plenty of B vitamins • Siberian ginseng
Pain (chemotherapy can sometimes damage nerves, which can produce a burning sensation or a tingling or shooting pain; and peripheral neuropathy (*see p.127*)	• Acupuncture • Imagery, visualisation and other mind–body techniques (*see p.100*) • Hypnotherapy and meditation (*see p.98*) • Psychological support, e.g. counselling • Relaxing herbal remedies, e.g. valerian
Lymphoedema (swelling of arms, legs or other body parts due to build-up of lymph fluid)	• Exercises • Massage • Lymphatic drainage
Damage to fertility	• Cryopreservation of sperm or ovarian tissue
Depression, anxiety	• Talking to supportive friends, family and clergy • Counselling, prayer, healing • Herbal remedies, e.g. St John's wort
Radiotherapy	
Skin problems (red, blotchy, itchy and irritated, like sunburn)	• Aloe vera gel • Comfrey or pine ointment
Internal burning sensation	• Sage extract • *Belladonna* 6x • Liquorice

PRIMARY TREATMENT **OTHER TREATMENTS** may be given to relieve symptoms caused by cancer; for example, analgesics such as morphine relieve pain caused by the spread of cancer to the bone.

CAUTION

Drugs used in cancer treatment can cause a range of side-effects: ask your doctor to explain these to you.

Nutritional Therapy

For cancer to grow and spread in the body it must penetrate a mesh of tissue fibres known as the extra-cellular matrix. Cancer cells have the ability to secrete certain enzymes that allow them to spread. Several nutrients have the potential to block the action of these enzymes, which can help inhibit the growth and spread of cancerous tumours. Foods that may help include citrus fruits and soy-containing foods such as soya milk, tofu and miso.

Cancer cells also need a blood supply to survive. Certain compounds known as angiostats can help to prevent the formation of new blood vessels and "starve" existing tumours. Soy foods contain a substance called genistein, which has angiostatic properties.

Certain nutrients also seem to have the capacity to inhibit the growth of cancer cells. Some of these nutrients also seem to help convert abnormal cancerous cells into normal cells (a process known as re-differentiation). Some of the most important of these nutrients are carotenoid nutrients such as beta-carotene, alpha-carotene and lycopene. Foods rich in carotenoid nutrients include yellow, pink, orange and red fruits and vegetables such as tomatoes, carrots, apricot, red peppers and squash.

ANTIOXIDANTS AND CANCER Evidence suggests that the development of cancer can be related to damaging, destructive molecules called free radicals. Certain nutrients, including beta-carotene, vitamins A, C and E and the minerals zinc and selenium have the ability to quell free radicals through what is known as antioxidant action. In theory, higher levels of antioxidants might help combat cancer. In one study, a group taking high doses of nutrients including vitamins A, C, E, and zinc had half the risk of bladder cancer recurrence compared to a group not taking these nutrients. In another study, 200mcg of selenium, compared to placebo (inactive medication), halved the risk of dying from cancer in a group of individuals with a history of skin cancer.

> **CAUTION**
>
> Specific advice about dietary approaches to cancer should be sought from a practitioner experienced in the area.

Homeopathy

Homeopathy has been most investigated as a therapy for breast cancer. It has been researched for hot flushes due to tamoxifen, a drug used in the treatment of breast cancer, as a therapy for improving cancer patients' quality of life and for its ability to reduce the adverse effects of radiotherapy.

Hot flushes due to tamoxifen are a common symptom for women taking this drug. Cancer patients commonly experience a number of symptoms, including depression, anxiety and fatigue. *Amyl nitrosum*, *Lachesis*, *Calcarea carbonica*, *Natrum muriaticum*, *Sepia*, *Pulsatilla* and *Sulphur* are often prescribed medicines for hot flushes and maintaining quality of life. You should see a homeopath for treatment.

AMYL NITROSUM AND LACHESIS *Amyl nitrosum* is specifically prescribed for hot flushes. Women who respond to it have a sensation of blood surging to the head, sometimes with a throbbing headache, followed by profuse sweating and chilliness. Women who respond to *Lachesis* usually have hot flushes too, but they also have migraines, particularly left-sided ones. In fact, in women who respond to *Lachesis* all symptoms tend to be worse on the left, and they are also intolerant of tight clothes. They may also bruise easily.

CALCAREA CARBONICA Women who respond to *Calcarea carbonica* may also have hot flushes, but even without them, these women sweat, particularly on the head and neck at night. They are anxious and tend to niggle over little things. They may be woken regularly by bad dreams.

NATRUM MURIATICUM Women who respond to *Natrum muriaticum* are usually depressed, although this may be well hidden. These women have a "stiff upper lip", and do not like to talk about their problems. They often have vaginal dryness. Other possible symptoms include recurrent cold sores on the lips.

SEPIA Women who respond to *Sepia* may also have these features, including the depression and vaginal dryness. However, while women who respond to *Natrum muriaticum* are generally caring and sympathetic to those around them, women who respond to *Sepia* may be bad-tempered and less affectionate to their families.

PULSATILLA AND SULPHUR In women who respond to *Pulsatilla* there is great changeability, both in mood and symptoms. These women are typically soft-spoken and easily moved to tears. Patients who respond to *Sulphur* may become lethargic and depressed but are usually strong-willed and hot (both in temperature and temperament). Their feet are especially hot and may be smelly, and they kick off their shoes at every opportunity and may stick their feet out of the bed at night. They get burning pains at various sites and may have smelly discharges. They often have skin trouble, and any rash they develop is often very itchy.

BELLADONNA A clinical trial done in Italy showed that a combination of *Belladonna* and a homeopathic medicine that is made from water irradiated with X-rays reduced the side-effects of radiotherapy to the breast, which included swelling, heat and discoloration.

Western and Chinese Herbal Medicine

There is no evidence that herbal medicines can cure cancer. However, herbalists use three strategies to help people with cancer: support the immune system; inhibit cancer cell growth; and detoxify the body.

POLYSACCHARIDES AND SAPONINS Polysaccharides in medicinal mushrooms such as ganoderma (*Ganoderma lucidum*), also known as reishi or ling zhi, and shiitake (*Lentinus edodes*), as well as semi-purified polysaccharide extract (PSK and PSP) obtained from *Coriolus versicolor*, have immunostimulating properties.

Polysaccharides are an active constituent of Siberian ginseng (*Eleutherococcus senticosus*) and astragalus (*Astragalus membranaceus*), both of which have immune-supporting potential. In addition, ginseng has a non-specific tonic effect.

PHENOLS AND FLAVONOIDS A number of other Chinese herbs said to have anticancer activity are rich in phenolic compounds including flavonoids. *Scutellaria barbata*, a traditional Chinese herb, may have some anti-cancer activity, as might rhubarb root (*Rheum palmatum*).

Green tea and its polyphenolic components have demonstrated antimutagenic activity and can inhibit tumour growth in the laboratory. They may increase the effectiveness of chemotherapy drugs. Green tea consumption has been found to enhance the survival of women with ovarian cancer.

Western herbalists believe that herbs rich in phenols and flavonoids, such as garlic and onions, can reduce the risk of cancer. Milk thistle (*Silybum marianum*) is used to detoxify the liver. (*See also Nutritinal Therapy, above.*)

PROANTHOCYANIDINS AND PHYTO-OESTROGENS Opinion is divided as to whether taking herbal antioxidants rich in proanthocyanidins, such as grapeseed extract, interferes with chemotherapy and radiotherapy. There is recent evidence of beneficial interactions between the herbal and drug treatments.

The possibility that phyto-oestrogens found in medicinal plants such as black cohosh (*Cimicifuga racemosa*) and red clover (*Trifolium pratense*) may be contraindicated in women with pre-existing breast tumours is also contentious. It now appears that some phyto-oestrogens may help to protect against breast cancer.

> **CAUTION**
>
> • See p.62 before taking a herbal remedy.
>
> • Experimental evidence suggests that many plants have anti-cancer effects. However, we strongly emphasise that there is not yet enough evidence from clinical trials to make herbal treatment of cancer reliable.

TYPES OF CANCER

There are several hundred types of cancer. Doctors classify and name them according to the body tissue where they form. A few of the most common types are explained below.

TYPE AND LOCATION	NAME OF CANCER
Carcinomas Cancers of the epithelial cells. A thin layer of these cells covers the body; they also form skin. Epithelial cells line the gut, inside of the chest and other body cavities.	• Squamous cell carcinoma (Squamous cells are block-shaped cells that form skin, as well as mouth, gut and lung linings.) • Adenocarcinoma (Adenomatous cells are glandular cells that are found in stomach, breast and other organs that produce secretions.) • Transitional cell carcinoma (Transitional cells are layers of stretchy cells that line the bladder and urinary tract.) • Basal cell carcinoma (Basal cells form the lowest of the skin layers.)
Sarcomas Grow in supporting tissue, which include bones, ligaments, cartilage, tendons, fibrous (connective) tissues and fat.	• Fibrosarcoma (Fibrocytes make up fibrous tissue.) • Liposarcoma (Lipocytes are fat cells.) • Rhabdomyosarcoma (Mycocytes are muscle cells.) • Osteosarcoma (Osteocytes are bone cells.) • Chondrosarcoma (Chondroblasts are cartilage cells.)
Leukaemias Cancers of the white blood cells (leukocytes).	• Lymphocytic leukaemia (There are two groups of leukocytes: lymphocytes and granulocytes.) • Myeloid leukaemia (Granulocytes develop from blood-forming cells called myeloblasts.) • Lymphoblastic leukaemia (Blast cells, or blasts, are immature white blood cells.)
Lymphomas Arise in the lymphatic system. They may affect lymph tissues, lymph nodes, the spleen, bone marrow and the thymus gland.	• Hodgkin's disease (Affect lymphocytes, which are infection-fighting white blood cells found in lymph glands.) • Non-Hodgkin's lymphoma

Acupuncture

Acupuncture has a number of important uses in alleviating some of the symptoms associated with cancer, but it cannot treat or cure the disease. Some hospices offer acupuncture as part of their programme of palliative care (treatment to relieve symptoms). It is often difficult to judge how much acupuncture speeds up the resolution of acute symptoms and how effective it is as a constitutional "pick me up" in terminal illness.

RELIEF FROM NAUSEA There is good evidence to suggest that activating a specific acupuncture point just above the wrist on the inside of the arm (P6) will alleviate the nausea and vomiting that is frequently produced by anti-cancer drugs. Clinical trials have suggested that acupuncture is as effective as some of the modern and expensive antinausea drugs.

PAIN RELIEF Acupuncture has been used extensively to ameliorate pain associated with cancer. Sometimes pain can be caused by the cancer itself, or it may be the result of the tumour pressing on surrounding tissue. Acupuncture for cancer pain needs to be repeated frequently, but it can often provide a safe and effective form of treatment with few side-effects.

Sometimes the use of anti-cancer drugs or radiotherapy may cause pain which acupuncture can also relieve. Distressing symptoms, such as the suffocating breathlessness experienced by many patients dying from lung cancer, also appear to be helped by acupuncture.

If acupuncture is being used to treat acute pain, or post-chemotherapy nausea, then daily, or even twice daily, treatment is best. If it is used as a general treatment, a weekly session is perfectly acceptable.

Bodywork Therapies

LYMPHATIC DRAINAGE After surgery or radiotherapy, for example following partial or total mastectomy, the lymph glands under the arm may be damaged or removed. This can mean that normal lymph drainage from the region becomes impeded, leading to fluid accumulation and swelling (oedema) of the limb. If you have had such surgery, talk to a cancer care nurse about having manual lymphatic drainage. The methods used, involving very carefully targeted and light massage techniques, are capable of rapidly improving such conditions.

MASSAGE Living with cancer is often a stressful experience and, if massage appeals to you, it is to be recommended. Massage therapy, sometimes coupled with the use of various essential oils, has been shown in a number of research studies to be beneficial to cancer patients. It eases pain, reduces anxiety and depression, and helps to create a sense of well-being.

A study undertaken in 2000 looked at children with leukaemia who received massage from their parents (who were taught basic techniques). As a result, both the children and the parents had lower anxiety levels and fewer signs of stress. Parents felt less helpless in having an opportunity for greater participation in their children's recovery.

In another study, women in the early stages of breast cancer were given three massages weekly for five weeks. They reported much reduced anxiety levels and were found to have increased numbers of beneficial immune cells. The researchers reported, "The mechanisms underlying the improvement in immune function may be related to the decrease in cortisol levels, as cortisol stress hormones are suspected of destroying immune cells... These findings could result in improvement in quality of life and perhaps a longer survival rate."

ACUPRESSURE The nausea that often results from chemotherapy or anaesthetics can apparently be reduced by applying firm thumb pressure for several minutes to the acupressure point P6 on the front of each forearm (*see p.154*).

Exercise

Rest is apparently not the best medicine for the fatigue caused by treatment such as chemotherapy. A large study found that

Psychological Therapies

PRIMARY TREATMENT The use of "talking" therapies in the treatment of patients with cancer is aimed mainly at addressing the pain and subsequent depression associated with cancer. It has not been shown that psychological therapies can influence the progression of the disease itself.

However, a growing body of evidence supports the view that therapies can improve a patient's quality of life by improving their ability to cope with the illness. This in turn may have an effect on length of survival. In a study into breast cancer survival rates, women who had group therapy and learned pain-management techniques lived on average two years longer than those in the control group.

It is worth joining a group for mutual support, particularly if you do not have a partner or close network of family and friends. (*See below, and p.486*).

RELAXATION THERAPY There are few well-designed studies into the use of relaxation along with conventional medication for pain control. However, one study found that patients who received either relaxation or were trained in cognitive behavioural skills reported less pain than people in a control group who did not have training in these skills.

If you have cancer, it may be worthwhile practising daily relaxation (*see p.99 for details of a relaxation sequence*). You could also learn cognitive behavioural techniques.

Mind–Body Therapies

VISUALISATION Although much has been written and researched about the use of imagery to boost the body's power to destroy cancer tissue, its effects are not well established, scientifically speaking.

Nonetheless, when it is incorporated into a relaxation and group support programme, use of imagery may be an effective way of improving immune function or calming a tense and nervous body and mind. For some people with cancer, using imagery for relaxation and to help with focus can be a very important adjunct to some form of psychological treatment (*see left*).

The important point is that for many people, cancer becomes a turning point in their lives when they actively seek ways of working more effectively with their minds and bodies. Visualisation can be a significant component of rediscovering the link between the body and the mind.

Many cancers can now be cured, and others can be successfully controlled for many years

---

exercise improves physical functioning and well-being for many breast cancer patients. Researchers in Canada found that women undergoing treatment for early stage breast cancer who maintained a regular exercise programme of hour-long walking sessions three to five times per week for six months had a significant improvement in cardiac conditioning and overall functioning.

In contrast, the researchers found that inactivity contributed to the weakening of those patients who followed the traditional medical advice to take little or no exercise during cancer treatment. However, the researchers warn that this does not mean that more is better. Anyone with cancer beginning an exercise programme should first consult their doctor, along with someone, such as an exercise physiologist, who can evaluate their level of fitness.

Yoga

Gentle yoga exercise can help to calm the mind and the body, and may help to promote a sense of well-being.

GROUP THERAPY In a research study, 50 women with metastatic breast cancer (cancer that had spread to the breast from elsewhere in the body) who participated in professionally led support groups lived twice as long (36.6 months) as those women who did not participate. The researchers provided "supportive-expressive group therapy" where a time was allowed for the women to express their deepest fears and emotions. Patients in the support group also reported experiencing 50 per cent less pain than those not participating in the group.

COGNITIVE BEHAVIOURAL THERAPY Psycho-education, which is a type of cognitive behavioural therapy, teaches patients to become more aware of how they may develop anxiety or depression by how they think and behave. Meta-analysis of studies examining the use of psycho-education in cancer patients concluded that it was beneficial for patients with cancer and helped with anxiety, depression, mood swings, nausea, vomiting and pain.

PREVENTION PLAN

The following measures may help to reduce the likelihood of developing cancer:

- Eat a healthy, balanced diet, including at least five portions of fruit and vegetables each day (*for further nutritional advice, see p.44*).

- Avoid known environmental hazards, such as excessive sun exposure and tobacco smoke.

- Attend any screening appointments you are offered (such as cervical smears for women).

HIV AND AIDS

Infection with the human immunodeficiency virus (HIV) usually leads to the development of acquired immune deficiency syndrome (AIDS), in which the immune system becomes severely weakened. This allows serious infections to develop, often from organisms that do not usually pose a danger to health. At present, antiretroviral drugs can limit HIV infection for many years, but there is no cure for the disease or vaccine against it. Drug treatment may be supported by a variety of complementary approaches, aimed at boosting well-being and general health.

WHAT ARE THE SYMPTOMS?

Initial symptoms may include:
- Swollen lymph glands
- Fever
- Fatigue
- Rash
- Muscle aches
- Sore throat

Symptoms that may develop as the disease progresses include:
- Persistent swollen lymph glands
- Mouth ulcers and mouth infections, such as thrush (*see p.383*)
- Gum disease (gingivitis)
- Bouts of herpes simplex infections (*see p.162*), such as cold sores or genital herpes
- Extensive genital warts
- Itchy, dry skin
- Weight loss and diarrhoea

AIDS-defining illnesses include:
- Pneumocystis pneumonia
- Candidiasis affecting the respiratory tract or oesophagus
- Tuberculosis
- Herpes simplex infection, including infection of the lungs or oesophagus
- Infection of the brain with the toxoplasma organism
- Kaposi's sarcoma (a cancer that usually causes purplish skin lesions)
- Lymphoma (cancer of the lymph nodes)
- Cervical cancer

WHY MIGHT I HAVE THIS?

PREDISPOSING FACTORS
- Unprotected sexual intercourse (anal or vaginal)
- Intravenous drug use

WHY DOES IT OCCUR?

TRANSMISSION The HIV virus is transmitted through bodily fluids, including blood, semen, vaginal secretions and breast milk. It is most commonly transmitted through sexual intercourse (vaginal and anal), but can also be passed on through the sharing of contaminated needles by intravenous drug users. A woman infected with HIV can pass the infection on to her baby during pregnancy or, more often, at birth. It may also be transmitted through breast-feeding.

HIV infection is not caught from everyday contact, such as touching an infected person, or from coughs and sneezes from an infected person or by working or living with someone who has HIV or AIDS.

TREATMENT PLAN

PRIMARY TREATMENTS
- Antiretroviral drugs and treatment of specific symptoms
- Emotional and practical support

BACK-UP TREATMENTS
- Dietary changes and supplements
- Mind–body therapies

WORTH CONSIDERING
- Homeopathy
- Acupuncture

For an explanation of how treatments are rated, see p.111.

CD4 LYMPHOCYTES HIV enters the bloodstream and infects cells that have a structure known as a CD4 receptor on their surfaces. The cells include a type of white blood cell called a CD4 lymphocyte, which fights infection in the body. HIV reproduces in these cells and destroys them. At first, the immune system can still function normally despite the infection, and symptoms may not arise for years. However, eventually the number of CD4 lymphocytes in the body begins to fall, especially if the infection remains untreated. This increases susceptibility to other infections and also to certain types of cancer. A person with HIV infection is said to have developed AIDS if the CD4 lymphocyte count falls below a certain level or if he or she develops an AIDS-defining illness (*see below*).

DISEASE DEVELOPMENT The first symptoms of HIV may appear within four weeks of infection and may include vague, flu-like symptoms (*see left*), such as muscle aches and swollen glands. However, in many cases there are no symptoms at this stage. These symptoms usually clear up within a few weeks. Many people then feel perfectly healthy, often for years, but as the disease progresses further symptoms may develop (*see left*), such as persistent swollen glands and weight loss.

IMPORTANT

If you suspect you may have HIV, see your doctor or attend a clinic as soon as possible. Prompt diagnosis and early treatment are both essential.

The time between initial infection with HIV and the development of AIDS varies from person to person and can take from a few years to 15–20 years. Some people are unaware that they are infected until they develop one or more of the serious infections or cancers that are recognised as AIDS-defining illnesses (*see left*). Once AIDS develops, nerve damage may result in tingling, pain and numbness in the legs, feet and sometimes the hands. Dementia (*see p.133*) may also develop; symptoms vary from mild memory problems to personality changes and diminished intellectual ability in more severe cases.

SELF-HELP

If you are diagnosed with HIV, the following measures can help you to stay healthy.
- Even if you feel well, don't miss regular health checks.
- Take regular exercise, such as swimming or walking, three times a week.
- Eat nutritious, well-balanced meals and snacks (*see p.44*), even if you find that your appetite is poor.
- Keep the strain on your immune system to a minimum: as far as possible avoid other infections.
- Stay positive and if anxiety or depression become a factor, seek support (*see p.486 for organisations offering help*). Stress management or meditation can also help you deal with your feelings.

TREATMENTS IN DETAIL

Conventional Medicine

HIV infection is usually diagnosed by looking for the antibody to the virus in the blood. If the condition is diagnosed, referral to a specialist will be necessary for a full assessment. Regular reviews are carried out with blood tests to monitor the CD4 lymphocyte count and the number of viruses present.

Powerful antiretroviral drugs are now available that aim to keep the virus under control so that the development of AIDS is delayed, sometimes indefinitely.

If the CD4 count becomes low or is decreasing rapidly, drug therapy is likely to be recommended. It may also be considered in early infection when the first symptoms are present. Pregnant women

---

HOW ANTIRETROVIRAL DRUGS WORK

Antiretroviral drugs block enzymes (the chemical machinery) that the virus uses to reproduce. Different drugs work at different stages of the virus "production line". The HIV virus attaches to the CD4 cell, then empties its genetic material (RNA) into the cell. This RNA is converted into DNA by an enzyme called reverse transcriptase. Drugs called reverse transcriptase inhibitors stop this enzyme from working. Once the virus's RNA has been converted into DNA it can enter the cell's nucleus, where it combines with the cellular DNA. The virus then turns the cell into a "HIV factory", making billions of viral RNA particles. As these leave the cell, they are coated with protein to make them into complete viruses. The drugs called protease inhibitors work by blocking the protease enzyme, so the virus's protein coat does not form.

Preventing viral replication

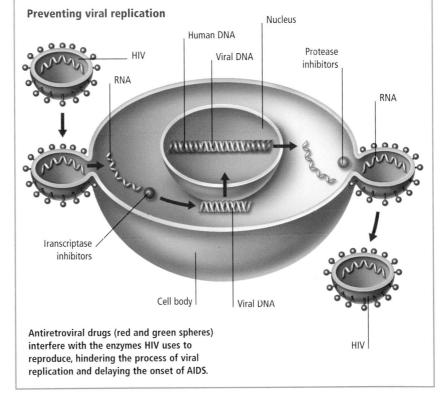

Antiretroviral drugs (red and green spheres) interfere with the enzymes HIV uses to reproduce, hindering the process of viral replication and delaying the onset of AIDS.

---

who are HIV positive may also take antiretroviral drugs that reduce the risk of transmission of HIV to the foetus. Caesarean section and avoiding breast-feeding are also likely to reduce the risk. A course of antiretroviral treatment is recommended for anyone following contact with HIV.

Drugs cannot eradicate the virus but aim to keep it under control by interfering with its replication (*see box, above*). Various drugs for HIV infection have been shown to be particularly beneficial when used in combination. Side-effects can be a problem, and regular monitoring with blood tests will be necessary. The drugs will need to be changed if side-effects are unaccept-

able or if there is not an adequate response, which may be due to resistance of the virus to one or more of the drugs.

PRIMARY TREATMENT **ANTIRETROVIRAL DRUGS** There are two main groups of antiretroviral drugs used, both of which aim to disrupt viral replication.

Reverse transcriptase inhibitors, such as zidovudine and lamiduvine, alter the genetic material both within the infected cell, which is needed by the virus to replicate, and within the virus itself.

Protease inhibitors, such as indanavir and ritonavir, prevent the production of the viral proteins that are necessary for the virus to replicate.

PRIMARY TREATMENT **OTHER TREATMENT** Treatments will be needed for specific problems and may include topical corticosteroids for mouth ulcers and antibiotic or antiviral drugs for infections. Kaposi's sarcoma or lymphoma may be treated with radiotherapy or in some cases chemotherapy.

PRIMARY TREATMENT **EMOTIONAL SUPPORT** is crucial, not only to help the affected individual come to terms with the disease but also for the individual's family, friends and carers. The many HIV and AIDS charities and support groups can give invaluable help and understanding.

> **CAUTION**
>
> Drugs for HIV and AIDS can cause a range of possible side-effects: ask your doctor to explain these to you.

Nutritional Therapy

NUTRITIONAL SUPPLEMENTS Wasting and weight loss are common and important complications of HIV infection and AIDS, and this seems to have a bearing on survival. Wasting is believed to worsen immune function and increase the risk of further infection. It is possible for HIV and AIDS patients to regain weight, and seems to help improve immune function. One study found that a protein-based liquid nutritional formula containing omega-3

dence that it is also linked to abnormal fat and protein metabolism in the body. People with HIV and AIDS can benefit from eating a nutritious diet based on whole, unprocessed foods. (*For more details, see p.44*).

OMEGA-3 FATTY ACIDS (found in oily fish such as mackerel, salmon and sardines) can influence immunological and inflammatory processes. Studies have shown that levels of omega-3 fatty acids are generally very low in AIDS patients. Eating extra omega-3 fatty acids may help those with AIDS and HIV. Either have at least three portions of oily fish a week or take 5–10g per day of fish oil.

VITAMINS AND MINERALS People with HIV or AIDS often have multiple nutritional deficiencies. One study found that developing a vitamin A and B12 deficiency was associated with a reduced CD4 count, and restoring levels of vitamin A, B12 and zinc to normal was associated with an increased CD4 count. The authors of this study concluded that nutrient deficiencies are associated with the progression of HIV.

Other research has found that low levels of vitamin B12, vitamin A, niacin (vitamin B3) and zinc are associated with faster HIV disease progression. Taking a broad-spectrum multivitamin and mineral supplement may help to prevent and/or reverse nutrient deficiencies and might also help to slow the progression of the disease. However, a study of vitamin A

from muscle and increase body weight and body cell mass in AIDS-related weight loss. One of the studies showed benefit from supplementation with 14g L-glutamine twice daily for eight weeks. If you have HIV or AIDS, taking 4–6g of L-glutamine each day may help maintain your weight and well-being.

N-ACETYL CYSTEINE The amino acid N-acetyl cysteine (NAC) may also be beneficial for people infected with HIV. NAC can inhibit the replication of the HIV virus in the test tube and studies show that supplementation may help people with HIV. NAC may work better in combination with glutamine, since these two amino acids promote the synthesis of glutathione, a naturally occurring antioxidant that may be protective in individuals with HIV. HIV-positive individuals may benefit from taking 600mg of NAC three times per day.

> **CAUTION**
>
> Consult your doctor before taking fish oil supplements with blood-thinning drugs, such as warfarin (*see p.46*).

Homeopathy

A clinical trial done in India suggests that homeopathy may have a favourable effect on CD4 count when used early in the development of AIDS. The mostly commonly used medicines were *Phosphorus*, *Pulsatilla*, *Sulphur* and *Lycopodium*.

COTRIMOXAZOLE AND HOMEOPATHIC MEDICINES Cotrimoxazole is an antibiotic often required to treat or prevent the severe infections that people with AIDS develop, and it is a serious problem if someone with AIDS is allergic to this drug. There is evidence that homeopathic treatment can help control this allergy, enabling AIDS patients who are allergic to cotrimoxazole to take it.

KALIUM CARBONICUM AND MERCURIUS SOLUBILIS In industrialised countries, homeopathy is more often used in a supportive role to treat HIV infection and AIDS. Among medicines that have been found helpful are *Kalium carbonicum*. Typically the patient is run down and tired,

> In developed countries where appropriate care is available, HIV can be seen as a chronic illness

fatty acids, taken as a 236ml dose three times per day, increased weight and CD4 count (an indicator of increased immunity) in HIV-infected patients. However, another study of supplements containing a large amount of omega-3 fatty acids and arginine found no improvement in immune function.

DIETARY CHANGES AIDS-related weight loss is thought to be partly due to reduced intake of food. However, there is some evi-

found no effect on CD4 count or viral load; another study of vitamin E and vitamin C found no difference in viral load between treatment and a placebo.

GLUTAMINE The amino acid glutamine appears to be important for optimal functioning of the immune system, especially in the critically ill. Taking glutamine-enriched supplements may maintain and improve immune function in AIDS patients. They may also reduce weight loss with a persistent wheezy cough, and often wakes up coughing at 3 or 4 am.

Mercurius solubilis may be given for infections, particularly for sore throats and tonsillitis, especially if the lymph glands in the neck are swollen. Excessive saliva in the mouth is a very characteristic feature in people who respond to *Mercurius solubilis*. In these people, the tongue feels sore and swollen and imprints of the teeth may be visible around its edge. Bad breath may also be a problem. These patients are said to be "human thermometers" because they are always too hot or cold and sweat very freely as soon as they get hot.

PHYTOLACCA AND THUJA OCCIDENTALIS may also be helpful for sore throats and other infections with a lot of rheumatic pain. *Thuja occidentalis* may be useful for recurrent infections and particularly for persistent urethritis in men or vaginal discharge in women. In people for whom it is suitable there is often widespread swelling of the lymph glands, numerous warts and polyps and stubborn nasal catarrh. These are sometimes accompanied by strange fixed ideas and obsessions.

PHOSPHORUS is sometimes helpful to aid general well-being and reduce the frequency of infections. People who respond to *Phosphorus* are tired and weak, although a bit better for rest and hence feel better in the morning. There may be hepatitis or a history of hepatitis, or diarrhoea, often with blood. They often bleed easily and may get bruises for no apparent reason. They may have a loss of appetite, although they are often thirsty, especially for cold, refreshing drinks. People who respond to *Phosphorus* are very sensitive, both to the physical and human environment. They are often emotionally volatile, as well as sympathetic and vivacious.

Acupuncture

Acupuncture cannot cure HIV infection and AIDS, but it is sometimes used to alleviate many of the symptoms associated with the disease. The traditional Chinese approach is to "balance the meridians" and hence provide immune balance, helping the immune system to perform to its maximum ability within the constraints of the illness.

There are specific complaints that may be associated with HIV infection or AIDS, such as tiredness, chest infections and irritable bowel, which acupuncture may help to alleviate and/or manage.

There are no specific randomised controlled trials in this area, but a number of studies have looked at whole treatment packages for HIV and AIDS, which include nutritional and herbal remedies and sometimes involve acupuncture. In general, these natural approaches to managing HIV and AIDS have been claimed to be of substantial benefit by proponents, but compared to sham acupuncture, true acupuncture was deemed to be no more effective for treating peripheral neuropathy (*see p.127*) related to HIV.

Probably the best way of using acupuncture is as part of such a programme, which is designed to maintain a healthy lifestyle. If acupuncture is for long-term health maintenance, a monthly session is best.

HIV and AIDS can be passed on by contaminated needles, and although safe disposal of needles used in acupuncture is well documented, particular attention should be paid to this issue by both the therapist and anyone receiving treatment.

Mind–Body Therapies

Mind–body therapies such as biofeedback and relaxation appear to be able to enhance the immune response by calming anxiety and stress.

Given the devastating psychological and biological impact of HIV and AIDS and the demonstrated effectiveness of mind–body therapies (*see below*) in helping people cope with these conditions, it is recommended that affected individuals take up regular relaxation (*see p.99 for a relaxation sequence*), yoga or meditation.

STRESS MANAGEMENT One of the earliest studies indicating that mind–body therapies might be useful for people who are HIV positive and/or have AIDS was conducted in 1995.

This study evaluated the effects of a stress-management programme on anxiety, mood, self-esteem and T-cell count in a group of HIV-positive men who had no symptoms except for T-cell counts below 400. This early, innovative programme consisted of 20 twice-weekly sessions of progressive muscle relaxation and electromyograph biofeedback-assisted relaxation training, meditation and hypnosis. The treatment group showed significant improvement when compared to a group that did not receive any mind–body treatment. All of the positive changes were maintained after a month.

Later studies also suggested that mind–body practices, such as relaxation exercises done at home, reduce stress levels and have a positive effect on immune response. Since stress is known to compromise the immune system, these results suggest that stress management to reduce arousal of the nervous system and anxiety is an important part of a treatment regime for HIV infection.

Infection with herpes simplex virus type 2 (HSV-2) is common in people with HIV and has negative implications for their health. A study examined the effect of a 10-week course of mind–body therapies on a group of men with mild HIV symptoms. Overall, those who practised the most relaxation had the greatest reduction in symptoms from herpes simplex.

Finally, in 2001 a study looked at the effects of a seven week self-management and coping skills training programme in people with HIV or AIDS. The study aimed to discover whether a self-management programme would have any impact on the mood and attitude of participants.

Those who completed the programme showed significant positive changes in terms of their mood, the way they coped with the disease and their attitudes. Treatment significantly improved participants' coping strategies and they became noticeably less pessimistic and anxious.

PREVENTION PLAN

The following may help:

- Do not have sex with multiple partners.
- Always use condoms during sex.
- Couples who wish to have unprotected sex should have an HIV test. Remember it can take three months after infection for the antibodies that are usually measured to be detectable.
- Never share needles if you use injectable drugs.

CHRONIC FATIGUE SYNDROME

People with chronic fatigue syndrome (CFS) have severe fatigue that has caused substantial disability for at least six months. The term CFS is now preferred to myalgic encephalomyelitis (ME), because in most cases of CFS no underlying disease of the muscles or nervous system can be found. The condition affects more women than men. There is no single treatment for CFS. Instead, improvement in symptoms often comes from a combination of approaches, including cognitive behavioural therapy, dietary changes, supplements and exercise.

WHAT ARE THE SYMPTOMS?

- Fatigue that is severe enough to interfere with work or home life and lasts at least six months
- Muscle aches and pains
- Irritability and mood changes
- Sleep disturbances
- Headaches
- Poor concentration
- Poor short-term memory
- Depression

WHY MIGHT I HAVE THIS?

PREDISPOSING FACTORS

- Low adrenal gland function
- Food sensitivity (see p.000)
- Candidiasis
- Magnesium deficiency
- Essential fatty acid deficiency
- Vitamin B deficiency

TREATMENT PLAN

PRIMARY TREATMENTS

- Self-help measures (*see left*)
- Graduated exercise
- Psychological therapy
- Nutritional therapy

BACK-UP TREATMENTS

- Drugs and other treatment for symptoms

WORTH CONSIDERING

- Homeopathy
- Western herbal medicine
- Breathing retraining
- Environmental health measures
- Massage
- Acupuncture

For an explanation of how treatments are rated, see p.111.

WHY DOES IT OCCUR?

One in five people consult their doctor about tiredness but only a small proportion will have CFS, which is profound fatigue that makes any physical and mental activity very difficult and is not improved by bed rest. There does not appear to be a single cause of the disease; instead, it seems to be the result of a combination of physical and psychological factors. It can follow a viral illness, such as glandular fever, in which case it may be known as post-viral fatigue syndrome. CFS usually begins suddenly, although the onset can sometimes be gradual.

SELF-HELP

PRIMARY TREATMENT Try the following measures to improve the condition:

- Find a sympathetic doctor. Try contacting the CFS charities (*see p.486*), some of whom keep databases of doctors with an interest in CFS.
- Join a CFS support group.
- Pace yourself: be prepared for good days and bad days.
- Take regular relaxation, follow a graded exercise programme to reduce stress.
- Practise cognitive behavioural techniques, which can help to reduce fears and pessimism.
- Compile a list of the things you want to achieve and break it down into phased, achievable goals. Keep goals manageable so that you do not become discouraged.
- Talk to your employer about a phased return to work.

TREATMENTS IN DETAIL

Conventional Medicine

The diagnosis of CFS is made by ruling out other causes of persistent fatigue, such as an underactive thyroid. (This is diagnosed by a blood test.) A programme aimed at gradually increasing physical activity is likely to be recommended to try to reduce the fatigue and improve quality of life (*see Exercise, p.477*). The doctor may also make a referral for psychotherapy, in particular cognitive behavioural therapy (*see Psychological Therapies, p.477*). Drugs may be prescribed to treat specific problems, such as depression.

Nutritional Therapy

Some of the most common underlying problems associated with CFS that nutritional therapists see include low adrenal gland function, food sensitivity (*see p.456*), low thyroid function (*see p.319*) and gut flora problems (*see p.40*). Identifying and correcting any underlying problem is often effective in restoring energy and combating fatigue.

PRIMARY TREATMENT **MAGNESIUM** There is some evidence that many CFS patients have low levels of magnesium. Studies also show that giving magnesium injections into the muscle can improve the symptoms in most people with CFS. In one study, 80 per cent of those receiving magnesium reported increased energy, better mood and a reduction in pain. Taking supplements can also improve symptoms. If you have CFS, you may benefit from taking 500–750mg of magnesium each day.

ESSENTIAL FATTY ACIDS Supplementation with essential fatty acids (EFAs) might also benefit people with CFS. Low levels of essential fatty acids, specifically the omega-3 type, may be found in people with CFS. One study found that taking high doses of omega-3 fatty acids over a three-month period brought about an improvement in 85 per cent of CFS patients. A diet rich in foods high in omega-3 fatty acids, such as oily fish (e.g. salmon, trout, mackerel, herring and sardines) and walnuts, may help reverse CFS symptoms in time. In addition, it may help to take essential fatty acid supplements. Taking 1g of concentrated fish oil once or twice a day might help in the long term.

PRIMARY TREATMENT **VITAMIN B** People who have CFS tend to be deficient in B vitamins. In practice, supplementation with a high-potency B-complex supplement that contains at least 25–50mg of vitamins B1, B2, B5 and B6 appears to be beneficial in improving symptoms of CFS, possibly because the B vitamins are involved in many metabolic pathways that generate energy in the body.

CARNITINE Carnitine, an amino acid, is required for energy production in the mitochondria of body cells (the parts of the cell concerned with generating energy). Deficiency of carnitine has been found in some people with CFS. Taking 1g of carnitine three times daily has been found to improve CFS symptoms in one study, although improvement generally takes 4–8 weeks to become apparent. Try taking 1,000mg once or twice a day.

CAUTION

Consult your doctor before taking fish oil and magnesium supplements with blood-thinning drugs, such as warfarin. (*See p.46*.)

Homeopathy

Evidence from clinical trials and case reports suggest that homeopathy can be helpful in treating CFS. However, CFS is a

---

CFS AND ADRENAL GLAND FUNCTION

Together the pituitary and adrenal glands determine how much energy the body uses and also how it responds to stress. Some experts link CFS to lowered adrenal gland function, but the evidence is far from clear. The adrenal glands produce several hormones that control energy levels, including cortisol and adrenaline. Cortisol is increased when the body is under stress.

Adrenaline alerts the nervous system and mobilises sugars and fats. However, in the long term, adrenal overload may deplete the body's energy reserves. Cortisol also reduces the normal immune system responses. It is possible that CFS patients develop a lowered "stress threshold", leading to overworked adrenal glands and eventual "adrenal exhaustion".

Hormonal feedback and the adrenal glands

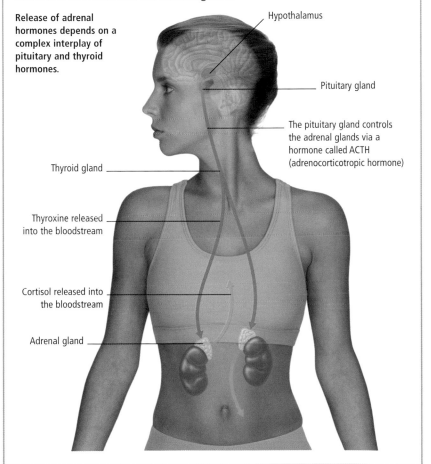

Release of adrenal hormones depends on a complex interplay of pituitary and thyroid hormones.

Hypothalamus

Pituitary gland

The pituitary gland controls the adrenal glands via a hormone called ACTH (adrenocorticotropic hormone)

Thyroid gland

Thyroxine released into the bloodstream

Cortisol released into the bloodstream

Adrenal gland

---

complex problem and often responds best to a combined approach including dietary changes, graded exercise programmes, lifestyle management, homeopathy and certain other therapies.

It is necessary to visit a homeopath for constitutional homeopathic treatment if you have CFS. Many medicines may be appropriate for treating this condition, including *Phosphorus* medicines, such as *Phosphoric acid, Kalium phosphoricum* and *Calcarea phosphorica.*

KALIUM PHOSPHORICUM is one of the most frequently given basic medicines for CFS. It is suitable when there is general weakness and weariness, possibly with blurring of vision and humming or buzzing noises in the ears, a tendency to be startled by sudden noises and a curious symptom of very yellow urine.

CALCAREA PHOSPHORICA may be appropriate when the person has a lot of aches and pains; it is useful for young people who seem to have developed CFS after a growth spurt. People who respond to *Calcarea phosphorica* may crave smoked or salted food, such as salami and kippers.

PHOSPHORIC ACID AND PICRIC ACID In people who respond to *Phosphoric acid*, the initial problem is mental exhaustion, evinced by weak memory, poor concentration and so forth. There is often diarrhoea or looseness of the bowels, which may be diagnosed as irritable bowel syndrome.

In people who respond to *Phosphoric acid*, CFS is often triggered by an emotional upset, such as divorce or an unhappy relationship, and in men there is often impotence. If impotence is a prominent feature, *Picric acid* may be another possible treatment.

spp.), ginkgo (*Ginkgo biloba*) and schisandra (*Schizandra chinensis*) in conditions such as this which are characterised by neurological and immune dysfunction.

Many people with CFS are highly sensitive to treatment, and it often needs to be started at a low dose, using well-tolerated remedies. Your precise treatment will depend of course on your symptoms, but it is likely to include the following herbs.

IMMUNE-STIMULATING HERBS To stimulate immune resistance and detoxification, you may be given astragalus (*Astralagus membranaceus*), burdock (*Arctium lappa*) and echinacea. If a viral cause is suspected, antiviral remedies such as St John's wort (*Hypericum perforatum*) and thuja (*Thuja occidentalis*) may be appropriate.

CAUTION

See p.69 before taking a herbal remedy and, if you are already taking prescribed medication, consult a medical herbalist first.

Environmental Medicine

There are many possible environmental triggers for chronic fatigue syndrome that are still being investigated and are the subject of some controversy. It is possible that individuals with sensitivities to certain environmental chemicals and/or a genetic predisposition to CFS may have an adverse reaction to paints and other chemicals at a level that would not normally be considered toxic.

Treatment for CFS involves identifying the likely cause and avoiding it. You may need the support of an expert who can take an environmental and occupational history looking for relevant environmental exposures (*see p.86*).

SICK BUILDING SYNDROME This causes a a set of general symptoms, similar to those of CFS, as a result of exposure to compounds from building materials. Your symptoms may improve with the use of low-emitting building materials, continuous ventilation, using non-toxic office supplies and careful storage of chemicals.

MERCURY People may be exposed to mercury by consuming fish; the US Food and Drug Administration recommends that pregnant women and other vulnerable groups do not consume suspect fish (*for details, see p.86*).

People who work in mining, ore smelting and in dental surgeries are at risk of mercury poisoning. If you work with dental amalgam, it is important to take precautions to prevent releasing mercury into the environment. You should ensure your workplace is adequately ventilated.

However, it is probably not necessary to remove dental amalgam fillings. Although leaching of mercury from them is often mentioned as a cause for a variety of health problems, this claim is doubted by many researchers.

It can be difficult to know if mercury is contributing to your CFS because some forms of mercury-level testing, such as hair

> CFS can affect people of all ages, but women are more frequently affected than men

SILICEA A number of other medicines may be prescribed for CFS, including *Silicea*. People who respond to *Silicea* are pale and weak, with fine hair. They are usually chilly and feel cold even in a warm room. Their hands and feet are cold yet clammy. They tend to catch infections easily; their immune systems are weak and their coughs and colds are very slow to clear up. If they get a boil or spot, it is very slow to resolve and usually does not burst. Although they may be very tired, they are determined and will push themselves hard.

ZINCUM METALLICUM is another possible medicine for CFS. A particularly characteristic feature of these people is that they have fidgety, twitchy feet.

Western Herbal Medicine

Herbal practitioners view CFS as a disease resulting from neuro-endocrine exhaustion – the body, mind and spirit lack the resources needed to restore normal immune and nervous function. There has been little formal research specifically into the use of herbal medicine for CFS, but herbalists traditionally use cayenne (*Capsicum frutescens*), echinacea (*Echinacea*

CIRCULATORY STIMULANTS Cayenne pepper, ginkgo and prickly ash (*Zanthoxylum spp.*) increase blood flow (and thus nutrient supply) to the peripheral parts of the body, especially to the head. They also have helpful antioxidant actions. Relatively large doses may be prescribed.

The use of ginkgo in CFS, due to its circulatory stimulant and neuroprotective actions within the brain, is particularly important. Cayenne – and in particular capsaicin, one of its key active constituents – has potent antioxidant and anti-inflammatory actions.

GLANDULAR TONICS Dandelion (*Taraxacum officinale*) root, kelp (*Luminaria spp.*) and liquorice (*Glycyrrhiza glabra*) support and strengthen the liver and endocrine glands, in particular the thyroid and adrenal glands.

ADAPTOGENS American ginseng (*Eleutherococcus senticosus*), Siberian ginseng (*Panax quinquefolius*) and schisandra (*Schizandra chinensis*) are important for people with CFS because they help the body to respond effectively (to adapt) to things that cause stress such as cold, chemical toxins and anxiety.

analysis and some urine tests, are unreliable. Some researchers also doubt the effectiveness of chelation therapy in removing mercury from the body.

DETOXIFICATION To improve the symptoms of chronic fatigue syndrome it is important to remove possible environmental toxins from the body (or "detoxify"). This can be done through changes in the diet (for example, following one of the many possible low-allergenic diets). It also is a good idea to take liver-tonic herbs such as milk thistle and supplements, such as vitamin C, vitamin E, selenium, green tea and mixed carotenes. (*For help with detoxification, consult a qualified herbalist or nutritionist.*)

LIGHT THERAPY When over 100 people with CFS were studied, it was found that major symptoms in about a third of the participants were strongly influenced by season. It appears that a sub-group of patients with CFS show seasonal variation in symptoms resembling those of seasonal affective disorder (*see p.432*), in which symptoms are worse in the winter. Light therapy has been found to provide some people with CFS with an effective alternative or additional treatment to anti-depressant drugs.

Acupuncture

CFS has many associated symptoms, in particular irritable bowel and muscle pain. While there are no rigorous clinical trials of acupuncture and the treatment of CFS, many individuals who experience this condition use acupuncture and report considerable benefit. There is no doubt that there is evidence for the treatment of individual symptoms, such as muscle pain, with acupuncture. There is also a clear case for the use of acupuncture within the context of a traditional Chinese approach to CFS, in that "re-balancing the body's energy" is likely to be of benefit. However, acupuncture alone will not prove effective and needs to be used in association with other approaches.

Acupuncture in general should be given weekly for six to eight weeks as the only new treatment, to enable both the patient and the therapist to judge whether it is having any real benefit.

Massage

Massage therapy, which is noted for its ability to improve well-being, has been found to be very helpful in the overall treatment of CFS. In one study, there was an immediate improvement in feelings of depression and anxiety after a single massage was given to participants. After 10 days of daily massage, researchers noted "fatigue-related symptoms, particularly emotional stress... were reduced, as were depression, difficulty sleeping and pain."

Breathing Retraining

Researchers have found that hyperventilation (shallow, fast breathing) is common in CFS patients. Such patterns of breathing can create or contribute to a variety of CFS symptoms, including anxiety, fatigue, poor stamina and muscle pain. Breathing retraining of one sort or another, often yoga-based, can be very helpful in easing these symptoms (*see p.62*).

Exercise

PRIMARY TREATMENT People with long-term CFS withdraw from all activity and lose fitness and muscle strength. A programme aimed at gradually increasing physical activity is likely to be recommended; research shows this helps to reduce fatigue and improves quality of life.

However, exercise needs to be carefully controlled for people with CFS. People with CFS respond poorly to anything more than exercise within current tolerance and can feel even more exhausted unless the process is carefully monitored.

In one study, the response to exercise of a group of 15 people with CFS was compared to that of a group of 15 healthy people of the same age and gender. The CFS patients had weaker heart function and respiratory responses during and after exercise compared to the control group.

On the positive side, in three trials involving 350 adults, patients with CFS had weekly exercise sessions for 3–4 months. They also had advice on coping with the condition and pacing themselves. The results suggest that graded exercise programmes reduce fatigue and improve quality of life, and may be as helpful for CFS as cognitive behavioural therapy.

Psychological Therapies

PRIMARY TREATMENT Psychological therapies are useful in treating CFS, but not because this illness is "all in the mind". The most successful treatment strategies for CFS involve cognitive behavioural therapy.

Treatment aims to overcome illness-perpetuating behaviours. The most important starting point is usually to promote a regular pattern of non-stressful activity, rest and sleep, with a gradual return to normal activity. At the same time, it is important to reduce anxiety and depression.

COGNITIVE BEHAVIOURAL THERAPY helps people to recognise their habitual reactions to the illness and then change negative patterns of thinking. It does not work for everyone: there is no satisfactory evidence for the effectiveness of CBT in patients with milder CFS or in patients who are so disabled by the condition that they are unable to come to treatment as outpatients. There is also no satisfactory evidence for the effectiveness of group cognitive behavioural therapy in treating CFS.

For some people, however, CBT can be very effective. A 1991 study showed it led to substantial improvements in overall disability, fatigue and physical and psychiatric symptoms. These improvements depended on the strength of the participants' belief that their symptoms were due exclusively to physical causes and were not influenced by the length of illness. The study also suggested that advice to avoid physical and mental activity in CFS is not appropriate.

A later study reviewed the psychological treatments for treating CFS. The results showed CBT significantly improved physical functioning in people with CFS compared to orthodox medical management or just relaxation therapy alone.

A recent study also showed that CBT was significantly more effective than guided support groups in relieving fatigue and functional impairment.

If you have CBT, you will probably attend weekly sessions, which last about 50 minutes each. How long initial treatment continues depends on the individual. It is generally necessary to continue with less frequent treatment for about six months after the end of the initial treatment. It is important to carry on practising the technique daily after regular treatment ends.

WHAT ARE THE SYMPTOMS?

- Insomnia
- Fatigue
- Headaches
- Irritability
- Problems concentrating

WHY MIGHT I HAVE THIS?

TRIGGERS

- Long-distance air travel in which time zones are crossed

TREATMENT PLAN

PRIMARY TREATMENTS

- Self-help measures (*see right*)

BACK-UP TREATMENTS

- Melatonin (not available in the UK)
- Light therapy

WORTH CONSIDERING

- Exercise
- Chiropractic
- Acupressure
- Acupuncture

For an explanation of how treatments are rated, see p.111.

JET LAG

The condition known as jet lag occurs as a result of long-distance air travel in which time zones are crossed. Many people find that jet lag is worse when they fly from the west to the east, or when they take an overnight flight. Some symptoms that are often associated with jet lag, such as a dry nose and throat or muscle aches, are probably due to being in the dry and often cramped atmosphere of the jet itself and not to crossing time zones. Many simple measures, such as lifestyle adjustments and exercise, can help make jet lag symptoms less severe.

WHY DOES IT OCCUR?

Within the hypothalamus in the brain is a tiny structure called the suprachiasmatic nucleus (SCN) which controls the body's sleep–wake cycle. In the morning when light is detected by the retina at the back of the eye, signals are transmitted to the SCN via the optic nerve. Messages are then relayed to the pineal gland to switch off production of melatonin, a hormone that induces drowsiness. When darkness falls, levels of melatonin start to rise again.

Jet lag arises because normal patterns of eating, sleeping and waking are not yet synchronised with the local time, giving rise to a range of symptoms that may include difficulty in sleeping, tiredness and headaches. It can take up to five days before the sleep–wake cycle is reset to the new time. It is not the length of the flight that determines whether jet lag, but how many time zones are passed through. Flying north to south within the same zone does not usually cause problems.

In addition, general health, age and lifestyle play a part in susceptibility to jet lag. Overeating, smoking and drinking alcohol tend to make it worse.

SELF-HELP

PRIMARY TREATMENT The following tips may help to keep jet lag to a minimum.

- Get plenty of sleep before you travel and take it easy when you arrive.
- When you board the flight, try to adjust your eating and sleeping patterns to the local time at the destination.
- Drink two glasses of water before the flight and plenty of fluids during it. Avoid alcohol and caffeinated drinks.
- Get up and walk around at regular intervals during the flight. This also helps to counter deep vein thrombosis.
- Make sure you get some exercise outside in daylight after you arrive at your destination and try to resist having a nap during the day.

TREATMENTS IN DETAIL

Conventional Medicine

ADVICE Your doctor may give you advice on how to minimise the effects of jet lag (*see Self-help, above*) and how you can cope if you have to take medication at regular intervals.

MELATONIN, the hormone that is largely responsible for regulating sleep, has been found to be useful for jet lag. It is not yet licensed in the UK. Research suggests that it may be helpful for people flying across five or more time zones, especially if they are flying east. Jet lag symptoms associated with crossing time zones have been found to be reduced with quick recovery of pre-flight energy and alertness levels.

Homeopathy

The homeopathic medicine most often recommended for jet lag is *Nux vomica*. This medicine is appropriate for sleep disturbance (especially when this involves waking too early), digestive disturbances and a dry, stuffy nose.

Other medicines that may help are *Kalium phosphoricum*, which is suitable when the person is exhausted, being too tired to sleep. Those whom it helps may also have disturbing dreams. *Arnica* is indicated when there are bruise-like aches and pains, which may be so severe that even the bed feels too hard.

Exercise

A study looked at the effect of exercising for a few hours on the day after a plane journey from Tokyo to Los Angeles (which is an eight-hour time difference). The researchers concluded that outdoor exercise hastens the resetting of the body's internal "clock", helping people to become synchronised to a new time zone.

In general, it is important to get as much exercise as you can during a flight. Walking up and down the aisle, standing for a while from time to time, and doing small twisting and stretching exercises in your seat can all help reduce discomfort, especially swelling of legs and feet. Get off the plane if possible at stopovers and do some exercises or take a walk. It is also helpful to get some exercise outside when you land.

Light Therapy

A most effective treatment for the general malaise of jet lag seems to be exposure to natural light, or exposure to the light from a natural full-spectrum light box or bulb. Stimulus from natural light is needed for the pineal gland to reduce secretion of melatonin, and a lack of light is a recognised cause of jet lag. Prolonged exposure to bright artificial daylight has proved effective in easing jet lag symptoms.

Acupuncture

While there are no clinical trials supporting the use of acupuncture in jet lag, acupuncturists believe that it appears to be effective and there are good theoretical reasons for supposing that this is the case. Acupuncture can be used to balance minor energetic dysfunctions, for example. It has also been used extensively in the treatment of insomnia and anxiety, symptoms that are frequently associated with jet lag. Acupuncture also has fundamental effects on neurotransmitters, the chemical messengers within the brain, and appears to balance and normalise the release and uptake of these chemicals within the brain.

Ideally, acupuncture should be given to balance the body a day or two before you

MELATONIN LEVELS AND JET LAG

Melatonin is a hormone produced in the pineal gland that is largely responsible for regulating the sleep–wake cycle. Melatonin is normally produced at night and seems to act as a signal to the body that it is dark. Levels of melatonin therefore tend to rise and fall with the hours of darkness and daylight. When people travel by plane across many time zones, their melatonin levels will initially be out of step with their new local time zone, making it difficult for them to sleep and wake at the right times.

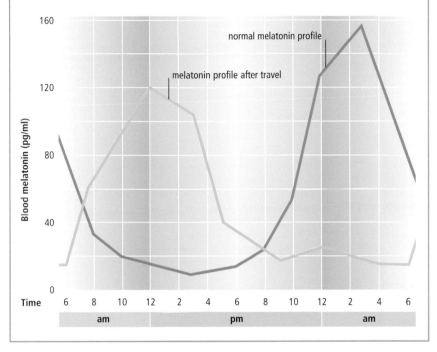

take a flight across several time zones, and then daily for three or four days after the flight. Often this will be part of a more generalised use of acupuncture to strengthen the body as a whole.

Bodywork Therapies

ACUPRESSURE Traditional Chinese Medicine has identified what it calls a horary cycle. In this cycle, energy circulates through the main acupuncture meridians, or energy pathways, in a very specific order. Acupressure on particular "horary [time-related] points" is used to treat or to prevent jet lag. An informal study has been reported that was conducted by a group of acupuncturists travelling from the United States to China. They divided into two groups, with one group acting as a control. The other group used acupressure treatments on their horary points while travelling.

After arrival, the control group experienced jet lag symptoms lasting from three days to two weeks. The group who treated themselves with acupressure experienced no jet lag symptoms. On the return trip, the groups switched and the results were similar, with those who used acupressure experiencing no jet lag symptoms.

CHIROPRACTIC It may be helpful to have a chiropractic session before and/or after you fly: one study evaluated the benefits of chiropractic treatment in relation to jet lag in athletes. One group of athletes received chiropractic treatment before flying, compared to two other groups, one of which received placebo (false) treatment and the other no treatment at all.

The results showed that the chiropractic care group had fewer jet lag symptoms and felt better overall than those in either of the other two groups. Those athletes who received chiropractic treatment also slept an average of one hour longer per night and experienced fewer disruptions in sleep patterns than athletes in either the placebo group or the control group.

GLOSSARY OF TERMS

A

Acupoint Term used in Traditional Chinese Medicine for a specific point on a meridian where the flow of *Qi* is accessible. Acupoints are stimulated by acupressure and acupuncture.

Acupressure Ancient Chinese massage that uses the thumbs and fingertips on acupoints to restore a healthy balance to an individual's energy.

Acupuncture Cornerstone therapy of Traditional Chinese Medicine in which ailments and disorders are treated by using needles to stimulate acupoints.

Acute A symptom or disorder that comes on suddenly.

Adaptogenic Restores balance within the body.

Adipose Relating to fat tissue, which is composed of cells called adipocytes.

Agglutination Term meaning sticking together – for example, sperm or red blood cells.

Aggravation A homeopathic term that means a worsening of symptoms.

Alexander technique Method of correcting imbalances in posture, with the aim of restoring health to both body and mind.

Alkaloids Organic compounds, such as nicotine and caffeine, that can be toxic yet are medicinally useful.

Allergen An environmental or dietary irritant which can trigger an allergic reaction in sensitive people.

Allergenic Sensitive to an environmental or dietary irritant.

Alpha blockers Drugs that interfere with nerve signals to the muscles. Used in the relief of urine retention, they work by relaxing the sphincter muscle of the bladder.

Alterative Term used in herbal medicine meaning restorative.

Amitriptyline Tricyclic antidepressant that is used to improve mood, activity levels and encourage sleep in long-term depression.

Anaemia Blood disease in which haemoglobin is deficient or abnormal.

Analgesics Drugs that relieve pain.

Androgen Male sex hormone.

Angiotensin-converting enzyme (ACE) inhibitors Powerful vasodilators that block an enzyme involved in blood-vessel constriction.

Antacids Mildly alkaline compounds that neutralise excess stomach acid.

Antibiotics Drugs that kill bacteria.

Antibody Protein in the blood responsible for destroying an invading substance or pathogen that the body considers to be harmful.

Anticonvulsants Drugs that inhibit excessive activity in the brain and are used to prevent and stop epileptic fits.

Antidepressants Drugs for treating moderate to severe depression.

Antifungals Drugs for killing fungi or inhibiting their growth.

Antigen Protein located on the surface of an invading micro-organism that stimulates the white blood cells to produce antibodies.

Antihistamines Drugs that counter the effects of histamine, a chemical released in the body during an allergic reaction.

Antihypertensives Drugs for reducing high blood pressure.

Anti-inflammatories Drugs, such as NSAIDs and corticosteroids, that relieve inflammation.

Antioxidants Chemicals that neutralise free radicals.

Aphthous ulcers Ulcers in the lining of the mouth; they may occur in oral thrush.

Aqueous Relating to water.

Arachidonic acid Derivative of an essential fatty acid that produces substances causing inflammation.

Arginine Amino acid essential for sperm formation.

Arrhythmia Disrupted heart rhythm.

Arterial plaque Deposit of fat on the inner wall of an artery.

Arteriosclerosis Hardening of the arteries.

Asana Physical posture in yoga.

Astringent Substance that contracts tissue and reduces a discharge or secretion.

ATP Adenosine triphosphate, a high-energy molecule in cells.

Atria The chambers of the upper heart chambers.

Autogenic training Relaxation therapy. Six mental exercises relieve stress and promote self-healing.

Autoimmune Term applied to disorders in which the body's immune system produces antibodies that attack its own tissues.

Autonomic nervous system Part of the nervous system that controls body functions such as breathing and heart rate which are not under conscious control.

Anxiolytic Term used to describe a chemical that relieves anxiety.

B

Balneotherapy Traditional spa therapy in which bathing improves well-being and helps to heal disorders of the skin, muscles and joints.

Benign Of no danger to health i.e. cell growth is under control and non-cancerous.

Benzodiazepines Anti-anxiety drugs that reduce excessive activity in the part of the brain that controls emotion.

Beta-blockers Drugs to reduce heart rate and prevent dilation of blood vessels by blocking the action of the neurotransmitter noradrenaline in the sympathetic nervous system.

Beta-endorphin Pain-relieving chemical found in the brain.

Biofeedback Interactive relaxation therapy in which feedback machines enable individuals to control their own body functions, such as muscle tension, brainwave patterns and electrical skin resistance.

Bioflavonoid Chemical that aids the absorption of vitamin C by the body.

Biphosphonates Drugs that treat bone disorders, such as osteoporosis.

Bodywork Term used to describe manipulative therapies or techniques, such as massage.

Bone mineral density (BMD) Measure of bone mass, often tested in osteoporosis.

Breathing retraining Learning to control the rate of abdominal breathing.

Bronchiectasis Permanent widening of the airways associated with a persistent productive cough and eventually shortness of breath.

C

Calcium-channel blockers Drugs that block the entry of calcium into muscle cells, allowing blood vessels to dilate.

Candida albicans A yeast-like micro-organism that occurs naturally in the mouth, gut and vagina, and on the skin. It is normally controlled by "friendly" bacteria.

Cardiorespiratory Relating to the heart and respiration.

Cardiovascular Relating to the heart and circulation.

Carminative A herb or drug that calms cramp or induces gas expulsion from the stomach or the intestines.

Cauda equina The array of nerves at the bottom of the spinal cord.

Chelation Binding of a metal and filtering it from the bloodstream by chemical means.

Chemonucleolysis Chemical breakdown of the nucleus of a vertebral disc.

Chiropractic Manipulation therapy that diagnoses and treats disorders of the spine and other joints of the body.

Cholesterol One of the major fats found in the blood and most tissues

Chronic Term to describe symptoms and conditions that are long-lasting and slow to change.

Chronic venous insufficiency Persistent lack of blood in the veins.

Clinical trial A scientific study to assess the safety and effectiveness of a medical treatment.

Clot Semi-solid mass of blood, also called a thrombus.

Co-enzyme Q10 An antioxidant nutrient, also known as ubiquinone, that the body makes to help it release energy from food. Also available as a supplement.

Cognitive behavioural therapy (CBT) Form of psychotherapy pioneered in the 1960s and based on a belief in the ability of the mind to change negative patterns of thinking and behaviour.

Collagen Tough protein found in bone and cartilage.

Compress Pad of fabric (usually cold) for relieving pain or inflammation.

Coronary Relating to the arteries that supply the muscles of the heart.

Coronary thrombosis Blood clot in a coronary artery.

Corticosteroids (or steroids) Anti-inflammatory drugs that suppress allergic responses and the immune system, and help in the treatment of conditions caused by deficiency of adrenal gland hormones.

Cranial osteopathy Otheopathy that focuses on correcting distortions in the bones of the skull (cranium) and face.

Craniosacral therapy Form of cranial osteopathy that adjusts the pressure on the membranes and fluids surrounding the brain and spinal cord.

Crossover trial A form of clinical trial in which patients receive both treatments in sequence, half taking one treatment first, and the other half the other treatment first.

CT (Computer Tomography) scans Diagnostic technique that combines X-rays and computers to produce a cross-section of a tissue under examination. Also called CAT (Computer Axial Tomography) scans.

Cyst Small, benign tumour filled with fluid or soft tissue.

Cytokine Drug that stimulates the immune system to attack the cells of certain cancers.

Cytotoxic test Diagnostic technique in which damage to white blood cells when mixed with extracts of a possible allergen is said to suggest sensitivity.

D

Decoction Brew obtained from boiling a herb in water.

Deep vein thrombosis Blood clot in a deep-lying vein, usually in the leg.

Demulcent Substance that soothes irritated membranes and tissues.

Dermatologist A medical practitioner who specialises in conditions of the skin

Diastolic blood pressure Lower of the two figures when blood pressure is measured.

Diuretic Chemical that stimulates urine production.

Dorsal root ganglia Groups of cells clustered at the point where the 12 dorsal nerves emerge from the spinal cord.

E

Eicosanoids Chemicals, derived from omega-6 fatty acids, that help to regulate inflammation and the flow of blood.

Echocardiography Ultrasound scanning of the heart.

Electromyographic (EMG) biofeedback Relaxation therapy in which biofeedback sensors, when placed on back or shoulder muscles, emit a rhythmic sound or flashing light in response to the strength of the muscle tension.

Embrocation Lotion for soothing a sore or pulled muscle.

Emollient Softening or smoothing the skin.

Endorphins Morphine-like substances produced by the body to relieve pain. Also known as the body's natural opiates.

Endoscopy Examination of a body cavity, such as the stomach, by means of a tube-like viewing instrument called an endoscope.

Endotoxin Toxin produced inside the body.

Enzyme Protein that speeds up a biochemical reaction.

Enthesitis Inflammation where a tendon attaches to a bone.

Epidermal (relating to the epidermis, or the outer layer of skin).

Epididymides Tightly coiled tubes that lie above and behind each testes where sperm are stored and mature.

Epidural space Space surrounding the membranes that envelop the spinal cord.

Essential fatty acid Polyunsaturated fatty acids that must be supplied in the diet because they are not made in the body. Two main types are omega-6 and omega-3.

Erythrocyte Red blood cell.

Etiology Cause of a particular disease.

Exfoliant Skin remover.

Exposure therapy Psychological technique designed to help a patient overcome the anxiety of a trauma or fear by carefully managed exposure to the trauma or fear.

Eye movement desensitisation and reprocessing (EMDR) Psychological technique that combines elements of exposure therapy and cognitive behaviour therapy.

F

Fistula An abnormal channel between organs or body cavities that normally do not connect, or between an organ or cavity and the skin.

Fatty acid The basic chemical building block of fats and oils.

Flavonoids Antioxidant chemicals thought to help prevent certain forms of cancer. In nature, flavonoids are found in fruits such as lemons, plums and blackcurrants.

Fluorescein angiography Photographic technique that makes use of a fluorescent dye (fluorescein) to study the blood vessels of the eye.

Food allergen Food that initiates an immune reaction.

Free radical Potentially harmful molecules produced by the body which can damage DNA and cause a range of physiological problems.

G

Ganglion Cluster of nerve cells.

Gastric Relating to or involving the stomach.

Gestalt therapy Method of psychotherapy that helps clients to gain self-awareness through analysing their thoughts, feelings and behaviour with the therapist in a variety of situations and scenarios.

Glycaemic Relating to the level of sugar in the blood.

Guided imagery Psychological technique that involves a patient concentrating their imagination on a particular part of their body.

H

H2 blockers Anti-ulcer drugs that help healing by preventing the release of histamine in the stomach, so reducing acid production.

Hatha yoga A form of yoga that uses physical postures (*asanas*) and breathing.

Heberden's nodes Bony spurs on the end joints of the fingers.

Hernia/herniation Protrusion of an internal organ through a ruptured cavity wall.

Histamine Chemical that is essential to the body's immune system and is central to the body's allergic reactions.

Holistic Term used to describe an approach to treatment in which the "whole" person is taken into account, rather than just the symptoms.

Homeostasis Constant state of the body's functions, such as the temperature and acidity of the blood, which feedback mechanisms restore to normal if they are disturbed.

Hydrogenation Process by which edible oils are treated to become solid.

Hydrolysates Protein molecules within milk.

Hydrotherapy Techniques in which water is used to stimulate the body and promote self-healing.

Hyperventilation Breathing too deeply or too rapidly so that the carbon dioxide level of the blood falls. It causes numbness of the hands and feet, faintness, muscle spasms and twitches.

Hypnotherapy Technique in which a patient is hypnotised and temporarily hands over control to a therapist, who initiates mental and physical changes in the patient.

Hypo-allergenic Containing minimal levels of potential allergens

Hypoglycaemia Low blood sugar.

I

Imagery Psychological technique that uses positive images and thought processes to invoke the senses and bring about healing.

Immunosuppressants Drugs that suppress the activity of the immune system.

Infusion Herbal tea.

Interpersonal therapy Psychological technique in which individuals are encouraged to examine and change the way they relate to other people.

Ischaemic Lack of blood supply.

IU (International Unit) A unit of potency for a vitamin or other biologically active substance accepted as an international standard.

KL

Keratolytic Loosening of dead and hardened cells on the surface of the skin.

Kinesiology Method of detecting body system imbalances, as well as food and environmental sensitivities, by testing muscle resistance.

Lactose A form of sugar found in milk.

Lens capsule Thin layer that encloses the lens.

Lesion Change in a tissue or organ due to a disease.

Leukocyte White blood cell.

Libido Sexual urge.

Lidocaine (lignocaine) Anaesthetic that is also used to combat arrhythmia and itching.

Liniment Oily cream for soothing muscle pain.

Liposuction A surgical procedure in which fatty tissue is removed through an incision in the skin.

Liver-tonifying Invigorating the liver.

Loin perineum Region between the anus and the scrotum in men.

Lutein One of a group of yellow carotenoid pigments.

Lymphatic pump techniques Gentle manipulation techniques used by massage and other therapists to encourage the flow of lymph fluid through the body's lymphatic system.

Lymphocytes White blood cells that recognise the antigens of invading bacteria and then produce antibodies to them.

Lymphocytes (T, or T-cells) White blood cells that recognise the antigens of viruses, parasites and cancer cells, and then multiply to fight them.

Lysine An essential amino acid that the body needs to extract from food. Thought to help prevent and treat cold sores and herpes infections.

M

McKenzie-concept exercises Self-treatment exercises to relieve back pain, particularly of the low back. Developed by Robin McKenzie, they focus on improving the structure and metabolism of the soft tissues, such as the discs between the vertebrae of the spine.

Magnetic resonance imaging *See* MRI scans.

Meditation Self-help technique for mastering your thoughts and feelings, bringing relaxation and refreshment to both mind and body.

Meninges Membranes that cover the brain and spinal cord.

Mensendieck exercises Exercises developed by Bess Mensendieck to train the musculoskeletal system.

Meridians Term used in Traditional Chinese Medicine. The meridians are the energy channels in the body through which *Qi* (energy) flows.

Meta-analysis Systematic review of a number of research studies and clinical trials that provide a more accurate picture of the total evidence available.

Metabolism General term for the chemical processes that govern all the functions of the body.

Microflora Term to describe the "friendly" bacteria in the intestine.

Mind–body therapies Techniques and approaches that harness thoughts, feelings, imagination and actions in order to influence biochemical and structural processes.

Mono-amine oxidase inhibitors (MAOIs) Antidepressant drugs that increase levels of serotonin and other mood-enhancing brain chemicals.

Motility Term applied to the ability of sperm to swim along.

MRI (Magnetic Resonance Imaging) scans Diagnostic technique that uses high-frequency radio waves to examine the structures of the body, particularly the central nervous system.

Mucilage Gum-like substance found in plants that becomes slippery and viscous in water. Used to soothe tissues.

Myocardial infarction Medical term for a heart attack.

Myofascial Relating to deep muscle tissues.

N

Nebuliser Device which turns a liquid drug into a fine spray, or aerosol. Used in asthma.

Neonate Newborn child.

Neurological Relating to the nerves.

Neuromuscular therapy (NMT) Manipulation therapy that enhances the mechanics of the body, releases endorphins and restores the healthy relationship between nerves and the musculoskeletal system.

Neuropathy Disrupted function of one or more nerves.

Neurotransmitter A chemical that is released from the end of a nerve which transmits impulses to another nerve or to a muscle cell.

Neurotoxic Poisonous to nerves.

Nodules Small, red swellings.

Nosodes Homeopathic remedy made from a disease product.

NSAIDs Non-steroidal anti-inflammatory drugs that relieve pain, stiffness and painful inflammation in the muscles, bones and joints.

O

Oedema Tissue swollen with fluid.

Oestrogenic Describe chemicals that have oestrogen-like action.

Oral Relating to or involving the mouth.

Orthodontic Relating to the alignment of teeth and jaws.

Orthotic Shock-absorbing foot support device.

Ossicles Tiny bones of the middle ear.

Osteopathy Manipulation therapy that diagnoses and treats structural and biomechanical problems in the body's musculoskeletal framework.

Oxidative attack Damage by free radicals.

P

Papules Inflamed spots.

Pathogenic Disease-causing.

PENS (Percutaneous Electrical Nerve Stimulation) Similar to TENS, except the pulses of low-voltage electricity are delivered into the soft tissue via needles that puncture the skin.

PET (Positron Emission Tomography) scans Diagnostic technique in conventional medicine that uses injected radioactive substances to detect the chemical activity in a tissue or organ and also to assess blood flow.

Photochemical Relating to a reaction that either needs light or UV radiation or else produces light.

Phytoestrogens Chemicals from plants, such as the soya bean and other pulses, with properties similar to oestrogen.

Pilates Conditioning technique that increases the body's flexibility and strength.

Placebo Chemically inert substance given in place of a drug. Used in medical drug trials as a control.

Plantar fasciitis Injury to the sole of the foot.

Platelets Blood-cell fragments involved in clotting.

Postpartum primapara Term used to describe a woman who has just given birth to her first child.

Probiotics "Friendly", disease-destroying bacteria in the gut that help in the manufacture of vitamins and enzymes, and so aid digestion.

Progressive relaxation (also Jacobson's Progressive Relaxation) Technique developed by Edmund Jacobson that alternately tenses and relaxes muscles of the body in an orderly sequence from the toes to the head.

Prophylaxis Preventative measures.

Prostaglandins Drugs or naturally occurring substances within the body that cause muscle contractions and produce mucus in the lining of the stomach.

Prosthesis Artificial body part.

Proteolytic Protein-digesting.

Psychodynamic therapy Psychological technique which encourages an individual to actively bring their true painful feelings from their subconscious and to consciously face them.

Psycho-education Psychological technique aimed at increasing an individual's knowledge and insight into their particular mental illness.

Psychotherapy Psychological technique in which an individual discusses their personal feelings, experiences, behaviour with a counsellor trained to help draw out and resolve any mental problems.

Psychotropic Term used to describe a substance that influences behaviour by affecting the mind.

Pulse-testing Traditional Chinese diagnostic technique in which nine pulse points are monitored to check the quality of *Qi* (energy).

Pustules Raised, pus-filled spots with a white centre.

QR

Qi (also chi) Life energy force of Traditional Chinese Medicine that flows through the body along meridians and can be accessed at acupoints. It is said to be inherited at conception and to be derived from fresh food and air.

Radiotherapy Use of radioactivity to treat cancer and, occasionally, other diseases.

Range of motion The normal amount that joint can be moved in certain directions

Referred pain Sensation experienced as a result of spinal problems that can affect nerves and muscles linked to other parts of the body, causing problems in those areas.

Reflexology Therapy that treats various ailments by massaging particular "reflex areas" on the feet (or, more rarely, the hands) with thumb or finger.

Renal Relating to the kidney.

Resorption Breaking down and absorbing a substance.

S

Sensitiser Chemical that sensitises the immune system to a specific allergen.

Serotonin Neurotransmitter that calms the mind and helps to induce sleep.

Selective serotonin uptake inhibitors (SSRIs) Antidepressants that keep serotonin levels high.

Sick building syndrome Condition in which fatigue, lack of concentration and recurrent infections are attributed to poor ventilation and chemical fumes from furnishings and office machines.

Sleep apnoea Temporary yet repeated interruption of breathing during sleep.

Sp. Abbreviation for species.

Spondylolisthesis Condition in which one vertebra slips forwards over the vertebra beneath.

Statins Drugs that lower blood cholesterol. Used to prevent stroke and heart attack.

Stagnation Term applied to *Qi* (energy) when it ceases to flow.

Steroidal Relating to a steroid.

Stress hormones Hormones, such as adrenaline and cortisol, which are released under stress.

Stroke Interruption in the brain's blood supply.

Sub-fertile Term applied to men when they are unable to produce normal sperm.

Supplements Nutrients, such as vitamins, minerals and trace elements, which can be taken to supplement the diet.

Synovial Relating to the fluid secreted by the lining of a joint.

Systematic desensitisation Psychological technique that combines relaxation and exposure to images of a feared object (e.g. a picture of a spider) to help the person conquer their fears.

Systemic therapy Class of talking therapies that combine cybernetics and anthropology to help resolve psychological problems within a "system", such as a family or group.

T

Tendinitis Painful inflammation of a tendon.

Tenosynovitis Painful swelling of a tendon and the synovial membrane of a joint.

TENS (Transcutaneous Electrical Nerve Stimulation) Stimulation of body tissue with pulses of low-voltage electricity for relieving pain.

Thrombolytic Breaking down a thrombus, or blood clot.

Tincture Herb extract in alcohol.

Topical Applied externally to the skin.

Traction Steady extension of a limb or muscle.

Trans-fatty acids Fats that occur naturally in meat and dairy products, and also in man-made foods such as margarines, where edible oils are treated to become solid (hydrogenation).

Trial, clinical Research which is used to establish scientific proof of a therapy or treatment – for example, the efficacy and safety of a new pharmaceutical drug or herbal remedy.

Trial, controlled A method of testing a treatment in which an experimental group receives the treatment and the control group receives none.

Trial, placebo controlled A method of testing a drug or a treatment in which the treatment must be shown to make a significant difference compared to a placebo (an inactive medicine or treatment).

Trial, randomised A clinical scientific trial in which large numbers of patients participate in order to cancel out individual differences.

Trial, randomised double-blind In this type of randomised trial neither the patients nor the practitioners know who is receiving the treatment and who is not.

Tricyclic antidepressants Drugs that raise the levels of neurotransmitters, such as serotonin and noradrenaline, involved in mood.

Triglyceride One of the major fats in the blood and in the cells of fat (adipose) tissue.

Trigger point A knot of tense muscle, which feels like a hard nodule when pressed. Trigger point may caused by pain from the spine and connective tissue.

UV

Ultrasound High-frequency sound technique used to scan internal organs and the foetus in the womb, and to treat soft-tissue injuries.

UV light Light containing ultraviolet wavelengths, which has antiviral, antifungal and antibacterial properties.

Vasa deferentia Tubes that transport sperm away from the epididymides towards the urethra.

Vascular disease Disease of the blood vessels.

Vasodilators Drugs that widen blood vessels. They are used to treat angina and high blood pressure.

Ventricles The lower heart chambers.

Vesicles Small blisters containing serum.

Viability Ability of sperm to fertilise the egg.

Visualisation Psychological therapy in which an individual is encouraged to consciously imagine particularly positive and beneficial events as a way of preventing self-fulfilling, negative patterns of behaviour.

WXYZ

Yin and yang Opposing but complementary energies in Traditional Chinese Medicine. All things are said to be a manifestation of *yin* and *yang*.

FINDING A PRACTITIONER

Being able to trust your practitioner and feeling a sense of rapport with him or her are vital factors in the healing process and should be considered when looking for a complementary practitioner. Competence is another key factor. Finding a good practitioner can be a matter of trial and error, so many people prefer word-of-mouth recommendations. Establishing adequate standards of training, ethical practice and disciplinary procedures for complementary therapies has always proved a problem. Although some practitioners complete three to four years of full or part-time degree studies, others have only had a weekend correspondence course.

This lack of regulation means you have little means of redress should anything go wrong or should you be dissatisfied with your treatment. At the very least, you need to feel confident that any undiagnosed serious condition would be recognised and that you would be advised to seek medical help if your practitioner suspected the problem lay beyond his or her expertise.

If you are considering trying chiropractic, osteopathy, acupuncture, psychotherapy, counselling or hypnotherapy, it is worth asking your doctor whether he or she can recommend a practitioner, as these therapies are becoming more accepted in mainstream medicine. Some GP practices even include practitioners from these fields. Additionally, some conventional health professionals may be qualified in acupuncture or homeopathy.

If you are choosing a complementary practitioner for yourself, you should consider the following issues. The list below is based on a checklist drawn up by the Royal College of Nursing and also includes suggestions from the British Medical Association.

Training and credentials

Always ensure that the practitioner is adequately trained and reputable, especially if the therapy involves the use of either physical manipulation or invasive techniques (e.g. if you swallow medication or have needles inserted into you). Ask the following questions:

- What are the practitioner's qualifications?

- What sort of training was undertaken, and for how long?

- For how many years has the practitioner been in practice?

- Will the practitioner advise your doctor of any treatment?

Professional organisations

Some disciplines have professional associations that regulate training and practice. These associations provide a code of conduct and maintain a register of members. For other disciplines, particularly non-invasive therapies, standards vary greatly and there may not be a single representative body. In the case of these therapies, you should be sure to ask the following questions:

- Is the practitioner registered with a recognised organisation, and does this organisation have a public register of practitioners?

- Does the organisation have a code of practice specifying the professional conduct required?

- Does the organisation have a complaints system and an effective disciplinary procedure and sanctions?

- Can the practitioner give you the address and telephone number of his or her professional organisation?

Financial considerations

When choosing any healthcare, financial considerations are important. A length course of therapy could be very expensive. Is the treatment available at little or no personal cost on referral by your doctor? Note that some therapies, such as chiropractic, osteopathy, homeopathy, acupuncture and psychotherapy, may be available through a limited number of mainstream health practices.

- Can you claim for the treatment through your private health insurance scheme if you have one?

- What is the cost (both short- and long-term) of the treatment?

- How many treatments might you expect to require?

- Does the practitioner have professional indemnity insurance so that you receive compensation if he or she is negligent?

Precautions

Avoid any practitioner with whom you feel uncomfortable. Trust and empathy are important when you are being treated by someone, and indeed treatment is unlikely to succeed without them. Treatment is often conducted on a one-to-one basis, and may involve removing clothes and being touched. You should also avoid any practitioner who seems to be making excessive claims about the treatment or who guarantees that a particular treatment will bring about a cure. No form of treatment – either conventional or complementary – is perfect, and miracles should neither be expected by the client nor promised by the practitioner. After your initial consultation, you should ask yourself the following questions:

- Was the practitioner's conduct and demeanour entirely professional?

- Did the practitioner answer any questions clearly and thoroughly?

- Were you given further information to read in your own time?

- Were you told how many treatments you might need?

- What was the practitioner's attitude towards any conventional medical treatment you may be receiving? You should avoid any practitioner who suggests changing (or abandoning) your conventional medicine without first consulting your doctor.

USEFUL WEBSITES AND ADDRESSES

Knowing where to go for information and help enables you to become more actively involved in your own healthcare. When you understand the causes of illness, the meaning of symptoms and what treatment options are available, you may feel more in control of your well-being – and this is therapeutic in itself.

Hundreds of associations and organisations are dedicated to helping people deal with medical and emotional conditions. Sources of information range from government agencies, such as the Department of Health, to nonprofit organisations, such as the Red Cross. Only a limited sample could be included in this list. Most listings are the headquarters of national groups and organisations. Information on a wide range of such organisations is usually available from libraries as well as from your local hospital and your own GP and health clinic.

Most organisations provide information about resources for the management of specific conditions. Many have support groups to help people with a medical or emotional condition, or they can provide information about local groups in your area. Online sites are given for the UK self-help groups and for some of the most useful US sites. Most online sites provide links to related sites.

Although the web is brimming with advice on health matters, much of it can be ill-informed, biased or downright wrong. This is especially true of interactive sites. If you put a health question to an "expert", make sure you check their credentials and know how much privacy you can expect. You should always be suspicious of "miracle cures" and should note any sponsorship or advertising deals that could indicate a bias in the advice that is given.

Caution
The publishers cannot accept responsibility for the quality of any information that may be provided by the organisations listed below.

General health information

Aetna Intelihealth
www.intelihealth.com

Alternative Health News Online
www.altmedicine.com

American Medical Association
www.ama-assn.org

Bandolier
www.jr2.ox.ac.uk/bandolier

BBC Online Health and Fitness
www.bbc.co.uk/health

British Medical Association
www.bma.org.uk
BMA House
Tavistock Square
London WC1H 9JP
(020) 7387 4499

Centers for Disease Control
and Prevention (US)
www.cdc.gov
1-800-311-3435

Centre for Reviews and Dissemination (CRD)
www.york.ac.uk/inst/crd
University of York
York YO10 5DD
(01904) 321040
crd@york.ac.uk

Consumer Health Information Centre
www.chic.org.uk
medicine advice line: (020) 8742 7042

Department of Health
www.dh.gov.uk
Richmond House
79 Whitehall
London SW1A 2NL
(020) 7210 4850
dhmail@dh.gsi.gov.uk

eBMJ (Electronic British Medical Journal)
www.bmj.com

Health Information Service
0800 665544

Health On the Net Foundation
www.hon.ch
Info@healthonnet.org

Healthfinder®
www.healthfinder.gov
healthfinder@nhic.org

Healthnet
www.healthnet.org.uk

Health Protection Agency
www.phls.co.uk
020 7339 1300

Health Supplement Information Service
www.hsis.org

Internet Health Library
www.internethealthlibrary.com

Medicines and Healthcare products Regulatory Agency (MHRA)
www.mca.gov.uk
Market Towers
1 Nine Elms Lane
London SW8 5NQ
(020) 7084 2000
info@mhra.gsi.gov.uk

National Institutes of Health (US)
www.nih.gov

National Library of Medicine (US)
www.ncbi.nlm.nih.gov/pubmed

Netdoctor
www.netdoctor.co.uk

NHS Direct
www.nhsdirect.nhs.uk
0845 4647

NHS Direct Best Treatments
www.besttreatments.co.uk

NHS Health Scotland
www.hebs.scot.nhs.uk
0131 536 5500

Office of Rare Diseases (US)
www.rarediseases.info.nih.gov

OMNI
www.omni.ac.uk

BIOME
University of Nottingham
Greenfield Medical Library
Queens Medical Centre
Nottingham NG7 2UH
0115 849 3251
help@omni.ac.uk

Patient UK
www.patient.co.uk
info@patient.co.uk

Royal College of General Practitioners
www.rcgp.org.uk
14 Princes Gate
Hyde Park
London SW7 1PU
(020) 7581 3232
info@rcgp.org.uk

Self Help UK
www.self-help.org.uk
selfhelp@intuition-comms.co.uk

Wired for Health
www.wiredforhealth.gov.uk

World Health Organization
www.who.int

Alcohol, smoking and drug dependence

Action on Smoking and Health
www.ash.org.uk
102 Clifton Street
London EC2A 4HW
(020) 7739 5902
enquiries@ash.org.uk

Addiction Recovery Agency
www.addictionrecovery.org.uk
King's Court, King's Street
Bristol BS1 4EE
(0117) 930 0282
info@addictionrecovery.org

Al-Anon Family Groups
Website www.al-anonuk.org.uk
61 Great Dover Street
London SE1 4YF
(020) 7403 0888
alanonuk@aol.com

Alcohol Concern
www.alcoholconcern.org.uk
Waterbridge House
32–36 Loman Street
London SE1 0EE
(020) 7928 7377
contact@alcoholconcern.org.uk

Alcoholics Anonymous
www.alcoholics-anonymous.org.uk
0845 769 7555

Drinksense
www.gurney.co.uk/drinksense
79A Eastfield Road
Peterborough PE1 4AS
(01733) 347105
drinksense@netcom.co.uk

Institute of Alcohol Studies
www.ias.org.uk
1 The Quay
St. Ives
Cambridgeshire PE27 5AR
(01480) 466766
info@ias.org.uk

National Association for Children of Alcoholics
www.nacoa.org.uk
PO Box 64
Fishponds
Bristol BS16 2UH
0800 358 3456
helpline@nacoa.org.uk

National Drugs Helpline
0800 776600

ADHD

The National Attention Deficit Disorder Information and Support Service
addiss.co.uk
10 Station Road
Mill Hill
London NW7 2JU
(020) 8906 9068
info@addiss.co.uk

Other websites:
www.chadd.org
www.add.org

Allergies

Anaphylaxis Campaign
www.anaphylaxis.org.uk
PO Box 275
Farnborough
Hampshire GU14 6SX
(01252) 542029
info@anaphylaxis.org.uk

Asthma and Allergy Foundation of America (US)
www.aafa.org

Asthma and Allergy Information and Research
www.users.globalnet.co.uk/~aair
Department of Respiratory Medicine

Glenfield Hospital
Groby Road
Leicester LE3 9QP
(0116) 270 7557
aair@globalnet.co.uk

Allergy UK
www.allergyuk.org
3 White Oak Square
London Road
Swanley
Kent BR8 7AG
helpline (allergy); 01322 619864
helpline (chemical sensitivity): 01322 619898
info@allergyuk.org

European Federation of Allergy and Airways Diseases Patients' Associations
www.efanet.org

Food Allergy and Anaphylaxis Alliance
www.foodallergyalliance.org

Alzheimer's disease

Alzheimer's Disease Society
www.alzheimers.org.uk
10 Greencoat Place
London SW1P 1PH
0845 300 0336
enquiries@alzheimers.org.uk

Ankylosing spondylitis

National Ankylosing Spondylitis Society
www.nass.co.uk
PO Box 179
Mayfield
East Sussex TN20 6ZL
(01435) 873527
nass@nass.co.uk

Other websites:
www.spondylitis.org

Arthritis and rheumatism

Arthritis Care
www.arthritiscare.org.uk
18 Stephenson Way
London NW1 2HD
0808 800 4050
helplines@arthritiscare.org.uk

Arthritis Research Campaign
www.arc.org.uk
Copeman House
St Mary's Court, St Mary's Gate
Chesterfield
Derbyshire S41 7TD
0870 850 5000
info@arc.org.uk

British Society for Rheumatology
www.rheumatology.org.uk
41 Eagle Street
London WC1R 4TL
(020) 7242 3313
bsr@rheumatology.org.uk

National Rheumatoid Arthritis Society
www.rheumatoid.org.uk
Unit B4 Westacot Business Centre
Westacott Way
Littlewick Green
Maidenhead
Berkshire LS6 3RT
0845 458 3969
enquiries@rheumatoid.org.uk

Asthma

**Asthma and Allergy
Foundation of America (US)**
www.aafa.org

**Asthma and Allergy
Information and Research**
www.users.globalnet.co.uk/~aair
Department of Respiratory Medicine
Glenfield Hospital
Groby Road
Leicester LE3 9QP
(0116) 270 7557
aair@globalnet.co.uk

British Lung Foundation
Website www.britishlungfoundation.org
73–75 Goswell Road
London EC1V 7ER
0845 850 5020
enquiries@blf-uk.org

National Asthma Campaign
www.asthma.org.uk
Providence House
Providence Place
London N1 0NT
08457 010203
(020) 7226 2260
enquiries@asthma.org.uk

Back pain

BackCare
www.backcare.org.uk
16 Elmtree Road
Teddington
Middlesex TW11 8ST
0870 950 0275

Other websites:
www.allaboutbackandneckpain.com
www.backandneck.about.com
www.spine-health.com
www.spineuniverse.com

Bereavement

Cruse Bereavement Care
www.crusebereavementcare.org.uk
126 Sheen Road
Richmond
Surrey TW9 1UR
0870 167 1677
(020) 8939 9530

Brain and nervous system

British Brain and Spine Foundation
www.bbsf.org.uk
7 Winchester House
Cranmer Road
Kennington Park
London SW9 6EJ
0808 808 1000
(020) 7793 5900

Dementia Research Centre
www.dementia.ion.ucl.ac.uk

**The National Hospital for
Neurology and Neurosurgery**
Queen Square
London WC1N 3BG
(020) 7829 8773

The Stroke Association
www.stroke.org.uk
240 City Road
London EC1V 2PR
0845 30 33 100
(020) 7566 0300
info@stroke.org.uk

See also
Alzheimer's disease
Headache and Migraine
Pain
Chronic Fatigue Syndrome/ME
Multiple Sclerosis

Care and support

Carers National Association
20–25 Glasshouse Yard
London EC1A 4JT
0345 573369
(020) 7490 8818

Hospice Information Service
www.hospiceinformation.info
St. Christopher's Hospice
51–59 Lawrie Park Road
Sydenham
London SE26 6DZ
0870 903 3903

Princess Royal Trust for Carers
www.carers.org
142 Minories

London EC3N 1LB
(020) 7480 7788
help@carers.org

Private Healthcare UK
www.privatehealth.co.uk
Intuition Communication
Concept House
271 High Street
Berkhamsted
Hertfordshire HP4 1AA
(01442) 385019

Cancer

American Cancer Society (US)
www.cancer.org

Breast Cancer Care
www.breastcancercare.org.uk
210 New Kings Road
London SW6 4NZ
0808 800 6000
(020) 7384 2984
info@breastcancercare.org.uk

CancerBACUP
www.cancerbacup.org.uk
3 Bath Place
Rivington Street
London EC2A 3JR
0808 800 1234
(020) 7696 9003

Cancer and Leukaemia in Childhood
www.clic.uk.com
Abbeywood Business Park
Filton
Bristol BS34 7JU
0845 301 0031
info@clic.org.uk

Cancer Research UK
www.cancerresearchuk.org
PO Box 123
Lincoln's Inn Fields
London WC2A 3PX
(020) 7242 0200

Everyman, Action Against Male Cancer
www.icr.ac.uk/everyman

Institute of Cancer Research
www.icr.ac.uk
123 Old Brompton Road
London SW7 3RP
(020) 7352 8133

Macmillan Cancer Relief
www.macmillan.org.uk
89 Albert Embankment
London SE1 7UQ
0808 808 2020
cancerline@macmillan.org.uk

National Cancer Institute (US)
www.cancer.gov

Oncolink (US)
www.oncolink.com

Ovacome (Ovarian Cancer)
www.ovacome.org.uk
Elizabeth Garrett Anderson Hospital
Huntley Street
London WC2E 6DH
(020) 7380 9589

Prostate Cancer Charity
www.prostate-cancer.org.uk
3 Angel Walk
London W6 9HX
0845 300 8383
(020) 8222 7622
info@prostate-cancer.org.uk

Children's health

Contact a Family
www.cafamily.org.uk
209–211 City Road
London EC1V 1JN
0808 808 3555
(020) 7608 8700
info@cafamily.org.uk

Great Ormond Street Hospital for Children NHS Trust
www.gosh.nhs.uk
Great Ormond Street
London WC1N 3JH
(020) 7405 9200

Institute of Child Health
www.ich.ucl.ac.uk
30 Guilford Street
London WC1N 1EH
(020) 7242 9789

Chronic fatigue syndrome

Action for ME
www.afme.org.uk
PO Box 1302
Wells
Somerset BA5 1YE
Tel (lo-call): 0845 123 2380
admin@afme.org.uk

Complementary therapies

British Chiropractic Association
www.chiropractic-uk.co.uk
17 Blagrave Street
Reading
Berks RG1 1QB
(0118) 950 5950
enquiries@chiropractic-uk.co.uk

British Massage Therapy Council
01865 774123

British Medical Acupuncture Society
www.medical-acupuncture.co.uk
3 Winnington Court
Northwich
Cheshire CW8 1AQ
(01606) 786782
Admin@medical-acupuncture.org.uk

British Osteopathic Association
www.osteopathy.org
Langham House West
Mill Street, Luton
Bedfordshire LU1 2NA
(01582) 488455
enquiries@osteopathy.org

Feldenkrais Guild UK
www.feldenkrais.co.uk
0700 785 506

General Hypnotherapy Register
www.general.hypnotherapy-register.com
PO Box 204
Lymington
Hampshire SO41 6WP
01590 683770

General Osteopathic Council
www.osteopathy.org.uk
176 Tower Bridge Road
London SE1 3LU
(020) 7357 6655
info@osteopathy.org.uk

Homoeopathic Medical Association
www.the-hma.org
6 Livingstone Road
Gravesend
Kent DA12 5DZ
(01474) 560336
info@the-hma.org

Register of Chinese Herbal Medicine
www.rchm.co.uk
Office 5
1 Exeter Street
Norwich NR2 4QB
01603 623994
herbmed@rchm.co.uk

Society of Homeopaths
www.homeopathy-soh.org
11 Brookfield
Duncan Close, Moulton Park
Northampton NN3 6WL
0845 450 6611
info@homeopathy-soh.org

Society of Teachers of Alexander Technique
www.stat.org.uk
1st Floor, Linton House

39–51 Highgate Road
London NW5 1RS
0845 230 7828
office@stat.org.uk

The Sutherland Society
(UK organisation for cranial osteopathy)
www.cranial.org.uk

The UK Tai Chi Association
PO Box 159
Bromley
Kent BR1 3XX
uk-tai-chi@cheerful.com

Counselling and psychological therapies

Association for Psychological Therapies
www.apt.ac
1 Saxby Street
Leicester LE2 0ND
(0870 600 300
office@apt.ac

British Association for Behavioural and Cognitive Psychotherapies
www.babcp.org.uk
PO Box 9
Accrington, BB5 2GD
(01254) 875 277
babcp@babcp.com

British Association for Counselling and Psychotherapy
www.bacp.co.uk
35–37 Albert Street
Rugby
Warwickshire CV21 2SG
(0870) 443 5252
bacp@bacp.co.uk

British Psychological Society
www.bps.org.uk
St Andrews House
48 Princess Road East
Leicester LE1 7DR
(0116) 254 9568
enquiry@bps.org.uk

United Kingdom Council for Psychotherapy
www.psychotherapy.org.uk
167-169 Great Portland Street
London W1W 5PF
(020) 7436 3002
ukcp@psychotherapy.org.uk

Depression

Depression Alliance
www.depressionalliance.org
212 Spitfire Studios

63–71 Collier Street
London N1 9BE
0845 123 2320

Manic Depression Fellowship
www.mdf.org.uk
21 St George's Road
London SE1 6ES
08456 340 540
mdf@mdf.org.uk

Other websites:
www.depression.org

See also
Counselling and Psychological Therapies
Mind and Emotions

Diabetes

Diabetes UK
www.diabetes.org.uk
10 Parkway
London NW1M 7AA
careline: 0845 120 2960
(020) 7424 1000
info@diabetes.org.uk

Insulin Dependent Diabetes Trust
www.iddtinternational.org
enquiries@iddtinternational.org

Juvenile Diabetes Research Foundation
www.jdrf.org.uk
19 Angel Gate, City Road
London EC1V 2PT
(020) 7713 2030
info@jdrf.org.uk

Digestive disorders

British Society of Gastroenterology
www.bsg.org.uk
3 St Andrews Place
London NW1 4LB
(020) 7387 3534
bsg@mailbox.ulcc.ac.uk

Digestive Disorders Foundation (CORE)
www.digestivedisorders.org.uk
3 St Andrews Place
London NW1 4LB
(020) 7486 0341
info@corecharity.org.uk

National Association for Colitis and
Crohn's Disease
www.nacc.org.uk
4 Beaumont House
Sutton Road
St Albans
Herts AL1 5HH
0845 130 2233

IBS Network
www.ibsnetwork.org.uk
Unit 5
53 Mowbray Street
Sheffield S3 8EN
0114 272 3253
info@ibsnetwork.org.uk

See also
Nutrition

Ear and hearing disorders

British Tinnitus Association
www.tinnitus.org.uk
Ground Floor, Unit 5
Acorn Business Park
Woodseats Close
Sheffield S8 0TB
0800 018 0527
info@tinnitus.org.uk

RNID
www.rnid.org.uk
19-23 Featherstone Street
London EC1Y 8SL
0808 808 0123
information@rnid.org.uk

Eating disorders

Anorexia and Bulimia Care
www.anorexiabulimiacare.co.uk
PO Box 173
Letchworth
Herts SG6 1XQ
(01462) 423 351
anorexiabulimiacare@ntlworld.com

Eating Disorders Association
www.edauk.com
1st Floor Wensum House
103 Prince of Wales Road
Norwich NR1 1DW
adult (0845) 634 1414
youth (0845) 634 7650
helpmail@edauk.com

Exercise and fitness

Health-club.net
www.health-club.net

The Fitness League
www.thefitnessleague.com
The Fitness League
6 Station Parade
Sunningdale
Berkshire SL5 0EP
01344 874787

Keep Fit Association
www.keepfit.org.uk
Astra House, Suite 1.05

Arklow Road
London SE14 6EB
(020) 8692 9566
kfa@keepfit.org.uk

Sport England
www.sportengland.org
3rd Floor, Victoria House
Bloomsbury Square
London WC1B 4SE
(08458) 508 508
info@sportengland.org

Eye disorders

College of Optometrists
www.college-optometrists.org
42 Craven Street
London WC2N 5NG
(020) 7839 6000
optometry@college-optometrists.org

Institute of Ophthalmology
www.ucl.ac.uk/ioo
11–43 Bath Street
London EC1V 9EL
(020) 7608 6800

Royal College of Ophthalmologists
www.rcophth.ac.uk
17 Cornwall Terrace
London NW1 4QW
(020) 7935 0702

Moorfields Eye Hospital NHS
Foundation Trust
www.moorfields.org.uk
(020) 7253 3411

Other Websites:
www.ascrs.org
www.macular.org
www.mdsupport.org

Fibromyalgia

Fibromyalgia Association UK
www.fibromyalgia-associationuk.org
PO Box 206
Stourbridge DY9 8YL
0870 220 1232
fmauk@hotmail.com

Other websites:
www.fmnetnew.com
www.afsafund.org
www.fmaware.org

Gout

UK Gout Society
www.ukgoutsociety.org
PO Box 527
London WC1V 7YP
info@ukgoutsociety.org

Headache and migraine

Migraine Action Association
www.migraine.org.uk
Unit 6, Oakley Hay Lodge Business Park
Great Folds Road, Great Oakley
Northants NN18 9AS
(01536) 461333

Migraine Trust
www.migrainetrust.org
2nd Floor, 55–56 Russell Square
London WC1B 4HP
(020) 7436 1336
info@migrainetrust.org

National Headache Foundation (US)
www.headaches.org

Heart and circulation disorders

British Heart Foundation
www.bhf.org.uk
14 Fitzhardinge Street
London W1H 6DH
Heartline: 08450 70 80 70
(020) 7935 0185

High Blood Pressure Foundation
www.hbpf.org.uk
Department of Medical Sciences
Western General Hospital
Edinburgh EH4 2XU
(0131) 332 9211
hbpf@hbpf.org.uk

Blood Pressure Association
www.bpassoc.org.uk
60 Cranmer Terrace
London SW17 0QS
(020) 8772 4994

Raynaud's and Scleroderma Association
www.raynauds.org.uk
112 Crewe Road, Alsager
Cheshire ST7 2JA
(01270) 872776
info@raynauds.org.uk

British Vascular Foundation
www.bvf.org.uk
10 Chertsey Road
Woking
Surrey GU21 5AB
bvf@care4free.net

Other websites:
www.americanheart.org
www.circ.ahajournals.org
www.coronary-artery.com
www.heartpoint.com
www.nhlbi.nih.gov/hbp

HIV and AIDS

AIDSmap
www.aidsmap.com

AVERT
www.avert.org
4 Brighton Road
Horsham
West Sussex RH13 5BA
(01403) 210202
info@avert.org

Body Positive
www.bodypositive.org.uk

Children with AIDS Charity
www.cwac.org
Lion House
3 Plough Yard
London EC2A 3LP
(020) 7247 9115
info@cwac.org

Crusaid
www.crusaid.org.uk
1–5 Curtain Road
London EC2A 3JX
(020) 7539 3880
office@crusaid.org.uk

Terrence Higgins Trust
www.tht.org.uk
52–54 Grays Inn Road
London WC1X 8JU
0845 1221 200
info@tht.org.uk

Infertility

ISSUE, The National Fertility Association
www.issue.co.uk
(01922) 722888
info@issue.co.uk

FertilityUK
www.fertilityuk.org
Bury Knowle Health Centre
207 London Road,Headington
Oxford OX3 9JA
admin@fertilityuk.org

Internet Health Resources
www.ihr.com

Liver disorders
British Liver Trust
www.britishlivertrust.org.uk
44 High Street
Ringwood BH24 1AG
(01425) 463080
info@britishlivertrust.org.uk

Men's health

BBC Website Health and Fitness
www.bbc.co.uk/health/mens

Prostate Help Association
www.personal.u-net.com/~pha
PHA (2003) (W)
Langworth
Lincoln, LN3 5DF
philip@pro-state.co.uk

Everyman: Action Against Male Cancer
www.icr.ac.uk/everyman

Impotence: Your Questions Answered
www.impotence-help.co.uk

Prostate Cancer Charity
www.prostate-cancer.org.uk
3 Angel Walk
London W6 9HX
0845 300 8383
(020) 8222 7622
info@prostate-cancer.org.uk

See also
Infertility

Mind and emotions

Mental Health Foundation
www.mhf.org.uk
20 Upper Ground
London SE1 9QB
(020) 7803 1100
mhf@mhf.org.uk

MIND
www.mind.org.uk
15–19 Broadway
London E15 4BQ
0845 766 0163
contact@mind.org.uk

National Institute of Mental Health
nimh.nih.gov

Rethink – severe mental illness
www.rethink.org
30 Tabernacle Street
London EC2A 4DD
advice line: (020) 8974 6814
advice@rethink.org

Royal College of Psychiatrists
www.rcpsych.ac.uk
17 Belgrave Square
London SW1X 8PG
(020) 7235 2351
rcpsych@rcpsych.ac.uk

SANE
www.sane.org.uk
1st Floor, Cityside House
40 Adler Street
London E1 1EE
0845 767 8000
london@sane.org.uk

See also
Counselling and Psychological Therapies
Obsessive Compulsive Disorder (OCD)
Phobias
Post Traumatic Stress Disorder (PTSD)
Schizophrenia
Seasonal Affective Disorder
Stress

Multiple sclerosis (MS)

Multiple Sclerosis Society
www.mssociety.org.uk
372 Edware Road
London NW2 6ND
0808 800 8000
info@mssociety.org.uk

Nutrition

BANT –
British Association for Nutritonal Therapy
www.bant.org.uk
27 Old Gloucester Street
London W1N 3XX
08706 061284
theadministrator@bant.org.uk

British Nutrition Foundation
www.nutrition.org.uk
52–54 High Holborn
London WC1V 6RQ
(020) 7404 6504
postbox@nutrition.org.uk

Food and Drug Administration (US)
www.fda.gov

Obesity

BBC Website Health and Fitness
www.bbc.co.uk/health/fightingfat

Association for the Study of Obesity
www.aso.org.uk

National Obesity Forum
www.nationalobesityforum.org.uk
PO Box 6625
Nottingham NG2 5PA
(0115) 8462109
info@nationalobesityforum.org.uk

International Association for
the Study of Obesity
www.iotf.org

231 Gower Street
London NW1 2NS
(020) 7691 1900
obesity@iotf.org

Obsessive–compulsive disorder (OCD)

OCD Action
www.ocdaction.org.uk
@2–24 Highbury Grove
London N5 2EA
(020) 7226 4000
info@ocdation.org.uk

See also
Counselling and Psychological Therapies
Mind and Emodtions

Osteoporosis

National Osteoporosis Society
www.nos.org.uk
Camerton
Bath BA2 0PJ
0845 450 0230
(01761) 471771
info@nos.org.uk

Pain

Pain Concern
www.painconcern.org.uk
PO Box 13256
Haddington EH41 4YD
01620 822572
info@painconcern.org.uk

Pain Research Institute
www.liv.ac.uk/pri
Clinical Sciences Centre,
University Hospital Aintree
Lower Lane
Liverpool L9 7AL
(0151) 529 5820
pri@liv.ac.uk

See also
Brain and Nervous System
Fibromyalgia

Phobias

National Phobics Society
www.phobics-society.org.uk
339 Stretford Road, Hulme
Manchester M15 4ZY
0870 7700 456
nationalphobic@btconnect.com

See also
Counselling and Psychological Therapies
Mind and Emotions
Post-traumatic stress
disorder (PTSD)

ASSIST
www.traumatic-stress.freeserve.co.uk
11 Albert Street
Rugby CV21 2RX
(01788) 560800
help@assist-trauma-care.co.uk

Combat Stress
(Ex-Services Mental Welfare Society)
www.combatstress.org.uk
Tyrwhitt House
Oaklawn Road
Leatherhead
Surrey KT22 0BX
(01372) 841600
Email contactus@combatstress.org.uk

Trauma After Care Trust (TACT)
Buttfields
The Farthings
Withington
Gloucestershire GL54 4DF
0800 169 6814
tact@tacthq.demon.co.uk

See also
Counselling and Psychological Therapies
Mind and Emotions

Pregnancy and childbirth

Association of Breastfeeding Mothers
www.abm.me.uk
PO Box 207, Bridgwater
Somerset TA6 7YT
0870 401 7711
counselling@abm.me.uk

National Childbirth Trust
www.nctpregnancyandbabycare.com
Alexandra House
Oldham Terrace
London W3 6NH
0870 7703236
enquiries@national-childbirth-trust.co.uk

UKparents
www.ukparents.co.uk

Repetitive strain injury
RSI-UK
www.rsi-uk.org.uk

Safety and health

Health and Safety Executive
www.hse.gov.uk
00845 345 0055

Institute for Occupational Safety and Health
www.iosh.co.uk
The Grange
Highfield Drive, Wigston
Leicestershire LE18 1NN
(0116) 257 3100
enquiries@iosh.co.uk

**Royal Society for
the Prevention of Accidents**
www.rospa.org.uk
353 Bristol Road
Edgbaston
Birmingham B5 7ST
(0121) 248 2000
help@rospa.com

Schizophrenia

Rethink
www.rethink.org
30 Tabernacle Street
London EC2A 4DD
Advice line: (020) 8974 6814
0845 456 0455
info@rethink.org

Schizophrenia Association of Great Britain
www.sagb.co.uk
Bryn Hyfryd
The Crescent
Bangor
Gwynedd LL57 2AG
(01248) 354048
info@sagb.co.uk

See also
Counselling and Psychological Therapies
Mind and Emotions

Seasonal affective disorder

SADAssociation
www.sada.org.uk
PO Box 989
Steyning
West Sussex BN44 3HG

Skin disorders

Acne Support Group
www.m2w3.com/acne
PO Box 9
Newquay
Cornwall TR9 6WG
(0870) 870 2263

British Association of Dermatologists
www.bad.org.uk
4 Fitzroy Square
London W1T 5HQ
(020) 7383 0266
admin@bad.org.uk

Herpes Viruses Association
www.herpes.org.uk
41 North Road
London N7 9DP
0845 123 2305
info@herpes.org.uk

National Eczema Society
www.eczema.org
Hill House, Highgate Hill
London N19 5NA
0870 241 3604
helpline@eczema.org

Psoriasis Association
www.psoriasis-association.org.uk
7 Milton Street
Northampton NN2 7JG
08456 760076
mail@psoriasis.demon.co.uk

Shingles Support Society
www.herpes.org.uk/shingles

Skin Care Campaign
www.skincarecampaign.org

Sleep Disorders

**British Snoring and
Sleep Apnoea Association**
www.britishsnoring.co.uk
52 Albert Road North, Reigate
Surrey RH2 9EL
0800 085 1097
info@britishsnoring.co.uk

Other websites:
www.sleepnet.com
www.talkaboutsleep.com

Sports injuries

WorldOrtho
www.worldortho.com

Stammering

British Stammering Association
www.stammering.org
15 Old Ford Road
London E2 9PJ
0845 603 2001
(020) 8983 1003
mail@stammering.org

Stress

The Stress Management Society
www.stress.org.uk
PO Box 193
Harrow
Middlesex HA1 3ZE

**International Stress
Management Association**
www.isma.org.uk
PO Box 348
Waltham Cross EN8 8ZL
07000 780430

Other websites:
www.stress.org

Urinary system disorders
British Kidney Patient Association
www.britishkidney-pa.co.uk
Bordon
Hampshire GU35 9JZ
(01420) 472021/2

Cystitis and Overactive Bladder Foundation
www.interstitialcystitis.co.uk
76 High Street
Stony Stratford
Buckinghamshire MK11 1AH
(01908) 569 169
info@cobfoundation.org

National Kidney Research Fund
www.nkrf.org.uk
Kings Chambers
Priestgate
Peterborough PE1 1FG
0845 300 1499

Women's health

**National Association for
Premenstrual Syndrome**
www.pms.org.uk
41 Old Road
East Peckham
Kent TN12 5AP
0870 777 2178
contact@pms.org.uk

National Endometriosis Society
www.endo.org.uk
50 Westminster Palace Gardens
Artillery Row
London SW1P 1RR
0808 808 2227
nes@endo.org.uk

Ovacome (Ovarian Cancer)
www.ovacome.org.uk
Elizabeth Garrett Anderson Hospital
Huntley Street
London WC2E 6DH
(020) 7380 9589
gdq53@dial.pipex.com

See also
Infertility

PRIMARY TREATMENT REFERENCES

This is an evidence-based book and the authors haved cited scientific references wherever possible for all treatments. The references for the complementary primary treatments are as follows. The references for the conventional medical treatments were too numerous to list here. The authors of the conventional medicial text took the Cochrane Library's (www.cochrane.co.uk) reviews of scientific research and other medical databases into account when rating treatments. (For an explanation of how treatments are rated, see p.111.)

A full list of all the authors' references for the treaments in this book may be found by visiting our website at www.dk.com/newmedicine.

Brain and Nervous System

CARPAL TUNNEL SYNDROME

Dobrusin R. *Osteopathic approach to conservative management of thoracic outlet syndromes.* Journal American Osteopathic Association. 89:1046-1057.

Garfinkel M. *Yoga-based intervention for carpal tunnel syndrome: a randomized trial.* Journal American Medical Association. 1998;280:1601–1603.

Sequeira W. *Yoga in treatment of carpal-tunnel syndrome.* Lancet 1999; 353 (9154):689-690.

Sucher B. *Myofascial manipulative release of carpal tunnel syndrome: documentation with MRI.* Journal American Osteopathic Association. 1994;94:647-663

DIZZINESS AND VERTIGO

Jewell M.D., Young G. *Interventions for nausea and vomiting in early pregnancy.* 2001. The Cochrane Library Issue 3, Oxford.

HEADACHE

Mauskop, A. et al. *Intravenous magnesium sulfate rapidly alleviates headaches of various types.* Headache. 1996;36:154-160.

Savi L. et al. *Food and headache attacks. A comparison of patients with migraine and tension-type headache.* Panminerva Med. 2002;44(1):27-31.

Gauthier, J.G., Ivers, H., & Carrier, S. *Nonpharmacological approaches in the management of recurrent headache disorders and their comparison and combination with pharmacotherapy.* Clinical Psychology Review. 1996;16(6):543-571.

MEMORY IMPAIRMENT

Brush J. A. and Camp C. J. *Using spaced retrieval as an intervention during speech-language therapy.* Clinical Gerontologist. 1998;19:51-64.

Camp C. J. and Stevens A. B. *Spaced retrieval: A memory intervention for dementia of the Alzheimers type.* Clinical Gerontologist. 1990;10:58-61.

MIGRAINE

Egger J. et al. *Is migraine food allergy? A double-blind trial of oligoantigenic diet treatment.* Lancet. 1983;ii:865-869.

Grant E.C. *Food allergies and migraine.* Lancet. 1979:I:966-969.

Hughs E.C. et al. *Migraine: a diagnostic test for etiology of food sensitivity by a nutritionally supported fast and confirmed by long-term report.* Ann Allergy. 1985;55:28-32.

Monro J. et al. *Food allergy in migraine.* Lancet. 1980;ii:1-4.

MOTION SICKNESS

Jewell M.D. and Young G. *Interventions for nausea and vomiting in early pregnancy.* 2001. The Cochrane Library Issue 3, Oxford.

PERSISTENT PAIN

Kabat-Zinn J., Lipworth L. et al. *The clinical use of mindfulness medilation for the self-regulatlon of chronic pain.* J Behav Med 1985;8(2): 163-90.

Morley S., Eccleston C. et al. *Systematic review and meta-analysis of randomized controlled trials of cognitive behavior therapy and behavior therapy for chronic pain in adults, excluding headache.* Pain. 1999;80(1-2):1-13.

Torp S., Riise T. et al. *The impact of psychosocial work factors on musculoskeletal pain: a prospective study.* J Occup Environ Med. 2001;43(2): 120-126.

Wells N. *Perceived control over pain: relation to distress and disability.* Res Nurs Health. 1994;17(4):295-302.

STROKE

Hesse S. et al. *Treadmill training with partial body weight support after stroke.* Physical Medicine And Rehabilitation Clinics Of North America. 14(1, Suppl.):S111-S123.

MULTIPLE SCLEROSIS

Swank R.L. et al. *Effect of a low saturated fat diet in early and late cases of multiple sclerosis.* Lancet. 1990;336:37-39.

Skin Ailments

PSORIASIS

Clover, A. Br Hom J. 2000;89:68–72.

Spence D. Br Hom J. 2000;89(Sup.)1:44.

Rosenberg, E., Belew, P. *Microbial factors in psoriasis.* Arch Dermatol. 1982;118;1434–1444.

Kuwano, S., Yamauchi, K. *Effect of berberine on tyrosine decarboxylase activity of Streptococcus faecalis.* Chem Pharm Bull. 1960:8:491–496.

Thurmon, F.M. *The treatment of psoriasis with sarsaparilla compound.* New Eng J Med. 1942;227:128–133.

ECZEMA AND CONTACT DERMATITIS

Niggemann, B., et al. *Outcome of double-blind, placebo-controlled food challenge tests in 107 children with atopic dermatitis.* Clin Exp Allergy. 1999;29:91–96.

Atherton, D.J. *Diet and atopic eczema.* Clin Allerg. 1988;18:215–228.

Horrobin, D.F. *Essential fatty acid metabolism and its modification in atopic eczema.* Am J Clin Nutr. 2000;71(Sup.):367S–372S.

Gimenez-Arnau, A., et al. *Effects of linoleic acid supplements on atopic dermatitis.* Adv Exp Med Biol. 1997;443:285–289.

Sullivan, J.B, Krieger, G.R. *Clinical Environmental Health and Toxic Exposures.* 2nd Edition. Lippincott, Williams, & Wilkins, Philadelphia, Pennsylvania, 2001.

HIVES

Henz, B.M., Zuberbier, T. *Most chronic urticaria is food-dependent, and not idiopathic.* Exp Dermatol. 1998;7(4):139–142.

Lessof, M.H. *Reactions to food additives.* Clin Exp Allergy. DATE;25(Sup.1):27–28.

Juhlin, L. *Additives and chronic urticaria.* Ann Allergy. DATE;59:119–123.

Kulczycki, A. *Aspartame-induced urticaria.* Ann Int Med. 1986;104:207–208.

Eye Ailments

MACULAR DEGENERATION

Age-Related Eye Disease Study Research Group. *A randomized, placebo-controlled, clinical trial of high-dose supplementation with vitamins C and E, beta carotene, and zinc for age-related macular degeneration and vision loss: AREDS Report No. 8.* Arch Ophthalmol. 2001;119:1417–1436.

Respiratory Ailments

COLDS AND FLU

Anderson T.W. et al. *Vitamin C and the common cold: a double-blind trial.* Can Med Assoc J. 1972;107:503-508.

Eby G.A. et al. *Reduction in duration of common colds by zinc gluconate lozenges in a double-blind study.* Antimicrob Agents Chemother. 1984;25:20-24.

Garland M.L. and Hagmeyer K.O. *The role of zinc lozenges in treatment of the common cold.* Ann Pharmacother. 1998;32:63-69.

Gorton H.C. et al. *The effectiveness of vitamin C in preventing and relieving the symptoms of virus-induced respiratory infections.* J Manipulative Physiol Ther. 1999;22(8):530-533.

Hemila H. *Does vitamin C alleviate the symptoms of the common cold? - a review of current evidence.* Scand J Infect Dis. 1994;26(1):1-6.

McCarthy M. *Zinc Lozenges shorten duration of common cold.* Lancet. 1996;348:184.

Mossad S.B. et al. *Zinc gluconate lozenges for treating the common cold. A randomized, double-blind, placebo-controlled study.* Annals of Internal Medicine. 1996;125(2):81-88.

Petrus E.J. et al. *Randomized, double-masked, placebo-controlled clinical study of the effectiveness of zinc acetate lozenges on common cold symptoms in allergy-tested subjects.* Curr Ther Res. 1998;59:595–607.

Prasad A.S. et al. *Duration of symptoms and plasma cytokine levels in patients with the common cold treated with zinc acetate: a randomized, double-blind, placebo-controlled trial.* Ann Intern Med. 2000;133(4):245-252.

Van Straten M. and Josling P. *Preventing the common cold with a vitamin C supplement: a double-blind, placebo-controlled survey.* Adv Ther. 2002;19:151-159.

Melchart 1999 *(echinacea)*

Vickers and Smith 2000; Cochrane 2003 *(Oscillococcinum)*

ASTHMA

Bowler S., Green A., Mitchell C. *Buteyko breathing techniques in asthma : a blinded randomised controlled trial.* Medical Journal of Australia. 1998;169:575-578.

Tisp B., Burns M., Kro D. *Pursed Lip breathing using ear oximetry.* Chest. 1986;90:218-221.

Fluge T., Richter J., Fabel H., et al. *Long-term effects of breathing exercises and yoga in patients with bronchial asthma.* [In German]. Pneumologie. 1994;48:484–490.

Hockemeyer J., and Smyth J. *Evaluating the feasibility and efficacy of a self-administered manual-based stress management intervention for individuals with asthma: Results from a controlled study.* Behavioral Medicine,. 2002;27(4):161-172.

Kilpelainen M., Koskenvuo,M., Helenius H., and Terho E.O. *Stressful life events promote the manifestation of asthma and atopic diseases.* Clinical and Experimental Allergy. 2002;32(2): 256-263.

Liu L.Y., Coe C.L., Swenson C.A., Kelly E.A., Kita H., and Busse,W.W. *School examinations enhance airway inflammation to antigen challenge.* American Journal of Respiratory Critical Care Medicine. 2002;165(8): 1062-1067.

Rietveld. S., van Beest. I., and Everaerd W. *Stress-induced breathlessness in asthma.* Psychological Medicine. 1999; 29(6):1359-1366.

Stetter. F., and Kupper, S. *Autogenic training: A meta-analysis of clinical outcome studies.* Applied Psychophysiology and Biofeedback. 2002;27(1):45-98.

Wilson AF, Honsberger RW, Chiu JT and Novey SH. *Transcendental meditation and asthma.* Respiration. 1975;32:74–80.

Digestion and Urinary Systems

CROHN'S DISEASE

Brandes J.W. et al. *Sugar free diet: A new perspective in the treatment of Crohn's disease? Randomized, control study.* Z Gastroenterol. 1981;19(1):1-12.

Heaton K.W. et al. *Treatment of Crohn's disease with an unrefined carbohydrate, fibre rich diet.* BMJ. 1979;2:764-766.

Jones V.A. et al. *Crohn's disease: maintenance of remission by diet.* Lancet. 1985;2:177-180.

Riordan A.M., et al. *Treatment of active Crohn's disease by exclusion diet. East Anglian Multicentre Controlled Trial.* Lancet. 1993;342:1131-1134.

Timmons B .H., Ley R. eds. *Behavioral and pyschological approaches to breathing disorders.* Plenum, 1994:115.

Tisp B., Burns M., Kro D., Kao D., Madison R., Herrera J. *Pursed lip breathing using ear oximetry.* Chest. 1986;90:218-221.

ULCERATIVE COLITIS

Gionchetti P. et al. *Oral bacteriotherapy as maintenance treatment in patients with chronic pouchitis: a double-blind, placebo-controlled trial.* Gastroenterology. 2000;119(2):305-309.

Gionchetti P. et al. *Microflora in the IBD pathogenesis. Possible therapeutic use of probiotics.* Gastroenterol Internat. 1998;11:108-110.

CYSTITIS

Kingwatanakul P., Alon U.S. *Cranberries and urinary tract infection.* Child Hosp Q. 1996;8:69-62.

Reid G., Sobel J.D. *Bacterial adherence in*

the pathogenesis of urinary tract infections. J Urol. 1984;131:1013-1016.

Howell A.B. et al. *Inhibition of the adherence of P fimbriated Escherichia coli to uroepithelial-cell surfaces by proanthocyanidin extracts from cranberries.* New Engl J Med. 1998;339:1085-1086.

Jepson R.G., Mihaljevic L., Craig J. *Cranberries for treating urinary tract infections.* Cochrane Database Syst Rev. 2000;(2):CD001322. Review.

Jepson R.G., Mihaljevic L., Craig J. *Cranberries for preventing urinary tract infections.* Cochrane Database Syst Rev. 2001;(3):CD001321. Review.

Lowe F.C. and Fagelman, E. *Cranberry juice and urinary tract infections: what is the evidence?* Urology. 2001;57:407-413.

Stothers L. *A randomized trial to evaluate effectiveness and cost effectiveness of naturopathic cranberry products as prophylaxis against urinary tract infection in women.* Can J Urol. 2002 ;9(3):1558-1562.

Foo L.Y., Lu Y., Howell A.B., Vorsa N. *The structure of cranberry proanthocyanidins which inhibit adherence of uropathogenic P-fimbriated Escherichia coli in vitro.* Phytochemistry. 2000;54(2):173-181.

Kiel R.J., Nashelsky J., Robbins B. *Does cranberry juice prevent or treat urinary tract infection?* J Fam Pract. 2003;52(2):154-155.

Reid G. *The role of cranberry and probiotics in intestinal and urogenital tract health.* Crit Rev Food Sci Nutr. 2002;42(3 Suppl):293-300.

Muscle, Bone and Joint Ailments

SCIATICA

Cherkin, D., et al. *A comparison of physical therapy, chiropractic manipulation, and provision of an educational booklet for the treatment of patients with low back pain.* New England Journal Of Medicine. 1998;339(15):1021–1029.

SPORTS INJURIES

Allen, R. *Sports Medicine.* In: Foundations of Osteopathic Medicine (Ward, R., ed). Williams and Wilkins, Baltimore, 1997.

Feinberg, E. *Sports Chiropractic.* In: Contemporary Chiropractic (Redwood, D., ed). Churchill Livingstone, New York, 1997.

TEMPOROMANDIBULAR JOINT DISORDER

Nguyen, P., et al. *A randomized double-blind clinical trial of the effect of chondroitin sulfate and glucosamine hydrochloride on temporomandibular joint disorders: a pilot study.* Cranio. 2001;19(2):130–139.

Shankland, W.E. *The effects of glucosamine and chondroitin sulfate on osteoarthritis of the TMJ: a preliminary report of 50 patients.* Cranio. 1998;16(4):230–235.

FROZEN SHOULDER

Liebenson, C., (ed). *Rehabilitation of the Spine.* Williams & Wilkins, Baltimore

Simons, J., Travell, J., Simons, L. *Myofascial Pain and Dysfunction: The Trigger Point Manual* (Volume 1, Upper Body, 2nd edition, pp.604–612). Williams & Wilkins, Baltimore, 1999.

Strong, J., et al. *Pain: A textbook for therapists.* Churchill Livingstone, Edinburgh, 2002.

OSTEOPOROSIS

Eastell, R., Lambert, H. *Strategies for skeletal health in the elderly.* Proc Nutr Soc. 2002;61:173–180.

New, S.A., et al. *Positive associations between net endogenous non-carbonic acid production (NEAP) and bone health: further support for the importance of the skeleton to acid-base balance.* Bone. 2001;28:S94.

Feskanich, D., et al. *Calcium, vitamin D, milk consumption, and hip fractures: a prospective study among postmenopausal women.* Am J Clin Nutr. 2003;77(2):504–511.

Chapuy, M.C., et al. *Vitamin D and calcium to prevent hip fractures in elderly women.* New Eng J Med. 1992;327:1637–1642.

Dawson-Hughes, B., et al. *Effect of calcium and vitamin D supplementation on bone density in men and women 65 years of age or older.* New Eng J Med. 1997;337:670–676.

Minne, H.W., et al. *Vitamin D and calcium supplementation reduces falls in elderly women via improvement of body sway and normalisation of blood pressure: a prospective, randomised and double-blind study.* Osteoporosis International. 2000;11:S115.

Papadimitropoulos, E., et al. *Meta-analyses of therapies for postmenopausal osteoporosis. VIII: Meta-analysis of the efficacy of vitamin D treatment in preventing osteoporosis in postmenopausal women.* Endocr Rev. 2002;23(4):560–569.

OSTEOARTHRITIS

Qiu, G.X., et al. *Efficacy and safety of glucosamine sulfate versus ibuprofen in patients with knee osteoarthritis.* Arzneimittelforschung. 1998;48:469–474.

Leeb, B.F., et al. *A meta-analysis of chondroitin sulfate in the treatment of osteoarthritis.* J Rheumatol. 2000;27(1):205–211.

McAlindon, T.E., et al. *Glucosamine and chondroitin for treatment of osteoarthritis: a systematic quality assessment and meta-analysis.* JAMA. 2000;283:1469–1475.

Young, L.D., Bradley, L.A., Turner, R.A. *Decreases in health care resource utilization in patients with rheumatoid arthritis following a cognitive behavioral intervention.* Biofeedback and Self-Regulation. 1995(Sep);20(3):259–268.

Lorig, K., Mazonson, P., Holman, H.R. *Evidence suggesting that health education for self-management in patients with chronic arthritis has sustained health benefits while reducing health care costs.* Arthritis and Rheumatism. 1993;36(4r):439–446.

Mullen, P.D., et al. *Efficacy of psycho-educational interventions on pain, depression and disability with arthritic adults: a meta-analysis.* J of Rheumatology. 1987;14(15):33–39.

Stanford Patient Education Research Center. *The Chronic Disease Self-Management Workshop Leaders Manual.* Stanford University, 1999.

Lorig, K., et al. *The beneficial outcomes of the arthritis self-management course are inadequately explained by behavior change.* Arthritis and Rheumatism. 1989;31(1):91–95.

Marks, R. *Efficacy theory and its utility in arthritis rehabilitation: review and recommendations.* Disabil Rehabil. 2001(May10);23(7):271–280.

FIBROMYALGIA

Kaplan, K.H., Goldenberg, D.L., Galvin-Nadeau, M. *The Impact of a Meditation-based Stress Reducton Program on Fibromyalgia.* Gen Hosp Psychiatry. 1993(Sep);15(5):284–289.

Buckelew, S.P., Conway, R., et al. *Biofeedback/Relaxation Training and Exercise Interventions for Fibromyalgia: A Prospective Trial.* Arthritis Care Res. 1998(Jun);11(3):196–209.

Hadhazy, V.A., et al. *Mind-body Therapies for the Treatment of Fibromyalgia: A Systematic Review.* J Rheumatol. 2000(Dec);27(12):2922–2928.

Fisher, P., et al. *Effect of homoeopathic treatment on fibrositis (primary fibromyalgia).* BMJ. 1989;299:365–366.

Bell, I.R., et al. *Improved clinical status in fibromyalgia patients treated with individualized homeopathic remedies versus placebo.* Rheumatology. 2004;43:577–582.

ANKYLOSING SPONDYLITIS

Helliwell, P., Abbott, C.A., *Chamberlain, M.A. A randomised trial of three different physiotherapy regimes in ankylosing spondylitis.* Physiotherapy. 1996,82:85–90.

Women's Health

PREMENSTRUAL SYNDROME

Rossignol A.M. et al. *Prevalence and severity of the premenstrual syndrome. Effects of foods and beverages that are sweet or high in sugar content.* J Reprod Med. 1991;36:131-136.

Rossignol A.M. *Caffeine-containing beverages and premenstrual syndrome in young women.* Am J Public Health. 1985;75:1337.

MENOPAUSE

McKenna D.J., Jones K., Humphrey S., Hughes K. *Black cohosh: efficacy, safety, and use in clinical and preclinical applications.* Altern Ther Healt Med. 2001;7(3):93-100.

Men's Ailments

ERECTILE DYSFUNCTION

Li, T.B., et al. *Effects of ginsenosides, lectins and Momordica charantia insulin like peptide on corticosterone production by isolated rat adrenal cells.* J
Ethnopharmacol. 1987;21:21–29.

Hong, B., Ji, Y.H., Hong, J.H., et al. *A double-blind crossover study evaluating the efficacy of Korean red ginseng in patients with erectile dysfunction: a preliminary report.* J Urol. 2002;168:2070–2073.

Price, A., Gazewood, J. *Korean red ginseng effective for treatment of erectile dysfunction.* J Fam Pract. 2003(Jan);52(1):20–21.

Deyama, T., Nishibe, S., Nakazawa, Y. *Constituents and pharmacological effects of Eucommia and Siberian ginseng.* Review. Acta Pharmacol Sin. 2001(Dec);22(12):1057–1070.

Hawton, K., Catalan, J., Fagg, J. *Sex therapy for erectile dysfunction: Characteristics of couples, treatment outcome and prognostic factors.* Archives of Sexual Behviour. 1992;21:61–175.

Kilmann, P.R., Auerbach, R. *Treatments of premature ejaculation and psychogenic impotence: A critical review of the literature.* Archives of Sexual Behaviour. 1979;8:81–100.

Masters, W.H., Johnson, V.E. *Human sexual inadequacy.* Little, Brown, Boston, 1970.

De Amicis, M.P., Goldberg, D.C., LoPiccolo, J., Davies, L. *Clinical follow-up of couples treated for sexual dysfunction.* Archives of Sexual Behavior. 1985;14 467–489.

BENIGN PROSTATIC HYPERTROPHY (PROSTATE ENLARGEMENT)

McCaleb, R. *Phytomedicines outperform synthetics in treating enlarged prostate.* Herbalgram. 1997;40.

Gutrierez, M., et al. *Spasmolytic activity of lipid extract from Sabal serrulata fruits; further studies of the mechanisms underlying this activity.* Planta Med. 1996;62:507–511.

Wagner, H., Flachsbarth, H. *A new antiphlogistic principle from Sabal serrulata, 1.* Planta Med. 1966;14:402–407.

Koch, E. *Extracts from fruits of saw palmetto (Sabal serrulata) and roots of stinging nettle (Urtica dioica): viable alternatives in the medical treatment of benign prostatic hyperplasia and associated lower urinary tracts symptoms.* Planta Med. 2001(Aug);67(6):489–500.

Sokeland, J. *Combined sabal and urtica*
extract compared with finasteride in men with benign prostatic hyperplasia: analysis of prostate volume and therapeutic outcome.* BJU Int. 2000(Sep);86(4):439–442.

Children's Ailments

ADHD

Patterson, G.R. *Coercive Family Process.* Castalia Publishing Company, Eugene, Oregon, 1982.

Pisterman, S., et al. *The role of parent training in treatment of preschoolers with ADDH.* American Journal of Orthopsychiatry. 1992;62:397–408.

Barkley, R.A., et al. *A comparison of three family therapy programs for treating family conflicts in adolescents with attention-deficit hyperactivity disorders.* Journal of Consulting and Clinical Psychology. 1992;60:450–462.

Forehand, R., McMahon, R.J. *Helping the non compliant child.* Guilford, New York, 1981.

Webster-Stratton, C., Hammond, M. *Predictors of treatment outcome in parent training for families with conduct problem children.* Behavior Therapy. 1990;21:319–337.

Abikoff, H. *Cognitive training in ADHD children: less to it than meets the eye.* Journal of Learning Disability. 1991;24:205–209.

Pfiffner, L.J., McBurnett, K. *Social skills training with parent generalization: treatment effects for children with attention deficit disorder.* Journal of Consulting and Clinical Psychology. 1997;65:749–757.

Hinshaw, S.P., Henker, B., Whalen, C.K. *Self-control in hyperactive boys in anger-inducing situations: effects of cognitive-behavioral training and of methylphenidate.* Journal of Abnormal Child Psychology. 1984;12:55–77.

DuPaul, G., Eckert, T.L. *The effects of school-based Interventions for attention deficit hyperactivity disorder: a meta-analysis.* School Psychology Review. 1997;26:5–27.

Whalen, C.K, Henker, B. *Therapies for hyperactive children: comparisons, combinations, and compromises.* Journal of Consulting and Clinical Psychology. 1991;59:126–137.

COLIC

Lothe, L., et al. *Cow's milk as a cause of infantile colic: A double-blind study.* Pediatr. 1982;70(1):7–10

Lothe, L., et al. *Cow's milk whey protein elicits symptoms of infantile colic in colicky formula-fed infants: A double-blind crossover study.* Pediatr. 1989;83(2):262–266.

Jakobsson, I., et al. *Cow's milk proteins cause infantile colic in breast-fed infants: a double-blind crossover study.* Pediatr. 1983;71(2):268–271.

GLUE EAR

Arroyave, C.M. *Recurrent otitis media with effusion and food allergy in pediatric patients.* (Article in Spanish). Rev Alerg Mex. 2001;48:141–144.

Nsouli, T.M., et al. *Role of food allergy in serous otitis media.* Ann Allergy. 1994;73:215–219.

HEAD LICE

Puri, H. (Ed.) *Neem: Medicinal and Aromatic Plants – Industrial Profiles.* Taylor and Francis, London, 1999.

Charles, V., Charles, S.X. *The use and efficacy of Azadirachta indica ADR ("Neem") and Curcuma longa ("Turmeric") in scabies. A pilot study.* Trop Geogr Med. 1992;44(1–2):178–81.

Jensen, O., Nielsen, A.O., Bjerregaard, P. *Pediculosis capitis treated with quassia tincture.* Acta Derm Venereol. 1978;58(6):557–9.

TONSILLITIS

Kempe, C., Gruning, H., Stasche, N., Hormann, K. *[Icelandic moss lozenges in the prevention or treatment of oral mucosa irritation and dried out throat mucosa.]* (Article in German.) Laryngorhinootologie. 1997(Mar);76(3):186–188.

Mind and Emotions

ANXIETY

Borkoved, T.D., Ruscio, A.M. *Psychotherapy for generalized anxiety disorder.* J Clin Psychiatry. 2001;62Sup11:37–42; discussion 43–45.

Butler, G., et al. *Comparison of behavior therapy and cognitive behavior therapy in the treatment of generalized anxiety disorder.* J Consult Clin Psychol. 1991(Feb);59(1):167–175.

Lenz, G., Demal, U. *Quality of life in depression and anxiety disorders: an exploratory follow-up study after intensive inpatient cognitive behaviour therapy.* Psychopathology. 2000(Nov–Dec);33(6):297–302.

Silverman, W.K., et al. *Treating anxiety disorders in children with group cognitive-behavioral therapy: a randomized clinical trial.* J Consult Clin Psychol. 1999(Dec);67(6):995–1003.

Toren, P., et al. *Case series: brief parent-child group therapy for childhood anxiety disorders using a manual-based cognitive-behavioral technique.* J Am Acad Child Adolesc Psychiatry. 2000(Oct);39(10):1309–1312.

Basco, M.R., et al. *Cognitive-behavioral therapy for anxiety disorders: why and how it works.* Bull Menninger Clin. 2000(Summer);64(3Sup.A):A52–70.

Rees, B.L. *Effect of relaxation with guided imagery on anxiety, depression, and self-esteem in primiparas.* J Holist Nurs. DATE(Sep);13(3):255–267.

Tusek, D.L., Cwynar, R., Cosgrove, D.M. *Effect of guided imagery on length of stay, pain and anxiety in cardiac surgery patients.* J Cardiovasc Manag. 1999(Mar–Apr);10(2):22–28.

Aitken, J.R., Benson, J.W. *The use of relaxation/desensitization in treating anxiety associated with flying.* Aviat Space Environ Med. 1984(Mar);55(3):196–199.

Eppley, K.R., Abrams, A.I., Shear, J. *Differential effects of relaxation techniques on trait anxiety: a meta-analysis.* J Clin Psychol. 1989(Nov);45(6):957–974.

Mathew, R.J., et al. *Anxiety and platelet MAO levels after relaxation training.* Am J Psychiatry. 1981(Mar);138(3):371–373.

Pender, N.J. *Effects of progressive muscle relaxation training on anxiety and health locus of control among hypertensive adults.* Res Nurs Health. 1985(Mar);8(1):67–72.

Wachelka, D., Katz, R.C. *Reducing test anxiety and improving academic self-esteem in high school and college students with learning disabilities.* J Behav Ther Exp Psychiatry. 1999(Sep);30(3):191–198.

Weber, S. *The effects of relaxation exercises on anxiety levels in psychiatric inpatients.* J Holist Nurs. 1996(Sep);14(3):196–205.

Ashton, C. Jr, et al. *Self-hypnosis reduces anxiety following coronary artery bypass surgery. A prospective, randomized trial.* J Cardiovasc Surg (Torino). 1997(Feb);38(1):69–75.

Benson, H., et al. *Treatment of anxiety: A comparison of the usefulness of self-hypnosis and a meditational relaxation technique. An overview.* Psychother Psychosom. 1978;30(3–4):229–242.

Davidson, G.P., Farnbach, R.W., Richardson, B.A. *Self-hypnosis training in anxiety reduction.* Aust Fam Physician. 1978(Jul);7(7):905–910.

Stetter, F., et al. *Ambulatory short-term therapy of anxiety patients with autogenic training and hypnosis. Results of treatment and 3 month follow-up.* Psychother Psychosom Med Psychol. 1994(Jul);44(7):226–234.

Kabat-Zinn, J., et al. *Effectiveness of a meditation-based stress reduction program in the treatment of anxiety disorders.* Am J Psychiatry. 1992(Jul);149(7):936–943.

Reibel, D.K., et al. *Mindfulness-based stress reduction and health-related qualify of life in a heterogeneous patient population.* Gen Hosp Psychiatry. 2001(Jul–Aug);23(4):183–192.

Clark, M.E., Hirschman, R. *Effects of paced respiration on anxiety reduction in a clinical population.* Biofeedback Self Regul. 1990(Sep);15(3):273–284.

Rice, K.M., Blanchard, E.B., Purcell, M. *Biofeedback treatments of generalized anxiety disorder: preliminary results.* Biofeedback Self Regul. 1993(Jun);18(2):93–105.

DEPRESSION

Linde, INITIAL et al *St. John's Wort for depression – an overview and meta-analysis of randomised clinical trials.* BMJ. 1996;313:253–258.

Hiller, K., et al. TITLE *Forschende Komplementarmedezin.* 1995;2:123–132.

Liske, E., et al. *Menopause – Combination product for psycho-vegetative complaints.* TW-Gynakol. 1997;10;4:172–175.

EATING DISORDERS

Crisp, A.H., et al. *A controlled study of the effect of therapies aimed at adolescent and family psychopathology in anorexia nervosa.* The British Journal of Psychiatry. 1991;159:325–333.

Mitchell, K., Carr, A. *Anorexia and bulimia. In: What works with children and adolescents?: A critical review of psychological interventions with children, adolescents and their families.* (Carr, A. (Ed), pp.233–257). Taylor & Francis/Routledge, Florence, Kentucky, 2000.

Leung, N., Waller, G., Thomas, G. *Group cognitive-behavioural therapy for anorexia nervosa: A case for treatment?* European Eating Disorders Review. 1999;7(5):351–361.

Wilson, G.T, et al. *Cognitive behavioral therapy for bulimia nervosa: Time course and mechanisms of change.* Journal-of-Consulting-and-Clinical-Psychology. 2002;70(2):267–274.

Whittal, M.L., Agras, W.S., Gould, R.A. *Bulimia nervosa: A meta-analysis of psychosocial and pharmacological treatments.* Behavior Therapy. 1999;30(1):117–135.

Jaeger, B., et al. *Psychotherapy and bulimia nervosa: Evaluation and long-term follow-up of two conflict orientated treatment conditions.* Acta Psychiatrica Scandinavica. 1996;93(4):268–278.

Wilfley, D.E., et al. *A randomized comparison of group cognitive-behavioral therapy and group interpersonal psychotherapy for the treatment of overweight individuals with binge-eating disorder.* Archives of General Psychiatry. 2002;59(8):713–721.

OBESITY

Anderson, R., et al. *Effects of lifestyle activity vs structured aerobic exercise in obese women.* Journal American Medical Association. 1999;281(4):335–340.

Ramadan, J., et al. *Low-frequency physical activity insufficient for aerobic conditioning is associated with lower body fat than sedentary conditions.* Nutrition. 2001;17(3):225–229.

Riebe, D., et al. *Evaluation of a Healthy-Lifestyle Approach to Weight Management.* Preventive Medicine. 2003;36(1):45–54.

Votruba, S., et al. *The role of exercise in the treatment of obesity.* Nutrition. 2000;16(3)179–188.

McWhorter, J., et al. *The obese child: Motivation as a tool for exercise.* Journal of Pediatric Health Care. 2003;17(1):11–17.

OBSESSIVE–COMPULSIVE DISORDER (OCD)

Foa, E.B., Franklin, M.E. *Psychotherapies for obsessive–compulsive disorder: A review. In: Obsessive-compulsive disorder. WPA series evidence and experience in psychiatry, 4.* (Maj, M., Sartorius, N., Eds., pp.93–146). John Wiley & Sons Ltd, New York, New York, 2000.

Abramowitz, J.S., Brigidi, B.D., Roche, K.R. *Cognitive-behavioral therapy for obsessive–compulsive disorder: A review of the treatment literature.* Research on Social Work Practice. 2001;11(3):357–372.

Warren, R., Thomas, J.C. *Cognitive-behavior therapy of obsessive–compulsive disorder in private practice: An effectiveness study.* Journal of Anxiety Disorders. 2001;15(4):277–285.

PHOBIAS

Gilroy, L.J, et al. *Controlled comparison of computer-aided vicarious exposure versus live exposure in the treatment of spider phobia.* Behavior Therapy. 2003;31:733–744.

Wiederhold, B.K., et al. *An investigation into physiological responses in virtual environments: an objective measurement of presence.* In: Toward cyberpsychology: Mind, cognition and society in the internet age (Riva, G., Calimberti, C., Eds). IOS Press, Amsterdam, 2001.

Emmelkamp, P.M.G. *Behavior therapy with adults. In: Handbook of psychotherapy and behavior change* (Garfield, S.L., Bergin, A.E., Eds., 4th edition, pp. 79–427). John Wiley & Sons Ltd, New York, New York, 1994.

Marshall, W.L. *The effects of variable exposure in flooding therapy.* Behavior Therapy. 1985;16:117–135.

Marshall, W.L. *The treatment of agoraphobia.* Paper at the Australia Behavior Modification Association, Perth, Western Australia, March, 1985.

Smith, T.A., et al. *Evaluating a behavioral method to manage dental fear: A 2-year study of dental practices.* Journal of the American Dental Association. 1990;121:525–530.

Liddell, A., et al. *Long-term follow-up of treated dental phobics.* Behaviour Research And Therapy. 1994;32(6):605–610.

Ost, L.G. *Acquisition of blood ad injection phobia and anxiety response pattern in clinical patients.* Behaviour Research and Therapy. 1991;29(4):323–332.

SLEEPING DISORDERS

Backhaus, J., et al. *Long-term effectiveness of a short-term cognitive-behavioral group treatment for primary insomnia.* Eur Arch Psychiatry Clin Neurosci. 2001;251(1):35–41.

Dashevsky, B.A., Kramer, M. *Behavioral treatment of chronic insomnia in psychiatrically ill patients.* J Clin Psychiatry. 1998(Dec);59(12):693–699.

McClusky, H.Y., et al. *Efficacy of behavioral versus triazolam treatment in persistent sleep-onset insomnia.* Am J Psychiatry. 1991(Jan);148(1):121–126.

Morin, C.M., Mimeault, V., Gagne, A.J. *Nonpharmacological treatment of late-life insomnia.* Psychosom Res. 1999(Feb);46(2):103–116.

STRESS

Crowther, J.H.. *Stress management training and relaxation imagery in the treatment of essential hypertension.* Journal of Behavioral Medicine. 1983;6(2):169–187.

Wynd, C.A. *Relaxation imagery used for stress reduction in the prevention of smoking relapse.* Journal of Advanced Nursing. 1992;17:294–302.

Tsai, S.L., Crockett, M.S. *Effects of relaxation training combining imagery and meditation on the stress level of Chinese nurses working in modern hospitals in Taiwan.* Issues in Mental Health Nursing. 1993;14:51–56.

Holden-Lund, C. *Effects of relaxation with guided imagery on surgical stress and wound healing.* Research in Nursing and Health. 1988;11(4):235–244.

Baider, L., Uziely, B., De Nour, A.K. *Progressive muscle relaxation and guided imagery in cancer patients.* General Hospital Psychiatry. 1994;16:340–347.

Systemic Disorders

ALLERGIC RHINITIS

Ogle K.A. and Bullock J.D. *Children with allergic rhinitis and/or bronchial asthma treated with elimination diet.* Ann Allergy. 1977;39:8-11.

INDEX

Page numbers in **bold** type refer to main entries in the ailments section. These include details of the ailment, the factors causing it, the treatment options, suggestions for self-help and relevant case studies and precautions.

ACKNOWLEDGMENTS

Author Acknowledgments

This book has been a huge collaborative effort and has been a long time in the making. From the initial concept, the book grew and developed with the input and creativity of a great number of people. In particular, we would like to thank the following for their invaluable expert knowledge and assistance: Daniel Firer and Joshua Holexa, Research Assistants, Program in Integrative Medicine, University of Arizona College of Medicine; David Casson BA, MBBS, MRCPI; Austin McCormick MbChB MROpth; Sue Davidson MB BS MRCP, MRCGP. Many thanks are also due to Adriane Fugh-Berman MD and her team at Georgetown University.

This book would not have been possible without the hard work and combined design and editorial ingenuity of the team at Dorling Kindersley, for which an enormous thank you to everyone, in particular to Mary-Clare Jerram and Penny Warren.

Publisher Acknowledgments

Dorling Kindersley would like to thank Professor Irving Gottesman for permission to base the chart on p.426 on information from his book *Schizophrenia Genius* (1990); to Jennie Brand-Miller and Thomas Wolever for permission to base information on p.43 on information from their book *The Glucose Revolution*; and to NAM Publications for permission to base the illustration on p.471 on material from their website.

DK would also like to thank Laura Knox for specially commissioned photography; Sophia Atcha for hair and make up; Mark Cavanagh for design assistance and PhotoShop imaging; Nicola Erdpresser for DTP assistance; Daphne Razazan for editorial advice; Jenny Lane for editorial assistance; Alyson Lacewing for proofreading; and Sue Bosanko for the index.

Picture Credits

The publisher would like to thank the following for permission to reproduce images:

Alamy pp 78l/Martyn Vickery, 186/BananaStock; **Bubbles Photo Library** p 382/Lois Joy Thurston; Courtesy of Bruckhoff, Hannover p 189; **Getty Images** pp 50r /Peter Scholey, 82c/Tim Flach; **Nature Picture Library** p 15 /Aflo; **Pulse Picture Library** p 246; Punchstock/Photodisc 32l, 82, 104; **Science Photo Library** pp 12r/Tek Image, 12c/David Mack, 12l/Tek Image, 19/Andrew Syred, 22/Colin Cuthbert, 27/Andrew Syred, 29/ Tek Image, 30/BSIP, Laurent, 35/John Pacy, 46/Eye of Science, 48, 48/Biophoto Associates, 53t/Stefanie Reichelt, 59/SteveGschmeissner, 73/Chris Knapton, 76/Eye of Science, 92/Nasa, 96, 98/AJ Photo/Hop American, 110/Eamonn McNulty, 122/Dr Arthur Tucker, 134/Alfred Pasieka, 145/Faye Norman, 149/CNRI, 156/VVG, 172/Dr P.Marazzi, 173/Alexander Tsiaras, 176/Dr P.Marazzi, 178, 179/Eye of Science, 180/Ralph Eagle, 182/Western Opthalmic Hospital, 185/Omikron, 194/Innerspace Imaging, 201/NIBSC, 202/Dr Gary Settles, 210/Innerspace Imaging, 215/David McCarthy, 217, 228, 231/Dr M.A. Ansary, 232/Zephyr, 240/Dr Linda Stannard, UCT, 250/Zephyr, 264/Dr P.Marazzi, 266/Alfred Pasieka, 275/Sovereign ISM, 291r/CNRI, 291l/Zephyr, 297/CNRI, 303/Dr Gilbert Faure, 310l & r /Prof. P.Motta/Dept. of Anatomy/University "La Sapienza", Rome, 312/Alfred Pasieka, 322/Zephyr, 345/Dr E. Walker, 347/BSIP, DR LR, 354/Dr M.A. Ansary, 371/BSIP VEM, 374r/VVG, 374l/Manfred Kage, 380/CNRI, 383/Dr P.Marazzi, 386l/Sinclair Stammers, 386r/VVG, 395, 396/Lowell Georgia, 398/Dr P.Marazzi, 400/Eamonn McNulty, 406/Tim Beddow, 433/BSIP/Laurent/Laetitia, 454/Chris Bjornberg, 114-155/Volker Steger, 158-179/Andrew Syred, 182-193/Omikron, 196-209/CNRI, 212-241 /CNRI, 244-265/Susuma Nishinaga, 268-311/Dr P.Marazzi, 314-321/John Burbidge, 324-353/BSIP VEM, 356-367/CC Studio, 370-379/John Walsh, 382-405/CNRI, 456-479/Steve Gschmeissner

Illustration p. 91 by John Woodcock.

All other images © Dorling Kindersley
For further information see: www.dkimages.com